MOSBY'S 1999
FAMILY PRACTICE SOURCEBOOK

MOSBY'S 1999
FAMILY PRACTICE SOURCEBOOK

KENNETH G. MARSHALL, MD
Department of Family Medicine
University of Western Ontario
London, Ontario, Canada

Mosby

St. Louis Baltimore Boston Carlsbad Chicago Minneapolis New York Philadelphia Portland
London Milan Sydney Tokyo Toronto

Mosby
Dedicated to Publishing Excellence

Publisher: Susie H. Baxter
Editor: Liz Fathman
Senior Developmental Editor: Laura C. Berendson
Project Manager: Patricia Tannian
Book Design Manager: Gail Morey Hudson
Manufacturing Manager: Linda Ierardi
Cover Designer: Teresa Breckwoldt

Composition by Douglas & Gayle Limited
Printing/binding by R.R. Donnelley & Sons

Mosby–Year Book, Inc.
11830 Westline Industrial Drive
St. Louis, Missouri 63146

Library of Congress Cataloging in Publication Data

Marshall, Kenneth G.
Mosby's family practice sourcebook / Kenneth G. Marshall.—1st ed.
p. cm.
Includes bibliographical references and index.
ISBN 0-8151-2785-5
1. Family medicine—Handbooks, manuals, etc. I. Title. II. Title: Family practice sourcebook.
[DNLM: 1. Family Practice. WB 110 M368m 1999]
RC55.M278 1999
616—DC21
DNLM/DLC
for Library of Congress 98-15925

98 99 00 01 02 / 9 8 7 6 5 4 3 2 1

To the many

bright, enthusiastic, curious, skeptical,

challenging, and articulate family medicine residents

I have had the privilege of working with at

McGill and the University of Western Ontario

PREFACE

No family physician, no matter how competent and dedicated, can acquire or keep in his or her head the vast and changing body of medical data that is needed for adequate care of patients. My goal in writing this annual book is to supplement the already extensive knowledge and skills of practicing family physicians with an up-to-date database that can be accessed quickly and easily.

This book deals primarily with conditions seen and treated by family physicians in an outpatient setting. Some material on inpatient treatment is included, primarily so that office-based family physicians have information with which to counsel patients or their families. Community health issues are also part of the text because prevention of disease is an important part of our mandate.

The *Family Practice Sourcebook* is not a textbook, and only rarely is an attempt made to cover all aspects of any medical condition. Rather, this is an up-to-date, annual reference manual dealing with selected aspects of a wide variety of subjects chosen because of their usefulness or interest for family physicians. Many of the entries are practical therapeutic programs for disorders such as acne, Parkinson's disease, or sexually transmitted diseases, while others cover the background data required by family physicians for making rational decisions about controversial issues such as cholesterol or prostate-specific antigen screening. I hope this text will facilitate the practice of "evidence-based," or if that is not possible, at least "reference-based" office medicine. To help achieve this, almost all of the data in this text has been extracted from recent articles in the medical literature and in most cases the full citations appear at the end of each topic.

HOW TO USE THIS BOOK

Finding Your Way Around the Text

There are six ways of finding your way around the text:

1. Index. Using the index is the most efficient way of finding what you want quickly. Drugs are listed by both generic and trade names.
2. Table of contents. The table of contents lists the major subject areas covered.
3. Inside front and back covers. A more detailed table of contents is given that corresponds to the outlines described below.
4. Outlines. At the beginning of each subject area listed in the table of contents is an outline of topics covered in that section.
5. Cross references. Related subjects are listed beneath the section and topic headings ("See also . . .").
6. Random perusal. This is the most fun. It requires a bit of time and if possible a winter evening in front of a crackling fire.

Organization of the Text

The overall organization is alphabetical as in a glossary. First-level headings as listed in the table of contents are based on anatomical systems ("Cardiovascular System," "Gastrointestinal System,") or specialties ("Gynecology," "Ophthalmology"), although a few important medical problems such as "Alcohol" and "Smoking" are also included at this level. Subheadings also tend to be in alphabetical order, but exceptions are made when the natural flow of content makes this inappropriate.

Topics that do not easily fit into one of the first-level headings are listed alphabetically under the major heading "Miscellaneous." Examples are "Bed Rest Complications," "Bites," "Informed Consent," "Leg Cramps," and "Multiple Chemical Sensitivities."

Where drugs are available in Canada but not the United States, or where the trade names in Canada differ from those in the United States, the proprietary names are underlined.

Errors

I have tried to minimize errors in this volume, but I cannot guarantee that none are present. Therefore anyone using this book should verify the accuracy of the contents, particularly in terms of drugs and dosages, before basing patient treatment on them.

Kenneth G. Marshall, M.D.

ACKNOWLEDGMENTS

Many family physicians from across Canada have reviewed part or all of an earlier draft of this manuscript. As a result of their critiques, I have revised or added many topics. For their help in this respect, I thank Drs. John Carsley of Montreal, Quebec, Jean De Serres of Chelsea, Quebec, John Eby of Victoria, British Columbia, Robert Hirzer of Coquitlam, British Columbia, Ken Hook of Tavistock, Ontario, Michael Klein of Vancouver, British Columbia, Kate Marshall of Montreal, Quebec, Jean Maskey of Vernon, British Columbia, Christine Myer of Montreal, Quebec, Michael Rondilla of London, Ontario, Heather Rubinstein of Montreal, Quebec, Barry Slapkoff of Montreal, Quebec, and Graydon Thorne of Thunder Bay, Ontario.

A text with as many references as this could not have been written without the help of good medical librarians. I was fortunate in having such support from Susan Mullan and Gérard Vanier, librarians at the Queen Elizabeth Hospital in Montreal, and later from Lynn Dunikowski and her dedicated staff—Bethany McLachlin, David LeSauvage, Lorraine Schoel, and Trixie Usselman—at the Canadian Library of Family Medicine in London, Ontario.

Academic pursuits such as writing textbooks are possible only in a milieu that fosters such activities. For their unstinting support, my thanks go to Drs. Bill Davis and Louise Nasmith, who held the chair of family medicine during my time at McGill, and Dr. Brian Hennen, who is chairman at the University of Western Ontario, where I am now located.

I am indebted to Jim Shanahan of Mosby, whose enthusiasm for evidence-based medicine played a big part in getting this work approved for publication. Jane Ryley and Laura Berendson, my editors at Mosby, have always been available for advice, consultation, and metaphorical hand-holding as I tried to pare this volume to an acceptable length without losing too much of the content. Trish Tannian, Mosby Project Manager, has done a superb job of copyediting, shaping my manuscript into a finished format, and overseeing the transition from manuscript to the printed text. I am very grateful to them all.

A special thanks goes to Owen Teo for his extraordinary patience and equanimity during the hundreds of hours he spent setting up my computer and teaching this middle-aged computer-illiterate family physician how to use it.

CONTENTS

MOSBY'S 1999
FAMILY PRACTICE SOURCEBOOK

ALCOHOL

(See also alcoholic hepatitis)

Topics covered in this section

EPIDEMIOLOGY AND NATURAL HISTORY OF EXCESSIVE ALCOHOL INTAKE

Between 5% and 7% of Canadians are considered to be dependent on alcohol, and another 20% are thought to be consuming enough to be at risk for problems arising from drinking[1]; it has been estimated that 15% of family medicine patients imbibe harmful amounts of alcohol.[2] A U.S. survey of college students found that 84% drank and that 44% met the criteria for binge drinking (five or more drinks in a row at least once in the last 2 weeks). Nineteen percent of the students were frequent binge drinkers, and half of these reported alcohol-related problems such as injuries and participation in unplanned sex.[3]

A long-term follow-up of two cohorts of white men from Boston sheds light on the natural history of alcoholism. One group were from working class and welfare families of inner-city Boston, and the other were Harvard sophomores. By age 60, 33% of the core city men and 21% of the Harvard graduates had at some point during their lives met the criteria of alcohol abuse given in the *Diagnostic and Statistical Manual of Mental Disorders,* ed. 3 (DSM-III). Prognosis for permanent abstinence was excellent after 5 to 6 years of teetotalism, but the relapse rate after 2 years of abstinence was 41%. The odds of returning to controlled drinking were poor. Although the incidence of alcohol abuse was greater in working class men than in university graduates, the rate of abstinence by the age of 60 was twice as great in the working class men as in the Harvard alumni. The natural history of alcohol abuse was not one of relentless progression, but rather one of persistence with fluctuations.[4]

REFERENCES

1. Ontario Ministry of Health: *A framework for the response to alchol and drug problems in Ontario,* Toronto, 1988, Queen's Park Printers.
2. Malla A, Merskey H: Screening for alcoholism in general practice, *Fam Pract Res J* 6:138-147, 1987.
3. Wechsler H, Davenport A, Dowdall G, et al: Health and behavioral consequences of binge drinking in college—a national survey of students at 140 campuses, *JAMA* 272:1672-1677, 1994.
4. Vaillant GE: A long-term follow-up of male alcohol abuse, *Arch Gen Psychiatry* 53:243-249, 1996.

DEFINITION OF HIGH-RISK DRINKING

Some workers in alcohol abuse divide "excessive" drinking into two categories: problem drinking and alcohol dependence.[1] The dividing line between these two is not well defined, but in general patients with alcohol dependence imbibe more than 50 drinks per week, drink excessively every day, have withdrawal symptoms with abstinence, and experience social and physical consequences. Problem drinkers usually consume 20 to 30 drinks weekly, have no withdrawal symptoms with abstinence, do not drink excessively daily, and do not suffer major social or physical consequences.[1]

According to a joint policy statement by the Addiction Research Foundation of Ontario and the Canadian Center on Substance Abuse, no one should drink more than two standard drinks per day.[2] The recommendations of the Alcohol Risk Assessment and Intervention (ARAI) program of the College of Family Physicians of Canada are similar. Low-risk drinkers are defined as those who have at least one alcohol-free day per week, who never take more than three drinks per day if they are female or four drinks per day if they are male, and who never have more than 12 drinks per week.[3] A British working group put the upper limit of sensible drinking at three to four drinks per day for men and two to three per day for women.[4]

REFERENCES

1. Kahan M: Identifying and managing problem drinkers, *Can Fam Physician* 42:661-667, 1996.
2. Ashley MF, Ferrence R, Room R, et al: Moderate drinking and health: report of an international symposium, *Can Med Assoc J* 151:809-828, 1994.
3. Alcohol Risk Assessment and Intervention (ARAI): *Resource manual for family physicians,* Toronto, 1994, College of Family Physicians.
4. Interdepartmental Working Group: *Sensible drinking,* London, 1995, Department of Health.

DEFINITIONS OF STANDARD DRINKS

A standard drink contains approximately 13.6 grams of alcohol and is the equivalent of:

12 ounces (360 ml) of regular strength beer	5% alcohol
5 ounces (150 ml) of table wine	12% alcohol
1.5 ounces (45 ml) of spirits	40% alcohol

CAGE, ARAI, AND OTHER QUESTIONNAIRES FOR ALCOHOL RISK ASSESSMENT

The CAGE questionnaire is a simple screening test for problem drinking.

C Have you ever felt the need to **CUT** down on your drinking?
A Has anyone ever **ANGERED** you by criticizing your drinking?
G Have you ever felt **GUILTY** over consequences of drinking?
E Have you ever had an **EYE OPENER** (morning drink)?

In one study a "yes" answer to at least one of the CAGE questions identified nearly 50% of excessive drinkers,[1] while other studies found that two or more "yes" answers had a sensitivity of 90% for detecting heavy drinkers.[2] A 1994 Canadian study reported that the false-positive rate was significant, 53% for females and 21% for males,[3] whereas a 1996 American study of elderly patients found few false-positive results (high specificity) but that half of binge drinkers (six or more drinks at one time) or regular heavy drinkers (more than 21 drinks per week) were not detected.[4]

A number of other questionnaires, some quite complex, relate to alcoholic intake. The best known in this category is the Michigan Alcohol Screening Test (MAST), which contains 25 items. AUDIT, an acronym for Alcohol Use Disorder Identification Test, is a 10-question form developed by the World Health Organization.[5,6] The ARAI program of the College of Family Physicians of Canada[7] suggests that an initial screening question be, "Has alcohol ever caused a problem for you or your family?" If a positive response is obtained, the CAGE questionnaire should be administered followed by specific questions to elicit the quantity of alcohol taken[7]:

Number of drinks taken on the days when the patient drinks
Number of days per week the patient drinks
Total weekly number of drinks
Maximum number of drinks taken in any 24-hour period in the previous month

Both the Canadian Task Force on the Periodic Health Examination[8] and the U.S. Preventive Services Task Force[9] give a "B" recommendation for screening adolescents and adults for alcohol intake.

REFERENCES

1. Wallace P, Cutler S, Haines A: Randomized controlled trial of general practitioner intervention in patients with excessive alcohol consumption, *BMJ* 297:663-668, 1988.
2. King M: At risk drinking among general practice attenders: validation of the CAGE questionnaire, *Psychol Med* 16:213-217, 1986.
3. McIntosh MC, Leigh G, Baldwin NJ: Screening for hazardous drinking, *Can Fam Physician* 40:1546-1553, 1994.
4. Adams WL, Barry KL, Fleming MF: Screening for problem drinking in older primary care patients, *JAMA* 276:1964-1967, 1996.
5. Saunders FB, Aasland OG, Amundsen A, et al: Alcohol consumption and related problems among primary health care patients: WHO Collaborative Project on Early Detection of Persons with Harmful Alcohol Consumption—I, *Addiction* 88:349-362, 1993.
6. Saunders JB, Aasland OG, Babor TF, et al: Development of the Alcohol Use Disorders Identification Test (AUDIT): WHO Collaborative Project on Early Detection of Persons with Harmful Alcohol Consumption—II, *Addiction* 88:791-804, 1993.
7. Alcohol Risk Assessment and Intervention (ARAI): *Resource manual for family physicians,* Toronto, 1994, College of Family Physicians.
8. Canadian Task Force on the Periodic Health Examination: *Canadian guide to clinical preventive health care,* Ottawa, 1994, Canada Communication Group—Publishing, pp 488-498.
9. US Preventive Services Task Force: *Guide to clinical preventive services,* ed 2, Baltimore, 1996, Williams & Wilkins, pp 567-582.

DETRIMENTAL EFFECTS OF ALCOHOL

(See also abuse; alcoholic hepatitis; alcohol and hypertension; beneficial effects of alcohol; fetal alcohol syndrome; homicide; motor vehicle accidents; poverty; suicide)

Several studies of drinking and mortality have reported a J-curve with a shallow dip in total mortality at lower amounts of drinking and increases in total mortality at higher levels of alcohol intake.[1,2] The reduction is due to a decrease in cardiovascular disease (see beneficial effects of alcohol below), while the increase is due to accidents, violence (including homicide and suicide), certain cancers, cirrhosis, and hemorrhagic strokes. Alcohol-induced morbidity includes social disruption,[3] hallucinations, delirium tremens, personality changes, violence, accidents, cirrhosis of the liver, pancreatitis, gastritis, hypertension,[4] cardiomyopathy, dysrhythmias, strokes,[5] subarachnoid hemorrhages, degenerative diseases of the nervous system, seizures, community-acquired pneumonias,[6] adult respiratory distress syndrome,[7] fetal abnormalities, and cancers of the mouth, pharynx, larynx, esophagus, and liver. The incidence of breast and colon cancer may also be increased in those who drink alcohol.[1,2] Most of these conditions are discussed elsewhere in the text.

Women who drink alcohol are particularly prone to liver disease. An increased risk of cirrhosis is found with an alcohol intake only half that which increases the risk of cirrhosis in men.[8]

A strong correlation exists between smoking and heavy drinking.[9,10] Much of the excess mortality of alcohol abusers is actually related to tobacco abuse.[9]

A 9-year follow-up of World War II veterans in Australia found no evidence that regular lifelong alcohol consumption was associated with impaired cognitive functioning in this geriatric population.[11]

Hangovers are probably not directly related to ethanol itself but rather to other constituents of alcoholic beverages, such as methanol. Between 25% and 50% of drinkers who have become intoxicated do not get hangovers.[12] The incidence of hangovers varies with the beverage drunk. In one study from the 1970s volunteers drank equal concentrations of alcohol but in different types of drinks. The severity of hangovers was related in decreasing order to brandy, red wine, rum, whisky, white wine, gin, vodka, and pure ethanol.[13] Some amelioration of hangovers is achieved by rehydration and by nonsteroidal antiinflammatory drugs, particularly if they are taken before retiring at night.[12]

REFERENCES

1. Ashley MF, Ferrence R, Room R, et al: Moderate drinking and health: report of an international symposium, *Can Med Assoc J* 151:809-828, 1994.
2. Friedman GK, Klatsky AL: Is alcohol good for your health? (editorial), *N Engl J Med* 329:1882-1883, 1993.
3. Room R: Alcohol consumption and social harm, *Contemp Drug Probl* 23:373-388, 1996.
4. Marmot MG, Elliott P, Shipley MJ, et al: Alcohol and blood pressure: the INTERSALT study, *BMJ* 308:1263-1267, 1994.
5. Gill JS, Zezulka AV, Shipley MJ, et al: Stroke and alcohol consumption, *N Engl J Med* 315:1041-1046, 1986.
6. Fernandez-Sola J, Junque A, Estruch R, et al: High alcohol intake as a risk and prognostic factor for community-acquired pneumonia, *Arch Intern Med* 155:1649-1654, 1995.
7. Moss M, Bucher B, Moore FA, et al: The role of chronic alcohol abuse in the development of acute respiratory distress syndrome in adults, *JAMA* 275:50-54, 1996.
8. Lieber CS: Medical disorders of alcoholism, *N Engl J Med* 333:1058-1065, 1995.
9. Hurt RD, Offord KP, Croghan IT, et al: Mortality following inpatient addictions treatment: role of tobacco use in a community-based cohort, *JAMA* 275:1097-1103, 1996.
10. Valiant GE, Schnurr PP, Baron JA, et al: A prospective study of the effects of cigarette smoking and alcohol abuse on mortality, *J Gen Intern Med* 6:299-304, 1991.
11. Dent OF, Sulway MR, Broe GA, et al: Alcohol consumption and cognitive performance in a random sample of Australian soldiers who served in the Second World War, *BMJ* 314:1655-1657, 1997.
12. Calder I: Hangovers: not the ethanol—perhaps the methanol (editorial), *BMJ* 314:2-3, 1997.
13. Pawan GL: Alcoholic drinks and hangover effects, *Proc Nutr Soc* 32:15A, 1973.

BENEFICIAL EFFECTS OF ALCOHOL

(See also detrimental effects of alcohol; fetal alcohol syndrome)

Epidemiological evidence suggests that moderate drinking is associated with a relative reduction of coronary artery disease risk in the order of 40% to 60%.[1-6] This effect is present in women[3,4] and men[4-6] of all age groups; it is more apparent in older persons because the risk of coronary artery disease is greater in that population. The beneficial effect has been reported with as little as one drink every second day and is associated with alcohol in any form: red wine, white wine, beer, or spirits.[1,4,5,7] A study of male British physicians found that those who drank 8 to 14 drinks per week had a relative mortality rate 30% lower than that of nondrinkers, while the heaviest drinkers had about the same mortality as the nondrinkers.[4] In a Danish trial of men without overt ischemic heart disease the risk of an initial cardiac event was greatest in abstainers, intermediate for those taking 1 to 21 drinks per week, and lowest among those imbibing more than 22 drinks per week.[8] An Australian study found that regular ingestion of 1 to 4 drinks per day for men or 1 to 2 drinks per day for women was protective, whereas the same number of weekly drinks taken in the form of binges was not. The authors postulated that that was because an important part of the protective effect of alcohol is a favorable alteration of the fibrinolytic system, an effect that wears off within 24 hours.[4]

Aside from activating fibrinolytic systems,[4,9] alcohol is thought to protect against vascular disease by raising concentrations of HDL_2 and HDL_3[10] or by enhancing insulin sensitivity, which helps prevent the development of syndrome X (insulin resistance, hypertension, dyslipidemia, central obesity, and vascular disease).[11]

Because of the potential for abuse, few workers in the field recommend that abstainers be advised to drink moderately or that very occasional drinkers be advised to increase their alcohol consumption in order to decrease their risk of coronary artery disease. This view is supported by the finding that on a population basis, a higher average mean consumption of alcohol is associated with higher rates of problem drinking.[12] This may be too rigid a perspective; Pearson and Terry[13] suggest that modest alcohol consumption might be recommended on a case-by-case basis after careful evaluation of contraindications, including the potential for abuse, and Victor and Hansen[14] state that in the absence of alcohol-related illnesses a drink or two a day "seems safe and advisable from a cardiovascular standpoint."Ashley and associates[15] point out that cardiovascular benefits are achieved only in the middle-aged and elderly and that very few drinks per week are required for this purpose. Younger individuals receive no cardiovascular benefit at all, whereas risks are linear with no known lower limits.

Moderate alcohol consumption appears to help protect against peripheral vascular disease[16] and non-insulin-dependent diabetes.[17,18] A probable mechanism for the latter is that alcohol improves insulin sensitivity.[11] Moderate drinking is also associated with a decreased incidence of the common cold.[19]

REFERENCES

1. Ashley MF, Ferrence R, Room R, et al: Moderate drinking and health: report of an international symposium, *Can Med Assoc J* 151:809-828, 1994.
2. Friedman GK, Klatsky AL: Is alcohol good for your health? (editorial), *N Engl J Med* 329:1882-1883, 1993.
3. Fuchs CS, Stampfer MJ, Colditz GA, et al: Alcohol consumption and mortality among women, *N Engl J Med* 332:1245-1250, 1995.
4. McElduff P, Dobson AJ: How much alcohol and how often? Population based case-control study of alcohol consumption and risk of a major coronary event, *BMJ* 314:1159-1164, 1997.
5. Doll R, Peto R, Hall E, et al: Mortality in relation to consumption of alcohol: 13 years' observation on male British doctors, *BMJ* 309:911-918, 1994.
6. Camargo CA, Hennekens CH, Gaziano JM, et al: Prospective study of moderate alcohol consumption and mortality in US male physicians, *Arch Intern Med* 157:79-85, 1997.
7. Rimm EB, Klatsky A, Grobbee D, et al: Review of moderate alcohol consumption and reduced risk of coronary heart

disease: is the effect due to beer, wine, or spirits? *BMJ* 312: 731-735, 1996.
8. Hein HO, Suadicani P, Gyntelberg F: Alcohol consumption, serum low density lipoprotein cholesterol concentration, and risk of ischaemic heart disease: six year follow up in the Copenhagen male study, *BMJ* 312:736-741, 1996.
9. Ridker PM, Vaughan DE, Stampfer MJ, et al: Association of moderate alcohol consumption and plasma concentration of endogenous tissue-type plasminogen activator, *JAMA* 272:929-933, 1994.
10. Gaziano JM, Buring JE, Breslow JL, et al: Moderate alcohol intake, increased levels of high-density lipoprotein and its subfractions, and decreased risk of myocardial infarction, *N Engl J Med* 329:1829-1834, 1993.
11. Kiechl S, Willeit J, Poewe W, et al: Insulin sensitivity and regular alcohol consumption: large, prospective, cross sectional population study (Bruneck study), *BMJ* 313:1040-1044, 1996.
12. Colhoun H, Ben-Shlomo Y, Dong W, et al: Ecological analysis of collectivity of alcohol consumption in England: importance of average drinker, *BMJ* 324:1164-1168, 1997.
13. Pearson TA, Terry P: What to advise patients about drinking alcohol: the clinician's conundrum (editorial), *JAMA* 272:967-968, 1994.
14. Victor RG, Hansen J: Alcohol and blood pressure—a drink a day . . . (editorial), *N Engl J Med* 332:1782-1783, 1995.
15. Ashley MJ, Ferrence R, Room R, et al: Moderate drinking and health: implications of recent evidence, *Can Fam Physician* 43:687-694, 1997.
16. Camargo CA Jr, Stampfer MJ, Glynn RJ, et al: Prospective study of moderate alcohol consumption and risk of peripheral arterial disease in US male physicians, *Circulation* 95:577-580, 1997.
17. Rimm EB, Chan J, Stampfer MJ, et al: Prospective study of cigarette smoking, alcohol use, and the risk of diabetes in men, *BMJ* 210:545-546, 1995.
18. Perry IF, Wannamethee SG, Walker MK, et al: Prospective study of risk factors for development of non-insulin dependent diabetes in middle aged British men, *BMJ* 310:560-564, 1995.
19. Cohen S, Doyle WJ, Skoner DP, et al: Social ties and susceptibility to the common cold, *JAMA* 277:1940-1944, 1997.

EFFECTS OF ALCOHOL ON LABORATORY TESTS

(See also laboratory findings in alcoholic hepatitis)

Increased gamma-glutamyl transferase (g-GT) often occurs when two to five or more drinks per day are taken regularly over 7 or more days. However, the sensitivity is poor, especially among young alcohol-dependent adults and non-alcohol-dependent heavy drinkers.[1] With abstinence or diminution of drinking, the g-GT concentration usually reverts to normal after 2 to 6 weeks.[2] g-GT levels are not reliable indicators of the quantity of alcohol imbibed by those who continue to drink.[2]

The mean corpuscular volume is raised in between one fourth and three fourths of alcohol-dependent drinkers.[1] The serum aspartate aminotransferase (AST) and serum alanine aminotransferase (ALT) levels are increased in about the same proportion of alcohol-dependent drinkers.[1] If some degree of alcoholic hepatitis is present, both the AST and ALT levels are elevated but rarely more than five times normal. Usually the elevation of AST is greater than that of ALT.

REFERENCES

1. Alcohol Risk Assessment and Intervention (ARAI): *Resource manual for family physicians,* Toronto, 1994, College of Family Physicians.
2. Kahan M: Identifying and managing problem drinkers, *Can Fam Physician* 42:661-667, 1996.

TREATMENT OF ALCOHOLISM

(See also epidemiology; natural history of excessive alcohol intake; seizures)

For most problem drinkers brief interventions by family physicians are the first line of management.[1,2] Even asking patients about their drinking habits has been reported to change behavior in 5% of patients at risk.[3] Two 10- to 15-minute counseling sessions by physicians significantly reduced the alcohol consumption of both male and female problem drinkers.[4]

An opiate receptor antagonist, naltrexone (ReVia), helps prevent relapses in alcoholic patients who have become abstinent. It decreases alcohol craving but does not induce a disulfiram reaction, and its beneficial effects appear to persist after a short-term (12-week) treatment program.[5] The usual dose is 50 mg once daily. The role of disulfiram (Antabuse) is controversial, although there is fair evidence that it is effective.[6] Important adverse effects include hepatitis and neuropathies. The usual dose is 250 to 500 mg each morning.

Depression has long been known to be associated with alcoholism, but whether the alcoholism causes the depression, or whether depression leads to alcoholism, is uncertain. In one study of depressed alcoholics who had been abstinent for a median of 8 days, desipramine (Norpramin, Pertofrane) was compared with placebo.[7] The desipramine-treated group had a significant amelioration of depression compared with the control subjects; whether this resulted in a decreased recidivism rate for drinking could not be determined. A specific problem encountered in this study was that some patients were encouraged to discontinue desipramine by the Alcoholics Anonymous groups in which they were participating.[7] Imipramine (Tofranil) has been shown to be safe and effective in relieving symptoms of depression in actively drinking alcoholics.[8]

Acute alcohol withdrawal syndromes require specific management. These syndromes can be classified as follows[9]:

1. *Minor withdrawal symptoms.* Symptoms often develop within 3 to 6 hours of the beginning of abstinence and include anxiety, tremulousness, insomnia, and in some patients tachycardia, sweating, gastrointestinal distress, and headaches. Symptoms usually abate within 24 to 36 hours.

2. *Delirium tremens.* Delirium tremens affects only 4% to 5% of alcoholics who abstain from drinking. The syndrome consists of disorientation, agitation, hallucinations that are usually visual, diaphoresis, hypertension, and mild fever. The illness has its onset 2 to 4 days after the last episode of drinking and usually lasts 2 to 5 days. It is rare in persons under the age of 30 and is seen mainly in those who have had more than five or six drinks per day over a prolonged period. The death rate is about 5%.
3. *Alcohol hallucinations.* Some alcoholics experience hallucinations (usually visual) without having delirium tremens. The onset is usually during the first day of abstinence, and the hallucinations resolve within 48 hours. Patients remain oriented.
4. *Alcoholic withdrawal seizures.* About 3% of abstaining alcoholics have withdrawal seizures. These are usually generalized and come on 12 to 24 hours after withdrawal.

The mainstay of management of all the withdrawal syndromes is an adequate dose of a long-acting benzodiazepine. This prevents some of the more serious syndromes if given early. The most commonly used drugs are diazepam (Valium) and chlordiazepoxide (Librium). Oral doses vary according to the clinical situation but traditionally range from 20 to 100 mg q6h for chlordiazepoxide and from 5 to 20 mg q6h for diazepam.[9]

Diazepam is probably the preferred drug for managing acute alcohol withdrawal because it is more rapidly absorbed than is chlordiazepoxide. Diazepam loading is a useful technique for supervised outpatients.[10] Patients are given 20 mg of diazepam po every hour for three doses if they weigh less than 76.5 kg (168 lb), 20 mg every hour for four doses if they weigh 76.5 kg (168 lb) to 90 kg (198 lb), and 20 mg every hour for five doses if they weigh more than 90 kg (198 lb). If the patient has had major withdrawal symptoms in the past, these doses may be doubled. Usually no further diazepam is needed, although in a few cases the procedure must be repeated the next day. Thiamin 100 mg should be given intramuscularly (poor gastric absorption in alcoholics) before withdrawal.[10]

REFERENCES

1. Kahan M: Identifying and managing problem drinkers, *Can Fam Physician* 42:661-667, 1996.
2. Peters C, Wilson D, Bruneau A, et al: Alcohol risk assessment and intervention for family physicians: project of the College of Family Physicians of Canada, *Can Fam Physician* 42:681-689, 1996.
3. Anderson P, Scott E: The effect of general practitioners' advice to heavy drinking men, *Br J Addict* 87:891-900, 1992.
4. Fleming MF, Barry KL, Manwell LB, et al: Brief physician advice for problem alcohol drinkers: a randomized controlled trial in community-based primary care practices, *JAMA* 277:1039-1045, 1997.
5. O'Malley SS, Jaffe AJ, Chang G, et al: Six-month follow-up of naltrexone and psychotherapy for alcohol dependence, *Arch Gen Psychiatry* 53:217-224, 1996.
6. Gallant DM: Recent advances in research and treatment of alcoholism and drug abuse. In Geller A, ed: *ASAM review course manual,* Washington, DC, 1990, American Society of Addiction Medicine, p 589.
7. Mason BJ, Kocsis JH, Ritvo EC, et al: A double-blind, placebo-controlled trial of desipramine for primary alcohol dependence stratified on the presence or absence of major depression, *JAMA* 275:761-767, 1996.
8. McGrath PJ, Nunes EV, Stewart JW, et al: Imipramine treatment of alcoholics with primary depression. a placebo-controlled clinical trial, *Arch Gen Psychiatry* 53:232-240, 1996.
9. Yost DA: Alcohol withdrawal syndrome, *Am Fam Physician* 54:657-664, 1996.
10. Mezciems PE: Withdrawal strategies for outpatients: alcohol, benzodiazepine, barbiturate, and opiate addictions, *Can Fam Physician* 42:1745-1752, 1996.

ANTIBACTERIALS

Topics covered in this section

Antibiotic Resistance
Pediatric Doses
Antibacterials, Oral and Intramuscular

ANTIBIOTIC RESISTANCE

It is well known that antibiotic use in hospitals facilitates the emergence of resistant strains of microorganisms. A study from Iceland suggests that the same phenomenon occurs outside of the hospital. Nasopharyngeal swabs from children in five different communities were cultured for pneumococcal carriage. Organisms resistant to penicillin were far more likely to be found in communities where total antibiotic sales for children as recorded in pharmacies were high than in those where they were low.[1] A concerted effort was made in Finland to decrease the use of macrolides because of emerging resistance of group A streptococci to these antibiotics. The effort was successful, and the frequency of resistant strains decreased.[2] Inappropriate antibiotic prescription for upper respiratory tract infections and bronchitis is rampant in the United States. In one survey more than 50% of patients with these diagnoses who sought medical care from primary care physicians received antibiotics.[3]

REFERENCES

1. Arason VA, Kristinsson KG, Sigurdsson JA, et al: Do antimicrobials increase the carriage rate of penicillin resistant pneumococci in children? Cross sectional prevalence study, *BMJ* 313: 387-391, 1996.

2. Seppälä H, Klaukka T, Vuopio-Varkila J, et al: The effect of changes in the consumption of macrolide antibiotics on erythromycin resistance in group A streptococci in Finland, *N Engl J Med* 337:441-446, 1997.
3. Gonzales R, Steiner JF, Sande MA: Antibiotic prescribing for adults with colds, upper respiratory tract infections, and bronchitis by ambulatory care physicians, *JAMA* 278:901-904, 1997.

PEDIATRIC DOSES

The usual method of calculating pediatric doses is as follows: If weight is given in pounds, divided by 2.2 to obtain weight in kilograms. Multiply weight in kg by recommended daily dose. Divide daily dose by frequency of dosage (e.g., by 3 if dosage is tid).

A shortcut for determining an antibiotic dose when the recommended dosage is 40 mg/kg/day is the rule of 6. For example, if you want to give 40 mg/kg/day in three divided doses (e.g., of amoxicillin, amoxicillin-clavulanate [Augmentin, Clavulin], erythromycin-sulfisoxazole [Pediazole], penicillin V, or cefaclor [Ceclor]), multiply the child's weight in pounds by 6, and the result is the number of milligrams required for each of the three daily doses.[1]

REFERENCES

1. Reynolds RD: Shortcuts for calculating the dose of pediatric medications, *Am Fam Physician* 54:878, 1996.

ANTIBACTERIALS, ORAL AND INTRAMUSCULAR

Tables 1 to 6 list the generic names, some of the trade names, and usual doses of selected antibiotics used in the care of ambulatory patients. Optimal doses vary with different clinical conditions, and these are not always indicated in the tables. A reputable drug reference should be consulted before prescribing.

Cephalosporins

Selected cephalosporins are listed in Table 1.

Fluoroquinolones (Table 2)

Quinolones are contraindicated in pediatric patients because studies in immature experimental animals have shown damage to the cartilage of weight-bearing joints. Tendon ruptures (shoulder, hand, and Achilles) have been reported as complications of treatment with quinolones.[1]

Fosfomycin

Fosfomycin (Monurol) is a broad-spectrum antibiotic that is generally used as a single-dose (3-g) treatment for uncom-

Table 1 Cephalosporins

Name	Usual adult dose	Usual child dose
First Generation		
Cephalexin monohydrate (Keflex)	250-500 mg qid	20-50 mg/kg/day in 4 divided doses
Second Generation		
Cefaclor (Ceclor)	250-500 mg tid	20-40 mg/kg/day in 2-3 divided doses
Cefuroxime axetil (Ceftin)	250-500 mg bid	20-30 mg/kg/day in 2 divided doses
Cefprozil (Cefzil)	250-500 mg bid	15-30 mg/kg/day in 2 divided doses
Third Generation		
Cefixime (Suprax)	400 mg once daily	8 mg/kg/day as a single dose
Cefpodoxime (Vantin)	100-200 mg bid	10 mg/kg/day in 2 divided doses
Ceftibuten (Cedax)	400 mg once daily	9 mg/kg/day as single dose

Table 2 Fluoroquinolones

Name	Usual adult dose	Usual child dose
Ciprofloxacin (Cipro)	250-500 mg (occasionally 750 mg) bid; 100 mg bid for 3 days for uncomplicated urinary tract infections	Not indicated
Levofloxacin (Levaquin)	500 mg once daily	Not indicated
Norfloxacin (Noroxin)	400 mg bid	Not indicated
Ofloxacin (Floxin)	200-400 mg bid	Not indicated
Sparfloxacin (Zagam)	200 mg once a day	Not indicated

Table 3 Macrolides

Name	Usual adult dose	Usual child dose
Azithromycin (Zithromax)	500 mg as single dose on day 1 followed by 250 mg daily on days 2-5; 1 g as single dose for *Chlamydia*	10 mg/kg/day on day 1 as single dose followed by 5 mg/kg/day on days 2-5 for otitis media; 12 mg/kg/day as single dose for 5 days for pharyngitis or tonsillitis
Clarithromycin (Biaxin)	250-500 mg bid	15 mg/kg/day in 2 divided doses
Dirithromycin (Dynabac)	500 mg once daily	Age 12 years and older only
Erythromycin base	250-500 mg qid or 333 mg tid	30-50 mg/kg/day in 3-4 divided doses
Erythromycin ethylsuccinate-sulfisoxazole (Pediazole)		30-50 mg/kg/day of erythromycin in 3-4 divided doses

plicated urinary tract infections. The product comes in a single 3-g dose sachet containing the granules, which are dissolved in 1/2 cup of water before the medication is taken.

Lincosamide

The most frequently used lincosamide is clindamycin (Cleocin, Dalacin). It is particularly effective against aerobic gram-positive organisms such as streptococci and staphylococci and also against anaerobes. The usual oral dosage is 150 to 300 mg q6h.

Macrolides (Table 3)

Erythromycin can raise to toxic levels the serum concentrations of a variety of drugs metabolized by the cytochrome P450 system. These include theophylline (Theo-Dur, Uniphyl), the antihistamines astemizole (Hismanal) and terfenadine (Seldane), digoxin, carbamazepine (Tegretol), warfarin (Coumadin), and cisapride (Prepulsid).

The reputed advantages of azithromycin are once a day doses, fewer gastrointestinal side effects than erythromycin, and better coverage of gram-negative organisms, particularly *Haemophilus influenzae* and *Moraxella catarrhalis,* including beta-lactamase-producing strains. It is effective against gram-positive organisms but is slightly less potent than other macrolides.

Penicillins

Penicillins are listed in Table 4.

Table 4 Penicillins

Name	Usual adult dose	Usual child dose
Benzathine penicillin G	2.4 million units IM as a single dose for primary or secondary syphilis	
Penicillin G (benzylpenicillin)	For IM and IV use only	
Penicillin V potassium, phenoxymethyl-penicillin (Pen-Vee)	300 mg (500,000 units) tid-qid	25-50 mg/kg/day (40 000-90,000 units/kg/day) given in 3 or 4 divided doses
Penicillinase Resistant		
Cloxacillin (Tegopen, Orbenin)	250-500 mg qid	25-50 mg/kg/day in 4 divided doses
Dicloxacillin (Dycill, Dynapen, Pathocil)	125-250 mg qid	12.5-25 mg/kg/day in 4 divided doses
Aminopenicillins		
Amoxicillin (Amoxil)	250-500 mg q8h	25-50 mg/kg/day in 3 divided doses
Amoxicillin plus clavulanate potassium (Augmentin, Clavulin)	250-500 mg of amoxicillin q8h	25-50 mg/kg/day of amoxicillin in 3 divided doses

Sulfonamides (Table 5)

A frequently prescribed sulfonamide is trimethoprim-sulfamethoxazole (Septra, Bactrim). The usual pediatric dose is 6 mg/kg/day of trimethoprim and 30 mg/kg/day of sulfamethoxazole in 2 divided doses. This translates roughly into:

Under 2 years	2.5 ml of pediatric suspension bid
2-5 years	2.5-5 ml of pediatric suspension bid
6-12 years	5-10 ml of pediatric suspension or 2-4 pediatric tablets bid

Tetracyclines (Table 6)

Tetracyclines may be partly inactivated by iron preparations and by bismuth subsalicylate. Because they are deposited in growing bones and teeth, they are contraindicated in pregnancy and during lactation and in general should not be given to children under the age of 13 (Canadian recommendations) or the age of 8 (American recommendations).

REFERENCES

1. Nightingale SL: New fluoroquinolone warning label, *JAMA* 276:774, 1996.

Table 5 Sulfonamides

Name	Usual adult dose	Usual child dose
Trimethoprim-sulfamethoxazole (TMP-SMX) (Septra, Bactrim)	One DS tablet bid	6 mg/kg/day of trimethoprim and 30 mg/kg/day of sulfamethoxazole in 2 divided doses
Erythromycin ethylsuccinate-sulfisoxazole (Pediazole)		30-50 mg/kg/day of erythromycin in 3-4 divided doses

Table 6 Tetracyclines

Name	Usual adult dose	Usual child dose
Tetracycline hydrochloride (Achromycin V)	250-500 mg qid	25-50 mg/kg/day in 4 divided doses (over the ages of 8-12)
Doxycycline (Vibramycin)	100 mg bid on day 1 followed by 100 mg daily	4.4 mg/kg/day on day 1 in 2 divided doses followed by 2.2 mg/kg/day as a single daily dose (over the ages of 8-12)
Minocycline (Minocin)	200 mg on day 1 followed by 100 mg daily	4 mg/kg/day on day 1 followed by 2 mg/kg/day (over the ages of 8-12)

BREAST DISEASES

Topics covered in this section

BREAST, BENIGN

Breast Pain

Mastalgia can be divided into the two broad categories of cyclical premenstrual breast pain and noncyclical breast pain. Two thirds of women with mastalgia have cyclical pain. Many women with breast pain are worried that this is a symptom of cancer. Reassurance after a careful examination is often the only therapy required. Three drugs that have been used for cyclical breast pain are gamma linolenic acid (Evening Primrose Oil), bromocriptine (Parlodel), and danazol (Cyclomen).[1]

Evening Primrose Oil is extracted from the seeds of the evening primrose (a flower that opens its blooms in the evening) and contains gamma linolenic acid, linoleic acid, and vitamin E. It is available without prescription. The usual dosage is 6 to 8 capsules daily in divided doses. Three small randomized trials of this compound for patients with mastalgia have shown favorable results with few reported adverse effects.[2] However, a certain amount of skepticism is in order because Evening Primrose Oil has been promoted as beneficial for a wide variety of ailments aside from mastalgia, including atopic dermatitis, rheumatoid arthritis, diabetic neuropathy, multiple sclerosis, various cancers, Raynaud's phenomenon, ulcerative colitis, preeclampsia, premenstrual syndrome, hot flushes, Sjögren's syndrome, schizophrenia, and hyperactivity.[3]

Bromocriptine is usually started as a single daily dose of 1.25 mg and is increased by 2.5 mg every 2 to 4 weeks as necessary. The usual dosage for mastalgia is 2.5 mg bid. The initial dose of danazol is 100 to 150 mg bid with reduction to about 100 mg/day once symptoms are controlled. Therapy with danazol is usually continued for 6 to 9 months. Both bromocriptine and danazol have significant side effects. The major one for bromocriptine is nausea, while for danazol the adverse effects are related to the medication's androgenic effects and include weight gain, fluid retention, fatigue, decrease in breast size, hirsutism, atrophic vaginitis, hot flushes, acne, greasy skin, depression, and hoarse voice. All except hoarseness are said to be reversible when the medication is discontinued.

REFERENCES

1. Mansel RE: Breast pain, *BMJ* 309:866-868, 1994.
2. Mansel RE, Pye JK, Hughes LE: Effects of essential fatty acids on cyclical mastalgia and non-cyclical breast disorders. In Horrobin DF, ed: *Omega-6 essential fatty acids: pathophysiology and roles in clinical medicine,* New York, 1990, Wiley-Liss, pp 557-566.
3. Kleijnen J: Evening primrose oil: currently used in many conditions with little justification (editorial), *BMJ* 309:824-825, 1994.

Breast Implants

Both a 1994 population-based retrospective study[1] and a 1995 follow-up report of the Nurses' Health Study[2] were unable to find any association between breast implants and connective tissue diseases. A number of other studies have failed to show any correlation between breast implants and specific connective tissue diseases such as rheumatoid arthritis,[3] scleroderma,[4] and systemic lupus erythematosus.[5] The only study to date showing a correlation between implants and connective tissue diseases was a retrospective cohort study of women self-reporting both implants and the diagnosis of connective tissue disease; the relative risk was 1.24.[6] In this study the diagnoses were not verified,[6] which is particularly important because the assessment was made after the widely publicized U.S. Food and Drug Administration ban on breast implants.[7] Despite the lack of scientific evidence, courts have awarded huge settlements to plaintiffs. This has widespread implications for the future of health care in the United States, both because it fosters an antiscientific approach to medical issues and because companies are increasingly unwilling to produce medical devices under the current product liability system.[7]

REFERENCES

1. Gabriel SE, O'Fallon WM, Kurland LT, et al: Risk of connective-tissue diseases and other disorders after breast implantation, *N Engl J Med* 330:1697-1702, 1994.
2. Sánchez-Guerrero J, Colditz GA, Karlson EW, et al: Silicone breast implants and the risk of connective-tissue diseases and symptoms, *N Engl J Med* 332:1666-1670, 1995.
3. Dugowson CE, Daling J, Koepsell T, et al: Silicone breast implants and risk for rheumatoid arthritis (abstract), *Arthritis Rheum* 35(suppl):S66, 1992.
4. Hochberg MC, Miller R, Wigley FM: Frequency of augmentation mammoplasty in patients with systemic sclerosis: data from the Johns Hopkins–University of Maryland Scleroderma Center, *J Clin Epidemiol* 48:565-569, 1995.
5. Strom BL, Reidenberg MM, Freundlich B, et al: Breast silicone implants and risk of systemic lupus erythematosus, *J Clin Epidemiol* 47:1211-1214, 1994.
6. Hennekens CH, Lee I-M, Cook NR, et al: Self-reported breast implants and connective-tissue diseases in female health professionals: a retrospective cohort study, *JAMA* 275:616-621, 1996.
7. Angell M: Shattuck Lecture—evaluating the health risks of breast implants: the interplay of medical science, the law, and public opinion, *N Engl J Med* 334:1513-1518, 1996.

BREAST CANCER

Breast Cancer Risk Factors

(See also breast cancer risk in patients receiving hormone replacement therapy; oral contraceptives and the risk of breast cancer)

Table 7 lists some of the established and probable risk factors for breast cancer.[1-12]

Table 7 Breast Cancer Risk Factors

Risk factor	Relative risk
Family history of breast cancer[1]	
Mother	1.8
Sister	2.5
Mother and sister	5.6
First pregnancy over 30 years of age[1]	2.0-5.0
Failure to breast feed*[,2]	1.2
Menarche before 12 years of age[1]	2.0
History of fibroadenoma[3]	2.2
Hyperplastic or proliferative breast dysplasia[1]	1.4-2.7
Geographical location (West versus Asia)[1]	5.0
Oral contraceptives[4]	1.3
Hormone replacement therapy for ≥5 years[5]	1.5
Premenopausal body mass index >35[1]	0.7
Postmenopausal body mass index >35[1]	2.0
Elevated bone density[6]	1.3-3.5
Alcohol[7]	?
Diet[8,9]	?
Smoking[10]	?
Exercise[11]	?
Radiation[12-15]	?

*Elevated risk reported only for breast cancer developing in premenopausal women.

The breast cancer rate in the West is five to seven times that in Asia. However, it has been shown that women of Japanese origin whose families moved to Hawaii acquired Western rates within two generations.[1]

A small risk factor for premenopausal (but not postmenopausal) breast cancer is failure to breast feed. The major beneficial effect of breast feeding is found in women who first lactate before 20 years of age and who breast feed their infants for 6 months or more.[2]

A history of fibroadenoma increases the relative risk of acquiring breast cancer by 2.17. The risk varies according to the histological features of the fibroadenoma.[3]

A 1996 systematic review of 54 case-controlled studies found that the odds ratio for development of breast cancer among current users of oral contraceptives was 1.24, whereas for women who had stopped the pill 1 to 4 years before it was 1.16. Women who had stopped the pill 10 years before had no increased risk.[4]

Among women between 47 and 80 years of age, those with the highest bone densities are at the highest relative risk for breast cancer. The reason for this may be a higher cumulative exposure to estrogen.[6]

Whether alcohol is a risk factor for breast cancer is uncertain. The initial report of a relationship between moderate drinking and breast cancer appeared in 1974. Close to 50 articles on the subject have appeared in the ensuing 20 years, and there has been no consensus on whether alcohol ingestion is causally related to breast cancer.[7]

It has been suggested that high-fat diets are a risk factor for breast cancer, but this has not been substantiated in a pooled analysis of seven cohort studies.[8] Case-control studies suggest that lack of vegetables in the diet may predispose to premenopausal breast cancer.[9]

A 1995 report found that women who had smoked for 30 years had a significantly increased risk of breast cancer.[10]

An epidemiological study of more than 25,000 Norwegian women found that regular exercise was associated with a decreased risk of breast cancer. This was more marked in lean than obese women and in premenopausal than postmenopausal women. The mechanism of this protection is speculative; it could be a hormonal change or simply a decrease in obesity.[11]

A rare but important risk factor for breast cancer is previous radiation exposure such as is used in the treatment of childhood Hodgkin's disease.[12,13] Finnish airline cabin attendants have been found to have an increased incidence of breast cancer, which is hypothesized to result from excessive exposure to ionizing radiation.[14] However, a study of U.S. radiology technologists found no excess incidence of breast cancer.[15]

Some studies have indicated that induced abortion is associated with an increased risk of breast cancer.[16] That this is unlikely is suggested by a 1997 report of the entire at-risk female population of Denmark, where population registries were used to determine the rates of induced abortion and breast cancer; no increased risk from induced abortion was detected.[17]

REFERENCES

1. McPherson K, Steel CM, Dixon JM: Breast cancer—epidemiology, risk factors and genetics, *BMJ* 309:1003-1006, 1994.
2. Newcomb PA, Storer BE, Longnecker MP: Lactation and a reduced risk of premenopausal breast cancer, *N Engl J Med* 330: 81-87, 1994.
3. Dupont WD, Page DL, Parl FF, et al: Long-term risk of breast cancer in women with fibroadenoma, *N Engl J Med* 331:10-15, 1994.
4. Collaborative Group on Hormonal Factors in Breast Cancer: Breast cancer and hormonal contraceptives: collaborative reanalysis of individual data on 53,297 women with and 100,239 women without breast cancer from 54 epidemiological studies, *Lancet* 347:1713-1727, 1996.
5. Colditz GA, Hankinson SE, Hunter DJ, et al: The use of estrogens and progestins and the risk of breast cancer in postmenopausal women, *N Engl J Med* 332:1589-1593, 1995.
6. Zhang Y, Kiel DP, Kreger BE, et al: Bone mass and the risk of breast cancer among postmenopausal women, *N Engl J Med* 336:611-617, 1997.
7. Ashley, MF, Ferrence R, Room R, et al: Moderate drinking and health: report of an international symposium, *Can Med Assoc J* 151:809-828, 1994.
8. Hunter DJ, Spiegelman D, Adami H-O, et al: Cohort studies of fat intake and the risk of breast cancer—a pooled analysis, *N Engl J Med* 334:356-361, 1996.
9. Freudenheim JL, Marshall JR, Laughlin R, et al: Premenopausal breast cancer risk and intake of vegetables, fruits, and related nutrients, *J Natl Cancer Inst* 88:340-348, 1996.
10. Bennicke K, Carsten C, Sabroe S, et al: Cigarette smoking and breast cancer, *BMJ* 310:1431-1432, 1995.

11. Thune I, Brenn T, Lund E, et al: Physical activity and the risk of breast cancer, *N Engl J Med* 336:1269-1275, 1997.
12. Bhatia S, Robison LL, Oberlin O, et al: Breast cancer and other second neoplasms after childhood Hodgkin's disease, *N Engl J Med* 334:745-751, 1996.
13. Donaldson SS, Hancock SL: Second cancers after Hodgkin's disease in childhood (editorial), *N Engl J Med* 334:792-793, 1996.
14. Pukkala E, Auvinen A, Wahlberg G: Incidence of cancer among Finnish airline cabin attendants, 1967-92, *BMJ* 311: 649-652, 1995.
15. Boice JD Jr, Mandel JS, Doody MM: Breast cancer among radiologic technologists, *JAMA* 274:394-401, 1995.
16. Brind J, Chichilli VM, Severs WB, et al: Induced abortion as an independent risk factor for breast cancer: a comprehensive review and meta-analysis, *J Epidemiol Community Health* 50: 481-496, 1996.
17. Melbye M, Wohlfahrt J, Olsen J, et al: Induced abortion and the risk of breast cancer, *N Engl J Med* 336:81-85, 1997.

Lifetime Risk of Acquiring Breast Cancer

(See also clinical significance of detecting small lesions in a screening program)

The estimated lifetime risk of acquiring breast cancer in Canada by 80 years of age is 9.3% and by 90 years of age is 10.7%. Seventy-five percent of cases are found in women over 50 years of age.[1] The annual incidence of breast cancer increases progressively with each decade; at age 30, the 10-year risk of acquiring breast cancer is 0.4%, at age 50 it is 2%, and at age 70, 3%.[2] The lifetime risk of dying of breast cancer is 4.1%.[1]

REFERENCES

1. National Cancer Institute of Canada: *Canadian cancer statistics 1997,* Toronto, 1997, The Institute.
2. Bryant HE, Brasher PMA: Risks and probabilities of breast cancer: short-term versus lifetime probabilities, *Can Med Assoc J* 150:211-216, 1994.

Breast Self-Examination

(See also breast examination by health professionals; guidelines for mammographic screening; prevention; screening)

The importance of teaching breast self-examination has been almost universally accepted. However, the evidence that it is beneficial is inconclusive, and it may even be detrimental:

1. The overall positive predictive value of breast self-examination has been reported to be 12% (88% false-positive rate). Breast self-examination reveals many benign lesions, leading to anxiety, anesthesia, and surgery.[1]
2. Younger women are much more likely to practice breast self-examination than are older women, yet older women are at far higher risk for breast cancer.[2]
3. Breast self-examination leads to earlier detection and more favorable nodal status and tumor size, but no evidence has shown that it prevents death from breast cancer.[3]

Both the Canadian Task Force on the Periodic Health Examination[4] and the U.S. Preventive Services Task Force[5] have concluded that insufficient evidence exists to make a clear recommendation about teaching breast self-examination ("C" recommendations). The American Academy of Family Physicians[6] recommends the procedure.

REFERENCES

1. Frank JW, Mai V: Breast self-examination in young women: more harm than good? *Lancet* ii:654-657, 1985.
2. Phillips AJ, Brennan ME: Reactions of Canadian women to Pap tests and breast self-examination, *Can Family Physician* 22:1271-1274, 1976.
3. Baines CJ: Searching for the truth about breast cancer screening, *Can J Diagn* 95-104, June 1993.
4. Canadian Task Force on the Periodic Health Examination: *Canadian guide to clinical preventive health care,* Ottawa, 1994, Canada Communication Group—Publishing, pp 788-795.
5. US Preventive Services Task Force: *Guide to clinical preventive services,* ed 2, Baltimore, 1996, Williams & Wilkins, pp 73-87.
6. American Academy of Family Physicians: *Age charts for periodic health examination,* Kansas City, Mo, 1994, The Academy (reprint no 510).

Breast Examinations by Health Professionals

(See also breast self-examination; controversies and uncertainties about mammographic screening; guidelines for mammographic screening; clinical practice guidelines for screening or case finding)

Only one series of investigations, the Canadian National Breast Screening Studies (NBSS), has compared physical examination alone to mammography plus physical examination (in almost all cases, physical examination was performed by trained nurses). All other mammographic studies compared mammography plus physical examination to no systematic examination. After 7 years of follow-up no decrease in death rates was found in the mammography plus physical examination cohorts compared with the physical examination only cohorts.[1,2]

Guidelines vary as to when physicians should perform breast examinations for cancer detection. The Canadian Task Force on the Periodic Health Examination gives a "D" recommendation to physician breast examination (and mammography) of women 40 to 49 years of age but an "A" recommendation to performing both these examinations on an annual basis in women 50 to 69 years of age.[3]

The U.S. Preventive Services Task Force gives a "C" recommendation for clinical breast examinations alone in women 40 to 69 years of age.[4] However, it gives an "A" recommendation to screening mammography every 1 to 2 years with or without annual clinical breast examinations for women 50 to 69 years of age.[4]

Annual physician breast examinations beginning at 40 years of age are recommended by many other U.S. organizations, including the American Cancer Society,[5] American College of Radiology,[6] American Medical Association,[7] American College of Obstetricians and Gynecologists.[8] The

American Academy of Family Physicians goes even further, recommending physician examination every 1 to 3 years beginning at age 30.[9]

In a study of women over 50 years of age, one third of those seen by male physicians had mammography but no clinical breast examination, whereas only 5% of those seen by female physicians had mammography and no clinical breast examination.[10] Since examination of the breasts by physicians may account for some or all of the apparent positive benefits of mammographic screening (see later discussion), the findings of this study are worrisome.

REFERENCES

1. Miller AB, Baines C, To T, et al: Canadian National Breast Screening Study. 1. Breast cancer detection and death rates among women aged 40-49 years, *Can Med Assoc J* 147:1459-1476, 1992.
2. Miller AB, Baines CJ, To T, et al: Canadian National Breast Screening Study. 2. Breast cancer detection and death rates among women aged 50 to 59 years, *Can Med Assoc J* 147:1477-1488, 1992.
3. Canadian Task Force on the Periodic Health Examination: *Canadian guide to clinical preventive health care,* Ottawa, 1994, Canada Communication Group—Publishing, pp 788-795.
4. US Preventive Services Task Force: *Guide to clinical preventive services,* ed 2, Baltimore, 1996, Williams & Wilkins, pp 73-87.
5. American Cancer Society: *Guidelines for the cancer-related checkup: an update,* Atlanta, 1993, The Society.
6. Dodd GD: Screening for breast cancer, *Cancer* 72:1038-1042, 1993.
7. Council on Scientific Affairs, American Medical Association: Mammographic screening in asymptomatic women aged 40 years and older, *JAMA* 261:2535-2542, 1989.
8. American College of Obstetricians and Gynecologists: *The obstetrician-gynecologist and primary-preventive health care,* Washington, DC, 1993, The College.
9. American Academy of Family Physicians: *Age charts for periodic health examination,* Kansas City, Mo, 1994, The Academy (reprint no 510).
10. Burns RB, Freund KM, Ash AS, et al: As mammography use increases, are some providers omitting clinical breast examination? *Arch Intern Med* 156:741-744, 1996.

Mammography

(See also breast examinations by physicians; breast self-examination; guidelines for mammographic screening; clinical significance of detecting small lesions in a screening program; detrimental effects of investigations; informed consent; patient preconceptions and informed consent; prevention; screening)

Mammographic techniques

(See also adverse effects of mammography)

Mammography may be performed with one view or two views, and use of two views has reportedly increased cancer detection significantly.[1] Whether technical improvements will actually change outcomes is controversial.[2,3] A comparison of mammographically detected cancers in the Swedish Two-Counties Study from 1977 to 1982 (using single view without a grid) and from 1989 to 1992 (using two views and a grid) showed no difference in type and size of cancers detected and their likely prognoses.[2] When only one film of two-view screening was read and compared with the results of reading both films, only one of 32 cancers was missed on the single film reading.[3]

Another way of improving the results of mammograms is to have them read by two radiologists.[4,5] This is because interpretation of the films often varies significantly.[6]

REFERENCES

1. Field S, Michell MJ, Wallis MG, et al: What should be done about interval breast cancers? Two view mammography and possibly a shorter screening interval (editorial), *BMJ* 310:203-204, 1995.
2. Tabár L, Duffy SW, Warren LW: New Swedish breast cancer detection results for women ages 40-49, *Cancer* 72:1437-1448, 1993.
3. Thurfjell E, Taube A, Tabár L: One- versus two-view mammography screening: a prospective population-based study, *Acta Radiol* 35:340-344, 1994.
4. Anderson ED, Muir BB, Walsh JS, et al: The efficacy of double reading mammograms in breast screening, *Clin Radiol* 49:248-251, 1994.
5. Thurfjell EL, Lernevall KA, Taube AA: Benefit of independent double reading in a population-based mammographic screening program, *Radiology* 91:241-244, 1994.
6. Beam CA, Layde PM, Sullivan DC: Variability in the interpretation of screening mammograms by US radiologists: findings from a national sample, *Arch Intern Med* 156:209-213, 1996.

Intervals between mammographic screenings

(See also efficacy of mammography; controversies and uncertainties about mammographic screening)

The intervals between mammographic screenings usually vary between 1 and 3 years. Cancers that are diagnosed in the intervals between screenings are called "interval cancers." One British report found that the number of interval cancers expressed as a percentage of the underlying incidence was 31% during the first year after screening, 52% in the second year, and 82% in the third year. On this basis the authors suggest that a 3-year interval is too long.[1] However, a 1995 metaanalysis of all the major studies found no difference in mortality between women screened annually and those screened every 2 to 2½ years.[2]

Mammography performed on women under 50 years of age is less sensitive than for women over 50. In one study the sensitivity of breast cancer detection by mammography in women over 50 years of age determined after 25 months of follow-up was 85.7% whereas that for women under 50 with the same length of follow-up was 71.4%.[3] The increased breast density of younger women, which makes the detection of cancers more difficult, has been offered as one explanation for this phenomenon, but a more likely explanation is that tumor growth in this younger population tends to be more rapid.[4] The particularly low screening sensitivity in women under 40 years of age who have a strong family history of breast cancer lends indirect support to this hypothesis. Whether screening women under 50 years of age is beneficial is controversial (see later discussion of controversies and uncertainties about mammographic screening), but if such a program were undertaken in this age group, annual screening would seem to be indicated.[4]

REFERENCES

1. Woodman CBJ, Threlfall AG, Boggis CR, et al: Is the three year breast screening interval too long—occurrence of interval cancers in NHS breast screening programmes North Western Region, *BMJ* 310(6974):224-226, 1995.
2. Kerlikowske K, Grady D, Rubin SM, et al: Efficacy of screening mammography: a meta-analysis, *JAMA* 273:149-154, 1995.
3. Kerlikowske K, Grady D, Barclay J, et al: Effect of age, breast density, and family history on the sensitivity of first screening mammography, *JAMA* 276:33-38, 1996.
4. Tabar L, Fagerberg G, Chen H, et al: Efficacy of breast cancer screening by age: new results from the Swedish Two-County trial, *Cancer* 75:2507-2517, 1995.

Major mammographic screening programs

Several good reviews of mammographic screening programs have been published.[1-9] Nine of the major randomized controlled trials with references are listed below. The reason for recording them here is that the effectiveness of mammographic screening is not settled. Family physicians have to keep up to date with the literature on the subject, and almost every article refers to one or more of these studies.

Health Insurance Plan of Greater New York (HIP)[10]	United States
Two-County[11,12]	Sweden
Malmo[13]	Sweden
Stockholm[14]	Sweden
Gothenburg[3,7]	Sweden
Edinburgh[15]	United Kingdom
National Breast Screening Study—1 (NBSS-1)[16]	Canada
National Breast Screening Study—2 (NBSS-2)[17]	Canada
Finland[18]	Finland

REFERENCES

1. Baines CJ: Searching for the truth about breast cancer screening, *Can J Diagn,* June 1993, pp 95-104.
2. Dixon T: Breast screening: time for translation? (editorial), *Can Fam Physician* 37:2544-2548, 1991.
3. Nyström L, Rutqvist LE, Wall S, et al: Breast cancer screening with mammography: overview of Swedish randomised trials, *Lancet* 341:973-978, 1993.
4. Miller AB: Mammography: reviewing the evidence; epidemiological aspect, *Can Fam Physician* 39:85-90, 1993.
5. US Preventive Services Task Force: Screening for breast cancer, *Am Fam Physician* 39:89-96, 1989.
6. Kerlikowske K, Grady D, Rubin SM, et al: Efficacy of screening mammography: a meta-analysis, *JAMA* 273:149-154, 1995.
7. Fletcher SW, Black W, Harris R, et al: Report of the International Workshop on Screening for Breast Cancer, *J Natl Cancer Inst* 85:1644-1656, 1993.
8. Glasziou PP, Woodward AJ, Mahon CM: Mammographic screening trials for women aged under 50: a quality assessment and meta-analysis, *Med J Aust* 162:625-629, 1995.
9. Smart CR, Hendrix RE, Rutledge JH, et al: Benefit of mammography screening in women ages 40-49, *Cancer* 75:1619-1626, 1995.
10. Shapiro S: *Periodic screening for breast cancer: the Health Insurance Plan Project and its sequelae, 1963-1986,* Baltimore, Md, 1988, Johns Hopkins University Press.
11. Tabar L, Fagerberg G, Duffy SW, et al: The Swedish Two-County trial of mammographic screening for breast cancer: recent results and calculation of benefit, *J Epidemiol Commun Health* 43:107-114, 1989.
12. Tabar L, Fagerberg G, Chen H, et al: Efficacy of breast cancer screening by age: new results from the Swedish Two-County trial, *Cancer* 75:2507-2517, 1995.
13. Andersson I, Aspegren K, Janzon L, et al: Mammographic screening and mortality from breast cancer: the Malmö Mammographic Screening trial, *BMJ* 297:943-948, 1988.
14. Rutqvist LE, Miller AB, Andersson I, et al: Reduced breast-cancer mortality with mammography screening—an assessment of currently available data, *Int J Cancer* (suppl 5):76-84, 1990.
15. Roberts MM, Alexander FE, Anderson TJ, et al: Edinburgh trial of screening for breast cancer: mortality at seven years, *Lancet* 335:241-246, 1990.
16. Miller AB, Baines CJ, To T, et al: Canadian National Breast Screening Study. 1. Breast cancer detection and death rates among women aged 40 to 49 years, *Can Med Assoc J* 147: 1459-1476. 1992.
17. Miller AB, Baines CJ, To T, et al: Canadian National Breast Screening Study. 2. Breast cancer detection and death rates among women aged 50 to 59 years, *Can Med Assoc J* 147: 1477-1488, 1992.
18. Hakama M, Pukkala E, Heikkilä M, et al: Effectiveness of the public health policy for breast cancer screening in Finland: population based cohort study, *BMJ* 314:864-867, 1997.

Efficacy of mammographic trials

(See also controversies and uncertainties about mammographic screening; evidence-based medicine; fallacies in the reporting of benefits of mammography; intervals between mammographic screenings; surrogate outcomes)

Whether screening mammography for women under 50 years of age is beneficial is controversial, mainly because no trial has yet demonstrated a significant decrease in mortality for women in this age group. An overview of five combined Swedish trials (including the Gothenburg trial) published in 1993 found a 13% mortality reduction in the 40- to 49-year age group, but this was not statistically significant.[1] A 1993 metaanalysis of eight randomized trials involving the same age group by Fletcher and associates[2] also failed to show any statistically significant decrease in mortality. In 1995 three metaanalyses of randomized trials of mammography in women under 50 years of age were published. The first reviewed seven randomized trials involving 160,000 women and found no benefit from the intervention.[3] The second concluded that there was a trend toward decreased mortality after 10 to 12 years of follow-up,[4] but in the opinion of the authors, even if this trend were to be verified with time and further studies, screening beginning at 50 years of age would probably achieve the same benefit.[4] In contrast, the third 1995 metaanalysis, that of Smart and associates,[5] concluded that the previous reports were erroneous and that mammographic screening indeed produced a statistically significant decrease in mortality in this age group, provided the Canadian National Breast Screening Study—1 (NBSS-1) was excluded.

The one study that has most upset proponents of mammography for women under 50 years of age is the Canadian NBSS-1 program, which showed an increase in breast cancer mortality in the screened group compared with the control group.[6] Various criticisms of this study have been put forth, and because of these, suggestions have made that the study should be excluded from metaanalyses.[5,7] Smart and associates[5] in their metaanalysis of mammographic studies in women 40 to 49 years of age gave results both with and without the NBSS-1 trial. They claimed there were a non–statistically significant 16% relative reduction in mortality if the NBSS-1 was included and a 23% statistically significant relative reduction in mortality if it was excluded. The validity of excluding the NBSS trial is discussed further in the later section on controversies and uncertainties about mammographic screening.

In contrast to the data for women less than 40 years of age, a significant decrease in mortality as a result of mammography has been documented among women between the ages of 50 and 69 years. Mortality for women aged 50 to 64 on entry to the Health Insurance Plan of Greater New York (HIP) study,[8] and for women aged 50 to 69 on entry to all the Swedish trials,[1] was significantly reduced. The relative mortality rates of women who had mammography in the combined Swedish studies were 0.72 for women 50 to 59 years of age and 0.69 for women 60 to 69.[2] The absolute mortality reduction rates were much smaller (see below). There was no decrease in mortality in the NBSS-2 study of Canadian women aged 50 to 59 at entry,[9] and there were statistically insignificant decreases in the Edinburgh[10] and Finnish trials.[11] A metaanalysis of all the major studies reported in 1995 concluded that mammography resulted in a decreased cancer death rate in women between the ages of 50 and 74 after a follow-up period of 7 to 9 years.[4]

No decrease in mortality was demonstrated in the combined five Swedish trials for women 70 to 74 years of age.[1] A 1995 report from San Francisco found that the detection rate of cancers by mammography was higher in women over 65 years of age than those under 65 and that on average the stage of the detected cancers was lower in the older than the younger group. However, because this is a surrogate outcome, there is no proof that mammography will result in a decreased mortality rate.[12]

REFERENCES

1. Nyström L, Rutqvist LE, Wall S, et al: Breast cancer screening with mammography: overview of Swedish randomised trials, *Lancet* 34:973-978, 1993.
2. Fletcher SW, Black W, Harris R, et al: Report of the International Workshop on Screening for Breast Cancer, *J Natl Cancer Inst* 85:1644-1656, 1993.
3. Glasziou PP, Woodward AJ, Mahon CM: Mammographic screening trials for women aged under 50: a quality assessment and meta-analysis, *Med J Aust* 162:625-629, 1995.
4. Kerlikowske K, Grady D, Rubin SM, et al: Efficacy of screening mammography: a meta-analysis, *JAMA* 273:149-154, 1995.
5. Smart CR, Hendrix RE, Rutledge JH, et al: Benefit of mammography screening in women ages 40-49, *Cancer* 75:1619-1626, 1995.
6. Miller AB, Baines CJ, To T, et al: Canadian National Breast Screening Study. 1. Breast cancer detection and death rates among women aged 40 to 49 years, *Can Med Assoc J* 147:1459-1476, 1992.
7. Leitch AM: Controversies in breast cancer screening, *Cancer* 76(suppl 10):2064-2069, 1995.
8. Shapiro S, Venet W, Strax P, et al: *Periodic screening for breast cancer: the Health Insurance Plan project and its sequelae, 1963-1986,* Baltimore, 1988, Johns Hopkins University Press.
9. Miller AB, Baines CJ, To T, et al: Canadian National Breast Screening Study. 2. Breast cancer detection and death rates among women aged 50 to 59 years, *Can Med Assoc J* 147:1477-1488, 1992.
10. Roberts MM, Alexander FE, Anderson TJ, et al: Edinburgh trial of screening for breast cancer: mortality at seven years, *Lancet* 335:241-246, 1990.
11. Hakama M, Pukkala E, Heikkilä M, et al: Effectiveness of the public health policy for breast cancer screening in Finland: population based cohort study, *BMJ* 314:864-867, 1997.
12. Faulk RM, Sickles EA, Sollitto RA, et al: Clinical efficacy of mammographic screening in the elderly, *Radiology* 194:193-197, 1995.

Effect of reporting methods on perception of benefits of mammography

(See also absolute risk reduction; efficacy of mammographic trials; numbers of patients who need to be screened or treated; relative risk reduction)

Although the reported relative reduction of death from breast cancer in women over 50 years of age who have had mammography looks impressive for many of these trials (14% to 40%), the absolute risk reduction is much smaller. For example, a relative mortality reduction of 35% in the HIP trial translates into an absolute reduction in breast cancer deaths of 0.02% (2 per 10,000). Put another way, in the HIP trial 5061 women would have had to be screened to prevent one breast cancer death.[1,2] In the five combined Swedish studies the overall relative decrease in breast cancer mortality for women 40 to 74 years of age was 24%. The absolute figures were 0.3:1000 at 6 years, 0.7:1000 at 9 years, and 1.2:1000 at 12 years.[3]

An evaluation of several randomized controlled studies of mammography by two Canadian surgeons that was published

Breast Diseases

in 1995 calculated the number of women who would have to be screened in each trial to save one life annually. Their figures are[4]:

Health Insurance Plan of New York	7,086
Swedish National Board of Health	13,665
Stockholm	15,703
Edinburgh	20,322
Malmo	63,264
Canadian National Breast Screening Study	No mortality reductions

The results of the Finnish breast screening program published in 1997 reported that 10,000 women had to be screened to save one life.[5]

REFERENCES

1. Dixon T: Breast screening: time for translation? (editorial), *Can Fam Physician* 37:2544-2548, 1991.
2. Scrabanek P: Mass mammography: the time for reappraisal, *Int J Technol Assess Health Care* 5:423-430, 1989.
3. Nyström L, Rutqvist LE, Wall S, et al: Breast cancer screening with mammography: overview of Swedish randomised trials, *Lancet* 341:973-978, 1993.
4. Wright CJ, Mueller CB: Screening mammography and public health policy: the need for perspective, *Lancet* 346:29-32, 1995.
5. Hakama M, Pukkala E, Heikkilä M, et al: Effectiveness of the public health policy for breast cancer screening in Finland: population based cohort study, *BMJ* 314:864-867, 1997.

Controversies and uncertainties about mammographic screening

(See also informed consent; ductal carcinoma in situ; guidelines for mammographic screening; intervals between mammographic screenings; efficacy of mammographic trials; prevention; screening)

One problem in assessing the efficacy of mammography is trying to determine whether any decrease of breast cancer deaths is due to early detection or to more effective treatment for all stages of the disease. For example, a study of breast cancer deaths from England and Wales found that the incidence of breast cancers in screened women increased sharply after the introduction of screening (an expected effect of this intervention) while the mortality from breast cancer had begun to level off before the introduction of screening and dropped sharply within 3 years of its institution. In the opinion of the authors the decline in death rates occurred too soon to be explained by screening and might be the result of an increasing use of tamoxifen.[1]

With the exception of the Canadian National Breast Screening Studies (NBSS), most of the major mammographic studies used a combination of mammography and physical examination of the breasts in the study group and no breast examinations in the control group. It is therefore uncertain how much of the decline in mortality rates in women over the age of 50 is attributable to physical examination of the breasts and how much to mammography.[2] In the NBSS, which showed no decrease in mortality after 7 years of follow-up, physical examination and mammography were used in the study group and physical examination in the control group.[2,3] If physical examination alone is an important modality for decreasing breast cancer mortality, this may account for the failure of the study to demonstrate a decreased mortality in women over the age of 50 who had mammography.

The NBSS has been criticized for its randomization process. An in-depth review by two independent epidemiologists (from McGill and Harvard) failed to find any evidence that problems with randomization altered the results.[4]

Another controversial issue about mammography is the clinical importance of diagnosing ductal carcinoma in situ. Carcinoma in situ accounts for nearly half of all mammographically diagnosed breast cancers, but whether the detection and treatment of this lesion decrease mortality is unknown (see later discussion of ductal carcinoma in situ). One possibility is that length bias accounts for much of the observed benefit of mammography. The argument here is that mammography preferentially detects tumors, such as ductal carcinoma in situ, that may have very slow growth rates and little or no propensity to spread even if untreated. A report from Yale gives some support to this. The recurrence and mortality rates were lower among women with breast cancers detected by mammography than among those with cancers detected by other means even when tumors of identical TNM stages were compared.[5]

One of the most controversial issues is whether mammography in women between 40 and 49 years of age decreases mortality. The conclusions of some relevant studies are summarized in the earlier discussion of the efficacy of mammographic trials. No individual trial has shown a statistically significant decrease in mortality, and the only metaanalysis to do so excluded the NBSS-1. This is an emotional and political issue (see guidelines for mammographic screening below). Some authors interpret the literature as showing a decrease in mortality, whereas others do not. Although the issue is certainly not resolved, what is clear is that even if future studies prove some benefit from screening in the 40 to 49 age group, this will be received by only a very small number of screened women.[6]

My view of the controversy over mammography for women between the ages of 40 and 49 is that since benefits are uncertain, since mammography is not innocuous (see adverse effect of mammographic screening procedures), and since the Canadian Task Force on the Periodic Health Examination gives the procedure a "D" recommendation and the U.S. Preventive Services Task Force gives it a "C," the odds are that the intervention will do more harm than good. Obviously, individual patients have the right to make up their own minds. To do so, they need to be informed of the pros and cons of this preventive modality. This is essentially the perspective of Pauker and Kassirer,[6] who consider the choice a "tossup."

REFERENCES

1. Quinn M, Allen E (United Kingdom Association of Cancer Registries): Changes in incidence of and mortality from breast cancer in England and Wales since introduction of screening, *BMJ* 311:1391-1395, 1995.
2. Miller AB, Baines CJ, To T, et al: Canadian National Breast Screening Study. 2. Breast cancer detection and death rates among women aged 50 to 59 years, *Can Med Assoc J* 147:1477-1488, 1992.
3. Miller AB, Baines C, To T, et al: Canadian National Breast Screening Study. 1. Breast cancer detection and death rates among women aged 40-49 years, *Can Med Assoc J* 147:1459-1476, 1992.
4. Bailar JC III, MacMahon B: Randomization in the Canadian National Breast Screening Study: a review for evidence of subversion, *Can Med Assoc J* 156:193-199, 1997.
5. Moody-Ayers SY, Wells CK, Feinstein AR: *Does the reduced breast cancer mortality after mammography screening represent cure, early detection or discovery of relatively "benign" tumors?* (abstract) Robert Wood Johnson-Clinical Scholars Program, 1996 National Meeting, Key Largo, Fla, November 1996.
6. Pauker SG, Kassirer JP: Contentious screening decisions: does the choice matter? (editorial), *N Engl J Med* 336:1243-1244, 1997.

Adverse effects of mammography

(See also attitudes, physician; prevention; screening)

According to some reports a proportion of women with suspect mammograms have psychological difficulties even after learning that they do not have cancer.[1] Other studies report temporary anxiety,[2] but this, by implication, is dismissed as unimportant because it is often no longer evident after 3 months.[3] (Just because a person recovers from a psychological trauma does not mean that it is not significant.)

How many women undergoing mammography receive false-positive reports? If only women who have biopsies are analyzed, the ratio is about 3:1.[3] From the psychological viewpoint a more realistic evaluation is the malignancy rate among all women who, as a result of a mammogram report, are recalled for further evaluation. Shades of gray and risk spectrum are not part of most people's conception of illness; to many, any recall means cancer.[4] In most studies 5% to 14% of women having mammograms are recalled.[5,6] As a specific example, in a 1991-1992 Scottish program in which the recall rate of 7.3% was on the low end of the spectrum, 8.6% of those recalled had cancer and 91.4% did not.[3] Similar results have been reported from a California study.[7,8]

The usual false-negative rate for mammograms is 10% to 15%.[9] The danger of a false-negative result is unwarranted reassurance of a patient who actually has cancer.

Failure to obtain fully informed consent for mammographic screening may also cause harm. Women under the age of 50 have been shown to overestimate their risk of dying of breast cancer in the next 10 years 20 fold and overestimate the benefit of screening 6 fold.[10] If women are not informed of the actual figures and the pros and cons of screening, they may have false assumptions when participating in a program and suffer adverse effects as a result. Patients must be involved in decisions about screening mammography.[11] Most articles on mammography downplay or avoid entirely the adverse effects of the process; as Dixon points out, it is the family physician, not the mammographer, who has to deal with the emotional havoc that this can induce.[12]

The major adverse physical effect of mammography is discomfort. In one study 35% of women stated that mammography caused physical discomfort and 6% described it as painful.[13]

REFERENCES

1. Lerman C, Trock B, Rimer BK, et al: Psychological and behavioral implications of abnormal mammograms, *Ann Intern Med* 114:657-661, 1991.
2. Ellman R, Angeli N, Chritians AM, et al: Psychiatric morbidity associated with screening for breast cancer, *Br J Cancer* 60:781-784, 1989.
3. Balmy WR, Wilson ARM, Pantoic J, et al: Screening for breast cancer, *BMJ* 309:1076-1079, 1994.
4. Wardle J, Pope R: The psychological costs of screening for cancer, *J Psychosom Res* 36:609-624, 1992.
5. Elmore JG, Wells CK, Lee CH, et al: Variability in radiologists' interpretations of mammograms, *N Engl J Med* 331:1493-1499, 1994.
6. Brown ML, Houn F, Sickles EA, et al: Screening mammography in community practice: positive predictive value of abnormal findings and yield of follow-up diagnostic procedures, *AJR Am J Roentgenol* 165:1373-1377, 1995.
7. Kerlikowske K, Grady D, Barclay J, et al: Positive predictive value of screening mammography by age and family history of breast cancer, *JAMA* 270:2444-2450, 1993.
8. Kerlikowske K, Grady D, Barclay J, et al: Likelihood ratios for modern screening mammography: risk of breast cancer based on age and mammographic interpretation, *JAMA* 276:39-43, 1996.
9. Kopans DB: The accuracy of mammographic interpretations (editorial), *N Engl J Med* 331:1521-1522, 1994.
10. Black WC, Nease RF, Tosteson AN: Perceptions of breast cancer risk and screening effectiveness in women younger than 50 years of age, *J Natl Cancer Inst* 87:720-731, 1995.
11. Harris R, Leininger L: Clinical strategies for breast cancer screening: weighing and using the evidence, *Ann Intern Med* 122:539-547, 1995.
12. Dixon T: Breast screening: time for translation? (editorial), *Can Fam Physician* 37:2544-2548, 1991.
13. Rutter DR, Calnan M, Vaile MS, et al: Discomfort and pain during mammography: description, prediction, and prevention, *BMJ* 305:443-445, 1992.

Guidelines for mammographic screening

(See also breast examination by health professionals; breast self-examination; clinical practice guidelines for screening or case finding; controversies and uncertainties about mammographic screening)

The recommendations of the Canadian Task Force on the Periodic Health Examination are that women aged 50 to 69 years should have annual physical examinations of the breast and annual mammography ("A" recommendation).[1] Screening by physical examination of the breasts and mammography is not recommended for women under 50 ("D" recommendation).[1] The recommendations of the U.S. Preventive Services Task Force are that women aged 50 to 69 should have screening mammography every 1 to 2 years with or without annual clinical breast examinations ("A" recommendation).[2] The Task Force gives a "C" recommendation for both mammography and clinical breast examination for women aged 40 to 49 and for those over 70.[2]

Most Canadian, British, and European organizations concur with the policy of not screening women under 50.[1] However, a number of U.S. organizations such as the American Cancer Society,[3] American College of Radiology,[4] American Medical Association,[5] and American College of Obstetricians and Gynecologists[6] have endorsed mammographic screening of women aged 40 to 59. In 1994 the American Cancer Society reaffirmed its recommendation that women in the age range of 40 to 49 have screening mammography,[7] whereas in the same year the U.S. National Cancer Institute withdrew such a recommendation and adopted a neutral stand, citing a lack of positive evidence of the efficacy of screening mammography in that age group.[8] In January 1997 the National Cancer Institute stated that available data did not justify recommending universal screening of women aged 40 to 49. This caused a furor among advocates of breast cancer screening, including politicians, and a few months later the National Cancer Institute reversed itself by accepting the recommendations of its advisory board that women age 40 to 49 at average risk of breast cancer have mammographic screening every 1 to 2 years.[9] At about the same time the American Cancer Society changed its recommendation for this age group from screening mammography every 1 to 2 years to annual screening mammography.[10]

REFERENCES

1. The Canadian Task Force on the Periodic Health Examination: *Canadian guide to clinical preventive health care,* Ottawa, 1994, Communication Group—Publishing, pp 788-795.
2. US Preventive Services Task Force: *Guide to clinical preventive services,* ed 2, Baltimore, 1996, Williams & Wilkins, pp 73-87.
3. American Cancer Society: *Guidelines for the cancer-related checkup: an update,* Atlanta, 1993, American Cancer Society.
4. Dodd GD: Screening for breast cancer, *Cancer* 72:1038-1042, 1993.
5. Council on Scientific Affairs, American Medical Association: Mammographic screening in asymptomatic women aged 40 years and older, *JAMA* 261:2535-2542, 1989.
6. American College of Obstetricians and Gynecologists: *The obstetrician-gynecologist and primary-preventive health care,* Washington, DC, 1993, American College of Obstetricians and Gynecologists.
7. Mettlin C, Smart CR: Breast cancer detection guidelines for women aged 40-49 years: rationale for the American Cancer Society Reaffirmation of Recommendations, *CA Cancer J Clin* 44:248-255, 1994.
8. Volkers N: NCI replaces guidelines with statement of evidence, *J Natl Cancer Inst* 86:14-15, 1994.
9. Marwick C: Final mammography recommendation? *JAMA* 277:1181, 1997.
10. Marwick C: Other voices weigh in on mammography decision, *JAMA* 277:1027-1028, 1997.

Prognosis

The most important factor determining the prognosis of breast cancer is the presence of positive axillary nodes. The more positive nodes present, the worse the prognosis.[1,2] However, even the presence of multiple positive nodes is not an immediate death sentence; in one study the actuarial 10-year survival of women with more than 10 positive nodes was 29%.[3] If nodes are negative, tumor size is the dominant factor in determining prognosis.[1] Other factors of prognostic importance include estrogen-receptor concentration and histological grade.[2]

Survival of women with metastatic breast cancer varies with the site of metastases. For those with bone or skin metastases it may be years, whereas for those with hepatic metastases or lymphangitic spread in the lungs it is months.[2]

REFERENCES

1. Berkowitz LD, Love N: Adjuvant systemic therapy for breast cancer: issues for primary care physicians, *Postgrad Med* 98:85-94, 1995.
2. Phillips DM, Balducci L: Current management of breast cancer, *Am Fam Physician* 53:657-665, 1996.
3. Walker MJ, Osborne MD, Young DC, et al: The natural history of breast cancer with more than 10 positive nodes, *Am J Surg* 169:575-579, 1995.

Ductal Carcinoma in Situ, Lobular Carcinoma in Situ

(See also controversies and uncertainties about mammographic screening; surrogate outcomes)

Ductal carcinoma in situ (DCIS) is an important disease because it is detectable by mammography and as a result the incidence of the disorder has skyrocketed in the past decade.[1,2] In 1992 DCIS accounted for about 12% of breast cancers diagnosed in the United States and between 30% and 40% of those cancers diagnosed by mammography.[1] Between 1985 and 1995, 43% of breast cancers diagnosed in women aged 40 to 49 were ductal carcinomas in situ, while for women aged 30 to 39 the percentage was 92%.[1]

DCIS is found in 6% to 18% of autopsies of women dying of other diseases.[1] Although it seems likely that some cases of DCIS will become invasive, it is unknown which will and which will not and whether detecting these lesions by mammography saves lives (see discussion of controversies and uncertainties about mammographic screening). Because the natural history is unknown, treatment is uncertain.

A decade ago it was thought that all cases were multicentric and therefore the usual treatment was mastectomy. Evidence is increasing that many are localized lesions, so more and more patients are being treated with limited procedures. U.S. figures from 1992 indicate that 43.8% of cases were treated by mastectomy, 23.3% by lumpectomy plus radiation, and 30.2% by lumpectomy alone.[1]

Lobular carcinoma in situ is a different entity from ductal carcinoma in situ. It cannot be detected by mammography and is an incidental finding in breast biopsies performed for other reasons. It is not an anatomical precursor of breast cancer but is a risk factor for breast cancer in either breast.

REFERENCES

1. Ernster VL, Barclay J, Kerlikowske K, et al: Incidence of and treatment for ductal carcinoma in situ of the breast, *JAMA* 275:913-918, 1996.
2. Page DL, Jensen RA: Ductal carcinoma in situ of the breast: understanding the misunderstood stepchild (editorial), *JAMA* 275:948-949, 1996.

Management of Breast Cancer

(See also follow-up of cancer patients who have had curative treatments)

Timing of surgery according to menstrual phase

In 1991 Badwe and associates[1] from Guy's Hospital in London performed a chart review of women who had surgery for breast cancer between 1975 and 1985. Survival at 10 years was 84% in the group operated on in the second half, or luteal phase, of the cycle but only 54% for those operated on in the first half, or follicular phase. This beneficial effect was noted primarily among node-positive women. A number of subsequent studies support this finding,[2,3] whereas others do not.[4,5] A metaanalysis of 21 papers on this issue found an average odds reduction of 16% for treatment in the luteal phase.[6] Postulated mechanisms for improved prognosis if the patient is operated on in the luteal phase relate to the influence of the hormonal milieu on cell division,[7] immune parameters,[7] and cell dissemination.[7,8]

REFERENCES

1. Badwe RA, Gregory WM, Chaudary MA, et al: Timing of surgery during menstrual cycle and survival of premenopausal women with operable breast cancer, *Lancet* 337:1261-1264, 1991.
2. Senie RT, Rosen PP, Rhodes P, et al: Timing of breast cancer excision during the menstrual cycle influences duration of disease-free survival, *Ann Intern Med* 115:401-403, 1991.
3. Veronesi U, Luini A, Mariani L, et al: Effect of menstrual phase on surgical treatment of breast cancer, *Lancet* 343:1545-1547, 1994.
4. Gnant MF, Seifert M, Jakesz R, et al: Breast cancer and timing of surgery during menstrual cycle: a 5-year analysis of 385 premenopausal women, *Int J Cancer* 52:707-712, 1992.
5. Wobbes T, Thomas CM, Segers MF, et al: The phase of the menstrual cycle has no influence on the disease-free survival of patients with mammary carcinoma, *Br J Cancer* 69:599-600, 1994.
6. Fentiman IS, Gregory WM, Richards MA: Effect of menstrual phase on surgical treatment of breast cancer (letter), *Lancet* 344:402, 1994.
7. Senie RT, Kinne DW: Menstrual timing of treatment for breast cancer, *Monogr Natl Cancer Inst* 16:85-90, 1994.
8. McCulloch P, Choy A: Effect of menstrual phase on surgical treatment of breast cancer (letter), *Lancet* 344:402-403, 1994.

Lumpectomy

(See also practice patterns)

A metaanalysis of a variety of treatment plans (limited surgery such as lumpectomy versus more extensive surgery such as mastectomy, either alone or with radiation therapy) found no differences in mortality with any of the treatment modalities after 10 years. The rate of local recurrence of breast cancer was decreased threefold in the radiation therapy groups, but this did not affect mortality. Patients receiving postoperative radiation therapy had a slightly lower death rate from breast cancer, but this was offset by an increased death rate from other causes.[1] A reanalysis of the data from the National Surgical Adjuvant Breast and Bowel Project (NSABP) found no difference in mortality after an average follow-up of 12 years among patients treated with total mastectomy, lumpectomy, or lumpectomy plus radiation.[2] Local resection is not necessarily limited to women with small tumors.[3]

Radiation therapy is a standard adjuvant therapy after lumpectomy because it dramatically reduces the incidence of local recurrences even though it may not affect mortality. There may be subsets of women who could be adequately treated by surgery alone, but at present surgery alone should probably be performed only in the context of randomized trials.[4] Rates of local resection and of mastectomy vary considerably from one geographical region to another (see discussion of practice patterns).

REFERENCES

1. Early Breast Cancer Trialists' Collaborative Group: Effects of radiotherapy and surgery in early breast cancer: an overview of randomized trials, *N Engl J Med* 333:1444-1455, 1995.
2. Fisher B, Anderson S, Redmond CK, et al: Reanalysis and results after 12 years of follow-up in a randomized clinical trial comparing total mastectomy with lumpectomy with or without irradiation in the treatment of breast cancer, *N Engl J Med* 333:1456-1461, 1995.
3. Khanna MM, Mark RJ, Silverstein MJ, et al: Breast conservation management of breast tumors 4 cm or larger, *Arch Surg* 127:1038-1041, 1992.
4. Recht A, Houlihan MJ: Conservative surgery without radiotherapy in the treatment of patients with early-stage invasive breast cancer: a review, *Ann Surg* 222:9-18, 1995.

Chemotherapy and tamoxifen

A 20-year follow-up of women who had radical mastectomy for breast cancer with positive axillary nodes compared those who had adjuvant combination chemotherapy with cyclophosphamide, methotrexate, and fluorouracil with those who had no chemotherapy. The total survival rates and the relapse-free survival rates were higher in the adjuvant chemotherapy group. An exception was the subgroup of postmenopausal women who received no demonstrable benefit from chemotherapy.[1] Other studies found that quality of life is improved in premenopausal or perimenopausal women with node-positive breast cancer who are treated with chemotherapy[2] but that it is not improved in postmenopausal patients with node-positive breast cancer who receive chemotherapy (other than tamoxifen).[3] The reason for the failure of chemotherapy in postmenopausal women is controversial. It may be because these women have been given lower, and thus inadequate, doses of chemotherapy or because the main benefit of chemotherapy in premenopausal women is its inhibition of ovarian function. In addition, whether chemotherapy actually cures or merely delays the progression of the disease is not clear.[4]

One form of adjuvant chemotherapy that is being used in some centers is high-dose chemotherapy with hematopoietic rescue using autologous stored marrow or peripheral blood stem cells. This allows much higher doses of chemotherapy than would otherwise be possible. It is used for high-risk patients with breast cancer, that is, those with multiple nodes involved or with inflammatory breast cancer. Long-term efficacy is unknown, but studies are in progress.[5]

Tamoxifen, which has an antiestrogen effect on breast tissue, is used for all stages of breast cancer in both postmenopausal and premenopausal women.[6] It has been shown to decrease the annual odds of death in postmenopausal women by about 25% and is most effective when the tumor is estrogen receptor positive.[7] In November 1995 the National Cancer Institute issued an advisory stating that tamoxifen should be given for only 5 years. The limitation is based on one American and one Scottish study showing no survival advantage in women taking the drug for more than 5 years.[8]

The usual dosage of tamoxifen (Nolvadex) is 20 mg/day. Side effects include hot flushes and irregular periods. The incidence of endometrial cancer is slightly increased, and the risk of thromboembolism is elevated to about that seen in women taking oral contraceptive pills.

REFERENCES

1. Bonadonna G, Valagussa P, Moliterni A, et al: Adjuvant cyclophosphamide, methotrexate, and fluorouracil in node-positive breast cancer: the results of 20 years of follow-up, *N Engl J Med* 332:901-906, 1995.
2. Hurny C, Bernhard J, Coates AS, et al: Impact of adjuvant therapy on quality of life in women with node-positive operable breast cancer, International Breast Cancer Study Group, *Lancet* 347:1279-1284, 1996.
3. Gelber RD, Cole BF, Goldhirsch A, et al: Adjuvant chemotherapy plus tamoxifen compared with tamoxifen alone for postmenopausal breast cancer: metaanalysis of quality-adjusted survival, *Lancet* 20:347:1066-1071, 1996.
4. Henderson IC: Paradigmatic shifts in the management of breast cancer (editorial), *N Engl J Med* 332:951-952, 1995.
5. Goldberg SL, Klumpp TR, Mangan KF: Why consider bone marrow transplantation in breast cancer? (editorial), *Am Fam Physician* 54:856-863, 1996.
6. Jordan VC: The strategic use of antiestrogens to control the development and growth of breast cancer, *Cancer* 70(suppl 4):977-982, 1992.
7. Henderson IC: Adjuvant systemic therapy for early breast cancer, *Cancer* 74:(suppl 1):401-409, 1994.
8. National Cancer Institute: NCI issues clinical announcement about long-term use of tamoxifen in breast cancer treatment, URL http://wwwicic.nci.hih.gov/ "late-breaking information".

Metastatic breast cancer

(See also adrenal insufficiency; bisphosphonates in the treatment of established osteoporosis; bisphosphonates for bone pain)

Drugs commonly used for metastatic breast cancer included tamoxifen (Nolvadex), megestrol (Megace), leuprolide (Lupron), and more recently anastrozole (Arimidex).[1] Adrenal insufficiency associated with megestrol therapy has been reported.[2]

Monthly 2-hour intravenous infusions of the bisphosphonate pamidronate (Aredia) in patients with stage IV breast cancer with bone metastases who were receiving chemotherapy resulted in a later onset of skeletal complications, less bone pain, and better quality of life than in the control group. Few adverse effects were reported.[3]

REFERENCES

1. Anastrozole for metastatic breast cancer, *Med Lett* 38:61-62, 1996.
2. Subramanian S, Goker H, Kanji A, et al: Clinical adrenal insufficiency in patients receiving megestrol therapy, *Arch Intern Med* 157:1008-1011, 1997.
3. Hortobagyl GN, Theriault RL, Porter L, et al: Efficacy of pamidronate in reducing skeletal complications in patients with breast cancer and lytic bone metastases, *N Engl J Med* 335: 1785-1791, 1996.

CARDIOVASCULAR SYSTEM

(See also congenital anomalies—congenital heart disease)

Topics covered in this section

Cardiomyopathy
Cardiopulmonary Resuscitation
Congestive Heart Failure
Coronary Artery Disease
Electrocardiograms
Hypertension
Valvular Heart Disease
Vascular Disease

ABDOMINAL AORTIC ANEURYSM

(See also attitudes; informed consent; prevention; screening; screening and apparent prevalence rates)

Smoking is a major risk factor for the development of abdominal aortic aneurysms.[1]

The mortality rate of ruptured abdominal aortic aneurysm is maximal in men between 70 and 80 years of age.[2] The rate of rupture increases significantly for aneurysms greater than 5 cm in diameter. A rough figure for the rupture rate of aneurysms greater than 5 cm is 5% per year, while the rupture rate for aneurysms of 3.5 cm or less is virtually zero.[3] The rate at which small aneurysms reach the benchmark diameter of 5 cm is about 10% per year; 20% of such aneurysms do not grow at all.[4] The operative mortality for elective resection and graft replacement of aortic aneurysms is a little less than 5%.[5] If surgery is delayed until the aneurysm is symptomatic, the mortality rate is 5% to 33%,[5,6] and if it is delayed until rupture, mortality is about 50%.[2,5,6] Mason and co-workers[2] calculate that 72% of patients with untreated abdominal aortic aneurysms will die of other causes and that it is necessary to operate on three patients electively to prevent one rupture. Although a number of vascular surgeons have advocated abdominal ultrasound screening, evidence supporting this is controversial. Mason and associates[2] recommend against it, not only because of the physical morbidity and mortality of surgery, but also because of the possible psychological harm to patients who are told they have an aneurysm, even if it is too small to warrant surgery at the time of diagnosis. The Canadian Task Force on the Periodic Health Examination[6] and the U.S. Preventive Services Task Force[7] give screening abdominal physical examination and screening abdominal ultrasound a "C" recommendation.

REFERENCES

1. Lederle FA, Johnson GR, Wilson SE, et al: Prevalence and associations of abdominal aortic aneurysm detected through screening, *Ann Intern Med* 126:441-449, 1997.
2. Mason JM, Wakeman AP, Drummond MF, et al: Population screening for abdominal aortic aneurysm: do the benefits outweigh the costs? *J Public Health Med* 15:154-160, 1993.
3. Nevitt MP, Ballard DJ, Hallet JW Jr: Prognosis of abdominal aortic aneurysms: a population-based study, *N Engl J Med* 321:1009-1014, 1989.
4. Guirgis EM, Barber GG: The natural history of abdominal aortic aneurysms, *Am J Surg* 162:481-483, 1991.
5. Canadian Task Force on the Periodic Health Examination: The periodic health examination, 1991 update. 5. Screening for abdominal aortic aneurysm, *Can Med Assoc J* 145:783-789, 1991.
6. Canadian Task Force on the Periodic Health Examination: *Canadian guide to clinical preventive health care,* Ottawa, 1994, Canada Communication Group—Publishing, pp 672-678.
7. US Preventive Services Task Force: *Guide to clinical preventive services,* ed 2, Baltimore, 1996, Williams & Wilkins, pp 67-72.

ARRHYTHMIAS

Atrial Fibrillation

(See also anticoagulation; cerebrovascular accident; subclinical hyperthyroidism and atrial fibrillation; transient ischemic attacks)

Epidemiology

Atrial fibrillation increases with age. Figures vary, but in one study the disorder was found in 1.7% of persons 60 to 64 years of age and in 11.6% of those more than 75 years of age.[1] Although a few patients have isolated or lone atrial fibrillation (see later discussion), the vast majority have coexisting heart disease. The usual associated cardiac conditions in order of frequency are hypertension, congestive heart failure, and rheumatic heart disease.[2] Because hypertension is common among subjects in control groups, it is not as highly predictive of atrial fibrillation as are congestive failure and rheumatic heart disease. Other recognized causes of atrial fibrillation include thyrotoxicosis, subclinical hyperthyroidism, and heavy alcohol intake, especially binge drinking.

The mortality rate of patients with atrial fibrillation is about twice that of patients in normal sinus rhythm. This is probably a reflection of associated heart disease, which is present in 80% of cases.[3]

Atrial fibrillation of recent onset often reverts spontaneously to sinus rhythm.[3]

REFERENCES

1. Lake FR., McCall MG, Cullen KJ, et al: Atrial fibrillation and mortality in an elderly population, *Aust NZ J Med* 19:321-326, 1989.
2. Kannel WB, Abbott RD, Savage DD, et al: Epidemiologic features of chronic atrial fibrillation: the Framingham Study, *N Engl J Med* 306:1018-1022, 1982.
3. Cairns JA, Connolly SJ: Nonrheumatic atrial fibrillation: risk of stroke and role of antithrombotic therapy, *Circulation* 84:469-481, 1991.

Risk factors for stroke

(See also lone atrial fibrillation)

Patients with atrial fibrillation at the highest risk for stroke are those with prosthetic heart valves or those with mitral valve disease.[1] Other factors increasing the risk are increasing age, a history of previous stroke or transient ischemic attack, diabetes, hypertension, and coronary artery disease.[2] In the pooled data of five randomized trials of patients with atrial fibrillation, the annual risk of stroke in patients younger than 65 years of age with no risk factors was 1%, whereas it rose to 8.1% in patients older than 75 with one or more risk factors.[2] In the same study there was no difference in risk between patients with constant and those with paroxysmal atrial fibrillation.[2] The risk of stroke in patients with lone atrial fibrillation is very low (see later discussion).

REFERENCES

1. Laupacis A, Albers G, Dunn M, Feinberg W: Antithrombotic therapy in atrial fibrillation, *Chest* 102(suppl):426S-433S, 1992.
2. Atrial Fibrillation Investigators: Risk factors for stroke and efficacy of antithrombotic therapy in atrial fibrillation: analysis of pooled data from five randomized controlled trials, *Arch Intern Med* 154:1449-1457, 1994.

Rate control

Rate control in atrial fibrillation has traditionally been accomplished with digoxin. However, beta-blockers may be a better choice[1]; they act quickly, whereas digoxin acts slowly, and they may cause a reversion to sinus rhythm,[2] whereas digoxin does not.[3] The specific drug that many prefer is sotalol (Sotacor), which combines beta-blocking and type III antiarrhythmic effects; it is usually given as an oral dose of 80 to 160 mg bid.[4,5]

When beta-blockers are contraindicated, diltiazem or verapamil may be used.[4] Amiodarone (Cordarone) is a class III antiarrhythmic that is also effective in controlling the rate of atrial fibrillation with maintenance doses of about 200 mg/day. It is not widely used because of potential adverse effects, especially pulmonary toxicity.[5]

Quinidine is a class I antiarrhythmic that is effective in maintaining sinus rhythm after cardioversion. However, total mortality is increased in cohorts of patients treated with this drug, so except in unusual circumstances it is not used for this purpose.[5]

REFERENCES

1. Havranek EP: The management of atrial fibrillation: current perspectives, *Am Fam Physician* 50:959-968, 1994.
2. Platia EV, Michelson EL, Porterfield JK, et al: Esmolol versus verapamil in the acute treatment of atrial fibrillation or atrial flutter, *Am J Cardiol* 63:925-929, 1989.
3. Falk RH, Knowlton AA, Bernard SA, et al: Digoxin for converting recent-onset atrial fibrillation to sinus rhythm: a randomized, double-blinded trial, *Ann Intern Med* 106:503-506, 1987.
4. Burgess JH, Marshall KG: A treatment plan for atrial fibrillation, *Patient Care Can* 6:19-28, 1995.
5. Antman EM: Maintaining sinus rhythm with antifibrillatory drugs in atrial fibrillation, *Am J Cardiol* 78(suppl 4):67-72, 1996.

Cardioversion

If cardioversion is undertaken, the immediate success rate varies from about 75% to 100%. The most consistent predictor for maintenance of sinus rhythm once conversion has been achieved is a short duration of the fibrillation before conversion.[1]

Cardioversion should be considered for any patient who has had fibrillation for 6 months or less. A common pharmacological means of achieving this is sotalol 80 to 160 mg orally bid. If this is unsuccessful, electrical rhythm reversion should be considered. Patients who have had fibrillation for some time should receive anticoagulants for 3 weeks before rhythm reversion and for 4 weeks afterward if the medication is successful.[2]

To help maintain sinus rhythm once cardioversion has been achieved, sotalol is the current drug of choice.[2] Although antiarrhythmic drugs such as quinidine slightly improve the maintenance of sinus rhythm, they also increase the total mortality rate and should not be used.[2,3] Digoxin may actually increase the incidence of recurrent fibrillation through its vasotonic effects.[2]

REFERENCES

1. Cairns JA, Connolly SJ: Nonrheumatic atrial fibrillation: risk of stroke and role of antithrombotic therapy, *Circulation* 84:469-481, 1991.
2. Burgess JH, Marshall KG: A treatment plan for atrial fibrillation, *Patient Care Can* 6:19-28, 1995.
3. Coplen SE, Antman EM, Berlin JA, et al: Prevention of recurrent atrial fibrillation by quinidine: a meta-analysis of randomized trials (abstract), *Circulation* 80(suppl II):II-633, 1989.

Anticoagulation

(See also anticoagulants; cerebrovascular accidents)

There have been five recent randomized trials of warfarin use in patients in atrial fibrillation who did not have rheumatic heart disease or prosthetic heart valves.[1-5] In addition, a comprehensive collaborative analysis of pooled data from these five studies has been published.[6] Among patients receiving warfarin, there was a relative reduction in stroke rates of 68% (absolute annual reduction of 3.1%). When patients in the warfarin group who had strokes were analyzed, it was found that many were not taking the medication at the time of the incident. The frequency of hemorrhagic complications was low in the five combined studies (1% for the control group and 1.3% for the warfarin group).[6] Two studies published since then have confirmed that warfarin significantly decreased the incidence of ischemic stroke in patients with atrial fibrillation.[7,8]

The most feared complication of warfarin anticoagulation is intracranial hemorrhage. Known risk factors for this are excessive anticoagulation, poorly controlled hypertension, increasing age, cerebrovascular disease, and prosthetic heart valves.[9] In one study, prolonged prothrombin time was the dominant risk factor but age was a strong independent risk factor for subdural hematomas, with the relative risk doubling every decade.[9] These findings were duplicated in the European Atrial Fibrillation Trial Study Group; major bleeding events were slightly increased in patients with international normalized ratios (INRs) between 2.5 and 4 and were

Cardiovascular System

dramatically increased at levels greater than 5.[10] In this trial INR levels less than 2 were ineffective, and the fewest adverse events (combined ischemic and hemorrhagic events) occurred in patients with INRs between 2 and 2.4, although those with levels of 2.5 to 3 did almost as well; patients over 75 years of age had a 3.6 times greater risk of major bleeding independent of INR levels.[10]

The very elderly (over 75 years of age) were not assessed in the original five studies, but more than 400 such patients were recruited for a continuation of the Stroke Prevention in Atrial Fibrillation Study (SPAF II).[7,11] The results showed that warfarin was indeed effective in preventing ischemic strokes in this age group, but much of the benefit was lost because of a higher incidence of intracranial hemorrhage (0.6% per year for those under 75 and 1.8% per year for those over 75).[11] However, most of the patients who had this complication had an INR greater than 3 or a PT ratio greater than 1.5.[7]

The results of the above studies suggests that most patients with atrial fibrillation would benefit from warfarin therapy. It is clearly the drug of choice for patients with rheumatic heart disease, congestive heart failure, or mechanical prosthetic heart valves. Except in patients with prosthetic valves (see later discussion of prosthetic valves), the dose of warfarin should be adjusted to keep the INR under 3 and preferably as close to 2 as possible. The recommendation of the American College of Chest Physicians is that it be kept between 2 and 3.[12] This is particularly important in the very elderly.[13] Subtherapeutic doses (INR less than 2) are not effective; a 1996 case-controlled study of patients with atrial fibrillation who had had ischemic strokes found that the odds ratio of such an event occurring increased sharply with INR values less than 2.[14] In general, an INR of 2 is equivalent to a PT ratio of 1.3, an INR of 3 to a PT ratio of 1.5, and an INR of 4 to a PT ratio of 2.

Some patients, such as those with uncontrolled hypertension or those subject to frequent falls, are not candidates for warfarin. Many of these patients would receive at least some benefit from aspirin therapy (see below). Finally, some patients with lone atrial fibrillation have such a low risk of stroke that warfarin is not indicated for them (see later discussion).

If a patient is to receive anticoagulants as an outpatient, one method is to start with warfarin (Coumadin) 5 mg daily for 2 to 4 days with daily INR or PT readings. As control is achieved, the interval between INR readings is increased. For the elderly a lower initial dose might be advisable.[15]

REFERENCES

1. Petersen P, Boysen G, Godtfredsen J, et al: Placebo-controlled, randomised trial of warfarin and aspirin for prevention of thromboembolic complications in chronic atrial fibrillation: the Copenhagen AFASAK study, *Lancet* 1:175-179, 1989.
2. Stroke Prevention in Atrial Fibrillation Investigators: The stroke prevention in atrial fibrillation study: final results, *Circulation* 84:527-539, 1991.
3. Boston Area Anticoagulation Trial for Atrial Fibrillation Investigators: The effect of low-dose warfarin on the risk of stroke in patients with nonrheumatic atrial fibrillation, *N Engl J Med* 323:1505-1511, 1990.
4. Connolly S, Laupacis A, Gent M: Canadian Atrial Fibrillation Anticoagulation (CAFA) Study, *J Am Coll Cardiol* 18:349-355, 1991.
5. Ezekowitz M, Bridgers S, James K, et al (Veterans Affairs Stroke Prevention in Nonrheumatic Atrial Fibrillation Investigators): Warfarin in the prevention of stroke associated with nonrheumatic atrial fibrillation, *N Engl J Med* 327:1406-1412, 1992.
6. Atrial Fibrillation Investigators: Risk factors for stroke and efficacy of antithrombotic therapy in atrial fibrillation: analysis of pooled data from five randomized controlled trials, *Arch Intern Med* 154:1449-1457, 1994.
7. Stroke Prevention in Atrial Fibrillation Investigators: Warfarin versus aspirin for prevention of thromboembolism in atrial fibrillation: Stroke Prevention in Atrial Fibrillation II Study, *Lancet* 343:687-691, 1994.
8. European Atrial Fibrillation Trial Study Group: Secondary prevention in non-rheumatic atrial fibrillation after transient ischaemic attack or minor stroke, *Lancet* 342:1255-1262, 1993.
9. Hylek EM, Singer DE: Risk factors for intracranial hemorrhage in outpatients taking warfarin, *Ann Intern Med* 120:897-902, 1994.
10. European Atrial Fibrillation Trial Study Group: Optimal oral anticoagulant therapy in patients with nonrheumatic atrial fibrillation and recent cerebral ischemia, *N Engl J Med* 333:5-10, 1995.
11. Stroke Prevention in Atrial Fibrillation Investigators: Bleeding during antithrombotic therapy in patients with atrial fibrillation, *Arch Intern Med* 156:409-416, 1996.
12. Hirsh J, Dalen JE, Deykin D, et al: Oral anticoagulants: mechanism of action, clinical effectiveness and optimal therapeutic range, *Chest* 102(suppl):312S-326S, 1992.
13. Albers GW: Atrial fibrillation and stroke: three new studies, three remaining questions, *Arch Intern Med* 154:1443-1448, 1994.
14. Hylek EM, Skates SJ, Sheehan MA, et al: An analysis of the lowest effective intensity of prophylactic anticoagulation for patients with nonrheumatic atrial fibrillation, *N Engl J Med* 335:540-546, 1996.
15. Burgess JH, Marshall KG: A treatment plan for atrial fibrillation, *Patient Care Can* 6:19-28, 1995.

Aspirin

(See also transient ischemic attacks)

Only two of the five randomized trials discussed previously under "Anticoagulation" randomized patients to an aspirin group. The Copenhagen Atrial Fibrillation, Aspirin, Anticoagulation (AFASAK) trial used a 75-mg dose of aspirin, and no statistically significant benefit was observed.[1] The Stroke Prevention in Atrial Fibrillation Study (SPAF) used 325 mg of aspirin and demonstrated a statistically significant decrease in stroke,[2] but when those over 75 years of age were analyzed separately, this group did not appear to receive any benefit.[3] Subsequent studies included the Stroke Prevention in Atrial

Cardiovascular System

Fibrillation II Study (SPAF II)[4] and the European Atrial Fibrillation Trial (EAFT).[5] Both showed a non–statistically significant decline in strokes among patients taking aspirin.

When the studies just quoted and others are viewed as a whole, aspirin appears to decrease the risk of stroke by a relative rate of about 21% with no clear relationship to aspirin dose.[6] In virtually all studies comparing aspirin and warfarin, warfarin was more effective except in subgroups such as patients younger than 65 years with lone atrial fibrillation in whom the risk of stroke was so low that no treatment was required (see later discussion).

REFERENCES

1. Petersen P, Boysen G, Godtfredsen J, et al: Placebo-controlled, randomised trial of warfarin and aspirin for prevention of thromboembolic complications in chronic atrial fibrillation: the Copenhagen AFASAK study, *Lancet* 1:175-179, 1989.
2. Stroke Prevention in Atrial Fibrillation Investigators: The stroke prevention in atrial fibrillation study: final results, *Circulation* 84:527-539, 1991.
3. Stroke Prevention in Atrial Fibrillation Investigators: A differential effect of aspirin on prevention of stroke in atrial fibrillation, *J Stroke Cerebrovasc Dis* 3:181-188, 1993.
4. Stroke Prevention in Atrial Fibrillation Investigators: Warfarin versus aspirin for prevention of thromboembolism in atrial fibrillation: Stroke Prevention in Atrial Fibrillation II Study, *Lancet* 343:687-691, 1994.
5. European Atrial Fibrillation Trial Study Group: Secondary prevention in non-rheumatic atrial fibrillation after transient ischaemic attack or minor stroke, *Lancet* 342:1255-1262, 1993.
6. Atrial Fibrillation Investigators: The efficacy of aspirin in patients with atrial fibrillation, *Arch Intern Med* 157:1237-1240, 1997.

Lone atrial fibrillation

The term "lone auricular fibrillation" was coined by Evans and Swann[1] in 1954 for patients who had atrial fibrillation without associated cardiac disease. In a collaborative analysis of five studies of atrial fibrillation stroke prevention, the annual stroke rate in patients with lone atrial fibrillation was zero in those less than 60 years of age, 1.6% in those aged 60 to 69, and 2.1% in those aged 70 to 79.[2] The practical significance of this is that persons under the age of 60 with lone atrial fibrillation do not require antithrombotic therapy for stroke prevention and those aged 60 to 75 appear to be adequately protected by aspirin. For those over 75, warfarin may be indicated if the dose is kept low and there are no contraindications.[3]

REFERENCES

1. Evans W, Swann P: Lone auricular fibrillation, *Br Heart J* 16:189-194, 1954.
2. Atrial Fibrillation Investigators: Risk factors for stroke and efficacy of antithrombotic therapy in atrial fibrillation: analysis of pooled data from five randomized controlled trials, *Arch Intern Med* 154:1449-1457, 1994.
3. Albers GW: Atrial fibrillation and stroke: three new studies, three remaining questions, *Arch Intern Med* 154:1443-1448, 1994.

Paroxysmal atrial fibrillation

Paroxysmal atrial fibrillation makes up over 40% of cases of fibrillation, but it has not been as well studied as constant atrial fibrillation. From the evidence available it seems prudent to treat paroxysmal atrial fibrillation in a manner identical to persistent atrial fibrillation.[1] Digoxin is not the drug of first choice for paroxysmal atrial fibrillation, since it does not reduce the frequency of attacks[2] or reduce the heart rate during the attacks.[3]

REFERENCES

1. Aboaf AP, Wolf PS: Paroxysmal atrial fibrillation: a common but neglected entity, *Arch Intern Med* 156:362-367, 1996.
2. Rawles JM, Metcalfe MJ, Jennings K: Time of occurrence, duration, and ventricular rate of paroxysmal atrial fibrillation: the effect of digoxin, *Br Heart J* 63:225-227, 1990.
3. Galun E, Flugelman MY, Glickson M, et al: Failure of long-term digitalization to prevent rapid ventricular response in patients with paroxysmal atrial fibrillation, *Chest* 99:1038-1040, 1991.

Wolff-Parkinson-White Syndrome

(See also palpitations)

Typical electrocardiographic findings in the Wolff-Parkinson-White syndrome are a delta-wave configuration and a short PR interval. The definitive treatment for patients with this syndrome is catheter radiofrequency ablation of the accessory pathway.[1] Treatment of an acute episode of atrial fibrillation in a patient with Wolff-Parkinson-White syndrome is electrical cardioversion or procainamide (Pronestyl) 50 mg IV over 1 minute repeated at 5-minute intervals or propranolol 0.5 to 1 mg IV.[1] Use of digoxin, diltiazem, or verapamil should be avoided.[2]

REFERENCES

1. Ganz LI, Friedman PL: Supraventricular tachycardia, *N Engl J Med* 332:162-173, 1995.
2. Janeira LF: Differentiating wide complex tachycardias, *Am Fam Physician* 54:1573-1584, 1996.

PACEMAKERS

Cellular telephones held over implanted pacemakers can interfere with pacemaker functions. Such telephones held over the ear do not interfere with the pacemaker.[1]

REFERENCES

1. Hayes DL, Wang PJ, Reynolds DW, et al: Interference with cardiac pacemakers by cellular telephones, *N Engl J Med* 336:1473-1479, 1997.

PALPITATIONS

(See also Wolff-Parkinson-White syndrome)

Palpitations are common presenting complaints in primary care; in one general medical outpatient clinic they were noted in 16% of patients.[1] Psychiatric disorders are common in patients with palpitations. In a Harvard study of 130 patients who were referred for Holter monitoring because of palpitations, the group had a 28% lifetime prevalence of panic disorder (6 times the rate of control subjects with a *p* value of .004), a 22% lifetime prevalence of major depression (1.6 times the rate of control subjects with a *p* value of .30), and a 10% lifetime prevalence of dysthymia (3.4 times the rate of control subjects with a *p* value of 1.00).[2]

Although anxiety disorders may cause palpitations as indicated previously, paroxysmal supraventricular tachycardia may mimic the symptoms of panic disorder.[3] In one study of patients with confirmed supraventricular tachycardia, two thirds of the patients met the criteria of the *Diagnostic and Statistical Manual of Mental Disorders,* edition 4 (DSM-IV), for panic disorder. Frequent symptoms included dizziness, shortness of breath, sweating, chest pain, fear of dying, flushing, tremulousness, and numbness. After definitive therapy, usually radiofrequency ablation, only 11% of patients whose symptoms had originally fulfilled the diagnostic criteria of panic disorder continued to experience such symptoms.[3]

The diagnosis of paroxysmal supraventricular tachycardia is usually easy if an electrocardiogram can be obtained during an episode; otherwise it is difficult. The resting electrocardiogram of some patients may exhibit the delta wave typical of Wolff-Parkinson-White syndrome, but this is relatively uncommon. Holter monitoring detects only a few cases because most patients do not have episodes of tachycardia during the monitoring period.[3]

REFERENCES

1. Kroenke K, Arrington ME, Mangelsdorff AD: The prevalence of symptoms in medical outpatients and the adequacy of therapy, *Arch Intern Med* 150:1685-1689, 1990.
2. Barsky AJ, Cleary PD, Coeytaux RR, et al: The clinical course of palpitations in medical outpatients, *Arch Intern Med* 155:1782-1788, 1995.
3. Lessmeier TJ, Gamperling D, Johnson V, et al: Unrecognized paroxysmal supraventricular tachycardia: potential for misdiagnosis as panic disorder, *Arch Intern Med* 157:537-543, 1997.

CARDIOMYOPATHY

Hypertrophic Cardiomyopathy

In recent years it has become possible to diagnose asymptomatic hypertrophic cardiomyopathy through molecular genetic assays. As a result of such studies, it has become clear that the prevalence of the disorder is more common than was previously thought (1:500) and that most patients have no or only mild symptoms. When annual mortality rates are calculated for unselected patients (in contrast to those from tertiary referral centers), they are about 1% or less.[1]

The drugs of choice for patients in heart failure are beta-blockers or verapamil (Calan, Covera-HS, Isoptin). Both slow the heart, and the prolonged diastole allows increased filling of the ventricles. However, these drugs do not protect patients against sudden death.[1]

Prophylactic drugs have not shown value in asymptomatic or mildly symptomatic patients. These patients should be encouraged to lead normal lives, but intense physical training or competitive athletics should probably be discouraged.[1]

REFERENCES

1. Spirito P, Seidman CE, McKenna WJ, et al: The management of hypertrophic cardiomyopathy, *N Engl J Med* 336:775-785, 1997.

Idiopathic Dilated Cardiomyopathy

Idiopathic dilated cardiomyopathy is the major indication for heart transplantation in both adults and children. The condition is 2.5 times as common in males as in females, and 2.5 times as common in blacks as in whites. The disorder may develop in children or the elderly, but most patients are between 20 and 50 years of age. At the time of clinical presentation, heart failure is usually advanced. The prognosis is variable. Some patients remain stable for a number of years, and others have a progressively downhill course. The average 5-year mortality is about 20%.[1]

REFERENCES

1. Dec GW, Fuster V: Idiopathic dilated cardiomyopathy, *N Engl J Med* 331:1564-1575, 1994.

CARDIOPULMONARY RESUSCITATION

(See also cardiac arrest; cardiac arrest during exercise; flight emergencies; informed consent; sudden infant death syndrome; vegetative state)

Hospitalized elderly patients with acute medical problems have a 10% to 17% chance of surviving to discharge after cardiopulmonary resuscitation (CPR). If they have chronic illnesses associated with a life expectancy of less than 1 year, the chance is less than 5%.[1-3] Even after a successful resuscitation, nearly half the survivors have significant residual functional deficits.[4] Patients grossly overestimate their chances of recovery, so in requesting advance directives it is important to provide them with accurate data so they can give reasonable informed consent.[1,2] A contributing factor to their overly optimistic expectations of CPR may be the subliminal messages of such television programs as *ER, Chicago Hope,* and *Rescue 911* in which the success rate of resuscitation is inordinately high.[5]

The results of resuscitation in nursing homes are abysmal with virtually no long-term survivors; for the very few who survive to discharge, quality of life is awful.[6,7] One editorialist suggests that for this population the norm should be no CPR unless specifically requested rather than CPR unless "do not resuscitate" orders have been specifically requested.[8]

Cardiovascular System

Reported overall survival rates of cardiac arrests that occur outside of hospitals vary from 1.4% to 18%. Results are better if bystanders have initiated CPR.[9] A Scottish study found that about 40% of patients who were successfully resuscitated outside of the hospital were discharged without significant neurological sequelae.[10] Current evidence suggests that while both ventilation and external chest compression should be given in cases of arrest outside the hospital, chest compression alone can give good results.[9]

A recent advance in CPR is the development of the automatic external defibrillator. This device, which is applied to a patient with no clinically detected pulse, senses cardiac rhythm. If it detects rapid ventricular tachycardia or ventricular fibrillation, it automatically delivers a countershock.[9]

A study from the Hospital for Sick Children in Toronto found that only 15% of children with out-of-hospital cardiac or respiratory arrest who were resuscitated in the emergency room survived to discharge and that all the survivors were left with neurological deficits. The authors concluded that except for cases of severe hypothermia or episodes of recurrent (rather than persistent) arrest, continuation of resuscitation for out-of-hospital cardiac arrests is futile after 20 minutes or after the two doses of epinephrine have been administered.[11]

Most advance directives are inaccessible to the health care team when a patient is transferred to a hospital and are therefore not followed.[12]

REFERENCES

1. Murphy DJ, Burrows D, Santilli S, et al: The influence of the probability of survival on patients' preferences regarding cardiopulmonary resuscitation, *N Engl J Med* 330:545-549, 1994.
2. Murphy DJ, Murray AM, Robinson BE, et al: Outcomes of cardiopulmonary resuscitation in the elderly, *Ann Intern Med* 111:199-205, 1989.
3. Taffet GE, Teasdale TA: In-hospital cardiopulmonary resuscitation, *JAMA* 260:2069-2072, 1988.
4. FitzGerald JD, Wenger NS, Califf RM, et al: Functional status among survivors of in-hospital cardiopulmonary resuscitation, *Arch Intern Med* 156:72-76, 1996.
5. Diem SJ, Lantos JD, Tulsky JA: Cardiopulmonary resuscitation on television: miracles and misinformation, *N Engl J Med* 334:1578-1582, 1996.
6. Applebaum GE, King JE, Finucane TE: The outcome of CPR initiated in nursing homes, *J Am Geriatr Soc* 38:197-200, 1990.
7. Awoke S, Mouton CP, Parrott M: Outcomes of skilled cardiopulmonary resuscitation in a long-term-care facility: futile therapy? *J Am Geriatr Soc* 40:593-595, 1992.
8. Nazerali N: Cardiopulmonary resuscitation of elderly people in long-term care: time for a paradigm shift (editorial), *Can Fam Physician* 42:2320-2322, 1996.
9. Ballew KA: Cardiopulmonary resuscitation, *BMJ* 324:1462-1465, 1997.
10. Cobbe SM, Dalziel K, Ford I, et al: Survival of 1476 patients initially resuscitated from out of hospital cardiac arrest, *BMJ* 312:1633-1637, 1996.
11. Schindler MB, Bohn D, Cox PN, et al: Outcome of out-of-hospital cardiac or respiratory arrest in children, *N Engl J Med* 335:1473-1479, 1996.
12. Morrison RS, Olson E, Mertz KR, et al: The inaccessibility of advance directives on transfer from ambulatory to acute care settings, *JAMA* 274:478-482, 1995.

CONGESTIVE HEART FAILURE

The following is the New York Heart Association classification of congestive heart failure:

Class I	Symptoms with unusual activity (manual labor)
Class II	Symptoms with usual activity (light yard work, sexual intercourse)
Class III	Symptoms with self-care activity (dressing, making bed)
Class IV	Symptoms at rest and worse with activity

Prognosis

The overall 5-year survival rate of patients with congestive heart failure is about 50%.[1] The annual death rates for various degrees of heart failure based on the New York Heart Association classifications are estimated to be[2]:

Class II	5% to 10% per year
Class III	10% to 20% per year
Class IV	20% to 50% per year

About half of the deaths from cardiac causes are sudden, and one fourth of these occur without prior worsening of the heart failure.[2]

REFERENCES

1. Andersson B, Waagstein F: Spectrum and outcome of congestive heart failure in a hospitalized population, *Am Heart J* 126:632-640, 1993.
2. Dracup K, Baker DW, Dubar SB, et al: Management of heart failure. II. Counseling, education, and lifestyle modifications, *JAMA* 272:1442-1446, 1994.

Systolic and Diastolic Heart Failure

Systolic heart failure is caused by a decreased contractility of the heart and is associated with dilation, which is often seen as an enlarged heart on chest roentgenogram. It is the type of heart failure with which most people are familiar and is much more common than diastolic failure. In systolic failure the left ventricular ejection fraction is usually less than 40%.[1]

Diastolic heart failure is the inability of the heart to relax properly. The patient has decreased cardiac compliance and increased filling pressures. The chest roentgenogram may show no increase in heart size, and the left ventricular ejection fraction is often greater than 40%. In fact, pure diastolic dysfunction may be defined as an elevated end-diastolic pressure without chamber enlargement.[1] Some of the causes of diastolic failure are hypertrophic cardiomyopathy, aortic stenosis, hypertension, and conditions such as cardiac amyloidosis and extensive scarring from coronary artery disease in which cardiac interstitial tissue is increased. An element of diastolic failure is particularly common in elderly or hypertensive patients.[1] Diastolic failure is sometimes detected by noting the changes in the indices of ventricular filling during an echocardiogram, but its sensitivity and specificity are poor.[2] If a patient has evidence of systemic or pulmonary venous congestion in the absence of left ventricular enlargement, the odds are high that diastolic failure is a major component of the failure.[1]

A number of patients have a combination of systolic and diastolic failure. It is important that physicians not rule out heart failure in a patient with dyspnea on effort, orthopnea, and decreased energy just because the heart size is normal.[1] According to one set of clinical guidelines, any patient with symptoms suggestive of heart failure should probably have echocardiography or, as a second choice, radionuclide ventriculography.[2] This is because the history, physical examination, and chest roentgenogram may not allow differentiation among systolic or diastolic dysfunction, valvular disease, or even noncardiac causes of the patient's symptoms.

REFERENCES

1. Cohn JN: The management of chronic heart failure, *N Engl J Med* 335:490-498, 1996.
2. Heart Failure Guideline Panel: Heart failure: management of patients with left ventricular systolic dysfunction, *Am Fam Physician* 50:603-616, 1994.

Diet and Exercise

Except in severe failure the maximum salt intake should be 3 g per day, which can be achieved by avoiding salty food and by not adding salt to food after it has been cooked. Patients with severe failure (for example, those requiring 80 mg of furosemide or more per day) should limit their salt intake to 2 g per day. This involves avoiding milk products, prepared foods, and canned foods and is unpalatable for most patients.[1]

Data on alcohol in congestive heart failure are inconclusive. Alcohol is obviously contraindicated in alcoholic cardiomyopathy. In other cases expert opinion is that patients should take a maximum of one drink per day.[1]

Patients with stable heart failure should be encouraged to exercise on a regular basis by walking or bicycling (on flat terrain). In some patients this has been shown to improve functional status and decrease symptoms.[1,2]

REFERENCES

1. Dracup K, Baker DW, Dubar SB, et al: Management of heart failure. II. Counseling, education, and lifestyle modifications, *JAMA* 272:1442-1446, 1994.
2. Heart Failure Guideline Panel: Heart failure: management of patients with left ventricular systolic dysfunction, *Am Fam Physician* 50:603-616, 1994.

Pharmacotherapy of Congestive Heart Failure

(See also ACE inhibitors in hypertension; coronary artery bypass grafting and angioplasty)

ACE inhibitors in congestive heart failure

(See also urticaria and angioedema)

Angiotensin-converting enzyme (ACE) inhibitors are first-line therapy for congestive heart failure. Captopril given to post–myocardial infarction patients with ventricular dysfunction resulted in a decreased incidence of congestive heart failure and a decreased mortality.[1] Enalapril has been shown to decrease the incidence of congestive heart failure in asymptomatic patients with reduced ejection fractions[2] and to decrease the mortality rate in patients who had mild to moderate or severe congestive heart failure.[3,4] Both enalapril and captopril have been shown to improve the New York Heart Association functional class by 0.5 to 1 class.[4] A meta-analysis of a large number of studies using different ACE inhibitors in congestive heart failure showed them to reduce total mortality and hospitalization rates in a broad range of patients. Those who benefited the most were the patients with the lowest ejection fractions.[5] In most cases high doses of ACE inhibitors are necessary to relieve symptoms or increase exercise capacity.[6]

ACE inhibitors should be used with caution in patients who have diminished renal function. If the creatinine level is greater than 3 mg/dl (250 μmol/L), only half the usual dose of ACE inhibitor should be given and it should be titrated upward slowly. ACE inhibitors should not be given to patients whose potassium concentration is 5.5 mmol/L or greater.[4]

Cough is not always a reason for stopping an ACE inhibitor.[4] Cough is a common symptom of congestive heart failure, so it is not always caused by the drug. For example, in one trial 37% of patients receiving enalapril reported cough compared with 31% of patients taking placebo.[3] Even if an ACE inhibitor is the cause of cough, the benefits of the drug may outweigh the distress of this symptom.[4] If the cough is intolerable, it may decrease in intensity with a lower dose of the ACE inhibitor. Another alternative is sodium cromoglycate, which in one small study reduced the severity of ACE inhibitor-induced cough.[7] In some cases an angiotensin II receptor antagonist such as losartan (Cozaar) can be substituted, since this class of drugs is not known to cause cough (or angioedema)[8] and short-term trials have shown losartan to be effective in congestive heart failure.[9]

Some patients are at increased risk of hypotension when given the first dose of an ACE inhibitor. These include patients who are volume depleted from diuretics, those in severe failure, those with a systolic blood pressure less than 100 mm Hg, and those over 75 years of age. If a patient is volume depleted, diuretics should be withheld for 1 to 2 days before the ACE inhibitor is begun. In patients at risk an initial very low dose of a short-acting ACE inhibitor such as

Table 8 ACE Inhibitors

Drug	Usual dose
Benazepril (Lotensin)	10-20 mg/day as a single dose
Captopril (Capoten)	25-50 mg bid or tid
Cilazapril (Inhibace)	2.5-5 mg/day as a single dose
Enalapril (Vasotec)	5-40 mg/day as a single dose or bid
Fosinopril (Monopril)	20 mg/day as a single dose
Lisinopril (Zestril, Prinivil)	10-40 mg/day as a single dose
Moexipril (Univasc)	7.5-30 mg/day in 1 or 2 divided doses
Perindopril (Coversyl)	4-8 mg/day as a single dose
Quinapril (Accupril)	10-20 mg/day as a single dose
Ramipril (Altace)	2.5-10 mg/day as a single dose
Trandolapril (Mavik)	2-4 mg/day as a single dose

captopril 6.25 mg should be given and the patient kept under observation for 2 hours.[4] Thereafter, dosage should be 12.5 mg of captopril tid or equivalent doses of other ACE inhibitors with gradual increases as necessary. If the patient is hypertensive, the initial dose may be higher.

Other notable adverse reactions to ACE inhibitors are angioedema and abnormalities of taste. Angioedema does not necessarily develop during the early days of therapy.[10] Furthermore, the etiology of angioedema in patients taking ACE inhibitors may not be recognized, and if they continue taking the drug, they are at high risk of recurrent episodes of the disorder.[11]

Many of the available ACE inhibitors and their usual maintenance doses are listed in Table 8.

REFERENCES

1. Pfieffer MA, Braunwald E, Moye LA, et al: Effect of captopril on mortality and morbidity in patients with left ventricular dysfunction after myocardial infarction: results of the Survival and Ventricular Enlargement Trial, *N Engl J Med* 327:669-677, 1992.
2. SOLVD Investigators: Effect of enalapril on mortality and the development of heart failure in asymptomatic patients with reduced left ventricular ejection fractions, *N Engl J Med* 327: 685-691, 1992.
3. SOLVD Investigators: Effect of enalapril on survival in patients with reduced left ventricular ejection fraction and congestive heart failure, *N Engl J Med* 325:293-302, 1991.
4. Baker DW, Konstam MA, Bottoriff M, et al: Management of heart failure. I. Pharmacologic treatment, *JAMA* 272:1361-1366, 1994.
5. Garg R, Yusuf S: Overview of randomized trials of angiotensin-converting enzyme inhibitors on mortality and morbidity in patients with heart failure, *JAMA* 273:1450-1456, 1995.
6. Dzau V: Tissue renin-angiotensin system in myocardial hypertrophy and failure, *Arch Intern Med* 153:937-941, 1993.
7. Hargreaves MR, Benson MK: Inhaled sodium cromoglycate in angiotensin-converting enzyme inhibitor cough, *Lancet* 345: 13-16, 1995.
8. Rush JE, Rajfer SI: Theoretical basis for the use of angiotensin II antagonists in the treatment of heart failure, *J Hypertens* 11 (suppl):S69-S71, 1993.
9. Dickstein K, Chang P, Willenheimer R, et al: Comparison of the effects of losartan and enalapril on clinical status and exercise performance in patients with moderate or severe chronic heart failure, *J Am Coll Cardiol* 26:438-445, 1995.
10. Forslund T, Tohmo H, Weckstrom G, et al: Angio-oedema induced by enalapril, *J Intern Med* 238:179-181, 1995.
11. Brown NJ, Snowden M, Griffin MR: Recurrent angiotensin-converting enzyme inhibitor-associated angioedema, *JAMA* 278:232-233, 1997.

Angiotensin II antagonists

Angiotensin II receptor antagonists include losartan (Cozaar) and valsartan (Diovan). They are as effective as ACE inhibitors, but no evidence has yet been published that they prolong life in congestive heart failure or after a myocardial infarction or that they prevent nephropathy in diabetic patients. They do not cause cough, rarely cause angioedema, and occasionally cause hyperkalemia.[1-3] The usual dosage of losartan is 50 to 100 mg/day as a single dose and that for valsartan is 80 to 320 mg/day as a single dose.

REFERENCES

1. Losartan for hypertension, *Med Lett* 37:57-58, 1995.
2. Gradman AH, Arcuri KE, Goldberg AI, et al: A randomized, placebo-controlled, double-blind, parallel study of various doses of losartan potassium compared with enalapril maleate in patients with essential hypertension, *Hypertension* 25:1345-1350, 1995.
3. Valsartan for hypertension, *Med Lett* 39:43-44, 1997.

Diuretics

The standard diuretic used for the outpatient treatment of congestive heart failure is furosemide (Lasix).[1] The oral dosage varies from 20 to 240 mg/day, but few patients need more than 80 mg/day if the drug is combined with an ACE inhibitor or metolazone (Zaroxolyn) or both. If an increased dose of furosemide is needed, greater diuresis can be obtained by doubling the morning dose rather than giving the dose twice a day.[2] However, if more than 160 mg of furosemide is required daily, two doses should be given.[1] For mild congestive heart failure a thiazide rather than furosemide can sometimes be used.[3]

Volume depletion should be avoided because it makes titration of the dose of an ACE inhibitor difficult. Once the excess fluid volume is controlled, patients should weigh themselves every morning. If the weight changes by more than 1 to 2 kg, medication reassessment is indicated.[1] With the initiation of diuretics, potassium levels should be monitored. If the diuretic is given with an ACE inhibitor, potassium levels usually remain within normal limits.

Metolazone is added to the furosemide–ACE inhibitor regimen when necessary. Dosage is 2.5 to 5 mg po daily or every 2 days for a few days at a time. Metolazone is usually given 1 hour before the furosemide, and careful monitoring of potassium is required.[3] Only exceptionally does metolazone have to be continued on a long-term basis.

REFERENCES

1. Baker DW, Konstam MA, Bottoriff M, et al: Management of heart failure. I. Pharmacologic treatment, *JAMA* 272:1361-1366, 1994.
2. Vasko MR, Cartwright DB, Knochel JP, et al: Furosemide absorption altered in decompensated congestive heart failure, *Ann Intern Med* 102:314-318, 1985.
3. Cohn JN: The management of chronic heart failure, *N Engl J Med* 335:490-498, 1996.

Digoxin

The withdrawal of digoxin from patients with congestive heart failure who are receiving diuretics alone[1] or with ACE inhibitors[2] worsens the left ventricular ejection fraction, functional status, and exercise capacity. The Digitalis Investigation Group reported in 1997 that patients randomly assigned to receive digoxin in addition to diuretics and ACE inhibitors had the same mortality rate as but fewer hospitalizations than those not receiving digoxin.[3]

At present digoxin has the greatest value for patients with severe congestive heart failure. It is not indicated for patients who are in sinus rhythm and whose ejection fraction is greater than 0.40. A loading dose is not required. The usual adult dose is 0.125 to 0.25 mg/day, and in most cases 0.125 mg is adequate, especially in the elderly.

REFERENCES

1. Uretsky BF, Young JB, Shahidi FE, et al (PROVED Investigative Group): Randomized study assessing effect of digoxin withdrawal in patients with mild to moderate chronic congestive heart failure: results of the PROVED trial, *J Am Coll Cardiol* 22:955-962, 1993.
2. Packer M, Gheorghiade M, Young JB, et al: Withdrawal of digoxin from patients with chronic heart failure treated with angiotensin-converting enzyme inhibitors: RADIANCE Study, *N Engl J Med* 329:1-7, 1993.
3. Garg R, Gorlin R, Smith T, et al (Digitalis Investigation Group): The effect of digoxin on mortality and morbidity in patients with heart failure, *N Engl J Med* 336:525-533, 1997.

Vasodilators

In 1986 the combination of hydralazine (Apresoline) and isosorbide dinitrate (Isordil, Coradur) was found to reduce both morbidity and mortality in congestive heart failure.[1] This regimen has since been replaced by ACE inhibitors, which are more effective, but the combination is still used in patients who cannot tolerate ACE inhibitors.[2] If the combination is used, the maintenance doses are usually high. Hydralazine is given as 25 to 75 mg tid or qid with a maximum daily dose of 300 mg, and isosorbide dinitrate as 10 to 40 mg tid or qid with a maximum daily dose of 240 mg. At the higher doses of hydralazine, drug-induced lupus may be a complication. Clinical benefits of these regimens may not be apparent for the first few weeks of treatment.

REFERENCES

1. Cohn JN, Archibald DG, Ziesche S, et al: Effect of vasodilator therapy on mortality in chronic congestive heart failure: results of a Veterans Administration Cooperative Study, *N Engl J Med* 314:1547-1552, 1986.
2. Heart Failure Guideline Panel: Heart failure: management of patients with left ventricular systolic dysfunction, *Am Fam Physician* 50:603-616, 1994.

Beta-blockers

At present the use of beta-blockers for chronic systolic heart failure is experimental. However, evidence is growing that they decrease mortality and improve functional status.[1-5] Heart failure activates the adrenergic system, and this may be detrimental through a variety of mechanisms, including activation of the renin-angiotensin system, which causes sodium retention, and venous and arterial constriction, which increases preload and afterload. Beta-blockers counter these effects. If beta-blockers are used, initial doses should be very small and titrated upward at about weekly intervals. Full therapeutic benefit may take 1 to 3 months.[4] If fluid retention increases initially, this may be controllable with increased doses of diuretics.[1]

Carvedilol (Coreg) has combined beta-blocking and $alpha_1$-blocking functions as well as antioxidant effects. In a U.S. evaluation of more than 1000 patients with heart failure, those receiving carvedilol in addition to the standard background therapy of diuretics, ACE inhibitors, and digoxin had a decreased mortality rate at 6 to 12 months (3.2% versus 7.8%), as well as a decreased hospitalization rate for cardiovascular events compared with control subjects given background therapy only.[6] Similar results were reported from a study in Australia and New Zealand.[7] A metaanalysis of 17 studies of beta-blockers in congestive heart failure found a significant reduction in all-cause mortality regardless of the cause of the failure; carvedilol seemed to be more effective than other beta-blockers.[5] Carvedilol is usually started at a dose of 3.125 mg bid and increased gradually to 12.5 mg bid.

REFERENCES

1. Sackner-Bernstein JD, Mancini DM: Rationale for treatment of patients with chronic heart failure with adrenergic blockade, *JAMA* 274:1462-1467, 1995.
2. Packer M, Bristow MR, Cohn JN, et al: The effect of carvedilol on morbidity and mortality in patients with chronic heart failure, *N Engl J Med* 334:1349-1355, 1996.
3. Pfeffer MA, Stevenson LW: ß-Adrenergic blockers and survival in heart failure (editorial), *N Engl J Med* 334:1396-1397, 1996.
4. Drugs for chronic heart failure, *Med Lett* 38:92-94, 1996.
5. Heidenreich PA, Lee TT, Massie BM, et al: Effect of beta-blockade on mortality in patients with heart failure: a meta-analysis of randomized clinical trials, *J Am Coll Cardiol* 30:27-34, 1997.
6. Packer M, Bristow MR, Cohn JN, et al (US Carvedilol Heart Failure Study Group): The effect of carvedilol on morbidity and mortality in patients with chronic heart failure, *N Engl J Med* 334:1349-1355, 1996.

7. Australia/New Zealand Heart Failure Research Collaborative Group: Randomised, placebo-controlled trial of carvedilol in patients with congestive heart failure due to ischaemic heart disease, *Lancet* 349:375-380, 1997.

Sequence of drugs for the treatment of congestive heart failure

Mild cases of congestive heart failure can be managed by an ACE inhibitor alone or an ACE inhibitor combined with a diuretic. Moderately severe failure is managed by an ACE inhibitor combined with a diuretic and digoxin, and severe failure is managed as above plus a second diuretic (metolazone) and probably the addition of a second vasodilator (long-acting nitrates or hydralazine).[1] Many patients also benefit from the careful addition of carvedilol (Coreg).[2,3] Beta-blockers or calcium channel blockers may be helpful in diastolic failure.[1]

REFERENCES

1. Heart Failure Guideline Panel: Heart failure: management of patients with left ventricular systolic dysfunction, *Am Fam Physician* 50:603-616, 1994.
2. Packer M, Bristow MR, Cohn JN, et al (US Carvedilol Heart Failure Study Group): The effect of carvedilol on morbidity and mortality in patients with chronic heart failure, *N Engl J Med* 334:1349-1355, 1996.
3. Australia/New Zealand Heart Failure Research Collaborative Group: Randomised, placebo-controlled trial of carvedilol in patients with congestive heart failure due to ischaemic heart disease, *Lancet* 349:375-380, 1997.

CORONARY ARTERY DISEASE

(See also esophageal reflux)

Over the last three decades the mortality rate from coronary artery disease has decreased by 2% to 4% per year in the United States. About one fourth of the decline can be attributed to primary prevention and three fourths to secondary prevention and improved treatment.[1]

REFERENCES

1. Hunink MG, Goldman L, Tosteson AN, et al: The recent decline in mortality from coronary heart disease, 1980-1990: the effect of secular trends in risk factors and treatment, *JAMA* 277:535-542, 1997.

Risk Factors for Coronary Artery Disease

(See also detrimental effects of smoking; esophageal reflux; exercise; hypertension; menopause; lipids; myocardial infarction; obesity; poverty; vitamin E)

The major established risk factors for coronary artery disease are age, male sex, family history, smoking, obesity, hypertension, physical inactivity, diabetes mellitus, elevated cholesterol, elevated low-density lipoprotein-cholesterol (LDL-C), and reduced high-density lipoprotein-cholesterol (HDL-C).[1] Many of these plus a number of other proposed risk factors are discussed elsewhere in the text. Only a few are considered here.

The single biggest risk for coronary artery disease is being human. As Rose[2] pointed out, the most frequent cause of death in men with no apparent risk factors for coronary artery disease is coronary artery disease. Another important risk factor is poverty.[3,4] Epidemiological evidence suggests that additional risk factors may be diets low in fish[5] or fiber (fruits, vegetables, and particularly cereals),[6] peripheral vascular disease,[7] and elevated homocysteine levels.[8,9] Whether homocysteine is causally related to the atherogenic-thrombogenic process or whether homocysteine-lowering interventions (such as high intake of folates or pyridoxine) would be of any benefit is unknown.[8,9] The previously held view that high coffee intake was related to coronary artery disease has not been borne out by a recent metaanalysis[10] or a prospective study in women (Nurses' Health Study).[11] The absolute risk that intercourse will trigger an infarct in a healthy person is about 1 in 1 million, while for someone who has had a previous myocardial infarction it is about 20 per million. Regular exercise reduces these minimal risks even further for both healthy and post–myocardial infarction patients.[12]

A major problem for both physicians and patients is knowing the degree to which single or multiple risk factors increase the chance that an individual without known vascular disease will have a cardiovascular event over the next 5 or 10 years. Without these data rational decisions about preventive treatment cannot be made. Two recent attempts to address this problem have been the publication by Haq and associates[13] of the Sheffield Risk and Treatment Tables in the *Lancet* in 1995 and the publication of easily comprehensible nomograms by McCormack and co-workers[14] in the *Canadian Medical Association Journal* in 1997. An essential point in both these publications is that single risk factors such as elevated cholesterol level in the absence of other risk factors such as hypertension, smoking, or diabetes have relatively little import. They also make the point that even if treatment decreases overall statistical risk, only a very small percentage of those treated will benefit (the number of patients who must be treated to prevent one clinical event is large[14]).

REFERENCES

1. Hoeg JM: Evaluating coronary heart disease risk: tiles in the mosaic, *JAMA* 277:1387-1390, 1997.
2. Rose G: High-risk and population strategies of prevention: ethical considerations, *Ann Med* 21:409-413, 1989.
3. Morrison C, Woodward M, Leslie W, et al: Effect of socioeconomic group on incidence of, management of, and survival after myocardial infarction and coronary death: analysis of community coronary event register, *BMJ* 314:541-546, 1997.
4. Bosma H, Marmot MG, Hemingway H, et al: Low job control and risk of coronary heart disease in Whitehall II (prospective cohort) study, *BMJ* 314:558-565, 1997.
5. Daviglus ML, Stamler J, Orencia A, et al: Fish consumption and the 30-year risk of fatal myocardial infarction, *N Engl J Med* 336:1046-1053, 1997.

Cardiovascular System

6. Rimm EB, Ascherio A, Giovannucci E, et al: Vegetable, fruit, and cereal fiber intake and risk of coronary heart disease among men, *JAMA* 275:447-451, 1996.
7. McKenna M, Wolfson S, Kuller L: The ratio of ankle and arm arterial pressure as an independent predictor of mortality, *Atherosclerosis* 87:119-128, 1991.
8. Nygard O, Nordrehaug JE, Refsum H, et al: Plasma homocysteine levels and mortality in patients with coronary artery disease, *N Engl J Med* 337:230-236, 1997.
9. Graham IM, Daly LE, Refsum HM, et al (European Concerted Action Project): Plasma homocysteine as a risk factor for vascular disease, *JAMA* 277:1775-1781, 1997.
10. Kawachi I, Colditz GA, Stone CB: Does coffee drinking increase the risk of coronary heart disease? Results from a meta-analysis, *Br Heart J* 72:269-274, 1994.
11. Willett WC, Stampfer MJ, Manson JE, et al: Coffee consumption and coronary heart disease in women, *JAMA* 275:458-462, 1996.
12. Muller JE, Mittleman MA, Maclure M, et al (Determinants of Myocardial Infarction Onset Study Investigators): Triggering myocardial infarction by sexual activity: low absolute risk and prevention by regular physical exertion, *JAMA* 275:1405-1409, 1996.
13. Haq IU, Jackson PR, Yeo WW, et al: Sheffield Risk and Treatment Table for cholesterol lowering for primary prevention of coronary heart disease, *Lancet* 346:1467-1471, 1995.
14. McCormack JP, Levine M, Rangno RE: Primary prevention of heart disease and stroke: a simplified approach to estimating risk of events and making drug treatment decisions, *Can Med Assoc J* 157:422-428, 1997.

Primary Prevention of Coronary Artery Disease

(See also alcohol; aspirin—secondary prevention of coronary artery disease; exercise; hypertension; hormone replacement therapy; lipids; fish oil and coronary artery disease; obesity; relative risk reduction; smoking; vitamin E)

Well-established recommendations for the primary prevention of coronary artery disease include exercise, diet, avoidance of smoking, control of hypertension, avoidance of obesity, lipid-lowering strategies, and hormone replacement therapy.[1] Another suggested protocol is the regular ingestion of aspirin or vitamin E. Most of these modalities are discussed elsewhere in the text; the role of aspirin is reviewed in the ensuing paragraphs.

Aspirin

Two well-publicized studies of the preventive effects of aspirin on healthy physicians (primary prevention) have been published. The British Doctors' Trial compared male physicians between the ages of 50 and 78 taking 500 mg of aspirin daily over a 6-year period to a similar group who avoided aspirin-containing products.[2] No significant differences were found in the endpoints of myocardial infarction, strokes (except for slightly more disabling strokes in the acetylsalicylic acid [ASA]-treated group), and total cardiovascular mortality. In the Physicians' Health Study of U.S. male physicians ranging in age from 40 to 84 years, the treated group was given 325 mg of ASA every second day and the control group a placebo. At the end of 5 years there were no differences in cardiovascular mortality. The aspirin-treated group had a slight increase in hemorrhagic stroke and a 44% reduction in myocardial infarctions.[3] The latter figure, although statistically significant, represents a relative, not an absolute, risk reduction rate (see relative risk reduction). Because the overall incidence of cardiovascular disease was low in the studied population, the relative risk reduction for myocardial infarction of 44% translates into an absolute reduction rate of 0.4%.[4,5] In other words four nonfatal myocardial infarctions were prevented by treating 1000 men with aspirin for 5 years.[5] No primary prevention trials of aspirin in women have been reported to date.[6]

In addition to decreasing the incidence of myocardial infarctions, aspirin probably decreases the size of infarcts. In one study 65% of aspirin users had non-Q-wave infarcts compared with 49% of non–aspirin users.[7]

REFERENCES

1. Grundy SM, Balady GJ, Criqui MH, et al: Guide to primary prevention of cardiovascular disease: a statement for healthcare professionals from the Task Force on Risk Reduction, *Circulation* 95:2329-2331, 1997.
2. Peto R, Gray R, Collins R, et al: Randomised trial of prophylactic daily aspirin in British male doctors, *Br Med J Clin Res Ed* 296:313-316, 1988.
3. Steering Committee of the Physicians' Health Study Research Group: Final report on the aspirin component of the ongoing Physicians' Health Study, *N Engl J Med* 321:129-135, 1989.
4. Rees MK: Use of low-dose aspirin as a preventive measure (letter), *Am Fam Physician* 52:766, 768, 1995.
5. Marshall KG: Use of low-dose aspirin as a preventive measure (letter), *Am Fam Physician* 52:761, 766, 1995.
6. Rich-Edwards JW, Manson JE, Hennekens C, et al: The primary prevention of coronary heart disease in women, *N Engl J Med* 332:1758-1766, 1995.
7. Col NF, Yarzebski J, Gore JM, et al: Does aspirin consumption affect the presentation or severity of acute myocardial infarction? *Arch Intern Med* 155:1386-1389, 1995.

Secondary Prevention of Coronary Artery Disease

(See also aspirin—primary prevention of coronary artery disease; cholesterol-lowering studies in patients with coronary artery disease; efficacy of the treatment of hypertension; exercise; hormone replacement therapy; secondary prevention of myocardial infarction; smoking)

Secondary prevention strategies for coronary artery disease are numerous. Guidelines include such items as smoking cessation, diet, exercise, lipid-lowering agents, aspirin, beta-blockers, ACE inhibitors, postmenopausal hormone replacement therapy, and blood pressure control.[1] Most of these are discussed elsewhere in the text. Aspirin and beta-blockers are discussed in the ensuing paragraphs.

In the Swedish Angina Pectoris Aspirin Trial, patients with stable angina who had not had a myocardial infarction were treated with 75 mg of ASA or a placebo. Over a 4-year period there was a relative reduction of 34% in myocardial infarctions and sudden deaths in the aspirin-treated group. All cardiovascular events, including strokes, as well as total mortality, were reduced by 22% to 32%. The absolute rate reduction of cardiovascular events was 51:1000 over 4 years or 5.1%. This reduction is more than 10 times greater than that reported for asymptomatic men in the Physicians' Health Study mentioned previously.[2] Similar results have been reported from the Multicenter Myocardial Ischemia Research Group. Patients were enrolled in this study within 6 months of the development of myocardial infarction or unstable angina. Cardiac events, including cardiac deaths, were markedly reduced in patients taking aspirin (250 to 325 mg/day), and this protective effect was particularly pronounced among patients who had had thrombolysis. Cardiac mortality at 2 years was 1.6% for patients taking aspirin and 5.4% for nonusers. Total cohort mortality was also reduced in the aspirin users.[3]

Beta-blockers without intrinsic sympathomimetic activity are cardioprotective; they reduce mortality after infarction, limit infarct size, and decrease arrhythmias and sudden death.[4]

REFERENCES

1. Smith SC Jr, Blair SN, Criqui MH, et al: Preventing heart attack and death in patients with coronary disease: Consensus Panel statement of the American Heart Association, *Circulation* 92:2-4, 1995.
2. Juul-Möller S, Edvardsson N, Jahnmatz B, et al: Double-blind trial of aspirin in primary prevention of myocardial infarction in patients with stable chronic angina pectoris, *Lancet* 340:1421-1425, 1992.
3. Goldstein RE, Andrews M, Hall WJ, et al (Multicenter Myocardial Ischemia Research Group): Marked reduction in long-term cardiac deaths with aspirin after a coronary event, *J Am Coll Cardiol* 28:326-330, 1996.
4. Kendall MJ, Lynch KP, Hjalmarson A, et al: Beta-blockers and sudden cardiac death, *Ann Intern Med* 123:358-367, 1995.

Angina

(See also secondary prevention of coronary artery disease)

Stable angina

Regular aspirin use decreases morbidity and mortality in patients with stable angina (see discussion of secondary prevention of coronary artery disease).

Proper use of nitroglycerin improves quality of life in patients with stable angina through symptom control; it has no effect on mortality. Nitroglycerin should not be given to patients taking dihydropyridine-derivative calcium channel blockers (e.g., nifedipine, felodipine, amlodipine) because both drug classes cause reflex tachycardia. An exception may be made if the patient is also taking a beta-blocker that will control the heart rate. To prevent tolerance, the last daily dose of short-acting nitroglycerin products should be taken at about 6 to 7 PM and long-acting products should be taken once a day in the morning or twice a day provided the second dose is given no later than 2 PM.

Some of the nitroglycerin products available for treating angina are regular short-acting sublingual tablets, translingual spray (Nitrolingual), sustained release formulations of nitroglycerin (e.g., Nitrong), isosorbide dinitrate (Isordil) with a usual sublingual dose of 5 mg q2-4h or an oral dose of 10 to 30 mg q4h, isosorbide-5-mononitrate (Imdur) with a usual dose of 20 mg bid for the regular tablets or 30 to 60 mg bid for the long-acting tablets, and nitroglycerin patches (Nitro-Dur, Transderm-Nitro, Minitran) delivering 0.2, 0.4, 0.6, or 0.8 mg/hr.

Beta-blockers are excellent drugs for controlling angina, but if they are contraindicated, calcium channel blockers might be considered because they increase coronary blood flow and are effective in the symptomatic management of angina. However, because some of the shorter acting formulations have been associated with an increased incidence of myocardial infarction, calcium channel blockers are no longer considered first-line agents for the treatment of either angina or hypertension (see calcium channel blockers in the section on hypertension).[1]

Unstable angina

Braunwald classifies unstable angina as follows[2]:

Class I. New-onset severe or accelerated angina developing within the past 2 months. Frequency of anginal episodes three per day. For patients who had stable angina, the episodes have become more frequent, last longer, are more severe, or are brought on by lesser degrees of exercise. No rest pain.

Class II. Angina at rest within the last month but not the past 48 hours (angina at rest subacute).

Class III. Angina at rest within the last 48 hours (angina at rest acute).

A collaborative overview of 145 randomized trials of antiplatelet therapy showed a significant relative reduction of vascular events in men, women, and the elderly with unstable angina who were treated with aspirin in doses between 75 and 325 mg/day.[3]

Growing evidence indicates that the addition of unfractionated heparin (regular intravenous heparin)[4] or low–molecular weight heparin to aspirin in patients with unstable angina decreases both myocardial infarctions and death rates over the short term.[5,6] Unfractionated heparin plus aspirin is associated with an increased incidence of major bleeding episodes,[4] but so far this does not seem to be a significant problem with aspirin plus low–molecular weight heparin.[5,6]

REFERENCES

1. Canadian Health Protection Branch: *Safety of calcium channel blockers in the treatment of patients with hypertension and coronary artery disease,* CD No 44, January 23, 1996.

2. Braunwald E: Unstable angina: a classification, *Circulation* 80: 410-414, 1989.
3. Antiplatelet Trialists' Collaboration: Collaborative overview of randomised trials of antiplatelet therapy. I. Prevention of death, myocardial infarction, and stroke by prolonged antiplatelet therapy in various categories of patients, *BMJ* 308:81-106, 1994.
4. Oler A, Whooley MA, Oler J, et al: Adding heparin to aspirin reduces the incidence of myocardial infarction and death in patients with unstable angina: a meta-analysis, *JAMA* 276:811-815, 1996.
5. Gurfinkel EP, Manos EJ, Mejail RI, et al: Low molecular weight heparin versus regular heparin or aspirin in the treatment of unstable angina and silent ischemia, *J Am Coll Cardiol* 26:313-318, 1995.
6. Wallentin L, Ohlsson J, Swahn E, et al: Low-molecular-weight heparin during instability in coronary artery disease, *Lancet* 347: 561-568, 1996.

Coronary Artery Bypass Grafting and Angioplasty

(See also anesthesia; detrimental effects of investigations; myocardial infarction; practice patterns; performance reports)

The following are clear indications for coronary artery bypass (CABG) surgery[1]:

1. Left mainstem coronary artery disease
2. Multivessel disease involving the proximal left anterior descending artery
3. Three-vessel disease and impaired left ventricular function

For patients with angina who have single-vessel disease or multiple-vessel disease not involving the proximal left anterior descending coronary artery and whose left ventricular systolic function is normal, medical therapy, angioplasty, and bypass surgery have been shown to be equally effective, and therefore the choice for a particular patient can be individualized.[1-3] In this group of patients bypass is associated with greater initial morbidity but results in better control of angina and less need for repeat interventions. Angioplasty has a lower immediate morbidity, but there is a greater risk of recurrent angina requiring medical therapy or further interventions. In one study of patients with multivessel disease, 31% of patients who initially had percutaneous transluminal coronary angioplasty (PTCA) had a subsequent CABG within 5 years.[4]

Objective measurements of the degree of angina such as the threshold of activity that will precipitate an attack are not sufficient in themselves to determine the best therapeutic modality. Patients differ considerably in how they tolerate symptoms, so their preferences are an important factor to be considered in reaching a decision.[5,6] Since the perioperative mortality of CABG is as high as 4%,[5] even some patients with left mainstem coronary artery disease may refuse the operation on this basis alone.[6]

An important factor in deciding whether a patient should undergo angioplasty is the volume of procedures performed in the institution where the procedure will be performed. The rate of major complications and death appears to be much lower in centers performing 400 to 600 or more procedures per year compared with those performing fewer than 400.[7-9] Furthermore, both patient mortality and the need for same-day CABG surgery are greater for individual cardiologists performing fewer than 75 PTCA procedures per year.[9] However, this type of data can be misleading; the issue is discussed in more detail in the section on performance reports.

Cerebral complications from coronary artery bypass are common. In one multicenter study such adverse events occurred in 6.1% of patients. Half of them had either fatal cerebral injury or nonfatal strokes, and the other half had a new deterioration of intellectual function or new-onset seizures.[10]

Although evidence exists that revascularization improves function and survival in patients with both angina and left ventricular failure,[11,12] whether the procedure is beneficial in patients with failure but no angina is unknown.[11]

The optimal revascularization procedure for diabetic patients is uncertain.[4,13] Diabetic patients subject to PTCA have higher in-hospital mortality and nonfatal myocardial infarction rates than do nondiabetic patients having the same procedure. They also have twice the mortality rate after 9 years of follow-up.[13] The adverse effects are probably related to the greater degree of vascular disease in these patients. Preliminary evidence indicates that diabetic patients taking insulin or oral hypoglycemic agents do better after CABG than after PTCA.[4] In one study the mortality rate of this category of patients 5 years after CABG was 20% whereas it was 45% 5 years after PTCA.[4]

The technical aspects of percutaneous coronary revascularization are in a constant state of change. Atherectomy and laser angioplasty came into vogue in the late 1980s and are now declining in frequency, whereas the placement of intracoronary stents is increasing.[14]

REFERENCES

1. Hillis LK, Rutherford JD: Coronary angioplasty compared with bypass grafting, *N Engl J Med* 33:1086-1087, 1994.
2. Hamm CW, Reimers J, Ischinger T, et al: A randomized study of coronary angioplasty compared with bypass surgery in patients with symptomatic multivessel coronary disease, *N Engl J Med* 331:1037-1043, 1994.
3. King SB III, Lembo NJ, Weintraub WS, et al: A randomized trial comparing coronary angioplasty with coronary bypass surgery, *N Engl J Med* 331:1044-1050, 1994.
4. Bypass Angioplasty Revascularization Investigation (BARI) Investigators: Comparison of coronary bypass surgery with angioplasty in patients with multivessel disease, *N Engl J Med* 335:217-225, 1996.
5. Nease RF Jr, Kneeland T, O'Connor GT, et al: Variation in patient utilities for outcomes of the management of chronic stable angina: implications for clinical practice guidelines, *JAMA* 273:1185-1190, 1995.
6. Hlatky MA: Patient preferences and clinical guidelines (editorial), *JAMA* 273:1219-1220, 1995.
7. Kimmel SE, Berlin JA, Laskey WK: The relationship between coronary angioplasty procedure volume and major complications, *JAMA* 274:1137-1142, 1995.

8. Ryan TJ: The critical question of procedure volume minimums for coronary angioplasty (editorial), *JAMA* 274:1169-1170, 1995.
9. Hannan EL, Racz M, Ryan T, et al: Coronary angioplasty volume-outcome relationships for hospitals and cardiologists, *JAMA* 279:892-898, 1997.
10. Roach GW, Kanchuger M, Mangano M, et al: Adverse cerebral outcomes after coronary bypass surgery, *N Engl J Med* 335: 1857-1863, 1996.
11. Baker DW, Jones R, Hodges J, et al: Management of heart failure. III. The role of revascularization in the treatment of patients with moderate or severe left ventricular systolic dysfunction, *JAMA* 272:1528-1534, 1994.
12. Elefteriades JA, Tolis G Jr, Levi E, et al: Coronary artery bypass grafting in severe left ventricular dysfunction: excellent survival with improved ejection fraction and functional state, *J Am Coll Cardiol* 22:1411-1417, 1993.
13. Kip KE, Faxon DP, Detre KM, et al: Coronary angioplasty in diabetic patients—the National Heart, Lung, and Blood Institute Percutaneous Transluminal Corollary Angioplasty Registry, *Circulation* 94:1818-1825, 1996.
14. Hasdai D, Berger PB, Bell MR, et al: The changing face of coronary interventional practice: the Mayo Clinic experience, *Arch Intern Med* 157:677-682, 1997.

Cardiac Arrest

(See also cardiac arrest during exercise; cardiopulmonary resuscitation; preparticipation medical examinations)

Ventricular arrhythmia resulting from coronary artery disease is the cause of 80% of cases of sudden cardiac death. Beta-blockers have been shown to have a significant protective effect against this event both in hypertensive patients and in post–myocardial infarction patients.[1]

A population-based case-control study found that polyunsaturated fatty acids from seafood (the equivalent of one fatty fish meal per week) decreased the risk of a primary cardiac arrest by 50%.[2]

REFERENCES

1. Kendall MJ, Lynch KP, Hjalmarson A, et al: Beta-blockers and sudden cardiac death, *Ann Intern Med* 123:358-367, 1995.
2. Siscovick DS, Raghunathan E, King I, et al: Dietary intake and cell membrane levels of long-chain n-3 polyunsaturated fatty acids and the risk of primary cardiac arrest, *JAMA* 274:1363-1367, 1995.

Myocardial Infarction

(See also detrimental effects of smoking; risk factors for coronary artery disease; practice patterns)

Panic disorder presenting as possible myocardial infarction

A series of 441 consecutive consenting patients with chest pain seen in the emergency room of a major Montreal teaching hospital specializing in heart disease was evaluated as to etiology and underlying psychiatric disorders. One fourth of these patients met the criteria of the *Diagnostic and Statistical Manual of Mental Disorders,* edition 3 revised (DSM-III-R), for panic attacks, and of this group one fourth had suicidal thoughts in the week before being seen in the emergency room. In addition, close to 60% of patients with panic disorder had other Axis I psychiatric diagnoses, mainly generalized anxiety disorder, agoraphobia, major depression, and dysthymia. In only 2% of cases was the panic disorder recognized by the attending staff cardiologists in the emergency room. Seventy-five percent of the patients with panic disorder were discharged from the emergency room with the diagnosis "noncardiac chest pain."[1]

REFERENCES

1. Fleet RP, Dupuis G, Marchand A, et al: Panic disorder in emergency department chest pain patients—prevalence, comorbidity, suicidal ideation, and physician recognition, *Am J Med* 101:371-380, 1996.

Office or home management of suspected acute myocardial infarction

In cases of suspected myocardial infarction, rapid transfer to an emergency facility for consideration of thrombolytic therapy is paramount (in general, thrombolytic therapy is not given if symptoms have persisted for more than 12 hours). If time permits, an immediate electrocardiogram (ECG) should be obtained and sent with the patient along with previous ECGs if available. This is because changing ECG patterns, especially ST segment changes or new-onset left bundle-branch block, support the diagnosis of myocardial infarction and determine whether thrombolytic therapy is indicated (enzyme changes are often not seen for at least 3 to 4 hours). Aspirin has been shown to reduce mortality, so a half to one aspirin should be given stat.[1-4] Aspirin should not be omitted because of a vague history of allergy or a remote history of gastrointestinal bleeding. If absolute contraindications to aspirin exist such as recent gastrointestinal bleeding, a cerebral hemorrhage, or a clear-cut sensitivity reaction, ticlopidine (Ticlid) may be used.[4] The administration of aspirin does not interfere with subsequent thrombolytic therapy.[1,4]

A randomized double-blind study from Scotland showed a significant decrease in death rate measured at 30 months among patients with suspected acute myocardial infarctions who received intravenous thrombolytic therapy with 30 units of anistreplase (Eminase) at home from their general practitioners compared with patients who received similar therapy only after arrival at the hospital.[5]

REFERENCES

1. Gutman MB, Lee TF, Gin K, et al: Acute care of myocardial infarction, *Can Fam Physician* 42:1330-1339, 1996.
2. Eisenberg MJ, Topol EJ: Prehospital administration of aspirin in patients with unstable angina and acute myocardial infarction, *Arch Intern Med* 156:1506-1510, 1996.
3. Gavagan T, Reddy MJ: Myocardial infarction: the first 24 hours, *Am Fam Physician* 54:921-931,1996.

4. Collins R, Peto R, Baigent C, et al: Aspirin, heparin, and fibrinolytic therapy in suspected acute myocardial infarction, *N Engl J Med* 336:847-860, 1997.
5. Rawles J: Magnitude of benefit from earlier thrombolytic treatment in acute myocardial infarction: new evidence from Grampian Region Early Anistreplase Trial (GREAT), *BMJ* 312:212-215, 1996.

Secondary Prevention Of Myocardial Infarction

(See also anticoagulants listings in index; coronary artery disease; cholesterol-lowering studies in patients with coronary artery disease; efficacy of the treatment of hypertension; exercise; exercise listings in index; lipid-lowering drugs; lipids; secondary prevention of coronary artery disease; smoking; practice patterns)

Risk stratification. For optimal provision of secondary prevention measures, patients who have had a myocardial infarction should be stratified according to their degree of risk for further coronary events. This is best performed by testing left ventricular function with echocardiography and assessing ischemia with exercise testing.[1]

The first-year mortality rate after a myocardial infarction is zero to 2% if the post–myocardial infarction exercise stress test is negative, but if it is positive, the total cardiac event rate is about 25%.[1] The American Heart Association and the American College of Cardiology have accepted three strategies for stress testing patients who have not had thrombolytic therapy[2]:

1. A symptom-limited test at 10 to 14 days after myocardial infarction plus a symptom-limited test at 6 to 8 weeks if the patient's life-style is strenuous
2. A submaximal test before discharge from the hospital plus a symptom-limited test at 6 to 8 weeks
3. A symptom-limited test at 3 weeks

If thrombolytic therapy has been given, a submaximal test before discharge and a symptom-limited test at 6 to 8 weeks are recommended.[2]

Patients who have contraindications to exercise stress testing have a much higher mortality rate than those who are able to undergo the test.[3]

Left ventricular function as determined by echocardiography is the single most important determinant of risk after myocardial infarction. The 1-year mortality rate varies from 3% when the ejection fraction is greater than 50% to more than 40% when it is less than 30%.[1]

Management guidelines. Recent guidelines for management of patients after myocardial infarction include the following recommendations[1]:

1. Evaluate left ventricular function by echocardiography.
2. Evaluate residual ischemia by exercise testing if possible.
3. Start low-dose aspirin immediately if it is not contraindicated and continue it indefinitely.
4. Start beta-blockers immediately if they are not contraindicated and continue them indefinitely.
5. Start ACE inhibitors before discharge for all patients with a left ventricular ejection fraction less than 40%.
6. Give anticoagulants for at least 3 months if the patient has extensive abnormalities of left ventricular wall motion or demonstrable left ventricular thrombus.
7. Modify coronary risk factors through smoking cessation, exercise, control of hypertension, and control of dyslipidemia. The goals for the last mentioned are a low-density lipoprotein-C concentration less than 2.6 mmol/L (100 mg/dl), a high-density lipoprotein-C concentration greater than 0.9 mmol/L (35 mg/dl), and a triglyceride level less than 1.58 mmol/L (140 mg/dl).

Post-myocardial infarction exercise, beta-blockers, aspirin, anticoagulants, and ACE inhibitors are discussed in the ensuing paragraphs. The remaining recommendations are dealt with elsewhere in the text.

Exercise. Metaanalysis of randomized controlled studies of rehabilitation exercise in post–myocardial infarction patients has shown a 25% relative reduction in mortality during the first 3 years of follow-up.[4] Regular exercise also decreases the slightly raised relative risk of triggering myocardial infarction during sexual intercourse.[5]

Beta-blockers. If not contraindicated, beta-blockers should be prescribed for all post–myocardial infarction patients because they decrease mortality rates.[1,6,7] Any beta-blocker without intrinsic sympathomimetic activity (ISA) may be used. Examples are:

Metoprolol (Lopressor)	100 mg bid
Timolol (Blocadren)	10 mg bid
Propranolol (Inderal)	60-80 mg tid
Atenolol (Tenormin)	100 mg/day

Beta-blocker therapy should be continued for at least 2 years[6] and probably indefinitely.[1] Old age is not a contraindication to beta-blocker therapy after myocardial infarction, and diabetes is rarely so. Despite this, many elderly people who have had a myocardial infarction are not treated with beta-blockers.[7]

For patients with a history of myocadial infarction or at high risk of coronary artery disease, atenolol (Tenormin) given just before and immediately after noncardiac surgery decreases cardiac morbidity and mortality.[8]

Aspirin. Aspirin in doses of 75 to 325 mg/day has been well documented to decrease morbidity and mortality in old and young men and women who have had myocardial infarctions. Benefit has been noted even when aspirin was started weeks or years after the initial infarction (see discussion of secondary prevention of coronary artery disease).[9] However, not all patients receive this drug. A 1996 U.S. multicenter study of elderly post–myocardial infarction patients found that 24% were discharged without a prescription for aspirin; after 6 months their mortality rate was 17% compared with 8.4% for those prescribed aspirin.[10]

A nonrandomized study suggests that myocardial infarctions are smaller in patients taking aspirin than in patients not taking aspirin. Sixty-five percent of aspirin users had non-Q-wave infarction compared with 49% of nonusers, and

30% of users had small infarcts compared with 22% of nonusers.[11]

Anticoagulants. Anticoagulation has been shown to decrease morbidity and mortality in post–myocardial infarction patients.[12,13] Oral anticoagulants are widely used in Europe, whereas aspirin is the drug of choice in North America. There are no good recent comparisons of the two modalities.[14] Three months of anticoagulation is recommended for post–myocardial infarction patients who have significant abnormalities of left ventricular wall motion or who are shown to have a left ventricular thrombus.[1]

ACE inhibitors. Studies using captopril (Capoten) and enalapril (Vasotec) have shown decreased mortality in post–myocardial infarction patients who had left ventricular ejection fractions less than 30%. These drugs are also probably effective in post–myocardial infarction patients whose ejection fractions are 30% to 40%. The approximate relative risk reduction is 20%.[15]

That ACE inhibitors might have a more extensive use in patients with anterior myocardial infarctions is suggested by a 1995 Italian study. All patients were randomly assigned to receive a 6-week course of the ACE inhibitor zofenopril or a placebo beginning within 24 hours of infarction. At 6 weeks the death rate and the incidence of severe congestive failure were significantly reduced in the zofenopril group. A decreased death rate was also observed in the treatment group at 1 year (10% versus 14.1%), even though the ACE inhibitor was given for only 6 weeks.[16] A similar study using lisinopril (Prinivil, Zestril) found that the absolute rate of death or severe ventricular dysfunction at 6 months in the treated group was decreased by 1.2%.[17]

In the ISIS-4 trial, captopril was begun within 24 hours of myocardial infarction in doses of 6.25 mg/day, increased to 50 mg bid, and given at this dose for 1 month. Compared with the placebo control group, the treated group had a 7% relative reduction rate in the 5-week mortality rate, which translates into a 0.5% absolute mortality reduction. At 12 months there was a 0.54% absolute mortality reduction in the captopril group.[18]

At present the optimal use of ACE inhibitors in myocardial infarction is uncertain. Long-term therapy (at least 3 years) seems advisable for any patient with evidence of left ventricular dysfunction. Patients without left ventricular dysfunction would probably benefit from a short course (5 to 6 weeks) of an ACE inhibitor, begun within hours of the infarct.[6,19]

REFERENCES

1. Deedwania PC, Amsterdam EA, Vagelos RH (California Cardiology Working Group on Post-MI Management): Evidence-based, cost-effective risk stratification and management after myocardial infarction, *Arch Intern Med* 157:273-280, 1997.
2. Gunnar RM, Passamani ER, Bourdillon PD, et al: Guidelines for the early management of patients with acute myocardial infarction: a report of the American College of Cardiology/American Heart Association Task Force on Assessment of Diagnostic and Therapeutic Cardiovascular Procedures (Subcommittee to Develop Guidelines for the Early Management of Patients with Acute Myocardial Infarction), *J Am Coll Cardiol* 16:249-292, 1990.
3. Villella A: Prognostic significance of maximal exercise testing after myocardial infarction treated with thrombolytic agents—the GISSI-2 database, *Lancet* 346:523-529, 1995.
4. US Department of Health and Human Services, Public Health Service, Agency for Health Care Policy and Research: *Cardiac rehabilitation,* Clinical Practice Guideline No 17, 1995.
5. Muller JE, Mittleman MA, Maclure M, et al (Determinants of Myocardial Infarction Onset Study Investigators): Triggering myocardial infarction by sexual activity: low absolute risk and prevention by regular physical exertion, *JAMA* 275:1405-1409, 1996.
6. Hennekens CH, Albert CM, Godfried SL, et al: Adjunctive drug therapy of acute myocardial infarction—evidence from clinical trials, *N Engl J Med* 335:1660-1667, 1996.
7. Soumerai SB, McLauglin TJ, Spiegelman D, et al: Adverse outcomes of underuse of ß-blockers in elderly survivors of acute myocardial infarction, *JAMA* 277:115-121, 1997.
8. Mangano DT, Layug EL, Wallace A, et al (Multicenter Study of Perioperative Ischemia Research Group): Effect of atenolol on mortality and cardiovascular morbidity after noncardiac surgery, *N Engl J Med* 335:1713-1720, 1996.
9. Antiplatelet Trialists' Collaboration: Collaborative overview of randomised trials of antiplatelet therapy. I. Prevention of death, myocardial infarction, and stroke by prolonged antiplatelet therapy in various categories of patients, *BMJ* 308:81-106, 1994.
10. Krumholz HM, Radford MJ, Ellerbeck EF, et al: Aspirin for secondary prevention after acute myocardial infarction in the elderly: prescribed use and outcomes, *Ann Intern Med* 124:292-298, 1996.
11. Col NF, Yarzebski J, Gore JM, et al: Does aspirin consumption affect the presentation or severity of acute myocardial infarction? *Arch Intern Med* 155:1386-1389, 1995.
12. Smith P, Arnesen H, Holme I: The effect of warfarin on mortality and reinfarction after myocardial infarction, *N Engl J Med* 323:147-152, 1990.
13. ASPECT Research Group: Effect of long-term oral anticoagulant treatment on mortality and cardiovascular morbidity after myocardial infarction, *Lancet* 343:499-503, 1994.
14. Cairns JA, Markham BA: Economics and efficacy in choosing oral anticoagulants or aspirin after myocardial infarction (editorial), *JAMA* 273:965-967, 1995.
15. Pfieffer MA, Braunwald E, Moye LA, et al: Effect of captopril on mortality and morbidity in patients with left ventricular dysfunction after myocardial infarction: results of the Survival and Ventricular Enlargement Trial, *N Engl J Med* 327:669-677, 1992.
16. Ambrosioni E, Borghi C, Magnani B: The effect of the angiotensin-converting enzyme inhibitor zofenopril on mortality and morbidity after anterior myocardial infarction, *N Engl J Med* 332:80-85, 1995.
17. Gruppo Italiano per lo Studio della Sopravvivenza nell'Infarto Miocardicol: Six month effects of early treatment with lisinopril and transdermal glyceryl trinitrate singly and together withdrawn six weeks after acute myocardial infarctions: the GISSI-3 Trial, *J Am Coll Cardiol* 27:337-344, 1996.

18. Collins R, Peto R, Flather M, et al: ISIS-4: a randomised factorial trial assessing early oral captopril, oral mononitrate, and intravenous magnesium sulphate in 58,050 patients with suspected acute myocardial infarction, *Lancet* 345:669-685, 1995.
19. Pfeffer MA: ACE inhibition in acute myocardial infarction (editorial), *N Engl J Med* 332:118-120, 1995.

ELECTROCARDIOGRAMS

A long tradition in primary care holds that routine ECGs are a valuable part of the periodic health examination of middle-aged or elderly patients. This is a myth.[1] The cardiogram has poor sensitivity and specificity for Q-wave myocardial infarction in asymptomatic individuals, and the positive predictive value for this entity for 60-year-old men is calculated to be only 3%.[1] T-wave and ST segment changes are so common and so nonspecific that they do not help identify patients at risk of coronary artery disease. The U.S. Preventive Services Task Force gives screening ECGs for middle-aged elderly men and women a "C" recommendation. They give a "D" recommendation for routine periodic health visits or routine preparticipation examinations in adolescents or young adults.[2]

A common argument for performing electrocardiography is to have ECGs available as a baseline in case cardiac symptoms develop in the future. The assumption is that the ECG will be relatively recent and rapidly accessible at whatever emergency room the patient goes to when symptoms of coronary artery disease develop. If the ECG is available, it will probably be helpful, but if cardiograms are going to be taken for this reason, the possible benefits for the very few must be weighed against the significant number of false-positive findings that would inevitably cause distress for both patients and physicians.

REFERENCES

1. Health Services Utilization and Research Commission: Anatomy of a practice guideline: tradition, science, and consensus on using electrocardiograms in Saskatchewan, *Can Fam Physician* 41:37-48, 1995.
2. US Preventive Services Task Force: *Guide to clinical preventive services,* ed 2, Baltimore, Williams & Wilkins, 1996, pp 3-14.

HYPERTENSION

(See also hypertensive disorders of pregnancy)

Definition and Epidemiology

The definitions of hypertension according to the Fifth Report of the Joint National Committee on Detection, Evaluation, and Treatment of High Blood Pressure (JNC V) are recorded in Table 9. The blood pressure should be recorded with the patient in the sitting position with the arm at heart level, and the mean of two readings taken 2 minutes apart should be used. For the initial diagnosis of hypertension, readings should be obtained at three different visits 1 to several weeks apart and the average values of the three visits used to determine the patient's blood pressure. Treatment on the basis of the initial readings alone is indicated only if the values exceed 120 mm Hg diastolic and 210 mm Hg systolic or if evidence of end organ damage is found.[1]

It has been estimated that 25% of the adult U.S. population has hypertension. The prevalence is higher in blacks than whites and increases with age. The mean increase in blood pressure from ages 30 to 65 is 20 mm Hg systolic and 10 mm diastolic.[2] Seventy percent of untreated persons with hypertension die of congestive heart failure or coronary artery disease, 15% of cerebral hemorrhage, and 10% of uremia.[3]

Blood pressure has a circadian pattern. It plateaus at its highest level during the day, falls during the evening to reach its lowest level after midnight, and rises steeply again in the early morning before waking.[4]

REFERENCES

1. National Institutes of Health, National Heart, Lung, and Blood Institute: *Fifth report of the Joint National Committee on Detection, Evaluation, and Treatment of High Blood Pressure (JNC V),* NIH Publication No 93-1088, 1993.
2. Kannel WB: Blood pressure as a cardiovascular risk factor: prevention and treatment, *JAMA* 275:1571-1576, 1996.
3. Kligman EW: Hypertension. In Mengel MB, Schwiebert LP, eds: *Ambulatory medicine: the primary care of families,* Norwalk, Conn, 1993, Appleton & Lange, pp 415-425.
4. Wever MA: Hypertension as a risk factor syndrome: therapeutic implications, *Am J Med* 94(suppl 4 A):4A-24A, 1993.

Secondary Hypertension

Except among persons who drink alcohol to excess, secondary hypertension is rare. Investigations for secondary hypertension are necessary only when it is clinically suspected. The following areimportant causes of the condition[1]:

1. Alcohol
2. Medications (e.g., oral contraceptives, nonsteroidal antiinflammatory drugs, sympathomimetics such as appetite suppressants and decongestants)
3. Renal parenchymal disease

Table 9 Definition of Hypertension

	Systolic (mm Hg)	Diastolic (mm Hg)
Normal	<130	<85
High normal	130-139	85-89
Hypertension	140+	90+
Stage 1 (mild)	140-159	90-99
Stage 2 (moderate)	160-179	100-109
Stage 3 (severe)	180-209	110-119
Stage 4 (very severe)	≥210	≥120

Modified from National Institutes of Health, National Heart, Lung, and Blood Institute: *Fifth report of the Joint National Committee on Detection, Evaluation, and Treatment of High Blood Pressure (JNC V),* NIH Publication No 93-1088, 1993.

4. Renovascular disease
5. Coarctation of the aorta
6. Cushing's syndrome
7. Primary hyperaldosteronism
8. Pheochromocytoma
9. Thyroid dysfunction (hyperthyroidism or hypothyroidism)

Secondary hypertension may be suspected on the basis of the history, physical examination, or basic hypertensive investigations. It should be seriously considered in young patients or those with onset after the age of 55 years. Alcohol and drug use should be determined for all patients, as should the presence or absence of physical stigmata of Cushing's disease. The femoral artery pulsations and leg blood pressure should be checked as a screen for coarctation of the aorta in all young hypertensive patients. An abnormal urinalysis may point to renal disease, hypokalemia to primary hyperaldosteronism, and an abnormal thyroid-stimulating hormone level to thyroid disease.[1]

The following are other clues to secondary hypertension[1]:

1. Abrupt onset of hypertension
2. Severe hypertension (diastolic ≥110 mm Hg)
3. Rapid worsening of hypertension
4. Hypertension resistant to treatment

Although not formally recognized as a cause of secondary hypertension, hyperventilation (as is commonly seen in panic disorders) can raise blood pressure.[2,3] This diagnosis is often missed.[3]

REFERENCES

1. Adcock BB, Ireland RB Jr: Secondary hypertension: a practical diagnostic approach, *Am Fam Physician* 55:1263-1270, 1997.
2. Todd GP, Chadwick IG, Yeo WW, et al: Pressor effect of hyperventilation in healthy subjects, *J Hum Hypertens* 9:119-122, 1995.
3. Kaplan NM: Anxiety-induced hyperventilation: a common cause of symptoms in patients with hypertension (editorial), *Arch Intern Med* 157:945-948, 1997.

White Coat Hypertension

In patients with "white coat hypertension," blood pressure readings are elevated when taken by physicians in their offices but normal when recorded at home or by ambulatory blood pressure monitoring. Most studies have found that the incidence of white coat hypertension is about 20% in the population of patients with mild hypertension as recorded in physicians' offices. Although there is some controversy about this issue, most investigators have found that white coat hypertension is not associated with increased morbidity.[1]

Appel and Stason[2] reviewed the literature comparing office-based readings taken by physicians, office-based readings taken by nurses or technicians, ambulatory blood pressure monitoring, and patient self-monitoring. The most significant finding was that end organ damage correlated much better with ambulatory blood pressure readings than with office readings. Within the office, readings by physicians were higher than readings by nurses or technicians. Data were insufficient to make a definitive statement about the value of patient self-monitoring.

A 1994 Italian study prospectively followed 1187 "hypertensive" subjects and 205 normotensive control subjects for up to 7.5 years with a mean of 3.2 years using ambulatory blood pressure monitoring; 19.2% of the subjects met the criteria for white coat hypertension. The total number of cardiovascular events was increased in patients with sustained hypertension, but there was no increase among those with white coat hypertension when compared with the control group.[3]

Until further prospective studies on ambulatory monitoring and home self-monitoring are published, a commonsense approach as suggested by Appel and Stason[2] seems reasonable. Patients found to have hypertensive readings by a physician in the office should have several more readings taken by nurses or technicians (most of the studies of the beneficial effects of lowering blood pressure depended on nurse or technician readings). If the blood pressure is still elevated when measured by nurses or technicians, the patient should be assessed for end organ damage and other cardiovascular risk factors. If either is present, the patient should be treated; if neither is present, home self-measurements or ambulatory monitoring should be undertaken and treatment decisions should be based on these readings.

REFERENCES

1. Pickering TG: White coat hypertension: to treat or not to treat? (editorial), *Am Fam Physician* 52:48, 58, 1995.
2. Appel LJ, Stason WB: Ambulatory blood pressure monitoring and blood pressure self-measurement in the diagnosis and management of hypertension, *Ann Intern Med* 118:867-882, 1993.
3. Verdecchia P, Porcellati C, Schillaci G, et al: Ambulatory blood pressure: an independent predictor of prognosis in essential hypertension, *Hypertension* 24:793-801, 1994.

Pseudohypertension

Pseudohypertension is found in 2% to 5% of elderly patients and may raise both the systolic and diastolic readings by as much as 20 to 30 mm Hg.[1] The diagnosis may be suspected in patients with very high readings and no signs of end organ damage, in patients who do not respond to intensive pharmacological therapy, and in those who have postural hypotension after minimal therapy.[2] The traditional confirmatory test on physical examination is Osler's maneuver, which consists of inflating the blood pressure cuff above the systolic reading while palpating the radial or brachial artery. If the artery can still be felt as a nonpulsatile cord when the cuff is inflated above the systolic reading, Osler's maneuver is positive and the patient probably has pseudohypertension.[1] Not all workers agree that this is a sensitive or specific test; Belmin and associates[3] found it insensitive and also found that a significant number of normotensive patients were Osler test positive.

REFERENCES

1. Messerli FH, Ventura HO, Amodeo C: Osler's maneuver and pseudohypertension, *N Engl J Med* 312:1548-1551, 1985.
2. Fifth report of the Joint National Committee on Detection, Evaluation, and Treatment of High Blood Pressure (JNC V), *Arch Intern Med* 153:154-183, 1993.
3. Belmin J, Visintin J-M, Salvatore R, et al: Osler's maneuver: absence of usefulness for the detection of pseudohypertension in an elderly population, *Am J Med* 98:42-49, 1995.

Abdominal Bruits and Renovascular Hypertension

Between 7% and 31% of young individuals have abdominal bruits. Screening for such bruits in normotensive individuals is not indicated. However, about 80% of patients with angiographically documented renal artery stenosis have bruits; the specificity is particularly high if there is a systolic-diastolic bruit. The absence of a bruit does not rule out renovascular hypertension.[1]

REFERENCES

1. Turnbull JM: Is listening for abdominal bruits useful in the evaluation of hypertension? *JAMA* 274:1299-1301, 1995.

Efficacy of the Treatment of Hypertension

Metaanalysis of recent studies on the treatment of hypertension has shown a 16% decrease in the incidence of coronary artery disease and a 38% decrease in the incidence of stroke over 2 to 3 years of treatment. These results occurred with a mean lowering of the diastolic blood pressure of 5 to 6 mm Hg.[1,2] In addition, the control of hypertension has been shown to decrease the incidence of congestive heart failure[3,4] and the development of left ventricular hypertrophy.[3]

At present the major studies proving decreased mortality rates through the treatment of hypertension have involved diuretics and beta-blockers.[5] Studies using other drug groups are in progress.

Although only a few randomized trials have specifically assessed the benefits of treating women, they have shown a 9% to 30% decrease in cardiovascular events.[6]

REFERENCES

1. Hebert PR, Moser M, Mayer J, et al: Recent evidence on drug therapy of mild to moderate hypertension and decreased risk of coronary heart disease, *Arch Intern Med* 153:578-581, 1993.
2. Fifth report of the Joint National Committee on Detection, Evaluation, and Treatment of High Blood Pressure (JNC V), *Arch Intern Med* 153:154-183, 1993.
3. Moser M, Hebert PR: Prevention of disease progression, left ventricular hypertrophy and congestive heart failure in hypertension treatment trials, *J Am Coll Cardiol* 27:1214-1218, 1996.
4. Kostis JB, Davis BR, Cutler J, et al (SHEP Cooperative Research Group): Prevention of heart failure by antihypertensive drug treatment in older persons with isolated systolic hypertension, *JAMA* 278:212-216, 1997.
5. Blake GH: Primary hypertension: the role of individualized therapy, *Am Fam Physician* 50:138-146, 1994.
6. Rich-Edwards JW, Manson JE, Hennekens C, et al: The primary prevention of coronary heart disease in women, *N Engl J Med* 332:1758-1766, 1995.

Nonpharmacological Treatment of Hypertension

(See also detrimental effects of alcohol; exercise; nonsteroidal antiinflammatory drugs; obesity)

Some of the nonpharmacological treatment modalities for hypertension are listed in Table 10. Many of these are discussed more fully in the ensuing paragraphs.

Smoking and hypertension

Smoking is not a risk factor for hypertension as such, but because it is a major cardiovascular risk factor, quitting is particularly important for hypertensive patients.

Weight reduction and hypertension

In the Western world an estimated one third of cases of hypertension are due to obesity.[1] In obese patients weight reduction may have a marked effect on lowering blood pressure. Significant lowering of pressure has been recorded in patients losing 4.5 kg (10 lb),[2,3] and reductions of 26 mm Hg systolic and 20 mm Hg diastolic have been reported in patients losing 9 to 10 kg (20 to 22 lb).[4] The goal of weight reduction in obese hypertensive patients should be a body mass index (BMI) of 20 to 25 (BMI = Wt in kg/Ht in meters squared). This is difficult to achieve.

Exercise and hypertension

Regular aerobic exercise has been shown to reduce both systolic and diastolic blood pressure by about 7 to 10 mm Hg.[5,6] A comprehensive review of the subject concluded that in individuals with a systolic blood pressure of 160 mm Hg or more, exercise in the form of walking, jogging, running, or cycling would lower the systolic pressure by an average of 10 mm Hg and the diastolic pressure by 8 mm Hg.[6] This is about the same benefit that is achieved with medications. Furthermore, exercise is an essential component of any weight loss program and is cardioprotective.

Alcohol and hypertension

A 1994 study found that individuals who have less than three drinks per day did not show any elevation of blood pressure. However, drinking more than that, even if in the form of binge drinking, caused a rise in blood pressure.[7] The

Table 10 Nonpharmacological Treatment of Hypertension

Weight loss
Exercise
Discontinuation or diminishment of alcohol consumption
Discontinuation of NSAIDs if possible
Diet

NSAIDs, Nonsteroidal antiinflammatory drugs.

Cardiovascular System

pressor effect of alcohol begins within a few days of starting to drink and recedes within a few days of discontinuing alcohol; weekend binge drinkers have their highest readings on Mondays, and these become progressively lower throughout the week.[8] In Western nations an estimated 5% to 11% of hypertension in men is caused by alcohol excess.[9] If hypertension is caused by excessive alcohol intake, a drop in blood pressure is usually evident within a few days of discontinuing alcohol.[10]

Nonsteroidal antiinflammatory agents and hypertension

A large number of elderly patients with hypertension may have the disorder simply because they are taking, or have recently taken, nonsteroidal antiinflammatory drugs (NSAIDs). In one study 41% of elderly patients with hypertension had used NSAIDs in the previous year as compared with 26% of younger controls. The higher the dosage of NSAIDs, the more likely that the patients were started on antihypertensive therapy.[11] In a metaanalysis of a number of studies an Australian group found that on average NSAIDs elevated supine mean blood pressure by 5 mm Hg. Among NSAIDs, piroxicam (Feldene) raised the blood pressure the most and aspirin and sulindac (Clinoril) the least. Furthermore, NSAIDs antagonized the blood pressure–lowering effect of antihypertensive drugs, particularly beta-blockers. Diuretics and vasodilators were less affected.[12]

Diet and hypertension

Only a minority of hypertensive patients show a significant drop in blood pressure as a result of salt limitation.[13-15] However, lower salt intake often enhances the effect of antihypertensive medications.[13,14] Foods high in salt include canned soups, bouillon cubes, smoked meat, smoked fish, bacon, ham, marinades, commercial sauces (ketchup, Worcestershire, mustard), salt-covered snacks (chips, nuts), and some mineral waters. Some medications high in salt are Alka-Seltzer, Bromo-Seltzer, and Rolaids.

A short-term trial of normotensive individuals and patients with mild hypertension reported lower blood pressures with a diet high in fruits and vegetables (8 to 10 servings per day) and even lower values when such a diet was combined with a diet low in dairy fat.[16]

Excessive licorice ingestion can induce a hyperaldosterone-like syndrome with hypertension and hypokalemic metabolic alkalosis.[17]

REFERENCES

1. MacMahon SW, Blacket RB, Macdonald GJ, et al: Obesity, alcohol consumption and blood pressure in Australian men and women: the National Heart Foundation of Australia Risk Factor Prevalence Study, *J Hypertens* 2:85-91, 1984.
2. Schotte DE, Stunkard AJ: The effects of weight reduction on blood pressure in 301 obese patients, *Arch Intern Med* 150: 1701-1704, 1990.
3. Fifth report of the Joint National Committee on Detection, Evaluation, and Treatment of High Blood Pressure (JNC V), *Arch Intern Med* 153:154-183, 1993.
4. Reisin E, Abel R, Modan M, et al: Effect of weight loss without salt restriction on the reduction of blood pressure in overweight hypertensive patients, *N Engl J Med* 298:1-6, 1978.
5. Kokkinos PF, Narayan P, Colleran JA, et al: Effects of regular exercise on blood pressure and left ventricular hypertrophy in African-American men with severe hypertension, *N Engl J Med* 333:1462-1467, 1995.
6. Fagard RH, Tipton CM: Physical activity, fitness, and hypertension. In Bouchard et al (eds): *Physical activity, fitness and health: international proceedings and consensus statement,* Champaign, Ill, 1994, Human Kinetics.
7. Marmot MG, Elliott P, Shipley MJ, et al: Alcohol and blood pressure: the INTERSALT study, *BMJ* 308:1263-1267, 1994.
8. Wannamethee G, Shaper AG: Alcohol intake and variations in blood pressure by day of examination, *J Hum Hypertens* 5:59-67, 1991.
9. MacMahon S: Alcohol consumption and hypertension, *Hypertension* 9:111-121, 1987.
10. Maheswaran R, Beevers M, Beevers DG: Effectiveness of advice to reduce alcohol consumption in hypertensive patients, *Hypertension* 19:79-84, 1992.
11. Gurwitz FH, Avorn J, Bohn RL, et al: Initiation of antihypertensive treatment during nonsteroidal anti-inflammatory drug therapy, *JAMA* 272:781-786, 1994.
12. Johnson AG, Nguyen TV, Day RO: Do nonsteroidal anti-inflammatory drugs affect blood pressure? A meta-analysis, *Ann Intern Med* 121:289-300, 1994.
13. Weinberger MH, Cohen SJ, Miller JZ, et al: Dietary sodium restriction as adjunctive treatment of hypertension, *JAMA* 259: 2561-2565, 1988.
14. Huttunen JK, Pietinen P, Nissinen A, et al: Dietary factors and hypertension, *Acta Med Scand* 701(suppl):72-82, 1985.
15. Midgley JP, Matthew AG, Greenwood CM, et al: Effect of reduced dietary sodium on blood pressure: a meta-analysis of randomized controlled trials, *JAMA* 275:1590-1597, 1996.
16. Appel LF, Moore TJ, Obarzanek E, et al: A clinical trial of the effects of dietary patterns on blood pressure, *N Engl J Med* 336:1117-1124, 1997.
17. Heikens J, Fliers E, Endert E, et al: Liquorice-induced hypertension—a new understanding of an old disease: case report and brief review, *Netherlands J Med* 47:230-234, 1995.

Criteria for the Pharmacological Treatment of Hypertension

(See also consensus conferences)

Some of the recommendations of the 1993 Canadian Consensus Conference on hypertension are as follows[1]:

1. Overall, antihypertensive therapy does more good than harm for diastolic levels greater than 90 mm Hg.
2. Treat all patients with diastolic levels greater than 100 mm Hg.
3. Treat all patients with diastolic levels greater than 90 mm Hg if target organ damage is present. Target organ damage is defined as follows.[2]

a. Coronary artery disease (angina; history of myocardial infarction, electrocardiographic or radiological changes of CAD)
b. Left ventricular hypertrophy
c. Cerebrovascular disease
d. Peripheral vascular disease
e. Retinopathy
f. Renal disease

4. Treat isolated systolic hypertension (systolic greater than 160 mm Hg and diastolic less than 90 mm Hg) in those over 60 years of age.
5. Consider treating systolic levels of 140 to 159 mm Hg if target organ damage is present.

In general, nonpharmacological therapy should be tried before using drugs. However, if the blood pressure is greater than 200 mm Hg systolic or 115 mm Hg diastolic, immediate medication is indicated.[3]

REFERENCES

1. Report of the Canadian Hypertension Society Consensus Conference. 2. Diagnosis of hypertension in adults 1993, *Can Med Assoc J* 49:409-418, 1993.
2. Fifth report of the Joint National Committee on Detection, Evaluation, and Treatment of High Blood Pressure (JNC V), *Arch Intern Med* 153:154-183, 1993.
3. Kaplan NM, Gifford RW Jr: Choice of initial therapy for hypertension, *JAMA* 275:1577-1580, 1996.

Pharmacological Treatment of Hypertension

Optimal blood pressure levels

In the treatment of hypertension it may be dangerous to aim for too low a blood pressure. Several studies have shown a J-shaped curve with the risk of coronary heart disease (but not stroke) rising at very low levels.[1] In a study of hypertensive patients without known cardiac disease who were treated pharmacologically, an increased mortality from primary cardiac arrest was noted at diastolic levels less than 85 mm Hg and the odds ratio for this event increased progressively as diastolic levels were reduced further. The authors suggest that until further evidence becomes available, it may be wise not to lower the diastolic pressure below 85 mm Hg.[2] The Joint National Committee on the Detection, Evaluation and Treatment of High Blood Pressure commented that the effects of decreasing the diastolic pressure below 85 mm Hg are unclear.[3] Whether lowering blood pressure below 85 mm Hg affects other types of morbidity such as strokes is unknown, but studies of such conditions are in progress.

REFERENCES

1. Farnett L, Mulrow CD, Linn WD, et al: The J-curve phenomenon and the treatment of hypertension: is there a point beyond which pressure reduction is dangerous? *JAMA* 265:489-495, 1991.
2. Siscovick DS, Raghunathan TE, Psaty BM, et al: Diastolic blood pressure and the risk of primary cardiac arrest among pharmacologically treated hypertensive patients, *J Gen Intern Med* 11: 350-356, 1996.
3. Fifth report of the Joint National Committee on Detection, Evaluation, and Treatment of High Blood Pressure (JNC V), *Arch Intern Med* 153:154-183, 1993.

Single-drug versus multiple-drug treatment

Traditional teaching about the pharmacological management of hypertension is that the dose of a single drug should be raised to its maximum level and if an adequate therapeutic effect is not achieved, the drug should be discontinued and another one tried. However, since toxic effects increase with dose, an equally rational approach may be to use two drugs at lower doses if low doses of a single drug are ineffective.[1] In one study using this approach a combination of the beta-blocker bisoprolol (Zebeta) in doses of 2.5 to 10 mg combined with 6.25 mg of hydrochlorothiazide was slightly more effective in reducing both systolic and diastolic blood pressure than was the calcium channel blocker amlodipine (Norvasc) alone or the ACE inhibitor enalapril (Vasotec) alone. There were fewer adverse reactions with the combination therapy (29% versus 42% and 47% for the single agents).[2] If the blood pressure is greater than 200 mm Hg systolic or 115 mm Hg diastolic, a single agent will rarely give adequate control.[3]

REFERENCES

1. Fagan TC: Remembering the lessons of basic pharmacology (editorial), *Arch Intern Med* 154:1430-1431, 1994.
2. Prisant LM, Weir MR, Papademetriou V, et al: Low dose combination therapy: an alternative first-line approach to hypertension treatment, *Am Heart J* 130:359-366, 1995.
3. Kaplan NM, Gifford RW Jr: Choice of initial therapy for hypertension, *JAMA* 275:1577-1580, 1996.

Factors influencing the choice of drugs

Many factors influence the choice of antihypertensive drugs. Since all classes of antihypertensives have been shown equally effective in lowering blood pressure,[1,2] the JNC V recommendation is to use either a diuretic or a beta-blocker as initial treatment unless a specific clinical reason exists for choosing another class of drugs.[3] The rationale is that these drugs are known to decrease morbidity and mortality. Specifically, low-dose diuretics have been shown to decrease the incidence of strokes, congestive heart failure, and coronary artery disease, while beta-blockers have been shown to decrease the incidence of strokes and congestive failure.[4] Although studies have shown that ACE inhibitors and calcium channel blockers lower blood pressure, as yet no definitive proof has shown that in the general hypertensive population they decrease the risk of strokes, congestive failure, or coronary artery disease. Short-acting dihydropyridine calcium channel blockers may even be harmful (see later discussion of calcium channel blockers).[4]

Table 11 is an outline summary of additional factors that influence the choice of antihypertensives. This table should be considered as a broad guide with many exceptions. Most of these determinants are discussed in more detail in the ensuing text.

Reduction of left ventricular hypertrophy. A comparison of six classes of drugs used to treat men with mild to moderate hypertension found that among those who achieved a diastolic level of <90 mm Hg there was a reduction in left ventricular mass after 1 year in patients taking diuretics (hydrochlorothiazide), beta-blockers (atenolol), and ACE inhibitors (captopril), but no reduction in left ventricular mass in those taking calcium channel blockers (diltiazem), alpha$_1$-adrenergic blocking agents (prazosin), or centrally acting adrenergic agents (clonidine).[5] This may be significant because it appears that reducing left ventricular hypertrophy gives benefits over and above that of simply lowering blood pressure.[6]

Quality of life. No one class of antihypertensive agent is clearly superior to another in terms of quality of life.[7] A 4-year follow-up of patients with mild hypertension taking a placebo or low doses of one of five classes of drugs (beta-blockers [acebutolol]; calcium channel blockers [amlodipine]; diuretics [chlorthalidone]; alpha$_1$-blockers [doxazosin]; ACE inhibitors [enalapril]) found that quality of life improved in all groups including those taking placebo. Quality of life was highest in those taking acebutolol and chlorthalidone.[7]

Cost. Antihypertensive drugs vary greatly in cost. The least expensive in most cases is generic hydrochlorothiazide.[8]

Elderly. Isolated systolic hypertension is primarily a disease of the elderly and is much more prevalent in women; it is estimated that about one third of women over 65 years of age have this condition.[9] Low-dose diuretics such as hydrochlorothiazide 12.5 to 25 mg/day have been shown to decrease the morbidity and mortality of coronary artery disease in elderly hypertensive patients.[10-13] A 1994 study compared the results of antihypertensive trials involving the elderly with those involving younger adults. The treatment of the elderly resulted in a greater decrease in morbidity and mortality at 5 years than did the treatment of younger cohorts.[13]

The drug of first choice for the elderly is a low-dose thiazide diuretic such as hydrochlorothiazide 12.5 mg.[3] If 25 mg of hydrochlorothiazide is required, it should be combined with a potassium-sparing diuretic to decrease the risk of cardiac arrest.[14] Doses higher than 25 mg should almost never be necessary.

Race. Blacks may not respond as well as whites to beta-adrenergic blockers or ACE inhibitors.[15]

Concomitant medical conditions. About two thirds of hypertensive patients have other medical disorders. The common ones in descending order of frequency are arthritis, diabetes mellitus, angina pectoris, chronic obstructive pulmonary disease, congestive heart failure, back problems, and myocardial infarction.[16]

Table 11 Choice of Drugs in the Treatment of Hypertension

Clinical factor	Preferred drugs	Drugs of less value
Reduction of left ventricular hypertrophy	Thiazides, beta-blockers, ACE inhibitors	Calcium channel blockers, alpha$_1$-blocking agents
Quality of life	Low dose; few side effects	High dose; significant side effects
Cost	Thiazides	New drugs
Elderly	Thiazides	
Black race	Diuretics, calcium channel blockers,* alpha$_1$-blockers	Beta-blockers, ACE inhibitors
Concomitant Medical Conditions		
Arthritis		Discontinue NSAIDs or use aspirin or sulindac (Clinoril)
Angina	Beta-blockers, calcium channel blockers*	
History of myocardial infarction	Beta-blockers	
Congestive heart failure	ACE inhibitors	?Beta-blockers
Diabetes	ACE inhibitors, ?beta-blockers	?Thiazides, ?beta-blockers
Chronic renal failure	ACE inhibitors? diltiazem? verapamil?	
Hyperlipidemia	ACE inhibitors, calcium channel blockers,* alpha$_1$-blockers	?Thiazides, ?beta-blockers (except those with ISA and labetalol)
Chronic obstructive pulmonary disease		Beta-blockers
Benign prostatic hypertrophy	Alpha$_1$-blockers	
Peripheral vascular disease	?Beta-blockers	
Depression		?Beta-blockers

?, The indications or contraindications to these drugs are controversial. Some of these are discussed below under the specific drugs.

*Diltiazem (Cardizem, Tiazac) does not have as great a negative inotropic and chronotropic effect as verapamil (Isoptin), nor does it cause the reflex tachycardia associated with dihydropyridine derivatives such as nifedipine (Adalat), felodipine (Renedil, Plendil), and amlodipine (Norvasc) (see later discussion).

Angina. Angina or a history of a myocardial infarction is a strong indication for beta-blockers, whereas chronic obstructive lung disease and in some cases heart failure are usually contraindications for this class of drugs.

Arthritis. Arthritis is often treated with nonsteroidal anti-inflammatory drugs, but they tend either to cause hypertension or to counter the therapeutic effect of many antihypertensive drugs.

Diabetes mellitus. Because of the very high risk of cardiovascular and renal disease in patients with both diabetes and hypertension, the U.S. National Heart, Lung and Blood Institute has recommended that the target blood pressure for such individuals be 130/85 mm Hg.[17] Even though no controlled studies have validated this approach, it appears to be a sensible one.[18]

Antihypertensives may decrease glucose tolerance, and thiazide diuretics are commonly considered the worst offenders. They are not. All classes of antihypertensives decrease glucose tolerance over the short term, and multiple-drug regimens are more likely to do so than single-drug treatments.[19] However, the decreased glucose tolerance of thiazides seems to be self-limited and disappears with time.[20] Therefore low-dose thiazides are acceptable treatment for diabetic patients provided that glucose levels are carefully monitored.[21] Support for this comes from the Systolic Hypertension in the Elderly Program (SHEP), which found that both diabetic and nondiabetic patients treated with low-dose thiazides (chlorthalidone) had decreased rates of cardiovascular events (fatal and nonfatal strokes and fatal and nonfatal myocardial infarctions) compared with a control group receiving placebo. The absolute reduction rates were actually higher in diabetic than in nondiabetic patients because of their underlying high risk levels (see disease prevalence and risk reduction).[22]

Reduction of blood pressure has been shown to postpone the development of diabetic nephropathy. ACE inhibitors appear to be the optimal drugs for achieving this.[23,24]

Beta-blockers are the only class of antihypertensives that have been shown to be cardioprotective; since persons with diabetes are at high risk of coronary events, beta-blockers are probably one of the drugs of choice for these patients.[25] This view is strongly supported by a 1996 Israeli report of non-insulin-dependent diabetic patients with coronary artery disease. The 3-year mortality rate among those treated with beta-blockers was 7.8% compared with a 14% rate for those not taking beta-blockers.[26] Although these drugs may mask the symptoms of hypoglycemia in patients who are taking hypoglycemic agents, this is only a relative contraindication.

Hyperlipidemias. ACE inhibitors, calcium channel blockers, or alpha-blockers have often been recommended as drugs of first choice in patients with hyperlipidemias because they do not adversely affect lipid profiles. This is a moot point; although thiazides and beta-blockers without intrinsic sympathomimetic activity may initially have an adverse effect on lipid profiles, it is not sustained.[20,27] Furthermore, thiazides and beta-blockers are the drugs used in the vast majority of studies showing reduced morbidity and mortality from treating hypertension. In one 1996 study a combination of diet and exercise plus treatment with five classes of antihypertensives (thiazides, beta-blockers, calcium channel blockers, $alpha_1$-antagonists, and ACE inhibitors) improved both blood pressure control and lipid profiles.[2]

Since many hypertensive patients with hyperlipidemia also have coronary artery disease, the treatment of first choice is often a beta-blocker because of its cardioprotective effect.

Chronic renal failure. A study from France compared beta-blockers and enalapril in the treatment of nondiabetic hypertensive patients with chronic renal failure.[28] At the end of 3 years, end-stage renal failure had developed in 35% of the patients taking beta-blockers as compared with 19% of the enalapril group. There was no difference in the blood pressure levels of the two groups. If a patient has a creatinine level greater than 3 mg/dl (250 μmol/L), ACE inhibitors should be started at low doses and the creatinine monitored closely. ACE inhibitors should not be used if the potassium level is 5.5 mmol/L or greater.[29]

Congestive heart failure. ACE inhibitors are the drugs of first choice in hypertensive patients with congestive heart failure.[30]

Benign prostatic hyperplasia. The drug of first choice for hypertensive patients with symptomatic benign prostatic hyperplasia is an alpha-blocker such as terazosin (Hytrin).[31]

Peripheral vascular disease. Beta-blockers may be used safely in cases of mild peripheral vascular disease.[32] Indeed, since peripheral vascular disease is a marker for widespread atherosclerosis, it may be an indication for beta-blockers without ISA because of their cardioprotective effects.

Depression. Beta-blockers are commonly believed to cause or aggravate depression; however, several studies have failed to show such a correlation.[33,34] Use of beta-blockers should probably be avoided in clinically depressed patients, but there is no justification for not using them because of fear of inducing depression in patients who have no history of that disorder.

REFERENCES

1. Neaton JD, Grimm RH Jr, Prineas RJ, et al: Treatment of mild hypertension study: final results, *JAMA* 270:713-724, 1993.
2. Materson BJ, Reda DJ, Cushman WC, et al (Department of Veterans Affairs Cooperative Study Group on Antihypertensive Agents): Single-drug therapy for hypertension in men: a comparison of six antihypertensive agents with placebo, *N Engl J Med* 328:914-921, 1993.
3. Fifth report of the Joint National Committee on Detection, Evaluation, and Treatment of High Blood Pressure (JNC V), *Arch Intern Med* 153:154-183, 1993.
4. Psaty BM, Smith NL, Siscovick DS, et al: Health outcomes associated with antihypertensive therapies used as first-line agents: a systematic review and meta-analysis, *JAMA* 277:739-745, 1997.

Cardiovascular System

5. Gottdiener JS, Reda DJ, Massie BM, et al: Effect of single-drug therapy on reduction of left ventricular mass in mild to moderate hypertension: comparison of six antihypertensive agents, *Circulation* 95:2007-2014, 1997.
6. Levy D, Salomon M, D'Agostino R, et al: Prognostic implications of baseline electrocardiographic features and their serial changes in subjects with left ventricular hypertrophy, *Circulation* 90:1786-1793, 1994.
7. Grimm RH Jr, Grandits GA, Cutler FA, et al: Relationships of quality-of-life measures to long-term lifestyle and drug treatment in the treatment of mild hypertension study, *Arch Intern Med* 157:638-648, 1997.
8. Drugs for hypertension, *Med Lett* 35:55-60, 1993.
9. Saltzberg S, Stroh JA, Frishman WH: Isolated systolic hypertension in the elderly: pathophysiology and treatment, *Med Clin North Am* 72:523-547, 1988.
10. SHEP Cooperative Research Group: Prevention of stroke by antihypertensive drug treatment in older persons with isolated systolic hypertension: final results of the Systolic Hypertension in the Elderly Program (SHEP), *JAMA* 265:3255-3264, 1991.
11. Medical Research Council Working Party: Medical Research Council trial of treatment of hypertension in older adults: principal results, *BMJ* 304:405-412, 1992.
12. Pearce KA, Furberg CD, Rushing J: Does antihypertensive treatment of the elderly prevent cardiovascular events or prolong life? A meta-analysis of hypertension treatment trials, *Arch Fam Med* 4:943-950, 1995.
13. Mulrow CD, Cornell JA, Herrera CR, et al: Hypertension in the elderly: implications and generalizability of randomized trials, *JAMA* 272:1932-1938, 1994.
14. Siscovick DS, Raghunathan TE, Psaty BM, et al: Diuretic therapy for hypertension and the risk of primary cardiac arrest, *N Engl J Med* 330:1852-1857, 1994.
15. Houston MC: New insights and approaches to reduce end organ damage in the treatment of hypertension: subsets of hypertension approach, *Am Heart J* 123:1337-1367, 1992.
16. Stewart AL, Greenfield S, Hays RD, et al: Functional status and well-being of patients with chronic conditions: results from the Medical Outcomes Study, *JAMA* 262:907-913, 1989 [Erratum *JAMA* 262:2542, 1989].
17. National High Blood Pressure Education Program Working Group report on hypertension in diabetes, *Hypertension* 23: 145-158, 1994.
18. Siwek J: New guidelines on treating hypertension in diabetics (editorial), *Am Fam Physician* 53:1982-1984, 1996.
19. Gurwitz JH, Bohn RL, Glynn RJ, et al: Antihypertensive drug therapy and the initiation of treatment for diabetes mellitus, *Ann Intern Med* 118:273-278, 1993.
20. Freis ED: The efficacy and safety of diuretics in treating hypertension, *Ann Intern Med* 122:223-226, 1995.
21. Moser M: Management of hypertension, part I, *Am Fam Physician* 53:2295-2302, 1996.
22. Curb JD, Pressel SL, Cutler JA, et al: Effect of diuretic-based antihypertensive treatment on cardiovascular disease risk in older diabetic patients with isolated systolic hypertension, *JAMA* 276:1866-1892, 1996.
23. Lewis EJ, Hunsicker LG, Bain RP, et al (Collaborative Study Group): The effect of angiotensin-converting-enzyme inhibition on diabetic nephropathy, *N Engl J Med* 329:1456-1462, 1993.
24. Remuzzi G, Ruggenenti P: Slowing the progression of diabetic nephropathy (editorial), *N Engl J Med* 329:1496-1497, 1993.
25. Kendall MJ, Lynch KP, Hjalmarson A, et al: Beta-blockers and sudden cardiac death, *Ann Intern Med* 123:358-367, 1995.
26. Jonas M, Reicherreiss H, Boyko V, et al: Usefulness of beta-blocker therapy in patients with non-insulin-dependent diabetes mellitus and coronary artery disease, *Am J Cardiol* 77:1273-1277, 1996.
27. Grimm RH Jr, Flack JM, Grandits GA, et al: Long-term effects on plasma lipids of diet and drugs to treat hypertension, *JAMA* 275:1549-1556, 1996.
28. Hannedouche T, Landais P, Goldfarb B, et al: Randomized controlled trial of enalapril and ß blockers in non-diabetic chronic renal failure, *BMJ* 309:833-837, 1994.
29. Baker DW, Konstam MA, Bottoriff M, et al: Management of heart failure. I. Pharmacologic treatment, *JAMA* 272:1361-1366, 1994.
30. Garg R, Yusuf S: Overview of randomized trials of angiotensin-converting enzyme inhibitors on mortality and morbidity in patients with heart failure, *JAMA* 273:1450-1456, 1995.
31. Hill SJ, Lawrence SL, Lepor H: New use for alpha blockers: benign prostatic hyperplasia, *Am Fam Physician* 49:1885-1888, 1994.
32. Radack K, Deck C: Beta-adrenergic blocker therapy does not worsen intermittent claudication in subjects with peripheral arterial disease: a meta-analysis of randomized controlled trials, *Arch Intern Med* 151:1705-1707, 1991.
33. Wurzelmann J, Frishman WH, Aronson M, et al: Neuropsychological effects of antihypertensive drugs, *Cardiol Clin* 4: 689-701, 1987.
34. Prisant LM, Spruill WJ, Fincham JE, et al: Depression associated with antihypertensive drugs, *J Fam Practice* 33:481-485, 1991.

Step-down therapy

Twenty-five percent of patients with mild or even moderate hypertension that has been well controlled with drugs for a year or more can safely have the doses of their antihypertensive medications slowly diminished and in many cases discontinued. These patients should be followed closely.[1] Some will remain normotensive for years while others will gradually become hypertensive again; if they do, treatment can be restarted.

REFERENCES

1. Alderman MH, Lamport B: Withdrawal of drug therapy in the treatment of hypertension. In Kaplan NM, Brenner BM, Garagh JH (eds): *New therapeutic strategies in hypertension,* New York, 1989, Raven Press, p 171.

Specific antihypertensive drugs

(See also ACE inhibitors in congestive heart failure; detrusor overactivity; factors influencing the choice of drugs; urticaria and angioedema; medical treatment of benign prostatic hypertrophy; stress incontinence)

Diuretics and diuretics combined with potassium-sparing agents. Hypokalemia secondary to thiazide drugs is dose dependent[1] and is not usually a problem with doses less than 25 mg/day. One reason for treating even mild hypokalemia is that low potassium is associated with elevations of blood pressure.[2] Although oral supplements of potassium chloride are traditionally given to counter hypokalemia, the use of a potassium-sparing agent such as amiloride, triamterene, or spironolactone in conjunction with a thiazide should be considered for doses of hydrochlorothiazide of 25 mg/day or more (Table 12). There is evidence that this decreases the risk of primary cardiac arrest compared with control patients receiving equivalent doses of thiazides with or without potassium supplementation.[3,4] Some of the available combined products are Dyazide, Moduretic or Moduret, and Aldactazide.

Other reputed adverse effects of thiazides are elevated cholesterol and glucose levels. Both of these effects are short lived and disappear with long-term therapy.[5] Spironolactone (Aldactone) should generally be avoided in males because of its propensity to induce gynecomastia.

Potassium supplementation

If hypokalemia is induced by diuretics, it is often best to prescribe a combination of a thiazide and a potassium-sparing diuretic. See "Diuretics" above. Foods high in potassium include milk products, meat, fruits, and vegetables. The highest content is in milk products and meat. A large number of commercial potassium supplements are available; the usual dose for oral replacement is about 20 mEq/day.

Calcium channel blockers

Calcium channel blockers are divided into three classes (Table 13): benzothiazepine derivatives (diltiazem), papaverine-like compounds (verapamil), and dihydropyridine derivatives (nifedipine, felodipine, amlodipine, nisoldipine). All calcium channel blockers increase coronary artery flow and are therefore antianginal agents. Verapamil has the most marked negative inotropic effect of all these agents. Verapamil and to a lesser extent diltiazem decrease atrioventricular node conduction and are therefore useful in patients with paroxysmal supraventricular tachycardia or atrial fibrillation with a rapid ventricular response.[6] Both verapamil and diltiazem may be used in patients with angina who are taking nitrates because these agents do not tend to cause reflex tachycardia.

It has been known for some time that calcium channel blockers have no cardioprotective effects after myocardial infarction.[6] Of more concern are reports of an association between short-acting calcium channel blockers and an increased incidence of myocardial infarction.[7-9] There are also reports that these agents may lead to increased perioperative bleeding,[10] gastrointestinal hemorrhages,[11] and possibly an increased risk of cancer.[12] A less serious adverse effect is that up to 21%[13] of patients taking nifedipine have been reported to develop gingival hyperplasia.

At present a cautious approach to the use of calcium channel blockers is warranted. Furberg[14] recommends considering any calcium channel blocker a third-line drug until controlled trials prove the safety of the newer formulations. In January 1996 the Canadian Health Protection Branch advised physicians to use only calcium channel blockers as second-line drugs for patients with hypertension or angina.[15]

Beta-blockers (Table 14)

Beta-blockers decrease heart rate, systolic blood pressure, myocardial contractility, and myocardial oxygen demand. Beta-blockers without ISA are the only antihypertensive drugs shown to be cardioprotective; they reduce mortality after infarction, limit infarct size, and decrease arrhythmias and sudden death. Beta-blockers may mask some of the symptoms of hypoglycemia in diabetic patients taking hypoglycemic medications, but except for patients with recurrent hypoglycemic episodes this is not a contraindication to using

Table 12 Diuretics and Diuretics Combined with Potassium-Sparing Agents

Drug	Usual dose
Diuretics	
Hydrochlorothiazide (HydroDIURIL, HCTZ)	12.5-25 mg qam
Chlorthalidone (Hygroton)	25 mg qam
Indapamide (Lozide)	1.25-2.5 mg qam
Spironolactone (Aldactone)	25-100 mg qam
Diuretics Plus K^+ Sparing Agents	
Hydrochlorothiazide 50 mg plus amiloride 5 mg (Moduretic, Moduret)	1/2 tablet qam
Hydrochlorothiazide 25 mg plus triamterene 50 mg (Dyazide)	1/2 tablet qam
Spironolactone 25 mg plus hydrochlorothiazide 25 mg (Aldactazide)	1 tablet qam

Table 13 Calcium Channel Blockers

Drug	Usual dose
Benzothiazepine Derivatives	
Diltiazem (Cardizem, Tiazac)	30-60 mg tid-qid for short acting; 60-180 mg bid for SR; 180-360 mg as a single dose for CD
Papaverine-Like Compounds	
Verapamil (Isoptin, Calan, Covera-HS)	80 tid for short acting; 180-240 mg as single dose for extended release
Dihydropyridine Derivatives	
Amlodipine besylate (Norvasc)	5-10 mg daily as a single dose
Felodipine (Renedil, Plendil)	5-10 mg/ day as a single dose
Nifedipine (Adalat, Procardia)	10-20 mg bid for short acting; 30-90 mg/day as a single dose for extended release
Nisoldipine (Sular)	20-40 mg/day as a single dose

these agents, since the cardioprotective benefits far outweigh this adverse effect. Although beta-blockers without intrinsic ISA may cause a slight lowering of HDL-cholesterol and some elevation of triglycerides, the clinical significance of these changes is unknown; there are no human or animal data showing that beta-blockers promote atherogenesis. Beta-blockers with intrinsic ISA activity do not adversely affect lipid profiles, but since they are not a good choice for cardioprotection, they have little role in the treatment of hypertension. Heart failure is only a relative contraindication for beta-blocker drugs,[16] while peripheral vascular disease is not a contraindication.[17]

It is a common belief that beta-blockers cause or aggravate depression; however, several studies have failed to show such a correlation.[18,19]

Beta-blockers may lead to or aggravate urinary incontinence because of detrusor overactivity. This is because beta-adrenergic stimulation normally inhibits the detrusor muscle.[20]

Sotalol is not indicated for the treatment of hypertension.

ACE inhibitors and angiotensin II–blocking agents (Table 15)

ACE inhibitors may cause disorders of taste, cough in up to 25% of patients, and rarely angioedema. In a double-blind crossover study of 10 patients with ACE inhibitor–induced cough, inhaled sodium cromoglycate significantly reduced the severity of the cough. The authors postulated that this was due to suppression of afferent vagal activity.[21] An alternative for patients unable to tolerate ACE inhibitors is to try an angiotensin II–blocking agent such as losartan (Cozaar). A more complete discussion of ACE inhibitors may be found in the section on ACE inhibitors in congestive heart failure.

Angiotensin II receptor antagonists include losartan (Cozaar) and valsartan (Diovan). They are as effective as ACE inhibitors, but there is as yet no evidence that they prolong life in congestive heart failure or after a myocardial infarction or that they prevent nephropathy in diabetics. They do not cause cough, rarely cause angioedema, and occasionally cause hyperkalemia.[22-24]

Alpha$_1$-adrenergic blocking agents (Table 16)

Reflex tachycardia often occurs in patients treated with alpha$_1$-blocking agents who are not also taking beta-blockers. Alpha$_1$-blockers inhibit the alpha-adrenergic receptors of the internal bladder sphincter and may lead to incontinence. On the other hand, they may relieve the symptoms of benign prostatic hyperplasia.

REFERENCES

1. Knauf H: The role of low-dose diuretics in essential hypertension, *J Cardiovasc Pharmacol* 22(suppl 6):S1-S7, 1993.
2. Whelton PK, He J, Cutler JA, et al: Effects of oral potassium on blood pressure: meta-analysis of randomized controlled clinical trials, *JAMA* 277:1624-1632, 1997.
3. Siscovick DS, Raghunathan TE, Psaty BM, et al: Diuretic therapy for hypertension and the risk of primary cardiac arrest, *N Engl J Med* 330:1852-1857, 1994.
4. Bigger JT Jr: Diuretic therapy, hypertension, and cardiac arrest, *N Engl J Med* 330:1899-1900, 1994.

Table 14 Beta-Blockers

Drug	Usual dose
Nonselective, Without ISA	
Nadolol (Corgard)	80-240 mg daily as a single dose
Propranolol (Inderal)	40-160 mg bid for short acting; 80-320 mg once a day for extended release
Timolol (Blocadren)	5-30 mg bid
Selective, Without ISA	
Atenolol (Tenormin)	50-100 mg daily as a single dose
Metoprolol (Lopresor, Toprol-XL)	50-100 mg bid for short acting; 100 mg daily as a single dose for extended release
Nonselective, with ISA	
Pindolol (Visken)	5-15 mg bid
Selective, with ISA	
Acebutolol (Sectral)	100-200 mg bid
Beta-Adrenergic and Alpha$_1$-Blocking Agents	
Labetalol (Trandate)	200-400 mg bid
Carvedilol (Coreg)	12.5 mg bid

Table 15 ACE Inhibitors and Angiotensin II Antagonists

Drug	Usual dose
ACE Inhibitors	
Benazepril (Lotensin)	10-20 mg/day as a single dose
Captopril (Capoten)	25-50 mg bid or tid
Cilazapril (Inhibace)	2.5-5 mg/day as a single dose
Enalapril (Vasotec)	5-40 mg/day as a single dose or bid
Fosinopril (Monopril)	20 mg/day as a single dose
Lisinopril (Zestril, Prinivil)	10-40 mg/day as a single dose
Moexipril (Univasc)	7.5-30 mg/day in 1 or 2 divided doses
Perindopril (Coversyl)	4-8 mg/day as a single dose
Quinapril HCl (Accupril)	10-20 mg/day as a single dose
Ramipril (Altace)	2.5-10 mg/day as a single dose
Trandolapril (Mavik)	2-4 mg/day as a single dose
Angiotensin II Antagonists	
Losartan (Cozaar)	50-100 mg/day as a single dose
Valsartan (Diovan)	80-320 mg/day as a single dose

Table 16 Alpha$_1$-Adrenergic Blocking Agents

Drug	Usual dose
Terazosin (Hytrin)	1-5 mg/day as a single dose
Prazosin (Minipress)	2-5 mg tid
Doxazosin (Cardura)	1-8 mg/day as a single dose

5. Freis EDZ: The efficacy and safety of diuretics in treating hypertension, *Ann Intern Med* 122:223-226, 1995.
6. Raspa RF, Wilson CC: Calcium channel blockers in the treatment of hypertension, *Am Fam Physician* 48:461-470, 1993.
7. Psaty BM, Heckbert SR, Koepsell TD, et al: The risk of myocardial infarction associated with antihypertensive drug therapies, *JAMA* 274:620-625, 1995.
8. Furberg CD, Psaty BM, Meyer JV: Nifedipine: dose-related increase in mortality in patients with coronary heart disease, *Circulation* 92:1326-1331, 1995.
9. Borhani NO, Mercuri M, Borhani PA, et al: Final outcome results of the Multicenter Isradipine Diuretic Atherosclerosis Study (MIDAS): a randomized controlled trial, *JAMA* 276:785-791, 1996.
10. Zuccalà G, Pahor M, Landi F, et al: Use of calcium antagonists and need for perioperative transfusion in older patients with hip fracture: observational study. *BMJ* 643-644, 1997.
11. Pahor M, Guralnik JM, Furberg CD, et al: Risk of gastrointestinal hemorrhage with calcium antagonists in hypertensive patients over 67, *Lancet* 347:1061-1066, 1996.
12. Pahor M, Guralnik JM, Salive ME, et al: Do calcium channel blockers increase the risk of cancer? *Am J Hypertens* 9:695-699, 1996.
13. Barclay S, Seymour RA: The incidence and severity of nifedipine-induced gingival hyperplasia, *J Clin Periodontol* 18:49-52, 1991.
14. Furberg CD: Should dihydropyridines be used as first-line drugs in the treatment of hypertension? The con side, *Arch Intern Med* 155:2157-2161, 1995.
15. Canadian Health Protection Branch: *Safety of calcium channel blockers in the treatment of patients with hypertension and coronary artery disease,* CD No 44, January 23, 1996.
16. Kendall MJ, Lynch KP, Hjalmarson A, et al: Beta-blockers and sudden cardiac death, *Ann Intern Med* 123:358-367, 1995.
17. Radack K, Deck C: Beta-adrenergic blocker therapy does not worsen intermittent claudication in subjects with peripheral arterial disease: a meta-analysis of randomized controlled trials, *Arch Intern Med* 151:1705-1707, 1991.
18. Wurzelmann J, Frishman WH, Aronson M, et al: Neuropsychological effects of antihypertensive drugs, *Cardiol Clin* 4: 689-701, 1987.
19. Prisant LM, Spruill WJ, Fincham JE, et al: Depression associated with antihypertensive drugs, *J Fam Pract* 33:481-485, 1991.
20. Mold JW: Pharmacotherapy of urinary incontinence, *Am Fam Physician* 54:673-680, 1996.
21. Hargreaves MR, Benson MK: Inhaled sodium cromoglycate in angiotensin-converting enzyme inhibitor cough, *Lancet* 345: 13-16, 1995.
22. Losartan for hypertension, *Med Lett* 37:57-58, 1995.
23. Gradman AH, Arcuri KE, Goldberg AI, et al: A randomized, placebo-controlled, double-blind, parallel study of various doses of losartan potassium compared with enalapril maleate in patients with essential hypertension, *Hypertension* 25:1345-1350, 1995.
24. Valsartan for hypertension, *Med Lett* 39:43-44, 1997.

VALVULAR HEART DISEASE

(See also anticoagulants; endocarditis prophylaxis; screening)

Heart Murmurs in Children

The ability of pediatric cardiologists to differentiate functional from organic murmurs in children by history and physical examination alone is excellent. Features suggesting organic disease include pansystolic nature of murmur, intensity of grade 3 or more, and an abnormal second heart sound.[1]

Aortic Stenosis

A long latent period occurs during the presymptomatic phase of aortic stenosis. Once symptoms such as angina, syncope, or heart failure occur, the mortality rate is very high over the next 2 to 5 years. In general, stenotic aortic valves should be replaced as soon as the patient is symptomatic. Age is not a contraindication, and results are usually excellent.[2]

Aortic Insufficiency

In a 1994 study, nifedipine in doses of 20 mg bid was given to asymptomatic patients with aortic insufficiency who had normal left ventricular ejection fractions. This resulted in a significant delay in the need for valve replacement compared with the control group. The rationale for nifedipine is that arteriolar vasodilation increases forward flow and decreases the amount of aortic regurgitation.[3]

Mitral Stenosis

Percutaneous balloon valvuloplasty would seem to be at least as effective as open surgical commissurotomy for most patients with mitral stenosis.[4]

Prosthetic Valves

The two major types of prosthetic valves are mechanical valves and tissue valves. Mechanical valves may be caged-ball (Starr-Edwards), single-tilting-disk (e.g., Medtronic-Hall, Bjork-Shiley), or bileaflet-tilting-disk (e.g., St. Jude). The most common tissue valve is the porcine heterograft valve. Porcine heterograft valves are expected to last 10 to 15 years but do not require long-term anticoagulation; mechanical valves last longer but require anticoagulation. Failure of porcine valves is usually gradual, so the replacement surgery can be elective.[5,6]

The surgical mortality of valve replacement depends largely on the patient's individual risk factors. Isolated aortic valve replacement in an otherwise healthy person has a 30-day mortality rate of 1% to 5% while that for isolated mitral valve replacement is 2% to 8%.[5]

The risk of thrombosis depends on the type of mechanical valve; it is greatest for the caged-ball valves, least for the bileaflet-tilting-disk, and intermediate for the single-tilting-disk. One set of recommendations is that the INR should be maintained between 4 and 4.9 for patients with caged-ball valves or multiple prosthetic valves, between 3 and 3.9 for those with single-tilting-disk valves, and between 2.5 and 2.9 for those with bileaflet-tilting-disk valves. Patients with porcine heterografts may be given anticoagulants to achieve a ratio between 2 and 3 for first 3 months. Modifications of these recommendations are required for patients at risk of bleeding such as the very elderly.[6]

The authors of a French study concluded that INR levels of 2 to 3 are acceptable for patients with single St. Jude bileaflet-tilting-disk valves implanted in the aortic or mitral regions.[7]

REFERENCES

1. McCrindle BW, Shaffer KM, Kan JS, et al: Cardinal clinical signs in the differentiation of heart murmurs in children, *Arch Pediatr Adolesc Med* 150:169-174, 1996.
2. Carabello BA, Crawford FA Jr: Valvular heart disease, *N Engl J Med* 337:32-41, 1997.
3. Scognamiglio R, Rahimtoola SH, Fasoli G, et al: Nifedipine in asymptomatic patients with severe aortic regurgitation and normal left ventricular function, *N Engl J Med* 331:689-694, 1994.
4. Dean LS, Mickel M, Bonan R, et al: Four-year follow-up of patients undergoing percutaneous balloon mitral commissurotomy —a report from the National Heart, Lung, and Blood Institute Balloon Valvuloplasty Registry, *J Am Coll Cardiol* 28:1452-1457, 1996.
5. Katz NM: Current surgical treatment of valvular heart disease, *Am Fam Physician* 52:559-568, 1995.
6. Vongpatanasin W, Hillis D, Lange RA: Prosthetic heart valves, *N Engl J Med* 335:407-416, 1996.
7. Acar J, Iung B, Boissel JP, et al: AREVA: multicenter randomized comparison of low-dose versus standard-dose anticoagulation in patients with mechanical prosthetic heart valves, *Circulation* 94:2107-2112, 1996.

VASCULAR DISEASE

(See also transient ischemic attacks)

Noninvasive Blood Flow Tests

(See also thrombophlebitis, peripheral vascular disease)

Doppler flow analysis

Doppler flow analysis is based on the principle that the frequency of a sound wave reflected from a moving particle is changed. In assessing vessels, blood flow velocity is determined by the magnitude of frequency shifts reflected off moving blood cells.[1] A Doppler probe may be used at the bedside to help in the diagnosis of suspected thrombophlebitis. When the probe is held over the femoral vein in normal individuals, flow variations with respiration are detectable, a Valsalva maneuver obliterates these variations, and at the completion of a Valsalva maneuver a temporary increase in flow takes place. In addition, manual compression of the foot or calf causes a detectable increase in flow. In patients with occlusive deep venous thrombosis (DVT) proximal to the probe, there are no detectable variations in flow with respiration or with a Valsalva maneuver. If occlusive DVT is present distal to the probe, no augmentation of flow is seen with compression of the foot or calf.[1] This is the investigative procedure of choice for suspected DVT.[2]

Another use of the Doppler probe is to determine the ankle-brachial index in cases of suspected peripheral vascular disease. The Doppler probe is held over the posterior tibial artery or the dorsalis pedis artery. A blood pressure cuff is placed just above the malleoli and inflated until the Doppler signal disappears and the pressure is recorded. The cuff is then deflated until the Doppler signal reappears, and this pressure is also recorded. Ankle pressure is the mean of the two readings. It is reported as the ratio of the ankle pressure to the blood pressure obtained at the level of the brachial artery, which is called the ankle-brachial index (ABI). Normally the ankle pressure is higher than the brachial pressure, so in normal individuals the index is greater than 1.[1] For the clinical usefulness and interpretation of the test, see the later discussion of peripheral vascular disease.

B-mode ultrasonography

Real-time ultrasonography processes the images rapidly enough to to allow the examiner to appreciate what is going on at that instant, such as motion of the arterial wall. B-mode ultrasonography can give an estimate of the site and degree of stenosis of a vessel, in some cases the surface characteristics of a lesion (smooth, ulcerated), and sometimes the composition of a lesion (fibrous, hemorrhagic).[1]

Duplex scanning

Duplex scanning combines real time B-mode ultrasonography and Doppler flow signal analysis. Duplex scanning is frequently used for assessing the internal carotid artery. Its sensitivity is high for high-grade stenosis but low for total occlusion.[1] It is also used in the assessment of DVT. Its sensitivity and specificity for proximal deep venous thrombosis are excellent, but it misses many cases of calf vein thrombophlebitis.[2] The most sensitive way of detecting a DVT using a duplex scanner is to determine whether the vein being assessed can be compressed by the scanning probe. Normal veins are easily compressible, whereas thrombus-containing veins are not.[1] The efficacy of this procedure is discussed in the section on thrombophlebitis.

Impedance plethysmography

Plethysmography measures volume change. For detection of a deep venous thrombosis (DVT) of the lower limb, the leg is elevated 15 to 20 degrees to drain the veins and a baseline calf volume is measured through a transducer. A thigh cuff is then rapidly inflated to occlude venous return, and the calf volume is again measured. After 45 seconds the cuff is released and the calf volume is measured once again. In a normal individual the calf volume increases at a steady rate after inflation of the cuff and decreases rapidly when the cuff is released. When a thrombus occludes the proximal veins, the calf is already distended, so the volume curve remains flat both during thigh compression and after the release of thigh compression. With a nonocclusive DVT the rate of rise of the calf volume is diminished during compression and the rate of fall in volume after release of the cuff is also reduced.[1] IPG is a less sensitive test than Doppler examination.[3]

REFERENCES

1. Steinmetz OK, Cole CW: Noninvasive blood flow tests in vascular disease, *Can Fam Physician* 39:2405-2416, 1993.
2. Douketis JD, Ginsberg JS: Diagnosis of deep vein thrombosis, *Can Fam Physician* 42:497-503, 1996.
3. Ginsberg JS, Wells PS, Hirsh J, et al: Reevaluation of the sensitivity of impedance plethysmography for the detection of proximal deep vein thrombosis, *Arch Intern Med* 154:1930-1933, 1994.

Arterial Disease

Peripheral vascular disease

(See also noninvasive blood flow tests)

In patients with claudication the risk of death from all causes is four to seven times greater and the risk of dying of cardiovascular disease within 10 years is 15 times that of patients who do not have claudication. The 5-year mortality rate for this condition is 29%.[1] Claudication is not always a progressive disease. In one 5-year follow-up study 4% of patients required an amputation and 16% had worsening of their symptoms.[2]

An objective measurement of peripheral vascular disease is the ankle-brachial index (see earlier discussion of noninvasive blood flow tests). Any value less than 1 is abnormal, and patients with rest pain usually have values less than 0.5. Some patients with peripheral vascular disease have a normal ABI at rest but an abnormal one after exercising or taking a vasodilator drug such as papaverine (augmented ABI).[3] Most cases of peripheral vascular disease seen in family medicine are easily diagnosed on the basis of history and physical examination. I am unaware of any evidence that obtaining an ABI improves the clinical outcomes of these patients.

Exercise is an essential component of the management of intermittent claudication. Patients should walk for at least 30 minutes three times a week and continue walking to a point at which the claudication pain is near maximal. One study found that after 6 months of such a program the distance walked to the onset and to maximal claudication pain increased by 120% to 180%.[4] A randomized trial comparing exercise training to limb arterial angioplasty found that exercise gave better results.[5]

Pentoxifylline (Trental), usually given as 400 mg bid or tid, can increase pain-free walking distances.[6,7] However, in comparative studies it is not as effective as a walking program alone.[7] Verapamil (Isoptin, Calan, Covera-HS) in doses of 120 to 480 mg/day also gives some relief of symptoms.[8]

Prophylactic aspirin given over long periods to asymptomatic men decreases the need for vascular surgery,[9] but whether it or other antithrombotic agents such as ticlopidine (Ticlid) are beneficial for patients with proven peripheral vascular disease is unproved. However, given the high incidence of coronary artery disease in these patients, prescribing aspirin makes sense.

Chelation therapy is not beneficial.[10]

REFERENCES

1. Criqui MG, Langoer RD, Fronek A, et al: Mortality over a period of 10 years in patients with peripheral arterial disease, *N Engl J Med* 326:381-386, 1992.
2. Kannel WB, Skinner JJ Jr, Schwartz MJ, et al: Intermittent claudication: incidence in the Framingham Study, *Circulation* 41:875-883, 1970.
3. Steinmetz OK, Cole CW: Noninvasive blood flow tests in vascular disease, *Can Fam Physician* 39:2405-2416, 1993.
4. Gardner AW, Poehlman ET: Exercise rehabilitation programs for the treatment of claudication pain: a meta-analysis, *JAMA* 274:975-980, 1995.
5. Creasy TX, McMillan PJ, Fletcher EW, et al: Is percutaneous transluminal angioplasty better than exercise for claudication? Preliminary results from a prospective randomized trial, *Eur J Vasc Surg* 4:135-140, 1990.
6. Ernst E: Pentoxifylline for intermittent claudication: a critical review, *Angiology* 45:339-345, 1994.
7. Spitzer S, Bach R, Schieffer H: Walk training and drug treatment in patients with peripheral arterial occlusive disease stage II: a review, *Int J Angiol* 11:204-210, 1992.
8. Bagger JP, Helligsoe P, Randsbaek F, et al: Effect of verapamil in intermittent claudication: a randomized double-blind, placebo-controlled, cross-over study after individual dose-response assessment, *Circulation* 95:411-414, 1997.
9. Goldhaber SZ, Manson JE, Stampfer MJ, et al: Low-dose aspirin and subsequent peripheral arterial surgery in the Physicians' Health Study, *Lancet* 340:143-145, 1992.
10. van Rij AM, Solomon C, Packer SG, et al: Chelation therapy for intermittent claudication: a double-blind, randomized, controlled trial, *Circulation* 90:1194-1199, 1994.

Raynaud's phenomenon

Most cases of Raynaud's phenomenon are idiopathic and develop in women in their twenties and thirties. Underlying diseases to be ruled out include lupus, scleroderma and other types of vasculitis, myeloproliferative disorders, and cryoglobulinemia. Symptomatic treatment involves keeping both the patient and the extremities warm and in some cases administering long-acting calcium channel blockers such as long-acting nifedipine (Adalat XL) or felodipine (Renedil, Plendil).[1]

REFERENCES

1. Keystone EC: Appropriate management of Raynaud's disease, *Patient Care Can* 7:14. 1996.

Venous Disease

Thrombophlebitis

(See also cardiovascular events caused by oral contraceptives; noninvasive blood flow tests; pulmonary embolism; thrombophlebitis in women receiving hormone replacement therapy)

The distinction between proximal and distal (calf only) deep vein thrombosis is important because patients with thrombi limited to the calf rarely have pulmonary emboli, and if they do, the emboli are generally inconsequential. However, in 20% to 30% of cases of calf vein thrombosis, extension to the proximal veins occurs within 2 weeks of presentation. Since both impedance plethysmography (IPG) and duplex ultrasound (DU) fail to detect a number of cases of calf vein thrombosis (see discussion of noninvasive blood flow tests above), serial measurements to detect proximal extensions are often indicated if the initial reports are negative (see below).[1] Pulmonary emboli develop in approximately 50% of patients with untreated proximal deep vein thrombosis.[2]

The clinical diagnosis of deep vein thrombosis is notoriously difficult, and most patients have no suggestive signs or symptoms. Among patients who do have symptoms or signs suggestive of phlebitis, only half actually have the condition.[3]

Reversible risk factors for deep vein thrombosis include trauma, surgery, temporary immobilization, travel, estrogen treatment, infection, Baker's cyst, and pregnancy. Permanent risk factors include inherited disorders of coagulation, malignancy, permanent immobilization, and idiopathic recurrent thromboembolic episodes.[4,5]

Some of the inherited disorders of coagulation that predispose to thrombophlebitis are antithrombin III, protein C and protein S deficiencies, and activated protein C resistance (which is caused by inheriting factor V Leiden). In activated protein C resistance the normal coagulation factor V is altered by a single amino acid, making it resistant to inhibition by the anticoagulant protein C. Factor V Leiden is the most common cause of molecular hypercoagulable states.[6] It is found in about 5% of white Americans, 2% of Hispanic Americans, 1% of African and Native Americans, and 0.5% of Asian Americans.[7] The congenital disorders of coagulation are usually inherited in an autosomal dominant pattern, so a family history can often be elicited.[8]

The antiphospholipid antibody syndrome consists of recurrent venous or arterial thrombosis; recurrent spontaneous abortions, usually in the second trimester; and the presence of antiphospholipid antibodies (anticardiolipin antibodies or lupus anticoagulant). Many but not all cases are in patients with systemic lupus erythematosus.[9,10] One of the most serious complications of this disorder is stroke. Treatment is lifelong warfarin (Coumadin)[9,10] except during pregnancy, when aspirin, heparin, or a combination of the two is used.[11]

Patients with cancer have long been known to have an increased incidence of thromboembolic disease. This might suggest that a workup for malignancy is needed for patients with thromboembolic disease. One study of 142 patients with confirmed deep venous thrombosis found that 12% of the patients had cancer at the time of initial hospitalization. All of the patients with cancer had findings suggesting this diagnosis on the basis of history, physical examination, routine admission blood work, or chest x-ray examination. Among the remaining patients the risk of cancer in the 3 years after the diagnosis of deep vein thrombosis was no greater than was reported in control subjects. An extensive workup for malignancy is not indicated in patients who are otherwise well and have deep vein thrombosis.[12]

A study from Sunnybrook Hospital in Toronto using serial impedance plethysmography and lower extremity contrast venography has shown that deep vein thrombosis is extremely common after major trauma. Overall, 58% of trauma patients had deep vein thrombosis and 18% had proximal deep vein thrombosis. Only 3 (1.5%) of 201 patients had clinical symptoms or signs suggesting the disorder. None of the patients had received prophylaxis against thromboembolism at the time of the study.[13]

REFERENCES

1. Douketis JD, Ginsberg JS: Diagnosis of deep vein thrombosis, *Can Fam Physician* 42:497-503, 1996.
2. Moser KM, LeMoine JR: Is embolic risk conditioned by location of deep venous thrombosis? *Ann Intern Med* 94:439-444, 1981.
3. Weinmann EE, Salzman EW: Deep-vein thrombosis, *N Engl J Med* 331:1630-1641, 1994.
4. Hirsh J: The optimal duration of anticoagulant therapy for venous thrombosis (editorial), *N Engl J Med* 332:1710-1711, 1995.
5. Chesterman CN: After a first episode of venous thromboembolism: stop anticoagulant treatment after four to six weeks in patients with "reversible" risk factors (editorial), *BMJ* 311:700-701, 1995.
6. Dahlback B: Inherited thrombophilia: resistance to activated protein C as a pathogenic factor of venous thromboembolism, *Blood* 85:607-614, 1995.
7. Ridker PM, Miletich JP, Hennekens CH, et al: Ethnic distribution of factor V Leiden in 4047 men and women: implications for venous thromboembolism screening, *JAMA* 277:1305-1307, 1997.
8. Bauer KA: Case records of the Massachusetts General Hospital, *N Engl J Med* 334:1045-1051, 1996.
9. Khamashta MA, Cuadrado MJ, Mujic F, et al: The management of thrombosis in the antiphospholipid-antibody syndrome, *N Engl J Med* 332:993-997, 1995.
10. Lockshin MD: Answers to the antiphospholipid-antibody syndrome? (editorial), *N Engl J Med* 332:1025-1027, 1995.
11. Rai R, Cohen H, Dave M, et al: Randomised controlled trial of aspirin and aspirin plus heparin in pregnant women with recurrent miscarriage associated with phospholipid antibodies (or antiphospholipid antibodies), *BMJ* 314:253-257, 1997.
12. Cornuz J, Pearson SD, Creager MA, et al: Importance of findings on the initial evaluation for cancer in patients with symptomatic idiopathic deep venous thrombosis, *Ann Intern Med* 125:785-793, 1996.
13. Geerts WH, Code KI, Jay RM, et al: A prospective study of venous thromboembolism after major trauma, *N Engl J Med* 331:1601-1606, 1994.

Treatment and prevention of thrombophlebitis. A variety of methods have been used to prevent deep vein thrombosis in at-risk patients. Physical measures include graduated compression stockings and intermittent external pneumatic compression of the lower extremities. Commonly used drugs include warfarin, intravenous heparin, and low–molecular weight heparin.[1] Aspirin has been shown to reduce pulmonary embolism by about 60% and deep vein thrombosis by 30% to 40%,[2] but it is not as effective as other prevention modalities.[1,3]

Since thrombi limited to the calf veins are unlikely to embolize, immediate anticoagulation is not always necessary. It is often safe to wait and perform serial impedance plethysmography or serial duplex ultrasound if the diagnosis is not clear after the initial investigations. However, since in 20% to 30% of patients thrombophlebitis extends to the proximal veins, and since calf vein thrombophlebitis can also cause a postphlebitic syndrome, anticoagulation is indicated in most cases once the diagnosis is made.[4]

The traditional initial treatment of thrombophlebitis is 5 days of intravenous (unfractionated) heparinization followed by oral anticoagulation (warfarin) therapy for at least 3 months. Such therapy reduces the incidence of recurrent thrombosis from 25% to less than 4%. A newer, simpler, more cost-effective method of initiating therapy is to use subcutaneous low–molecular weight heparin (LMWH) administered on an outpatient basis (Table 17). Metaanalyses comparing LMWH with unfractionated heparin suggest not only that LMWH is more effective, but also that it results in fewer major bleeding episodes.[5-7]

LMWH does not normally alter the partial thromboplastin time, so this is not monitored during therapy; INR is monitored in the usual way to control the level of concomitantly given warfarin. Heparin can cause thrombocytopenia through the development of heparin-dependent IgG antibodies, usually after 5 days of treatment. This complication appears to be less common in patients treated with LMWH than in those treated with unfractionated heparin.[8]

An area of controversy is the optimal duration of anticoagulant therapy. The risk of recurrent thromboembolism is low in patients who have thrombosis limited to the calf veins and those who have a reversible risk factor such as previous surgery compared with those who have permanent risk factors such as cancer or those with idiopathic deep vein thrombosis. In the opinion of Hirsh,[9] anticoagulants should be administered for 6 weeks to patients with reversible risk factors and for 6 months to those with idiopathic thrombophlebitis. Bedridden patients with cancer or those with recurrent thromboembolic episodes might require indefinite anticoagulation. Similar views were expressed by Chesterman,[10] who recommends 4 to 6 weeks of anticoagulation for patients with reversible risk factors such as trauma, surgery, temporary immobilization, travel, estrogen treatment, infection, Baker's cyst, and pregnancy.

Table 17 Low–Molecular Weight Heparins

Drug	Usual dose for postoperative prophylaxis against deep vein thrombosis
Dalteparin (Fragmin)	2500 IU (0.2 ml) sc daily
Enoxaparin (Lovenox)	30 mg (0.3 ml) sc bid
Tinzaparin (Innohep)	3500 IU sc once daily (50 IU/kg)

Patients with permanent risk factors including malignancy, inherited disorders of coagulation inhibition (antithrombin III, protein C, and protein S deficiencies), and lupus-type antibodies (antiphospholipid-antibody syndrome) need at least 6 months of anticoagulation and perhaps indefinite treatment.[9] Whether carriers of factor V Leiden who have had a single thromboembolic event should receive long-term anticoagulant therapy can be determined only by long-term trials.[11] A Swedish study found that indefinite coagulation after a second episode of thromboembolism resulted in fewer recurrences than occurred in those given anticoagulants for 6 months.[12] On an empirical basis, Ginsberg[13] recommended 1 year of treatment for patients who had had two episodes of thromboembolism and lifetime treatment for those with three or more episodes.

A number of reasons exist for placing filters in the inferior vena cava of patients with thrombophlebitis. Two clear indications are failure of anticoagulation therapy and a contraindication to anticoagulation therapy.[14] Filters have also been placed for floating proximal vein thrombi (as opposed to obstructing thrombi). This is a tenuous indication because the risk of pulmonary embolism in patients receiving anticoagulants is no higher in those with free-floating emboli than in those with obstructing emboli.[14,15]

It is estimated that a postthrombotic syndrome develops in more than 50% of patients with symptomatic proximal deep vein thrombosis, usually within 2 years of the initial thrombotic episode. The regular use of made-to-measure below-knee compression stockings during the day over a 2-year period (two new stockings every 6 months) decreases the risk by 50%.[16]

REFERENCES

1. Weinmann EE, Salzman EW: Deep-vein thrombosis, *N Engl J Med* 331:1630-1641, 1994.
2. Antiplatelet Trialists' Collaboration: Collaborative overview of randomised trials of antiplatelet treatment. III. Reduction in venous thrombosis and pulmonary embolism by antiplatelet prophylaxis among surgical and medical patients, *BMJ* 308:235-246, 1994.
3. Underwood MJ, More RS: The aspirin papers (editorial), *BMJ* 308:71-72, 1994.
4. Douketis JD, Ginsberg JS: Diagnosis of deep vein thrombosis, *Can Fam Physician* 42:497-503, 1996.
5. Leizorovicz A, Simonneau G, Decousus H, et al: Comparison of efficacy and safety of low molecular weight heparins and unfractionated heparin in initial treatment of deep venous thrombosis: a meta-analysis, *BMJ* 309:299-304, 1994.
6. Lensing AW, Prins MH, Davidson BI, et al: Treatment of deep venous thrombosis with low-molecular-weight heparins: a meta-analysis, *Arch Intern Med* 155:601-607, 1995.

7. Siragusa S, Cosmi B, Piovella F, et al: Low-molecular-weight heparins and unfractionated heparin in the treatment of patients with acute venous thromboembolism: results of a meta-analysis, *Am J Med* 100:269-277, 1996.
8. Warkentin TE, Levine MN, Hirsh J, et al: Heparin-induced thrombocytopenia in patients treated with low-molecular-weight heparin or unfractionated heparin, *N Engl J Med* 332: 1330-1335, 1995.
9. Hirsh J: The optimal duration of anticoagulant therapy for venous thrombosis (editorial), *N Engl J Med* 332:1710-1711, 1995.
10. Chesterman CN: After a first episode of venous thromboembolism: stop anticoagulant treatment after four to six weeks in patients with "reversible" risk factors (editorial), *BMJ* 311:700-701, 1995.
11. Simioni A, Prandoni P, Lensing WA, et al: The risk of recurrent venous thromboembolism in patients with an Arg[506] Gln mutation in the gene for factor V (factor V Leiden), *N Engl J Med* 336:399-403, 1997.
12. Schulman S, Granqvist S, Holmström M, et al: The duration of oral anticoagulant therapy after a second episode of venous thromboembolism, *N Engl J Med* 336:393-398, 1997.
13. Ginsberg JS: Management of venous thromboembolism, *N Engl J Med* 335:1816-1828, 1996.
14. Goldhaber SZ: A free-floating approach to filters (editorial), *Arch Intern Med* 157:264-265, 1997.
15. Pacouret G, Alison D, Pottier J-M, et al: Free-floating thrombus and embolic risk in patients with angiographically confirmed proximal deep venous thrombosis: a prospective study, *Arch Intern Med* 157:305-308, 1997.
16. Brandjes PM, Büller HR, Heijboer H, et al: Randomised trial of effect of compression stockings in patients with symptomatic proximal-vein thrombosis, *Lancet* 349:759-762, 1997.

Pulmonary embolism

(See also thrombophlebitis)

The risk factors for pulmonary embolism are similar to those for thrombophlebitis and include trauma, surgery, congestive heart failure, immobilization, cancer, and inherited disorders of coagulation. Important additional risk factors are obesity, smoking, and hypertension.[1]

Symptoms of pulmonary embolism include tachypnea and tachycardia, which are quite nonspecific.[2] Blood gas concentrations are not sensitive enough to rule out pulmonary embolism. In one study 30% of patients with pulmonary emboli had a Pao_2 of more than 80 mm Hg,[3] while in another study between 8% and 23% had a normal A-a gradient.[4] In a third investigation 30% of patients with pulmonary embolism but no past history of cardiopulmonary disease had no diminution of the Pao_2 or the $Paco_2$ and also had normal A-a gradients.[5] Among patients with pulmonary emboli and a prior history of cardiopulmonary disease, 14% had all three values in the normal range.[5]

The best investigative technique for suspected pulmonary embolisms is a ventilation/perfusion (V/Q) lung scan.[2] This is a two-step procedure in which the pulmonary distribution of inhaled radioactive material (ventilation scan) is compared with the pulmonary distribution of intravenously injected radioactive material (technetium-99m). In a classic case of pulmonary embolism the ventilation scan is normal and the perfusion scan shows multiple perfusion defects. There is a "mismatch" between the ventilation and perfusion scans.[2]

V/Q scans are reported as "normal," "low probability, "intermediate," and "high probability." In one study a pulmonary embolus was found in none of the patients with a "normal" scan, only 5% of those with a " low-probability" scan, 30% of those with "intermediate" results, and 90% of those with a "high-probability" scan.[6] Unfortunately, 50% to 70% of reports are in the intermediate range.[2] A suggested algorithm for this type of report, or for a low-probability report in a case where the clinical probability of pulmonary embolism is high, is to perform duplex scanning of the leg veins; if this is negative and the patient's condition is stable, it is often safe simply to follow with serial duplex scanning or plethysmography of the leg veins because recurrent pulmonary embolism is extremely rare in the absence of proximal deep vein thrombosis.[2,7]

Subcutaneous low–molecular weight heparin has been shown to be as effective as intravenous unfractionated heparin in the treatment of pulmonary embolism.[8,9]

REFERENCES

1. Goldhaber SZ, Grodstein F, Stampfer MJ, et al: A prospective study of risk factors for pulmonary embolism in women, *JAMA* 277:642-645, 1997.
2. Bergus GU, Barloon TS, Kahn D: An approach to diagnostic imaging of suspected pulmonary embolism, *Am Fam Physician* 53;1259-1266, 1996.
3. Cvitanic O, Marino PL: Improved use of arterial blood gas analysis in suspected pulmonary embolism, *Chest* 95:48-51, 1989.
4. Stein PD, Goldhaber SZ, Henry JW: Alveolar-arterial oxygen gradient in the assessment of acute pulmonary embolism, *Chest* 107:139-143, 1995.
5. Stein PD, Goldhaber SZ, Henry JW, et al: Arterial blood gas analysis in the assessment of suspected acute pulmonary embolism, *Chest* 109:78-81, 1996.
6. Gottschalk A, Sostman HD, Coleman RE, et al: Ventilation-perfusion scintigraphy in the PIOPED study. II. Evaluation of the scintigraphic criteria and interpretations, *J Nucl Med* 34: 1119-1126, 1993.
7. Hull RD, Raskob GE, Ginsberg JS, et al: A noninvasive strategy for the treatment of patients with suspected pulmonary embolism, *Arch Intern Med* 154:289-297, 1994.
8. Büller HR, Gent M, Gallus AS, et al (Columbus Investigators): Low-molecular-weight heparin in the treatment of patients with venous thromboembolism, *N Engl J Med* 337:657-662, 1997.
9. Simmoneau G, Sors H, Charbonnier B, et al: A comparison of low-molecular-weight heparin with unfractionated heparin for acute pulmonary embolism, *N Engl J Med* 337:663-669, 1997.

Venous ulcers

(See also ulcer, dermal)

Chronic venous ulcers result from dysfunction of the venous valves, which allows reflux of blood, increasing the pressure in the venous system. In some but not all cases this is secondary to thrombophlebitis. If the valves of the perforating veins are also incompetent, the pressure is transmitted to the dermal capillaries with dilation of the capillaries and leakage of plasma and both red and white cells. Activation of the extruded white cells leads to the release of various toxic products that cause tissue destruction and ulceration.[1]

Venous ulcers are almost always located in an edematous limb in the region of the malleoli; the surrounding skin shows the typical pigmentation and induration of chronic venous insufficiency. Conservative treatment consists primarily of compression, which may be accomplished with graded elastic compression stockings (with a 30 to 40 Torr gradient), inelastic compression bands attached with Velcro (CircAid), or Unna gel paste gauze boots. Surgical interventions that can be used in selected cases consist of stripping superficial veins and at times interrupting perforating veins; the latter can be performed through an endoscope to decrease the degree of skin scarring.[1]

REFERENCES

1. Angle N, Bergan JJ: Chronic venous ulcer, *BMJ* 314:1019-1022, 1997.

CENTRAL NERVOUS SYSTEM

Topics covered in this section

AMAUROSIS FUGAX

(See also cerebrovascular accidents)

About half of all cases of amaurosis fugax are due to atherosclerosis, and in patients over 40 years of age it is the likely etiology. Spasm is a much more common cause in young individuals with no other evident disease or with a history of migraines; in these cases the course is usually benign. Lupus is a rare cause.[1,2] Effective symptomatic treatment of patients with amaurosis fugax caused by spasm is nifedipine 60 mg/day (20 mg of the regular formulations tid or Adalat XL 60 mg once daily).

REFERENCES

1. Winterkorn JMS, Kupersmith M, Wirtschafter JD, et al: Brief report: treatment of vasospastic amaurosis fugax with calcium-channel blockers, *N Engl J Med* 329:396-398, 1993.
2. Gautier J-C: Amaurosis fugax (editorial), *N Engl J Med* 329:426-427, 1993.

AMYOTROPHIC LATERAL SCLEROSIS

Motor neuron disease usually affects the middle aged. Before the age of 60 there is a male predominance, but in older individuals the sex ratio evens out. Most patients first notice muscle weakness, but muscle wasting or difficulty in speaking or walking may be the initial symptoms.[1] The median time from diagnosis to death is 2 to 2½ years.[1,2] The survival curve is better for progressive muscular atrophy and worse for progressive bulbar palsy.[2] No cure has been found, but some studies of the drug riluzole (Rilutek) have shown that it slows the progression.[3,4]

REFERENCES

1. Li T-M, Alberman E, Swash M: Clinical features and associations of 560 cases of motor neuron disease, *J Neurol Neurosurg Psychiatry* 53:1043-1045, 1990.
2. Schiffer D, Brignolio F, Chió A, et al: A study of prognostic factors in motor neuron disease, *Adv Exp Med Biol* 209:255-263, 1987.
3. Bensimon G, Lacomblez L, Meininger V: A controlled trial of riluzole in amyotrophic lateral sclerosis, *N Engl J Med* 330:585-589, 1994.
4. Lacomblez L, Bensimon G, Leigh PN, et al (Amyotrophic Lateral Sclerosis/Riluzole Study Group II): Dose-ranging study of riluzole in amyotrophic lateral sclerosis, *Lancet* 347:1425-1431, 1996.

CEREBRAL PALSY

In term infants cerebral palsy is unlikely to result from birth injury or hypoxia at the time of birth.[1]

REFERENCES

1. Kuban KCK, Leviton A: Cerebral palsy, *N Engl J Med* 330:188-195, 1994.

CEREBROVASCULAR ACCIDENTS

(See also amaurosis fugax; atrial fibrillation; subarachnoid hemorrhage; transient ischemic attacks)

Risk Factors for Stroke

Generally accepted risk factors for stroke include old age; family history of stroke; hypertension; smoking; lack of exercise, diabetes mellitus, associated heart disease, especially atrial fibrillation, transient ischemic attacks (TIAs), excessive alcohol use, and the antiphospholipid syndrome. Possible risk factors include migraines, oral contraceptives, and hormone replacement therapy.

The association between migraine and stroke is equivocal. One 1993 case-controlled study found no association except in a subgroup analysis in which women who suffered from migraines and were under the age of 45 had an odds ratio of 4.0 of having a stroke.[1]

Studies in the 1960s and 1970s showed an increased incidence of ischemic strokes and subarachnoid hemorrhages in women who used oral contraceptives. This was particularly marked if they were smokers and over the age of 35.[2] At present almost all oral contraceptives contain much lower estrogen concentrations than were used in the sixties and seventies, and the current evidence is that the risk of stroke is only slightly higher in nonsmoking, nonhypertensive women (even those over the age of 35) who are using or have used low-dose birth control pills.[3-5]

Hormone replacement therapy appears to be associated with a decreased, not an increased, incidence of stroke.[6,7]

McCormack and associates[8] have published an easily comprehensible nomogram integrating multiple risk factors so that the chances that any particular individual will have a CVA within 10 years can be calculated.

REFERENCES

1. Tzourio C, Iglesias S, Hulbert JB, et al: Migraine and risk of ischemic stroke: a case control study, *BMJ* 307:289-292, 1993.
2. Longstreth WT: Oral contraceptives and stroke, *Stroke* 15:747-750, 1984.
3. Petitti DB, Sidney S, Bernstein A, et al: Stroke in users of low-dose oral contraceptives, *N Engl J Med* 335:8-15, 1996.
4. Poulter NR, Chang CL, Farley TM, et al: Ischaemic stroke and combined oral contraceptives—results of an international, multicentre, case-control study, *Lancet* 348:498-505, 1996.
5. Poulter NR, Chang CL, Farley TM, et al: Haemorrhagic stroke, overall stroke risk, and combined oral contraceptives—results of an international, multicentre, case-control study, *Lancet* 348:505-510, 1996.
6. Finucane FF, Madans JH, Bush TL, et al: Decreased risk of stroke among postmenopausal hormone users, *Arch Intern Med* 153:73-79, 1993.
7. Faldeborn M, Persson I, Terent A, et al: Hormone replacement therapy and the risk of stroke: follow-up of a population-based cohort in Sweden, *Arch Intern Med* 153:1201-1209, 1993.
8. McCormack JP, Levine M, Rangno RE: Primary prevention of heart disease and stroke: a simplified approach to estimating risk of events and making drug treatment decisions, *Can Med Assoc J* 157:422-428, 1997.

Prevention and Management of Strokes

(See also atrial fibrillation; transient ischemic attacks; exercise; noninvasive blood flow tests; screening; lipids; smoking)

A decreased incidence of strokes has been reported from the adequate treatment of hypertension,[1,2] exercise,[3,4] discontinuation of smoking,[5] control of atrial fibrillation,[6] treatment of TIAs,[7] and diets high in fruits and vegetables.[8] Aspirin given to asymptomatic individuals is not an effective agent for stroke prevention.[9,10] A large metaanalysis of individuals on a variety of lipid-lowering regimens showed no decrease in stroke rate.[11] However, a metaanalysis of 12 trials using only 3-hydroxy-3-methylglutaryl coenzyme A (HMG CoA) reductase inhibitors for the reduction of cardiovascular events found a statistically significant reduction of stroke rates, which was more marked in secondary than primary prevention trials.[12]

Stroke prevention through screening for carotid bruits and treatment of asymptomatic individuals with carotid artery stenosis has been studied. In the Asymptomatic Carotid Atherosclerosis Study (ACAS), asymptomatic patients found to have carotid artery stenosis of 75% or greater at the lesion site were randomly assigned to medical therapy or carotid endarterectomy. After 5 years in the endarterectomy cohort the relative risk reduction of strokes was 53% and the absolute risk reduction was 6%.[13] However, since only half of the strokes were disabling, the absolute reduction for disabling strokes was 2.6%. The number of endarterectomies required to prevent one stroke per year was 85, while the number required to prevent one disabling stroke per year was close to 170. Women did not appear to benefit as much as men from the procedure.[14]

Far more patients with asymptomatic carotid artery stenosis have cardiac events than have cerebrovascular events. In a Toronto study 696 patients with asymptomatic carotid stenosis detected by auscultation for carotid bruit and confirmed by Doppler ultrasound were followed for a mean of 3.5 years. During this time 29 patients had a stroke and 132 a cardiac event (in most cases a myocardial infarction [MI]). There were 5 deaths from stroke and 59 from cardiac events. In other words, cardiac events outnumbered stroke by 4.5 to 1 while cardiac deaths outnumbered stroke deaths by 12 to 1.[15]

Carotid bruits are present in more than 5% of the population older than the age of 65. In one study the relative risk of stroke among individuals with asymptomatic carotid bruits was three times that of persons without carotid bruits. However, the absolute increased risk in this study was only 1.5% per year.[16] Overall, when strokes do supervene in patients with carotid bruits, only one third are in the vascular distribution of the vessel with the bruit, although the rate of ipsilateral strokes is higher in those with tight stenosis.[17] The sensitivity of carotid bruits for detecting carotid artery stenosis greater than 70% is low. In the ACAS 25% of the patients had no bruit on the affected side,[13] and in another study the false-negative rate for severe disease was 43%.[18] The positive predictive value for significant stenosis is also low. One group of workers reported it as 37%,[18] whereas another found that only 18% of patients with a bruit had a stenosis of 75% or more.[19]

The effectiveness of aspirin prophylaxis for asymptomatic carotid stenosis found as a result of screening for carotid bruits was studied in a double-blind placebo-controlled trial. The patients had asymptomatic carotid bruits, no neurological symptoms or signs, and stenosis of at least 50% in one or both carotid arteries as determined by duplex ultrasonography. Half the patients were assigned to aspirin 325 mg/day and half to a placebo. At the end of 2 years the two groups showed no differences in total mortality or ischemic events, which included TIAs, strokes, MIs, and unstable angina.[20]

Until recently no study had shown aspirin to be beneficial in patients who had had a completed ischemic stroke. Two recent, very large, multicenter studies have shown that daily aspirin in doses of 160 mg,[21] or 300 mg[22] given as soon as possible after the stroke, resulted in slightly fewer deaths or recurrent strokes in the first few weeks and fewer deaths or dependent patients after several months. No benefit was observed from subcutaneously administered heparin.[22]

The Canadian Task Force on the Periodic Health Examination gives a "D" recommendation both to screening for carotid artery bruits and to endarterectomy in asymptomatic patients. It gives a "C" recommendation to medical therapy for patients with asymptomatic carotid stenosis.[23] The U.S. Preventive Services Task Force gives a "C" recommendation to screening for carotid artery bruit but does not specifically give a recommendation for carotid endarterectomy in asymptomatic individuals.[24] The 35 members of the Canadian Stroke Consortium published a report in early 1997 stating that evidence was insufficient to recommend either screening for carotid disease or carotid endarterectomy for asymptomatic patients.[25]

REFERENCES

1. Meissner I, Whisnant JP, Garraway WM: Hypertension management and stroke recurrence in a community, *Stroke* 19:459-463, 1988.
2. SHEP Cooperative Research Group: Prevention of stroke by antihypertensive drug treatment in older persons with isolated systolic hypertension: final results of the Systolic Hypertension in the Elderly Program (SHEP), *JAMA* 265:3255-3264, 1991.
3. Wannamethee G, Shaper AG: Physical activity and stroke in British middle-aged men, *BMJ* 304:597-601, 1992.
4. Shinton R, Sagar G: Lifelong exercise and stroke, *BMJ* 307: 231-234, 1993.
5. Whisnant JP, Homer D, Ingall TJ, et al: Duration of smoking is the strongest predictor of severe extracranial carotid artery atherosclerosis, *Stroke* 21:707-714, 1990.
6. Atrial Fibrillation Investigators: Risk factors for stroke and efficacy of antithrombotic therapy in atrial fibrillation: analysis of pooled data from five randomized controlled trials, *Arch Intern Med* 154:1449-1457, 1994.
7. Antiplatelet Trialists' Collaboration: Collaborative overview of randomised trials of antiplatelet therapy. I. Prevention of death, myocardial infarction, and stroke by prolonged antiplatelet therapy in various categories of patients, *BMJ* 308:81-106, 1994.
8. Gillman MW, Cupples A, Gagnon D, et al: Protective effect of fruits and vegetables on development of stroke in men, *JAMA* 273:113-117, 1995.
9. Steering Committee of the Physicians' Health Study Research Group: Final report on the aspirin component of the ongoing Physicians' Health Study, *N Engl J Med* 321:129-135, 1989.
10. Manson JE, Stampfer MJ, Colditz GA, et al:. A prospective study of aspirin use and primary prevention of cardiovascular disease in women, *JAMA* 266:521-527, 1991.
11. Hebert PR, Gaziano M, Hennekens CH: An overview of trials of cholesterol lowering and risk of stroke, *Arch Intern Med* 155:50-55, 1995.
12. Crouse JR III, Byington RP, Hoen HM, et al: Reductase inhibitor monotherapy and stroke prevention, *Arch Intern Med* 157:1305-1310, 1997.
13. Executive Committee for the Asymptomatic Carotid Atherosclerosis Study: Endarterectomy for asymptomatic carotid artery stenosis, *JAMA* 273:1421-1428, 1995.
14. Warlow C: Endarterectomy for asymptomatic carotid stenosis? (editorial), *Lancet* 345:1254-1255, 1995.
15. Norris JW, Zhu CZ, Bornstein NM, et al: Vascular risks of asymptomatic carotid stenosis, *Stroke* 22:1485-1490, 1991.
16. Wiebers DO, Whisnant JP, Sandok BA, et al: Prospective comparison of a cohort with asymptomatic carotid bruit and a population-based cohort without carotid bruit, *Stroke* 21:984-988, 1990.
17. Shuaib A: Update on stroke prevention strategies, *Can J CME*, May 1994, pp 61-68.
18. Davies KN, Humphrey PR: Do carotid bruits predict disease of the internal carotid arteries? *Postgrad Med J* 70:433-435, 1994.
19. Endean ED, Steffen G, Chmura C, et al: Outcome of asymptomatic cervical bruits in a veteran population, *J Cardiovasc Surg* 32:620-626, 1991.
20. Cote R, Battista RN, Abrahamowicz M, et al: Lack of effect of aspirin in asymptomatic patients with carotid bruits and substantial carotid narrowing, *Ann Intern Med* 123:649-655, 1995.
21. CAST (Chinese Acute Stroke Trial) Collaborative Group: CAST: randomised placebo-controlled trial of early aspirin use in 20,000 patients with acute ischaemic stroke, *Lancet* 349: 1641-1649, 1997.
22. International Stroke Trial Collaborative Group: The International Stroke Trial (IST): a randomised trial of aspirin, subcutaneous heparin, both, or neither among 19,435 patients with acute ischaemic stroke, *Lancet* 349:1569-1581, 1997.
23. Canadian Task Force on the Periodic Health Examination: *Canadian guide to clinical preventive health care,* Ottawa, 1994, Canada Communication Group—Publishing, pp 691-704.
24. US Preventive Services Task Force: *Guide to clinical preventive services,* ed 2, Baltimore, 1996, Williams & Wilkins, pp 53-61.
25. Perry JR, Szalai JP, Norris JW (Canadian Stroke Consortium): Consensus against both endarterectomy and routine screening for asymptomatic carotid artery stenosis, *Arch Neurol* 54:25-28, 1997.

Transient ischemic attacks

(See also anticoagulants; atrial fibrillation; aspirin; patient preferences and informed consent; prevention and management of strokes; relative risk reduction)

Three drugs have been used for preventing strokes in patients who have had TIAs. They are acetylsalicylic acid (ASA), ticlopidine (Ticlid), and anticoagulants (warfarin and heparin). Endarterectomy is a surgical alternative to medical therapy.

Aspirin. In 1978 the Canadian Cooperative Study Group reported that 650 mg of ASA given bid to patients who had had TIAs or nondisabling strokes decreased the incidence of stroke in men but not in women.[1] The United Kingdom Transient Ischemic Attack Trial published in 1991 showed that 1300 mg of ASA daily was as effective as 600 mg bid and that women also benefited.[2] The Dutch Transient Ischemic Attack Trial Study Group found that 30 mg of ASA daily was as effective as 283 mg/day in decreasing mortality from all vascular causes, as well as the incidence of nonfatal strokes and nonfatal MIs,[3] and the Swedish Aspirin Low Dose Trial demonstrated the effectiveness of 75 mg of aspirin daily.[4] A collaborative overview of 145 randomized trials of antiplatelet therapy showed a 22% relative reduction of strokes in patients with prior strokes or TIAs.[5] This beneficial effect was noted with aspirin doses that averaged 75 to 325 mg/day and was present in men, women, and the elderly.

At present the optimal dose of ASA in patients with TIAs is controversial. Traditionally Europeans favor 30 to 75 mg/day, many Americans prefer 650 mg bid, and Canadians, as is their wont, vacillated between the two. A report of the American College of Physicians states that all aspirin doses are equally effective,[6] while a comprehensive and thoughtful review in the *New England Journal of Medicine* concludes that 650 mg of aspirin daily is optimal for patients with strokes of arterial origin.[7]

Ticlopidine. The Ticlopidine Aspirin Stroke Study involving 56 North American centers compared stroke prevention in patients with previous cerebrovascular events given ticlopidine (Ticlid) 250 mg bid or ASA 650 mg bid. After 3 years a 21% relative reduction of nonfatal strokes and death was seen in the ticlopidine group (see relative risk reduction). These combined events occurred in 10% of the ticlopidine group and 13% of the aspirin group, so the absolute reduction was only 3%.[8] Subsequent studies have confirmed that ticlopidine, usually taken as 250 mg bid, results in a 3% to 4% better absolute stroke risk reduction than does aspirin.[9]

Severe diarrhea develops in about 20% of patients taking ticlopidine. Neutropenia occurs in 1% and in a few cases has been irreversible and fatal. Patients taking ticlopidine should have white blood cell counts every 2 weeks for the first 3 months of therapy. Total cholesterol, HDL-C, LDL-C, and triglyceride levels are raised by 8% to 10% in patients taking ticlopidine. At present the major indication for ticlopidine seems to be ASA failure or ASA intolerance.

Anticoagulants. Warfarin has been shown to be effective in preventing strokes in patients with TIAs, but no more so than ASA.[10,11] Warfarin is the drug of choice for patients with atrial fibrillation caused by rheumatic heart disease (see discussion of atrial fibrillation) or for patients with prosthetic heart valves (see discussion of valvular heart disease). Anticoagulants are likely to be given to patients with progressive strokes, those who are threatening to become "locked in," or those with TIAs who do not respond to ASA. Although anticoagulation seems a reasonable course of action, little evidence is available to support its efficacy.[12]

Endarterectomy. The risk of stroke in patients who have had a TIA is 12% to 13% in the first year and 30% to 35% after 5 years. The risk of a subsequent stroke in a patient who has already had a stroke is between 25% and 45% after 5 years.[13] Three important prospective studies published in 1991 have reported an absolute decrease in ipsilateral strokes of about 15% to 17% over 2 years in selected patients undergoing carotid endarterectomy compared with a medically treated control group.[14-16] These patients had a carotid stenosis of greater than 70%; had had previous TIAs, amaurosis fugax, or a nondisabling stroke in the appropriate carotid territory; and were less that 80 years old. It has long been known that the operation is not beneficial if stenosis is less than 30%, and a 1996 report documented that it also had no value for patients with 30% to 70% stenosis.[17]

What is an acceptable morbidity and mortality rate for carotid endarterectomy in patients with TIAs? One set of widely accepted criteria is that any center undertaking carotid endarterectomies should have a mortality rate less than 2%, as well as a morbidity rate (including stroke) less than 5% if the patient had had previous TIAs or less than 7% if the patient had had a previous ischemic stroke.[18] Results of the consensus conference of the American Heart Association published in 1995 put the upper limit for combined death and stroke from the operative procedure at 6% for patients who have had TIAs or mild strokes and at 3% for asymptomatic individuals.[13] According to one recent review a perioperative incidence for stroke and death of 10% or more negates any benefit from surgery.[7]

Before patients subject themselves to carotid endarterectomies, it is important that they know the morbidity and mortality records of the surgeons and centers performing the procedures. Then, with the help of their family physicians, they can weigh the small but not insignificant risks of immediate mortality and morbidity from surgery against the risks of future mortality and morbidity with medical therapy alone. Some patients may be unwilling to accept the surgical risks involved even if the evidence favoring surgery is well established (see discussions of patient preferences and informed consent).

REFERENCES

1. Canadian Cooperative Study Group: A randomized trial of aspirin and sulfinpyrazone in threatened stroke, *N Engl J Med* 299:53-59, 1978.

2. Farrell B, Godwin J, Richards S, Warlow C: The United Kingdom transient ischaemic attack (UK-TIA) aspirin trial: final results, *J Neurol Neurosurg Psychiatry* 54:1044-1054, 1991.
3. Dutch TIA Trial Study Group: A comparison of two doses of aspirin (30 mg vs. 283 mg a day) in patients after a transient ischemic attack or minor ischemic stroke, *N Engl J Med* 325: 1261-1266, 1991.
4. SALT Collaborative Group: Swedish Aspirin Low-dose Trial (SALT) of 75 mg aspirin as secondary prophylaxis after cerebrovascular ischaemic events, *Lancet* 338:1345-1349, 1991.
5. Antiplatelet Trialists' Collaboration: Collaborative overview of randomised trials of antiplatelet therapy. I. Prevention of death, myocardial infarction, and stroke by prolonged antiplatelet therapy in various categories of patients, *BMJ* 308:81-106, 1994.
6. Matchar DB, McCrory DC, Barnett HJM, et al: Medical treatment for stroke prevention, *Ann Intern Med* 121:41-53, 1994.
7. Barnett HJ, Eliasziw M, Meldrum HE: Drugs and surgery in the prevention of ischemic stroke, *N Engl J Med* 332:238-248, 1995.
8. Hass WK, Easton JD, Adams HP Jr, et al (Ticlopidine Aspirin Stroke Study Group): A randomized trial comparing ticlopidine hydrochloride with aspirin for the prevention of stroke in high-risk patients, *N Engl J Med* 321:501-507, 1989.
9. Harbison JW: Ticlopidine versus aspirin for the prevention of recurrent stroke: analysis of patients with minor stroke from the Ticlopidine Aspirin Stroke Study Group, *Stroke* 23:1723-1727, 1992.
10. Olsson JE, Brechter C, Backlund H, et al: Anticoagulant vs antiplatelet therapy as prophylactic against cerebral infarction in transient ischemic attacks, *Stroke* 11:4-9, 1980.
11. Buren A, Ygge J: Treatment program and comparison between anticoagulants and platelet aggregation inhibitors after transient ischemic attack, *Stroke* 12:578-580, 1981.
12. Brown J, Bernstein M: Antithrombotic therapy for patients with stroke symptoms, *Can Fam Physician* 42:1724-1730, 1996.
13. Moore WS, Barnett HJ, Beebe HG, et al: Guidelines for carotid endarterectomy: a multidisciplinary consensus statement from the Ad Hoc Committee, American Heart Association, *Circulation* 91:566-579, 1995.
14. North American Symptomatic Carotid Endarterectomy Trial Collaborators: Beneficial effects of carotid endarterectomy in symptomatic patients with high-grade stenosis (NIH), *N Engl J Med* 325:445-453, 1991.
15. European Carotid Surgery Trialists' Collaborative Group: MRC European Carotid Surgery Trial: interim results for symptomatic patients with severe (70-99%) or with mild (0-29%) carotid stenosis, *Lancet* 337:1235-1243, 1991.
16. Mayberg MR, Wilson SE, Yatsu F, et al: Carotid endarterectomy and prevention of cerebral ischemia in symptomatic carotid stenosis: Veterans Affairs Cooperative Studies Program 309 Trialist Group, *JAMA* 266:3289-3294, 1991.
17. European Carotid Surgery Trialists' Collaborative Group: Endarterectomy for moderate symptomatic carotid stenosis: interim results from the MRC European Carotid Surgery Trial, *Lancet* 347:1591-1593, 1996.
18. Beebe HG, Clagett GP, DeWeese JA, et al: Assessing risk associated with carotid endarterectomy: a statement for health professionals by an Ad Hoc Committee on Carotid Surgery Standards of the Stroke Council, American Heart Association, *Circulation* 79:472-473, 1989.

CONCUSSION

(See also seizures)

Symptoms of postconcussional disorder may be physical, cognitive, or emotional. Short-term physical symptoms are nausea, vomiting, drowsiness, and blurred vision, while more persistent symptoms are headaches, dizziness, tinnitus, and sometimes anosmia. The major cognitive deficits involve memory, concentration, and attention, while the emotional sequelae include irritability, depression, and fatigue. In most patients symptoms resolve over 3 to 6 months. It is important to realize that cognitive deficits may be subtle and detected only by specific psychometric tests and that postconcussional disorder may follow head injury without loss of consciousness.[1,2] Students who have had a concussion may respond more slowly in activities requiring information-processing skills than control subjects without head injury.[3]

A study of 1382 patients from California who suffered head trauma with either loss of consciousness or amnesia for the event but who had a Glasgow Coma Scale score of 15 (no abnormalities) found that computed tomographic (CT) scans showed no significant clinical abnormalities in patients who did not have nausea or vomiting and who had no signs of depressed skull fracture such as lacerations, contusions, and swelling. Even among those with such symptoms and signs, abnormal CT scans leading to surgical intervention were rare. Only three patients (0.2%) in the entire study population required surgery.[4]

A little known but important condition is the second impact syndrome. This involves a mild head injury to someone who has already suffered a mild concussion within the previous few hours or days. Such an injury may result in severe brain swelling and death. This is one reason that athletes with head injuries resulting in any loss of consciousness or any mental status abnormality lasting longer than 15 minutes should be removed from the sport for at least a week.[5]

REFERENCES

1. Anderson SK: Postconcussional disorder: common result of head injury, *Can J Diagn* 12:77-86, 1995.
2. Katz RT, Deluca J: Sequelae of minor traumatic brain injury, *Am Fam Physician* 46:1491-1498, 1992.
3. McSherry JA: Cognitive impairment after head injury, *Am Fam Physician* 40:186-190, 1989.
4. Miller EC, Derlet RW, Kinser D: Minor head trauma: is computed tomography always necessary? *Ann Emerg Med* 27:290-294, 1996.
5. Centers for Disease Control and Prevention: Sports-related recurrent brain injuries—United States, *JAMA* 277:1190-1191, 1997.

CREUTZFELDT-JAKOB DISEASE AND BOVINE SPONGIFORM ENCEPHALOPATHY

(See also dementia)

Creutzfeldt-Jakob Disease (CJD) is one of the infectious diseases of the brain causing a spongiform encephalopathy.[1,2]

The usual clinical presentation is one of rapidly progressive dementia associated with myoclonus. The EEG often shows periodic sharp wave activity. The infectious agent has been labeled a "slow virus" or a "prion." About 10% of human cases of CJD have a familial autosomal-dominant inheritance pattern, but even in this subgroup, tissue from the patient can transmit the disease to nonhuman primates. In the past a number of children acquired the disease after repeated injections of human growth hormone obtained from human pituitary glands. There have been no confirmed cases of person-to-person transmission or transmission through transfusions.[2] Other human examples of this type of encephalopathy are kuru, described among cannibals in central New Guinea, and the familial Gerstmann-Sträussler-Scheinker syndrome. In animals similar disorders are scrapie in sheep and bovine spongiform encephalopathy ("mad cow disease") in cattle.

A major concern that surfaced in 1996 was the possibility that bovine spongiform encephalopathy (BSE) could be transmitted to humans through eating contaminated beef. This alarm was triggered by the reporting of 10 cases of CJD among young people in the United Kingdom. Not only was the disease unusual because of the age of the patients, but the initial manifestations were behavioral (psychiatric) rather than cognitive and the neuropathological findings were different. A World Health Organization consensus conference on the subject held in April 1996 concluded that no definite link had been established between BSE and this new form of CJD but that exposure to BSE was the most likely explanation.[3] This group also concluded that there was no danger of transmitting the disorder through milk or milk products.[3] Analysis of the strains of prion found in the brains of patients presenting with this new form of atypical CJD found them to be similar to the strains found in cattle with BSE and different from the strains found in the usual forms of CJD.[4]

REFERENCES

1. Corey L, Fleming TR: Prion disease (editorial), *N Engl J Med* 326:486-487, 1992.
2. MacKnight C, Rockwood K: Bovine spongiform encephalopathy and Creutzfeldt-Jakob disease: implications for physicians, *Can Med Assoc J* 155:529-536, 1996.
3. Centers for Disease Control and Prevention: World Health Organization consultation on public health issues related to bovine spongiform encephalopathy and the emergence of a new variant of Creutzfeldt-Jakob disease, *JAMA* 275:1305-1306, 1996.
4. Collinge J, Sidle KC, Meads J, et al: Molecular analysis of prion strain variation and the aetiology of new variant CJD, *Nature* 383:685-690, 1996.

DEMENTIA

(See also anesthesia; coronary artery bypass grafting and angioplasty; Creutzfeldt-Jakob disease; hormone replacement therapy)

A retrospective study of 100 autopsy-confirmed cases of Alzheimer's disease found the typical natural history to be as follows. Diagnosis was made about 3 years after the onset of symptoms, institutionalization took place around 2 years after diagnosis, and the patient died approximately 4 years after that. The mean total duration of disease in this series was 8.5 years. Subgroup analysis found that the course of disease was longer in patients whose Alzheimer's disease was diagnosed before the age of 65, those with a family history of the disease, and females.[1]

In a Canadian study the estimated prevalence of dementia in people over the age of 65 was 8%. The age-standardized rate varied from 2.4% in those aged 65 to 74 to 34.5% for those over the age of 85. Alzheimer's disease accounted for the majority of cases.[2] The male/female ratio of Alzheimer's disease is 3:1.[2] In a community study in Boston the estimated annual incidence of new-onset Alzheimer's disease was 0.6% for those 65 to 69, 3.3% for those 80 to 84, and 8.4% for those over 85.[3]

Persons with low educational achievement are at greater risk for Alzheimer's disease.[4,5] A study of nuns found an excellent correlation between "low idea density" and "low grammatical complexity" in autobiographies written when the women were in their early twenties and the development of Alzheimer's disease in old age.[6]

An important differential diagnosis of Alzheimer's disease is age-associated memory impairment. In this condition the main problems are remembering names and recall on demand. Patients often do not recall a word when they need it, but it comes to them later. If a patient with age-associated memory impairment is asked to describe the last thing he forgot, he can do so in some detail, whereas a person with Alzheimer's disease is unlikely to remember and often turns to a spouse for help ("head-turning sign"). In addition, patients with Alzheimer's disease often have difficulties in other areas such as banking, driving, and orientation.[7] Behavioral or noncognitive symptoms are also common in patients with Alzheimer's disease, and these often lead to extreme frustration on the part of caregivers. They include decreased initiative and increasing stubbornness and suspiciousness. Delusions, which are usually paranoid, develop in about half of patients, and one fourth of patients have hallucinations, which are often visual. Depression and anxiety are also common.[8]

A traditional screening test for dementia is the Folstein Mini-Mental State Examination (MMSE).[9] A newer self-administered test applicable to U.S. residents (because of several questions about U.S. presidents, senators, governors, and so on) is the Cognitive Assessment Screening Test (CAST). It appears to be as sensitive as the MMSE.[10]

Reversible causes of dementia are rare. Therefore multiple investigations are unnecessary, although one worker in the field suggests that the basic workup should be thyroid function tests and measurement of vitamin B_{12} and calcium levels.[8] A low serum vitamin B_{12} concentration is common in elderly persons without dementia.[11] Brain imaging to detect treatable causes of dementia is rarely positive in patients who do not have focal abnormalities on neurological examination.[12] If the decision is made to use computed tomography (CT), a scan without contrast medium is adequate unless neurological examination shows evidence of motor abnormalities, in which case magnetic resonance imaging (MRI) is the procedure of choice.[8]

Provocative studies suggest that estrogen is beneficial for cognitive functioning (see discussion of hormone replacement therapy). A number of studies have also suggested that nonsteroidal antiinflammatory drugs (NSAIDs) decrease both the incidence of Alzheimer's disease[13-15] and its rate of progression once it is established.[16,17]

Two centrally acting cholinesterase inhibitors, tacrine (THA, Cognex) and donepezil (Aricept), are available for the treatment of Alzheimer's disease. Tacrine has been the more extensively investigated; while a number of studies using this drug have shown a statistically significant improvement, such improvement is quantitatively small, is probably of no clinical significance, and is gained at the cost of significant numbers of adverse effects.[18] Only 25% of patients show improvement with tacrine, and on discontinuation of the medication, cognitive functioning reverts to the level that would be expected if no medication had been given.[19] Approximately 30% of patients receiving tacrine have a threefold or greater elevation of liver enzyme levels, usually in weeks 6 to 8 of treatment and affecting women more commonly than men. In some cases the patient can be returned to a previous lower dose with subsequent gradual increases if the alanine aminotransferase (ALT) level decreases.[20] Tacrine is usually given as 10 to 40 mg qid. Trials of other drugs in this class have also shown slight benefits.[21] For example, in a 14-week trial of donepezil given as a single daily dose of 5 mg, 20% of the patients in the placebo group showed a continuing clinical decline, whereas this occurred in only 11% of the treated cohort. Unlike the results of the tacrine trials, the incidence of adverse effects was no higher in the treated than in the control group.[21] Neither tacrine nor donepezil prevents progression of the disease.[22]

Several double-blind randomized studies have compared selegiline or L-deprenyl (Eldepryl) to placebo in the treatment of Alzheimer's disease. These medications have delayed progression of the disease over study periods ranging from 1 month to 2 years.[20,23] A multicenter placebo-controlled trial of vitamin E 1000 mg bid over a 2-year period found that the treated group had a significant delay in the progression of Alzheimer's disease.[23]

Agitation in patients with dementia may be due to a variety of causes, including medical conditions, constipation, pain, hunger, sleep deprivation, and change in the environment. Drugs are indicated if precipitating factors cannot be identified or rectified. The most frequently used agents are low-dose antipsychotics, usually given in the evenings to help sleep through their sedative effects and to counter evening agitation or "sundowning."[24] Typical doses are shown in Table 18.

Benzodiazepines may also be used. In comparative studies they are better than placebos but less effective than antipsychotics. For patients who do not respond to antipsychotics or benzodiazepines, carbamazepine (Tegretol) or valproic acid (Depakene) may be tried.[24]

Table 18 Low-Dose Antipsychotics

Drug	Starting dose (mg/day)	Maximum dose (mg/day)
Haloperidol (Haldol)	0.5	2-5
Thioridazine (Mellaril)	10-25	50-100
Risperidone (Risperdal)	0.5-1	4-6
Clozapine (Clozaril)	12.5	75-100

REFERENCES

1. Jost BC, Grossberg GT: The natural history of Alzheimer's disease: a brain bank study, *J Am Geriatr Soc* 43:1248-1255, 1995.
2. Canadian Study of Health and Aging Working Group: Canadian Study of Health and Aging: study methods and prevalence of dementia, *Can Med Assoc J* 150:899-912, 1994.
3. Hebert LE, Scherr PA, Beckett LA, et al: Age-specific incidence of Alzheimer's disease in a community population, *JAMA* 273:1354-1359, 1995.
4. D'Arcy C. Education and socio-economic status as risk factors for dementia: data from the Canadian Study of Health and Aging, *Neurobiol Aging* 15:S40, 1994.
5. Stern Y, Gurland B, Tatemichi TK, et al: Influence of education and occupation on the incidence of Alzheimer's disease, *JAMA* 271:1004-1010, 1994.
6. Snowdon DA, Kemper SJ, Mortimer JA, et al: Linguistic ability in early life and cognitive function and Alzheimer's disease in late life, *JAMA* 275:528-532, 1996.
7. Rockwood K: Forgetfulness: is dementia the cause? *Can J CME* 7:51-57, 1995.
8. Geldmacher DS, Whitehouse PJ: Evaluation of dementia, *N Engl J Med* 335:330-336, 1996.
9. Folstein MF, Folstein SE, McHugh PR: Mini-mental state: a practical method for grading the cognitive state of patients for the clinician, *J Psychiatr Res* 12:189-198, 1975.
10. Drachman DA, Swearer JM: Screening for dementia: Cognitive Assessment Screening Test (CAST), *Am Fam Physician* 54:1957-1962, 1996.
11. Crystal HA, Ortof E, Frishman WH, et al: Serum vitamin B_{12} levels and incidence of dementia in a healthy elderly population—a report from the Bronx Longitudinal Aging Study, *J Am Geriatr Soc* 42:933-936, 1994.
12. Alexander EM, Wagner EH, Buchner DM, et al: Do surgical brain lesions present as isolated dementia? A population-based study, *J Am Geriatr Soc* 45:957-962, 1995.
13. Stewart WF, Kawas C, Corrada M, et al: Risk of Alzheimer's disease and duration of NSAID use, *Neurology* 48:626-632, 1997.
14. Canadian Study of Health and Aging: risk factors for Alzheimer's disease in Canada, *Neurology* 44:2073-2080, 1994.
15. Andersen K, Launer LJ, Ott A, et al: Do nonsteroidal anti-inflammatory drugs decrease the risk for Alzheimer's disease? The Rotterdam Study, *Neurology* 45:1441-1445, 1995.
16. Rogers J, Kirby LC, Hempelman SR, et al: Clinical trial of indomethacin in Alzheimer's disease, *Neurology* 43:1609-1611, 1993.

17. Rich JB, Rasmusson DX, Folstein MF, et al: Nonsteroidal anti-inflammatory drugs in Alzheimer's disease, *Neurology* 45:51-55, 1995.
18. Manning FC: Tacrine therapy for the dementia of Alzheimer's disease, *Am Fam Physician* 50:819-823, 1994.
19. Smucker WD: Maximizing function in Alzheimer's disease: what role for tacrine? *Am Fam Physician* 54:645-652, 1996.
20. Rabins P, Blacker D, Bland W, et al: Practice guideline for the treatment of patients with Alzheimer's disease and other dementias of late life, *Am J Psychiatry* 154 (suppl):S1-S39, 1997.
21. Rogers SL, Friedhoff LT: The efficacy and safety of donepezil in patients with Alzheimer's disease: results of a US multicentre, randomized, double-blind, placebo-controlled trial, *Dementia* 7:293-303, 1996.
22. Donepezil (Aricept) for Alzheimer's disease, *Med Lett* 39:53-54, 1997.
23. Sano M, Ernesto C, Thomas RG, et al: A controlled trial of selegiline, alpha-tocopherol, or both as treatment for Alzheimer's disease, *N Engl J Med* 336:1216-1222, 1997
24. Rabins P, Blacker D, Bland W, et al: Practice guideline for the treatment of patients with Alzheimer's disease and other dementias of late life, *Am J Psychiatry* 154 (suppl):S1-S39, 1997.

HEADACHES

Investigations of Patients with Chronic Headaches

Should patients with the clinical diagnosis of migraines or other types of benign chronic headaches have a CT or MRI scan? An evaluation of CT scans of 373 patients referred to a chronic headache clinic in a tertiary care center in London, Ontario, found two osteomas, one low-grade glioma, and one aneurysm. The only lesion treated was the aneurysm. The authors state that this detection rate is the same as might be expected in the general population without headaches.[1] Similar findings were reported from Turkey; no clinically significant lesions were detected by CT scanning of 592 patients with chronic headaches and normal findings on neurological examination.[2] A study of imaging and headaches in children concluded that imaging was indicated only if neurological abnormalities were found, a good history could not be obtained, or the child was very young.[3]

REFERENCES

1. Dumas MD, Pexman JHW, Kreeft JH: Computed tomography evaluation of patients with chronic headache, *Can Med Assoc J* 151:1447-1452, 1994.
2. Akpek S, Arac M, Atilla S, et al: Cost-effectiveness of computed tomography in the evaluation of patients with headache, *Headache* 35:228-230, 1995.
3. Maytal J, Bienkowski RS, Patel M, et al: The value of brain imaging in children with headaches, *Pediatrics* 96:413-416, 1995.

Analgesic Overuse Headaches

Many patients with migraines or other headaches are frequent users of analgesic drugs. This in itself can lead to withdrawal headaches, and a vicious circle of headaches–drugs–more headaches is established.[1-4] Terms used to describe this type of headache are analgesic overuse headache, chronic daily headache, and transformed migraine.

Almost any antimigraine drug, including aspirin, NSAIDs, acetaminophen, codeine, ergotamine, and sumatriptan, may be responsible. Rapoport[3] reported that the syndrome could be induced by more than 14 tablets of ASA or acetaminophen per week. Diamond and Dalessio[5] estimated that more than 20 doses of codeine a week could initiate withdrawal headaches, as could a weekly dose of 10 mg or more of ergotamine.

Although analgesic overuse is not the only cause of chronic daily headaches, it is thought to account for about 75% of cases. The clinical features are variable. Patients have daily or almost daily headaches that have variable locations and may be throbbing or steady. Patients often wake up with a headache. The headaches are often precipitated by physical exertion or intellectual effort, and the patient may have nausea, irritability, and difficulty concentrating.

Treatment consists of withdrawal of the analgesics. This may be done rapidly or slowly, but if a barbiturate (e.g., Fiorinal) is involved, the withdrawal should be slow. Best results are obtained if a migraine prophylactic regimen is started at the same time. Although many patients improve within 1 week, it may take up to 3 months for the maximal effect of analgesic withdrawal to be noted. About 70% of patients have at least a 50% decrease in headache frequency after withdrawal of analgesics.

REFERENCES

1. Kudrow L: Paradoxical effects of frequent analgesic use, *Adv Neurol* 33:335-341, 1982.
2. Mathew NT: Transformed migraine, *Cephalalgia* 13(suppl 12):78-83, 1993.
3. Rapoport A, Weeks R, Shftell F, et al: Analgesic rebound headache: theoretical and practical implications, *Cephalalgia* 5(suppl 3):448-449, 1985.
4. Becker WJ: Chronic daily headache and analgesic overuse, *Can J CME* 6:77-81, 1994.
5. Diamond S, Dalessio DJ: *The practicing physician's approach to headache,* ed 3, Baltimore, 1982, Williams & Wilkins, pp 114-121.

Caffeine Withdrawal Headaches

The caffeine content of various beverages is as follows[1]:

6 ounces of brewed coffee	85-100 mg
6 ounces of instant coffee	65 mg
6 ounces of tea	40 mg
12 ounces of caffeinated soft drink	45 mg

Caffeine withdrawal symptoms usually begin within 12 to 24 hours of the last caffeine intake, are at their maximum in 20 to 48 hours, and last for about a week.[2] In a Dutch study, individuals withdrawing from four to six cups of coffee per day had a high incidence of headaches beginning on day 1 and persisting as long as 6 days (mean 2.3 days).[3] A U.S. study found that even individuals taking an average of two and a half cups of coffee per day had withdrawal symptoms: 52% had moderate or severe headaches, and 8% to 11% had significant symptoms of anxiety or depression.[4]

REFERENCES

1. Hughes JR: Clinical importance of caffeine withdrawal, *N Engl J Med* 327:1160-1161, 1992.
2. Griffiths RR, Woodson PP: Caffeine physical dependence: a review of human and laboratory animal studies, *Psychopharmacology (Berl)* 94:437-451, 1988.
3. van Dusseldorp M, Katan MB: Headache caused by caffeine withdrawal among moderate coffee drinkers switched from ordinary to decaffeinated coffee: a 12 week double blind trial, *BMJ* 300:1558-1559, 1990.
4. Silverman K, Evans SM, Strain EC, et al: Withdrawal syndrome after the double-blind cessation of caffeine consumption, *N Engl J Med* 327:1109-1114, 1992.

Cluster Headaches

Men are affected by cluster headache six times as frequently as women. Alcohol is a frequent triggering factor. The pain is unilateral, is usually centered around the eye, is severe, comes on suddenly, and frequently awakens the patient from sleep. The usual attack lasts about 45 minutes.[1] In one study the most common behavior observed during attacks of cluster headaches was walking with the trunk bent slightly forward while clutching the head, or sitting and rocking back and forth with the hands pressed over the painful area. Some patients banged their heads against a hard object, and others pressed a finger or thumb into the affected eye.[2]

Drugs used for treatment of the acute attack include sumatriptan (Imitrex), dihydroergotamine (DHE, Migranal), ergotamine tartrate (Medihaler-ergotamine), ergotamine tablets or suppositories (Cafergot, Wigraine), inhaled oxygen at 8 L/min for 10 minutes, and 2% to 4% lidocaine (Xylocaine) by nasal instillation.[1] If lidocaine is used, it is administered by having the patient lie on the examining table with the head hanging over the edge so the neck is extended 45 degrees and the head is rotated 30 to 40 degrees toward the side of the headache. The lidocaine is slowly dropped into the nostril ipsilateral to the pain. If the nostril is plugged, a topical decongestant is given.[1,3] More information on the usual dosages of these drugs may be found in Table 19 in the section on migraines.

Lithium carbonate is often effective for the prophylaxis of cluster headaches in doses of 300 mg bid to qid. Serum lithium levels need be only between 0.4 and 0.8 mEq/L (0.4 to 0.8 mmol/L). Prednisone and methysergide (Sansert) are also effective prophylactic drugs. Prednisone is given in doses of 40 to 80 mg/day for 1 to 2 weeks and then tapered and discontinued over the following week, and methysergide is usually taken as 2 to 4 mg tid with meals. During cluster periods ergotamine may be given hs or on a regular basis bid to abort the headaches. For some patients indomethacin (Indocin, Indocid) 25 to 50 mg tid prevents attacks.[1]

REFERENCES

1. Walling AD: Cluster headache, *Am Fam Physician* 47:1457-1463, 1993.
2. Blau JN: Behaviour during a cluster headache, *Lancet* 342:723-725, 1993.
3. Kittrelle J, Grouse D, Seybold M: Cluster headache: local anesthetic abortive agents, *Arch Neurol* 42:496-498, 1985.

Migraines

(See also analgesic overuse headaches; caffeine withdrawal headaches; cluster headaches; investigations of patients with chronic headaches; risk factors for stroke)

Epidemiology

Eighteen percent of women and 6% of men in North America are estimated to suffer from migraines.[1] The association between migraines and stroke is equivocal (see discussion of risk factors for stroke). Many patients with migraines have superimposed withdrawal-type headaches from excessive use of medications to control the migraines (analgesic overuse headaches). Three fourths of women with migraines obtain relief with the onset of the menopause.[2]

Pathophysiology

The concept that the pain of migraine is directly caused by vascular hyperreactivity with initial vasoconstriction followed by vasodilation is no longer tenable. It is now thought that dysfunction of the serotonergic system in the brainstem activates trigeminal nerve fibers that supply blood vessels of the pia and dura mater. This results in the release of vasoactive substances (e.g., substance P, calcitonin gene–related polypeptide [CGRP]), causing inflammation and pain around the vessels. Vasoconstriction and vasodilation are secondary phenomena. Serotonin is central to this process, which may explain the efficacy of dihydroergotamine and sumatriptan, agents that act on serotonin receptors.[3]

Classification

Migraines are divided into two main classes. Between 10% and 20% of patients have migraine with aura (classic migraine), and most of the remainder have migraine without aura (common migraine). A few patients have complicated migraines defined as neurological symptoms lasting for the duration of the headache and occasionally causing permanent sequelae. Well-known variants of this type are basilar, hemiplegic, and ophthalmoplegic migraines, the last usually occurring in children. Although migraines are classically unilateral and pulsatile, they are bilateral in 40% of cases and may be nonpulsatile. The criteria of the International Headache Society for making a diagnosis of migraine without aura are that nothing in the history or physical examination suggests that the headaches are caused by another disease, that the patient has had at least five attacks of headache lasting 4 to 72 hours, and that these must have had at least two of the following characteristics[2-4]:

Central Nervous System

1. Unilateral
2. Pulsatile
3. Moderate to severe intensity
4. Aggravated by physical activity such as walking upstairs

In addition, the patient should experience at least one of the following associated symptoms[3,4]:

1. Nausea or vomiting
2. Photophobia, phonophobia

Treatment

Because of nausea, vomiting, and gastric stasis associated with migraines, metoclopramide (Maxeran) is a useful adjunct to ASA, acetaminophen, or NSAIDs.[3,5,6] In addition, preliminary evidence suggests that metoclopramide alone may be effective in relieving both the nausea and pain of migraines.[7]

Regardless of the drug chosen for treatment of an acute migraine attack, an important principle is to use an effective dose early in the attack.[3,5,6] In general acetaminophen or aspirin is tried first; if that does not work, NSAIDs are attempted; and if these fail, 5-HT_1 receptor agonists such as ergot derivatives or sumatriptan (Imitrex) are used. If the patient has nausea or vomiting, metoclopramide (Maxeran) may be added to any regimen (except sumatriptan with which it is unnecessary). Intense migraines persisting over many days may respond to a short course of oral steroids. Very severe migraines usually respond to intravenous neuroleptics, dexamethasone, or metoclopramide.[3,4]

Acetaminophen or aspirin should be given as soon as possible after the onset of the migraine with initial doses of 650 to 1000 mg[3] or 650 to 1300 mg.[4] These agents are often best combined with 10 mg of metoclopramide (Maxeran) or 10 to 20 mg of domperidone (Motilium).[6] Enteric-coated aspirin should not be used because this formulation delays absorption.[3] A single oral dose of acetaminophen (15 mg/kg) is often effective in controlling migraines in children, but a single oral dose of ibuprofen (10 mg/kg) is said to be better.[8]

A variety of NSAIDs have proved beneficial, including naproxen (Anaprox) with a maximal initial dose of 825 mg, ibuprofen (Motrin, Advil) with a maximal initial dose of 800 mg, ketorolac (Toradol) with a maximal initial intramuscular dose of 60 mg, indomethacin (Indocin, Indocid) with a maximal initial dose of 100 mg per rectum,[3] and mefenamic acid (Ponstan) with a maximal initial dose of 500 mg.[4] Capobianco and associates[3] favor naproxen if oral medications are tolerated or indomethacin suppositories if nausea and vomiting occur.

Sumatriptan (Imitrex) is available as tablets of 25 to 100 mg, as 6-mg prefilled syringes for subcutaneous injections, and as a nasal spray. It is a selective 5-HT_1 receptor agonist. The subcutaneous route gives rapid absorption and has been shown in controlled trials to alleviate both pain and nausea. There is no benefit to taking a second dose after an hour if the first one is ineffective. Forty percent of patients treated with sumatriptan get a recurrence of the headache, probably because of the short half-life of the drug. Sumatriptan is contraindicated in patients with coronary artery disease. It should not be repeated more than once subcutaneously or twice orally in 24 hours, or administered within 24 hours of taking an ergotamine preparation.[3,4] Daily use of sumatriptan may lead to a dependent state because withdrawal of the drug causes severe headache and anxiety.[9,10]

Ergot is an agonist of 5-HT_1 receptors but is less selective than sumatriptan. Ergotamine derivatives should be given as soon as possible after the onset of the migraine and are often best combined with 10 mg of metoclopramide (Maxeran) or 10 to 20 mg of domperidone (Motilium).[6] Oral absorption is relatively poor, so for some patients rectal suppositories may be more effective. Because ergotamine derivatives may cause nausea and vomiting, the dose must be adjusted (cutting refrigerated suppositories in half or even quarters) to avoid this reaction.[3] Ergotamine is available as tablets or suppositories combined with caffeine (Cafergot, Wigraine), as sublingual tablets (Ergomar), and as a metered dose inhaler (Medihaler-ergotamine). The usual initial dose of tablets or suppositories is 1 to 2 mg, and these may be repeated every half hour to a maximum dosage of 6 mg. Dihydroergotamine is available for intramuscular injection (DHE) and has recently been formulated as a nasal spray (Migranal). The usual initial dose is 1 to 3 mg intramuscularly or 1 spray of 0.5 mg in each nostril.

Drug combinations for migraines include acetaminophen or aspirin with codeine and often caffeine or aspirin, caffeine and the barbiturate butalbital with or without codeine (Fiorinal) or acetaminophen, and caffeine and butalbital (Esgic and Esgic Plus). Evidence supporting the efficacy of these drug combinations is poor, they may lead to addiction, and they are thought to be a major cause of rebound headaches that lead to chronic daily headaches.[4] Because of the risk of severe dependence, their use should be discouraged.[11]

Butorphanol (Stadol) is a mixed narcotic agonist-antagonist administered by nasal insufflation that is marketed for migraine treatment. Each spray contains about 1 mg of butorphanol, which has the analgesic equivalency of 5 mg of parenterally administered morphine. The median duration of pain relief in migraine is said to be 6 hours. A placebo-controlled study of 157 patients with migraine documented marked pain relief in 33% within 30 minutes, 47% within 1 hour, and 71% within 6 hours. Side effects were prominent, mainly dizziness, nausea, vomiting, and drowsiness. Some patients also experience confusion.[12] Butorphanol may be addictive and in some cases is sought by drug abusers.[13]

Intranasal lidocaine has been reported to relieve migraine in about half of the patients tested, but 42% of those who obtained relief had a relapse, usually within an hour. Overall, about one fourth of the patients had relief without relapse. The medication was administered by having the patient lie on a table with the head hyperextended 45 degrees and rotated 30 degrees toward the side of the headache; 1 ml of a 4% solution of the drug was dripped into the nose over 30 seconds.[14]

Central Nervous System 61

When other medications fail and the patient has had headaches for several days, a short course of oral prednisone often breaks a migraine cycle.[3,6]

A variety of drugs given IV or IM in the emergency room setting have aborted migraines. These include chlorpromazine (Thorazine, Largactil) 12.5 mg IV as an initial dose repeated every 30 minutes to a maximum of 37.5 mg,[3] prochlorperazine (Compazine, Stemetil) 7 to 10 mg IV stat,[15] metoclopramide (Maxeran) 7 to 10 mg IV stat,[7] dexamethasone 20 mg IV with or without 3.5 mg of prochlorperazine,[16] and ketorolac (Toradol), 60 mg IM.[17]

Table 19 lists some drugs and usual doses used in the treatment of acute migraine attacks.

Prophylaxis

Measures to prevent migraines focus on life-style modifications and, if necessary, pharmacotherapy (Table 20). Lifestyle factors that often contribute to migraines are fatigue, irregular sleeping patterns (sleeping in on weekends), stress, lack of exercise, missing meals, and specific dietary products. Some of the foods that have been reported to trigger migraines include alcohol, especially red wine, champagne, and beer; aged and processed cheese; sour cream; aged, cured, or processed meats, especially if they contain nitrates (hot dogs, bacon, smoked meat, many lunch meats); chicken livers; meat tenderizers; monosodium glutamate (Chinese food); soy sauce; yeast extracts; peanuts and peanut butter; chocolate; and caffeine-containing beverages.

Indications for pharmacological prophylaxis of migraines include more than two or three migraines a month, attacks lasting longer than 48 hours, severe attacks, and nonresponse to therapy. Between 55% and 65% of patients respond to prophylactic therapy, but amelioration of symptoms may be delayed for 1 to 2 months. In general it is wise to start with relatively low doses of prophylactic agents and raise them weekly if the response is inadequate.[3]

Beta-blockers are the agents of first choice. Established maintenance regimens are propranolol (Inderal) 40 to 320 mg/day, nadolol (Corgard) 40 to 240 mg/day, atenolol (Tenormin) 50 to 200 mg/day, and metoprolol (Lopressor) 100 to 200 mg/day.[3] Beta-blockers with intrinsic sympathomimetic activity such as pindolol (Visken) and acebutolol (Sectral) are not effective.[4]

Most calcium channel blockers are of questionable value in the prophylaxis of migraines. Verapamil (Calan, Isoptin)

Table 19 Treatment of Acute Migraine Attacks

Drug	Usual dose
Simple Analgesics	
Acetaminophen	650-1300 mg stat
Aspirin	650-1300 mg stat
NSAIDs	
Diclofenac (Voltaren)	50-100 mg stat
Flurbiprofen (Ansaid, Froben)	100 mg stat
Ibuprofen (Motrin, Advil)	400-800 mg stat (10 mg/kg for children)
Indomethacin (Indocin, Indocid)	100 mg stat po or pr
Ketorolac (Toradol)	60 mg IM stat
Mefenamic acid (Ponstan)	500 mg stat
Naproxen (Anaprox)	550-825 mg stat
Serotonin Agonists	
Sumatriptan (Imitrex)	25-100 mg po; 6 mg sc; 1 nasal insufflation
Ergot Derivatives	
Dihydroergotamine (Migranal)	1 spray (0.5 mg) each nostril; repeat once in 15 min prn
Dihydroergotamine (DHE)	1 mg IM stat; repeat q 1 hour × 2 prn
Ergotamine tartrate (Ergomar)	2 mg sc stat; repeat q 30 min × 2 prn
Ergotamine tartrate (Medihaler-ergotamine)	1 inhalation of 360 μg stat; repeat q 5 min × 5 prn
Ergotamine-caffeine (Cafergot)	2 tablets or 1 suppository stat; repeat with 1 tablet or 1/2 suppository q 30 min to maximum of 6 tablets or 2 suppositories
Ergotamine-caffeine-belladonna alkaloids (Wigraine)	1-2 tablets or 1 suppository stat; repeat q 30 min to maximum 6 tablets or 2 suppositories
Drug Combinations	
Butalbital-ASA-caffeine with or without codeine (Fiorinal)	Addictive; not recommended
Butalbital-acetaminophen-caffeine (Esgic Plus)	Addictive; not recommended
Narcotics—Agonist-Antagonist	
Butorphanol tartrate (Stadol)	1 spray in 1 nostril stat; repeat × 1 in 30-60 min prn
Topical Nasal Anesthetics	
Lidocaine (Xylocaine)	Nasal instillation of 1 ml of 4% solution
Antiemetics	
Metoclopramide (Maxeran)	10 mg po stat
Domperidone (Motilium)	10-20 mg po stat
Steroids	
Prednisone	Variable, e.g., 60 mg/day × 4 days with tapering over 10-14 days
Parenteral Drugs in Emergency Room	
Chlorpromazine (Largactil, Thorazine)	12.5 mg IV as an initial dose repeated q 30 min to a maximum of 37.5 mg
Prochlorperazine (Compazine, Stemetil)	7-10 mg IV stat
Metoclopramide (Maxeran)	7-10 mg IV stat
Dexamethasone	20 mg IV with or without 3.5 mg of prochlorperazine
Ketorolac (Toradol)	60 mg IM

NSAIDs, Nonsteroidal antiinflammatory drugs.

Table 20 Prophylaxis of Migraines

Drug	Usual dose
Beta-Blockers	
Atenolol (Tenormin)	50-200 mg/day
Metoprolol (Lopressor)	100-200 mg/day
Nadolol (Corgard)	40-240 mg/day
Propranolol (Inderal)	40-320 mg/day
Calcium Channel Blockers	
Flunarizine (Sibelium)	5-10 mg qhs
Verapamil (Calan, Isoptin)	240-480 mg/day
Tricyclic Antidepressants	
Amitriptyline (Elavil)	10-175 mg/day
Nortriptyline (Aventyl, Pamelor)	10-125 mg/day
Anticonvulsants	
Divalproex (Depakote)	250-1500 mg/day
Valproic acid (Depakene)	250-1500 mg/day
Nonsteroidal Antiinflammatory Drugs	
Naproxen sodium (Anaprox)	550 mg bid for 7 premenstrual days
Ergot Derivatives	
Methysergide (Sansert)	2-6 mg/day (drug holiday q 6 months)

seems to be marginally beneficial, the data for nifedipine are inconclusive, and diltiazem has not been adequately studied. If verapamil is used, the daily maintenance dose is 240 to 480 mg.[3] Flunarizine (Sibelium) has been effective at a usual maintenance dose of 5 to 10 mg qhs.[4]

Some patients respond well to tricyclic antidepressants such as amitriptyline (Elavil) with a usual daily maintenance dose of 10 to 175 mg or nortriptyline (Aventyl, Pamelor) in a daily maintenance dose of 10 to 125 mg.[3,4] An advantage of nortriptyline is that it has fewer anticholinergic side effects than amitriptyline.[4] Valproic acid (Depakene) and divalproex (Depakote) have been shown to be effective prophylactic agents for migraines with a daily maintenance dose of 250 to 1500 mg.[3,4] For some patients daily use of NSAIDs is an effective prophylactic regimen.[3] Naproxen sodium (Anaprox) 550 mg bid may be used for 1 week a month before the menstrual period as prophylaxis against premenstrual migraines.[4]

The semisynthetic ergot preparation methysergide (Sansert) is a serotonin antagonist and an effective prophylactic agent against migraines. The daily maintenance dose is 2 to 6 mg. The major problem with the drug is that it can induce retroperitoneal or pleuropulmonary fibrosis with continuous use in about 1:1500 patients. Because of this it should be reserved for patients in whom other prophylactic endeavors have failed. Patients must taper the drug and take a 3- to 4-week drug holiday every 6 months.[3]

Other drugs that have been used for migraine prophylaxis but have not been adequately studied are parthenolide (Tanacet 125 or "feverfew"), pizotyline (Sandomigran), and cyproheptadine (Periactin).[3]

REFERENCES

1. Stewart WF, Lipton RB, Celentano DD, et al: Prevalence of migraine headaches in the United States: relation to age, income, race, and other sociodemographic factors, *JAMA* 267:64-69 1992.
2. Kumar KL, Cooney TG: Headaches, *Med Clin North Am* 79:261-286, 1995.
3. Capobianco DJ, Cheshire WP, Campbell JK: An overview of the diagnosis and pharmacologic treatment of migraine, *Mayo Clin Proc* 71:1055-1066, 1996.
4. Pryse-Phillips WE, Dodick DW, Edmeads JG, et al. Guidelines for the diagnosis and management of migraine in clinical practice, *Can Med Assoc J* 156:1273-1287, 1997.
5. Tfelt-Hansen P, Henry P, Mulder LJ, et al: The effectiveness of combined oral lysine acetylsalicylate and metoclopramide compared with oral sumatriptan for migraine, *Lancet* 346:923-926, 1995.
6. Worthington I: Current migraine therapy, *Can J Clin Pharmacol* 3:39-51, 1996.
7. Ellis GL, Delaney J, DeHart DA, et al: The efficacy of metoclopramide in the treatment of migraine headache, *Ann Emerg Med* 22:191-195, 1993.
8. Hamalainen ML, Hoppu K, Valkeila E, et al: Ibuprofen or acetaminophen for the acute treatment of migraine in children—a double-blind, randomized, placebo-controlled, crossover study, *Neurology* 48:103-107, 1997.
9. Pini LA, Trenti T: Does chronic use of sumatriptan induce dependence? *Headache* 34:600, 1994.
10. Osborne MJ, Austin RC, Dawson KJ, et al: Is there a problem with long-term use of sumatriptan in migraine? *BMJ* 308:113, 1994.
11. Raja M, Altavista MC, Azzoni A, et al: Severe barbiturate withdrawal syndrome in migrainous patients, *Headache* 36:119-121, 1996.
12. Hoffert MJ, Couch JR, Diamond S, et al: Transnasal butorphanol in the treatment of acute migraine, *Headache* 35:65-69, 1995.
13. Canadian Adverse Drug Reaction Newsletter: Potential abuse of butorphanol nasal spray, *Can Med Assoc J* 156:1054-1056, 1997.
14. Maizels M, Scott B, Cohen W, et al: Intranasal lidocaine for treatment of migraine: a randomized, double-blind, controlled trial, *N Engl J Med* 276:319-321, 1996.
15. Coppola M, Yealy DM, Leibold RA: Randomized, placebo-controlled evaluation of prochlorperazine versus metoclopramide for emergency department treatment of migraine headache, *Ann Emerg Med* 26:541-546, 1995.
16. Saadah HA: Abortive migraine therapy in the office with dexamethasone and prochlorperazine, *Headache* 34:366-370, 1994.
17. Shrestha M, Singh R, Moreden J, et al: Ketorolac vs chlorpromazine in the treatment of acute migraine without aura: a prospective, randomized, double-blind trial, *Arch Intern Med* 156: 1725-1728, 1996.

MULTIPLE SCLEROSIS

(See also investigations; labeling; pets; spasticity)

Multiple sclerosis is primarily a disease of young white adults. Initial symptoms are usually noted in the third and fourth decades. About 60% of cases occur in women. The disease is more common in northern than in tropical regions, and over the past few decades the incidence has increased. There is often a family history of the disorder.[1,2]

Common initial symptoms of multiple sclerosis are isolated motor weakness, focal sensory losses or paresthesias, ataxia, diplopia, optic neuritis, and occasionally trigeminal neuralgia. A few patients have a positive Lhermitte's sign consisting of a sensation of electric shocks passing down the spine on flexion of the neck.[1,2]

MRI is the investigation of choice for confirming the diagnosis of multiple sclerosis when it is suspected clinically. However, MRI is negative in up to 10% of cases, and it is not 100% specific. In patients with multiple sclerosis, MRI almost always detects many more lesions than would be expected on the basis of clinical examination.[1,2] The presence of abnormal evoked potentials alone does not establish a diagnosis of multiple sclerosis. However, in the context of other clinical and laboratory findings, they may help confirm such a diagnosis. Visual evoked potentials and somatosensory evoked potentials are abnormal in more than three fourths of patients with multiple sclerosis, and brainstem auditory evoked responses are abnormal in more than half of such patients.[1] Somatosensory evoked potentials measure the integrity of the posterior columns and the projections to the sensory cortex, motor evoked potentials the integrity of the motor system, visual evoked potentials the delays in conduction of visual impulses to the visual cortex, and brainstem auditory evoked potentials the integrity of the central auditory systems.

False-positive results of evoked potentials may have devastating effects on a person's quality of life. I had one 60-year-old patient who was in excellent health but had had an episode of diplopia 6 years previously. At that time a neurologist told her that evoked potentials had shown that she had multiple sclerosis. Despite the subsequent reassurances of several neurologists that she did not have multiple sclerosis, and that such a diagnosis could not be based only on evoked potentials, she was an emotional wreck.

Both interferon beta-1a (Avonex)[3] and interferon beta-1b (Betaseron)[4] injections have been shown to decrease the number of relapses and the number of plaques found on MRI scanning in patients with relapsing-remitting multiple sclerosis. However, many patients have dropped out of the studies, often because their disease has worsened, and the long-term benefits in terms of decreased disability have not yet been determined.[5] Glatiramer (Copaxone) injections also look promising for relapsing-remitting multiple sclerosis.[6]

In a 1993 study of patients with optic neuritis, multiple sclerosis developed in only 7.5% of those given methylprednisolone 250 mg IV q6h for 3 days followed by prednisone 1 mg/kg orally for 11 days within 2 years, compared with a rate of 16.7% in the control group. Oral prednisone alone did not give this protective effect.[7] Whether all patients with optic neuritis should receive IV steroids is controversial.

REFERENCES

1. Brod SA, Lindsey JW, Wolinsky JS: Multiple sclerosis: clinical presentation, diagnosis and treatment, *Am Fam Physician* 54:1301-1311, 1996.
2. Rieumont MJ, Deluca SA: Neuroimaging evaluation in multiple sclerosis, *Am Fam Physician* 48:273-276, 1993.
3. Jacobs LD, Cookfair DL, Rudick RA, et al: Intramuscular interferon beta-1-alpha for disease progression in relapsing multiple sclerosis, *Ann Neurol* 39:285-294, 1996.
4. IFNB Multiple Sclerosis Study Group: Interferon beta-1b is effective in relapsing-remitting multiple sclerosis. I. Clinical results of a multicenter, randomized, double-blind, placebo-controlled trial, *Neurology* 43:655-661, 1993.
5. Richards RG: Interferon beta in multiple sclerosis: clinical cost effectiveness falls at the first hurdle (editorial), *BMJ* 313:1159, 1996.
6. Glatiramer acetate for relapsing multiple sclerosis, *Med Lett* 39: 61-62, 1997.
7. Beck RW, Cleary PA, Trobe JD: The effect of corticosteroids for acute optic neuritis on the subsequent development of multiple sclerosis, *N Engl J Med* 329:1764-1769, 1993.

MYASTHENIA GRAVIS

(See also paraneoplastic syndromes)

The incidence of myasthenia gravis occurs in two peaks, one in the second and third decades and involving mostly women and the second in the sixth and seventh decades and involving mostly men. The pathogenesis of myasthenia gravis is an autoantibody destruction of acetylcholine receptors at the neuromuscular junctions.[1]

The traditional diagnostic test for myasthenia gravis is to give the patient an IV dose of 2 mg of edrophonium (Tensilon) and see whether muscle strength improves. A positive result is usually seen within 30 to 60 seconds, and the effect lasts only about 5 minutes. Edrophonium inhibits the enzyme acetylcholinesterase, which normally inactivates acetylcholine. This allows the acetylcholine released into the neuromuscular junctions to act repeatedly with the acetylcholine receptors that still remain at the neuromuscular junctions. Another diagnostic test is the repetitive nerve stimulation test with action potentials being recorded from the innervated muscle. The most specific test is an assay for acetylcholine-receptor antibodies. However, antibodies are found in only 85% of all patients, and in only 50% of those whose only symptoms are ocular-muscle weakness.[1]

Treatment of myasthenia is effective, and the vast majority of patients are able to live normal lives. Thymectomy is indicated for any patient found to have a thymic tumor and for anyone with generalized myasthenia who is between the ages of puberty and 60. It has also been reported to be helpful in some patients with purely ocular myasthenia. Whether it is useful in those over the age of 60 who do not have a thymic tumor is uncertain. The standard medical treatment of myasthenia is pyridostigmine bromide (Mestinon). A few patients require long-term immunosuppressive therapy with drugs such as corticosteroids, azathioprine, or cyclosporine.

Intravenous immune globulin and plasma exchange are used to stabilize patients in myasthenic crisis or as perioperative therapy for patients undergoing thymectomy.[1]

REFERENCES

1. Drachman DB: Myasthenia gravis, *N Engl J Med* 330:1797-1810, 1994.

NEOPLASMS

The survival and quality of life of patients with single brain metastases were not improved with surgery plus radiation therapy compared with radiation therapy alone.[1]

REFERENCES

1. Mintz AH, Kestle J, Rathbone MP, et al: A randomized trial to assess the efficacy of surgery in addition to radiotherapy in patients with a single cerebral metastasis, *Cancer* 78:1470-1476, 1996.

NEUROPATHY

Bell's Palsy

Bell's palsy may be incomplete or complete; the prognosis is better for patients with the incomplete form and for those under 40 years of age. Recovery usually commences in 6 weeks, and the median time to complete resolution of paresis is 6 weeks.[1]

Whether steroids (prednisone) improve the recovery rates in patients with Bell's palsy is a matter of controversy. Recent studies suggest that they do if started within 48 or perhaps 72 hours.[1-4] Pryse-Phillips[4] recommends 1 mg/kg up to a maximum dose of 70 mg given as a single morning dose for 4 days; no tapering is necessary. From their review of the literature Williamson and Whelan[1] recommend treating only patients with complete paralysis. They suggest 1 mg/kg of prednisolone (maximum of 80 mg) given for a maximum of 10 days.

REFERENCES

1. Williamson IG, Whelan TR: The clinical problem of Bell's palsy: is treatment with steroids effective? *Br J Gen Pract* 46:743-747, 1996.
2. Shafshak TS, Essa AY, Bakey FA: The possible contributing factors for the success of steroid therapy in Bell's palsy: a clinical and electrophysiological study, *J Laryngol Otol* 108:940-943, 1994.
3. Austin JR, Peskind SP, Austin SG, Rice DH: Idiopathic facial nerve paralysis: a randomized double blind controlled study of placebo versus prednisone, *Laryngoscope* 103:1326-1333, 1993.
4. Pryse-Phillips W: Oral steroid use in Bell's palsy, *Patient Care Can* 6:12, 1995.

Carpal Tunnel Syndrome

The normal pressure within a limb compartment is 7 to 8 mm Hg. In carpal tunnel syndrome the pressure is often 30 mm Hg. With wrist flexion or extension it may be as high as 90 mm Hg.[1]

The most common cause of the carpal tunnel syndrome is nonspecific flexor tenosynovitis in the wrist, and probably the next most common is an old Colles' fracture. The more important medical conditions found in association with the disorder are diabetes, pregnancy, rheumatoid arthritis, and hypothyroidism. Rare medical causes are amyloidosis and acromegaly.[1] Whether some cases of carpal tunnel are occupationally related is controversial.[2]

Tinel's sign has a sensitivity of 60% and a specificity of 67%. Phalen's sign has a sensitivity of 75% and a specificity of 47%.[1]

First-line medical treatment of carpal tunnel syndrome consists of avoiding activities and wrist positions that aggravate the condition, wearing wrist splints, and taking NSAIDs. The pressure in the carpal tunnel is lowest with the wrist in the neutral position (not the position of function), and pressure is increased not only by flexion and extension of the wrist, but also by holding objects, making a fist, and flexing the fingers against resistance.[3] One minute of hand and wrist exercises (alternate flexion and extension of wrist and fingers 30 times in 1 minute) lowers the pressure and should be done every hour.[3] Splints that hold the wrist in the neutral position are particularly effective if worn at night.[1,4]

The role of steroid injections into the carpal tunnel is controversial. The two main reasons for this are the risk of damaging the median nerve[5] and the fact that although short-term improvement is common, long-term remissions are less frequent.[1,2,6,7] For example, in one British study of such injections short-term clinical improvement was recorded in half the patients but long-term improvement in only one fourth.[6] An Italian study found short-term improvement in most cases, but after 2 years the effect was evident in only 8% of those injected.[7] Surgery is more likely to be required if the patient is over 50 years of age, has had the disease longer than 10 months, and has constant paresthesias.[1]

A randomized double-blind placebo-controlled study of a small number of patients with mild to moderate carpal tunnel syndrome found that 20 mg of oral prednisone for 7 days followed by 10 mg for 7 days gave significant relief of symptoms but that the effect waned over a 2-month period.[8]

REFERENCES

1. Dawson DM: Entrapment neuropathies of the upper extremities, *N Engl J Med* 329:2013-2018, 1993.
2. Katz R: Carpal tunnel syndrome: a practical review, *Am Fam Physician* 49:1371-1379, 1994.
3. Seradge H, Jia YC, Owens W: In vivo measurement of carpal tunnel pressure in the functioning hand, *J Hand Surg* 20:855-859, 1995.
4. Weiss ND, Gordon L, Bloom T, et al: Position of the wrist associated with the lowest carpal-tunnel pressure—implications for splint design, *J Bone Joint Surg* 77A:1695-1699, 1995.
5. Kasten SJ, Louis DS: Carpal tunnel syndrome: a case of median nerve injection injury and a safe and effective method for injecting the carpal tunnel, *J Fam Pract* 43:79-82, 1996.
6. Irwin LR, Beckett R, Suman RK: Steroid injection for carpal tunnel syndrome, *J Hand Surgery (Br)* 21:355-357, 1996.

7. Girlanda P, Dattola R, Venuto C, et al: Local steroid treatment in idiopathic carpal tunnel syndrome: short- and long-term efficacy, *J Neurol* 240:187-190, 1993.
8. Herskovitz S, Berger AR, Lipton RB: Low-dose, short-term oral prednisone in the treatment of carpal tunnel syndrome, *Neurology* 45:1923-1925, 1995.

Guillain-Barré Syndrome

Guillain-Barré syndrome has traditionally been considered an immune-related inflammatory demyelinating polyneuropathy. However, many patients also have axonal degeneration. Symptoms of motor weakness (and often paresthesias) come on rapidly, and about one third of patients require treatment in the intensive care unit. The mortality rate is about 3%, maximum neurological deficits occur at 2 to 4 weeks, and 50% to 75% of patients recover completely within 6 to 12 months.[1,2]

In two thirds of cases a respiratory or gastrointestinal infection precedes the disease by 1 or 2 weeks.[1,2] A common precipitant of the syndrome is *Campylobacter jejuni* infection. In these situations patients often have axonal degeneration and recovery is slow, leaving residual deficits.[3]

Aside from supportive and rehabilitation care, therapeutic modalities that have been reported useful are plasma exchange and intravenous immune globulins with or without intravenous steroids.[2]

REFERENCES

1. Bolton CF: The changing concepts of Guillain-Barré syndrome (editorial), *N Engl J Med* 333:1415-1417, 1995.
2. Dematteis JA: Guillain-Barré syndrome: a team approach to diagnosis and treatment, *Am Fam Physician* 54:197-200, 1996.
3. Rees JH, Soudain SE, Gregson NA, et al: *Campylobacter jejuni* infection and Guillain-Barré syndrome, *N Engl J Med* 333:1374-1379, 1995.

Trigeminal Neuralgia

Trigeminal neuralgia usually affects otherwise healthy middle-aged adults, although in a few cases it is associated with multiple sclerosis or a tumor near the nerve root. The maxillary division of the trigeminal nerve is most often affected, and trigger sites are found on the face or in the mouth. Long-term spontaneous remissions are common, especially if they eventuate shortly after the onset of the disorder. Initial treatment is with carbamazepine (Tegretol), starting with a low dose and increasing as necessary until pain is relieved. This regimen is successful in 75% of cases. If control is not achieved, phenytoin (Dilantin) should be tried alone or along with carbamazepine. If control is still not achieved, baclofen (Lioresal) should be added.[1]

Surgery is indicated later in the course of the disease if symptoms remain. Various procedures are used, including neurectomy of trigeminal nerve branches and injury to the trigeminal ganglion by heat (radiofrequency thermal rhizotomy), mechanical pressure (trigeminal-ganglion balloon microcompression), or chemicals (retrogasserian glycerol rhizotomy).[2] A surgical procedure that appears to have an excellent outcome is microvascular decompression of the trigeminal nerve through a retromastoid craniectomy. A high percentage of affected patients have a nerve root compressed by a vessel and experience immediate pain relief after the decompression surgery.[1,2]

REFERENCES

1. Fields HL: Treatment of trigeminal neuralgia (editorial), *N Engl J Med* 334:1125-1126, 1996.
2. Barker FG II, Jannetta PJ, Bissonette DJ, et al: The long-term outcome of microvascular decompression for trigeminal neuralgia, *N Engl J Med* 334:1077-1083, 1996.

PARKINSON'S DISEASE

(See also extrapyramidal effects of neuroleptics; serotonin syndrome; tremors)

Parkinson's disease is a common condition in the elderly. In a study of 467 Boston residents over the age of 65 the prevalence of parkinsonian signs (bradykinesia, gait disturbance, rigidity, and tremor) was about 15% for ages 65 to 74, 30% for ages 75 to 84, and 52% for those over 85. The death rate in study subjects with parkinsonian signs was twice the rate of those without them.[1] The incidence of Parkinson's disease has been reported to be lower in smokers than in nonsmokers.[2]

Two recent population studies of patients with Parkinson's disease found rates of major depression to be 2.7%[3] and 7.7%.[4] Patients with significant cognitive deficits had higher rates than those without such deficits. Although major depression was relatively infrequent, almost half of the patients in a Norwegian community study had mild depressive symptoms.[4]

Initial symptoms of Parkinson's disease are often unilateral. As the disease progresses, the classic picture evolves with resting tremor, rigidity, hypokinesia (poverty of movement) or bradykinesia (slow movements), slow shuffling gait, stooped posture, masked facies, drooling, and micrographia. Postural instability with frequent falls is common, and in the later stages drooling is seen because of the stooped posture, decreased facial movements, and less frequent swallowing. Autonomic symptoms seen in the late stages are seborrhea, excessive perspiration, unstable temperature regulation, neurogenic bladder, and gastrointestinal hypomotility.[5]

The differential diagnosis of Parkinson's disease includes essential tremor, progressive supranuclear palsy (Steele-Richardson-Olszewski syndrome), neuroleptic drugs, certain antiemetics such as metoclopramide,[6] and Wilson's disease.[7] Wilson's disease should be ruled out in any young individual with parkinsonian-like symptoms (or for that matter other neurological symptoms or psychiatric symptoms associated with neurological symptoms). Investigations of such individuals include a slit-lamp examination for Kayser-Fleischer rings, liver function tests, and an assessment of plasma ceruloplasmin levels, which are usually less than 200 mg/L (20 mg/dl) in patients who have the disease.[7]

Central Nervous System

In North America the standard initial regimen for Parkinson's disease is a levodopa formulation (Sinemet, Prolopa) with or without selegiline (Eldepryl). A 1993 British study showed no significant differences in outcome in patients with early Parkinson's disease treated with levodopa-benserazide (Prolopa) alone, levodopa-benserazide plus selegiline (Eldepryl), or bromocriptine (Parlodel) alone; the incidence of adverse effects was higher in the group receiving selegiline.[8] A similar study from New York found no difference at 5 years between patients treated with L-dopa-carbidopa (Sinemet) alone and those treated with Sinemet plus selegiline, although patients taking selegiline required slightly lower doses of Sinemet.[9] A 1995 British study not only showed no clinical benefit from selegiline, but also demonstrated a higher mortality rate in the selegiline arm of the study.[10] Selegiline is now thought not to have "neuroprotective" properties, but rather to have some effect on symptom control. For mild cases of Parkinson's disease some physicians initiate therapy with amantadine (Symmetrel).

The major pathophysiological defect in Parkinson's disease is a deficit of dopamine in the substantia nigra and other basal ganglia. The reason levodopa is used in therapy is that dopamine does not cross the blood-brain barrier whereas levodopa does. In the body, levodopa is converted to dopamine by the enzyme aromatic-L-amino-acid decarboxylase. Dopamine is desirable in the central nervous system, but because of its side effects it is undesirable elsewhere in the body. For this reason levodopa is combined with inhibitors of aromatic-L-amino-acid decarboxylase that do not cross the blood-brain barrier (carbidopa in Sinemet and benserazide in Prolopa). The maximum required daily dose of carbidopa is 200 to 300 mg. Thus if a patient requires large doses of Sinemet, the 100/10 formulation should be given instead of the usual 100/25 form. The same principle applies for benserazide if Prolopa is used.

Levodopa/carbidopa (Sinemet) comes in both regular and controlled release formulations. As the disease progresses, the duration of symptom relief from each dose wanes ("wearing off" effect). This can often be ameliorated by switching to the controlled release formulation. In fact, evidence has been presented that constant levels of levodopa may lead to a lower incidence of the "on-off" phenomenon, and for this reason many neurologists recommend starting patients on controlled release formulations. Another way of controlling the "wearing off" effect or the "on-off" phenomenon is to add a small dose of a dopaminergic agonist such as bromocriptine (Parlodel) or pergolide (Permax).[5]

Dyskinesias develop in 30% to 80% of patients on prolonged levodopa therapy.[11] They are usually choreiform but may be dystonic or myoclonic; some amelioration comes about with lowering the dose of levodopa, but this may aggravate the parkinsonian symptoms.[12] Pallidotomy is usually effective in controlling the dystonias.[13]

Nausea is a major side effect of levodopa (and bromocriptine) and may be controlled with domperidone (Motilium) 10 to 20 mg 30 to 60 minutes before each dose. This may be necessary only when the patient starts taking the drug.[14]

Once a patient is taking levodopa 600 mg/day, it is preferable to add a dopamine agonist such as bromocriptine rather than just continue to increase the dose of levodopa.[15] Some neurologists advocate adding dopamine agonists even earlier in the disease on the grounds that lower levels of levodopa will be required and there will therefore be less fluctuation of benefits and a reduced incidence of dyskinesias.[14]

Anticholinergics such as trihexyphenidyl (Artane) or benztropine mesylate (Cogentin) may decrease tremor but are seldom useful for rigidity or bradykinesia. These drugs may cause confusion. They should be avoided or used with caution.

For patients who no longer respond to pharmacotherapy, pallidotomy, a stereotactic neurosurgical operation that destroys the globus pallidum, may give significant relief. The globus pallidum is thought to respond to the decreased dopamine secretion of the substantia nigra by increasing its production of neurotransmitters, which probably account for much of the bradykinesia, rigidity, and tremor.[13,16] Pallidotomy also is used to diminish or abolish the abnormal involuntary movements or dyskinesias that tend to develop in Parkinsonian patients receiving long-term levodopa therapy.[16]

Table 21 Drugs for Parkinson's Disease

Drug	Usual dose
Dopamine Precursors	
Levodopa/carbidopa (Sinemet)	100/25 tid-qid; maximum 1000 mg levodopa per day; controlled release formulations have about 70% bioavailability of regular tablets
Levodopa/benserazide (Prolopa)	100/25 tid-qid; maximum 1000 mg levodopa per day
Dopamine Agonists	
Bromocriptine (Parlodel)	1.25-40 mg/day in 2-3 divided doses
Pergolide mesylate (Permax)	0.05-3 mg/day in 3 divided doses
Dopaminergic Agents	
Amantadine (Symmetrel)	100 mg bid-tid
Selective MAO Inhibitory Drugs (Type B)	
Selegiline or L-Deprenyl (Eldepryl)	5 mg bid with breakfast and lunch
Anticholinergic Agents	
Trihexyphenidyl (Artane)	1-3 mg tid
Benztropine mesylate (Cogentin)	1-4 mg/day as a single or two divided doses
Antiemetics	
Domperidone (Motilium)	10-20 mg 30-60 min before medications causing nausea

Drugs used for the treatment of Parkinson's disease are listed in Table 21. In general the regimen starts with a low dose of whatever drug or drugs are chosen and a gradual buildup. Before treatment begins, the practitioner should ensure that the clinical syndrome has not been induced by drugs such as metoclopramide (Maxeran) or a neuroleptic.

REFERENCES

1. Bennett DA, Beckett LA, Murray AM, et al: Prevalence of Parkinsonian signs and associated mortality in a community population of older people, *N Engl J Med* 334:71-76, 1996.
2. Doll R, Peto R, Wheatley K, et al: Mortality in relation to smoking: 40 years' observations on male British doctors, *BMJ* 309: 901-911, 1994.
3. Hantz P, Caradoc-Davies G, Caradoc-Davies T, et al: Depression in Parkinson's disease, *Am J Psychiatry* 151:1010-1014, 1994.
4. Tandberg E, Larsen JP, Aarsland D, et al: The occurrence of depression in Parkinson's disease: a community-based study, *Arch Neurol* 53:175-179, 1996.
5. Martin WRW: How do I approach Parkinson's disease? *Can J CME* 8(3):21-27, 1996.
6. Avorn J, Gurwitz JH, Bohn RL, et al: Increased incidence of levodopa therapy following metoclopramide use, *JAMA* 274: 1780-1782, 1995.
7. Walshe JM, Yealland M: Wilson's disease: the problem of delayed diagnosis, *J Neurol Neurosurg Psychiatry* 55:692-696, 1992.
8. Parkinson's Disease Research Group in the United Kingdom: Comparisons of therapeutic effects of levodopa, levodopa and selegiline, and bromocriptine in patients with early, mild Parkinson's disease: three year interim report, *BMJ* 307:469-472, 1993.
9. Brannan T, Yahr MD: Comparative study of selegiline plus L-dopa-carbidopa versus L-dopa-carbidopa alone in the treatment of Parkinson's disease, *Ann Neurol* 37:95-98, 1995.
10. Lees AJ (Parkinson's Disease Research Group of the United Kingdom): Comparison of therapeutic effects and mortality data of levodopa and levodopa combined with selegiline in patients with early, mild Parkinson's disease, *BMJ* 311:1602-1606, 1995.
11. Nutt JG:Levodopa-induced dyskinesia: review, observations, and speculations, *Neurology* 2:340-345, 1990.
12. Olanow CW: A 61-year-old man with Parkinson's disease, *JAMA* 275:716-722, 1996.
13. Lozano AM, Lang AE, Galvez-Jinenez, et al: Effect of Gpi pallidotomy on motor function in Parkinson's disease, *Lancet* 346: 1383-1387, 1995.
14. Kishore A, Snow BJ: Drug management of Parkinson's disease, *Can Fam Physician* 42:946-952, 1996.
15. Calne DB: Treatment of Parkinson's disease, *N Engl J Med* 329: 1021-1028, 1993.
16. Salzman EW: Living with Parkinson's disease, *N Engl J Med* 334:114-116, 1996.

RESTLESS LEGS SYNDROME

(See also insomnia)

Patients with the restless legs syndrome complain of a sensation of formications or other paresthesias often described as an aching, cramping, or crawling sensation deep in the legs, usually the calves. These occur at rest, generally at night, and are relieved by moving or walking. Associated symptoms include periodic movements during sleep (bed partners may complain of being kicked) and myoclonic jerks when awake. Insomnia is common and often the initial symptom, and in many cases the underlying restless legs syndrome is not diagnosed. The disorder is intermittent and may have prolonged remissions. An estimated 5% of the general population is affected, and there is sometimes a family history. The incidence of the disorder is higher in patients with iron deficiency anemia (25%) and in patients undergoing dialysis (30% to 40%). Other reported associated conditions are pregnancy, diabetes mellitus, polyneuropathy, and rheumatoid arthritis. The pathophysiology is unknown but is thought to be related to disorders of the central and peripheral nervous systems.[1,2]

Many drugs have been used to treat the restless legs syndrome, an indication that none is terribly successful. The most effective seem to be levodopa-carbidopa (Sinemet),[1-4] bromocriptine (Parlodel),[1,2,4,5] clonazepam (Rivotril),[1,2,4] opioids,[2,4,6] and clonidine (Catapres).[2,7] One of the problems with drug treatment of this disorder is that after a period of successful use, tolerance develops and patients fail to respond. One solution is to rotate drug classes on a weekly or biweekly basis.[4] When prescribing medications for this condition the practitioner should start with low doses and increase them gradually. The usual dose of Sinemet 100/25 is ½ to 2 tablets hs, repeated during the night prn; that of bromocriptine is 1.25 to 7.5 mg hs; clonazepam 0.5 mg hs; and clonidine 0.1 to 0.3 mg hs.

In view of the generally poor response to drugs it is desirable to avoid them entirely if possible. If pharmacotherapy is necessary, it is probably wise to reserve opioids and benzodiazepines for patients who fail to respond to other treatment modalities. I would start with Sinemet.

REFERENCES

1. Feigen A: Restless leg syndrome, *JAMA* 274:1191-1192, 1995.
2. O'Keeffe ST: Restless legs syndrome: a review, *Arch Intern Med* 156:243-248, 1996.
3. Brodeur C, Montplaisir J, Godbout R, et al: Treatment of restless legs syndrome and periodic movements during sleep with L-dopa: a double-blind controlled study, *Neurology* 38:145-148, 1988.
4. Kreuger BR: Restless legs syndrome and periodic movements of sleep, *Mayo Clin Proc* 65:999-1006, 1990.
5. Walters AS, Hening WA, Kavey N, et al: A double-blind randomized crossover trial of bromocriptine and placebo in restless legs syndrome, *Ann Neurol* 24:455-458, 1988.
6. Hening WA, Walters AS: Successful long-term therapy of the restless legs syndrome with opioid medication, *Sleep Res* 18: 241, 1989.
7. Wagner ML, Walters AS, Coleman R, et al: A double-blind study of clonidine in restless legs syndrome, *Neurology* 44 (suppl 2): A218, 1994, Abstract 365P.

Central Nervous System

SEIZURES

(See also anticonvulsants in pregnancy; febrile seizures; anticonvulsants in the treatment of bipolar disorder; febrile seizures; syncope; treatment of alcoholism)

Seizures are classified as follows:

1. Partial seizures (focal seizures). Partial seizures begin in one part of a cerebral hemisphere and may or may not become generalized. Simple partial seizures have preserved consciousness and may be manifested by motor, somatosensory or special sensory, autonomic, or psychic symptoms. Complex partial seizures (temporal lobe seizures, psychomotor seizures) may start as simple partial seizures that are followed by impaired consciousness, or consciousness may be impaired from the onset.
2. Generalized-onset seizures. Generalized-onset seizures have involvement of both cerebral hemispheres from the beginning. They are subcategorized as tonic-clonic (grand mal), absence (petit mal), atypical absence, myoclonic, tonic, and atonic.

Recognized precipitating factors for seizures include alcohol, drug abuse, medications (e.g., neuroleptics, tricyclics), neoplasms, neurocysticercosis, previous head injury, and previous CVA.

The major causes of spontaneous loss of consciousness are seizures, pseudoseizures (conversion reactions), and syncope.[1,2] Multifocal and generalized myoclonic jerks are commonly seen in syncope.[1] However, recovery of consciousness is rapid, usually occurring within a minute, and incontinence is rare. Patients with syncope often have prodromal sensations of lightheadedness, nausea, dizziness, ringing in the ears, and a sense that the vision is "going gray." Syncope rarely occurs in the recumbent position, and is often precipitated by triggers such as prolonged standing, quick rising, pain, micturition, or cough.[1]

One study found that tongue biting (lacerations observed by a physician) had a sensitivity of 24% and a specificity of 99% for epilepsy. Lateral tongue biting was 100% specific for tonic-clonic seizures.[2]

Brief convulsive episodes immediately following head injury with rapid recovery are usually called posttraumatic seizures. However, the prognosis is excellent and they are probably not true epileptic reactions.[1,3]

The rate of recurrence after an unprovoked seizure is variable. Recurrence is thought to be more likely if there was a previous serious central nervous system injury, if the patient has a family history of seizures, if the seizure was of the complex partial type, or if the electroencephalogram (EEG) is abnormal.[4-7] In a study of 407 New York children with unprovoked seizures followed for a mean of 6.3 years, the overall recurrence rate by 8 years was 44%. Of the recurrences, 53% occurred within 6 months and 88% within 2 years. Among children with cryptogenic (idiopathic) seizures, major risk factors for recurrence were the occurrence of the seizure when asleep, an abnormal EEG, Todd's paralysis (temporary postseizure paralysis of a limb), and older age. The best prognosis was among children who experienced their seizures while awake and who had normal EEGs. Status epilepticus at the time of the initial seizure, having more than one seizure within 24 hours of the initial seizure, or a past history of febrile seizures did not increase the risk of recurrences.[7]

Whether all patients who have had an unprovoked seizure require therapy is controversial. It has been established that treatment will decrease the frequency of recurrent seizures.[8-10] For example, in an Israeli study of adults between the ages of 18 and 50 with the new onset of a single unprovoked generalized tonic-clonic seizure, 45 patients were treated with carbamazepine (Tegretol) and 42 were given no antiseizure medications. At the end of 3 years 71% of the untreated patients had recurrent seizures compared with 22% of the treated patients.[10] However, treatment does not alter the long-term prognosis,[11,12] and therefore, if the risk of recurrence is low, the adverse effects of treatment may outweigh the benefits.[8]

Drug treatment of seizures should begin with a single drug because 70% to 80% of patients treated with medications respond to such a regimen. If adequate control is not achieved with full therapeutic doses of a single drug in a compliant patient, a second drug is added. Initial doses are low and are increased gradually as necessary.[4-6]

Carbamazepine (Tegretol), phenytoin (Dilantin), and valproate (Depakene, Depakote, Epival) are the first-line drugs for both partial seizures and generalized tonic-clonic seizures.[4,5] Valproate is the preferred drug for myoclonic and atonic-type seizures, whereas absence seizures should be treated with ethosuximide (Zarontin) or valproate.[4-6]

A number of new antiepileptic drugs are used primarily as add-on treatments for patients with treatment-resistant partial seizures. They are more effective than placebos,[13,14] but whether they have a major role in the management of seizures remains controversial.[15] Some of these drugs are listed in Table 22.

When serum levels of antiepileptic drugs are drawn to determine whether therapeutic levels have been achieved, they should be obtained only after steady-state conditions have been reached. For phenytoin this is 6 days after starting or changing the dose, for carbamazepine and valproic acid it is 3 days, and for phenobarbital it is 20 days. Except for phenobarbital, which has an extremely long half-life, trough levels should be obtained. Immediate serum levels are indicated within 6 hours of a seizure or when toxicity or noncompliance is suspected.[16] In some patients seizures are controlled with subtherapeutic levels.[6]

If antiepileptic medications are withdrawn after a few years of good control, about 60% of patients remain seizure free.[6] Patients may have to avoid driving for 6 to 12 months after withdrawal of medications.

Table 22 Antiepileptic Drugs

Generic names	Trade names
Standard Drugs	
Carbamazepine	Tegretol
Ethosuximide	Zarontin
Phenobarbital	
Phenytoin	Dilantin
Primidone	Mysoline
Valproate (valproic acid, divalproex)	Depakene (valproic acid); Depakote, Epival (divalproex)
New Add-On Drugs	
Clobazam	Frisium
Felbamate	Felbatol
Gabapentin	Neurontin
Lamotrigine	Lamictal
Topiramate	Topamax
Vigabatrin	Sabril

REFERENCES

1. Sander JW, O'Donoghue MF: Epilepsy: getting the diagnosis right; all that convulses is not epilepsy (editorial), *BMJ* 314: 158-159, 1997.
2. Benbadis SR, Wolgamuth BR, Goren H, et al: Value of tongue biting in the diagnosis of seizures, *Arch Intern Med* 155:2346-2349, 1995.
3. McCrory PR, Bladin PF, Berkovic SF: Retrospective study of concussive convulsions in elite Australian rules and rugby league footballers: phenomenology, aetiology, and outcome, *BMJ* 314:171-174, 1997.
4. Parks BR Jr, Dostrow VG, Noble SL: Drug therapy for epilepsy, *Am Fam Physician* 50:639-648, 1994.
5. Drugs for epilepsy, *Med Lett* 37:37-40, 1995.
6. Brodie MJ, Dichter MA: Antiepileptic drugs, *N Engl J Med* 334:168-175, 1996.
7. Shinnar S, Berg AT, Moshe SL, et al: The risk of seizure recurrence after a first unprovoked afebrile seizure in childhood—an extended follow-up, *Pediatrics* 98:216-225, 1996.
8. Camfield P, Camfield C, Dooley J, et al: A randomized study of carbamazepine versus no medication following a first unprovoked seizure in childhood, *Neurology* 39:851-852, 1989.
9. First Seizure Trial Group: Randomized clinical trial on the efficacy of antiepileptic drugs in reducing the risk of relapse after a first unprovoked tonic-clonic seizure, *Neurology* 43:478-483, 1993.
10. Gilad R, Lampl Y, Gabbay U, et al: Early treatment of a single generalized tonic-clonic seizure to prevent recurrence, *Arch Neurol* 53:1149-1152, 1996.
11. Musicco M, Beghi E, Solari A: First seizure Trial Group: effect of antiepileptic treatment initiated after the first unprovoked seizure on the long-term prognosis of epilepsy, *Neurology* 44(suppl 2):A337-A338, 1994.
12. Shinnar S, Berg AT: Does antiepileptic drug therapy alter the prognosis of childhood seizures and prevent the development of chronic epilepsy? *Semin Pediatr Neurol* 1:111-117, 1994.
13. Dichter MA, Brodie MJ: New antiepileptic drugs, *N Engl J Med* 334:1583-1590, 1996.
14. Marson AG, Kadir ZA, Chadwick N: New antiepileptic drugs; a systematic review of their efficacy and tolerability, *BMJ* 313: 1169-1174, 1996.
15. Mignot G: Drug trials in epilepsy: new drugs have been poorly assessed (editorial), *BMJ* 313:1158, 1996.
16. Schoenenberger RA, Tanasijevic MJ, Jha A, et al: Appropriateness of antiepileptic drug level monitoring, *JAMA* 274:1622-1626, 1995.

SPASTICITY

Three of the drugs used to decrease spasticity in patients with upper motor neuron disease, especially those with spinal cord transections and multiple sclerosis, are baclofen (Lioresal), tizanidine (Zanaflex), and dantrolene (Dantrium). The initial dosages should be low and increased gradually to the usual maintenance dosages, which for baclofen is 40 to 80 mg/day in 3 or 4 divided doses, for tizanidine 12 to 36 mg tid, and for dantrolene 25 for 100 mg qid. Dantrolene is less effective than baclofen or tizanidine.[1]

REFERENCES

1. Tizanidine for spasticity, *Med Lett* 39:62-63, 1997.

SUBARACHNOID HEMORRHAGE

(See also cerebrovascular accidents; prevention; screening)

Subarachnoid hemorrhage is a relatively common neurological condition with a greater prevalence rate than that of primary brain tumors or multiple sclerosis. Risk factors are personal history of a previous intracerebral aneurysm; family history of aneurysm; smoking; hypertension; excessive alcohol intake, particularly binge drinking; and certain heritable connective tissue disorders such as autosomal dominant polycystic kidney disease, Ehlers-Danlos syndrome, and Marfan's syndrome.[1]

The characteristic symptom of a subarachnoid hemorrhage is the sudden onset of severe headache. In some patients severe lower back pain with bilateral radicular pain develops as a result of the irritating properties of blood that has descended into the subarachnoid space surrounding the lower spinal cord. Between one third and one half of patients in whom a significant subarachnoid hemorrhage is found have had an unusual headache in the preceding days or weeks that was caused by a "warning leak"; physicians usually miss the significance of these. Classic physical findings are meningismus and subhyaloid fundal hemorrhages, with the latter found in about a quarter of the patients. CT scans without contrast medium identify 90% to 95% of patients with subarachnoid hemorrhages if obtained within 24 hours, but because blood is rapidly absorbed, the sensitivity of CT detection drops to 80% at 3 days and 70% at 5 days. MRI is not a sensitive way of diagnosing an acute subarachnoid hemorrhage but is useful for detecting intracranial aneurysms.[1]

Whether asymptomatic relatives of individuals who have had a subarachnoid hemorrhage should be screened for intracerebral aneurysms is controversial. Although aneurysms may be detected and treated, not all aneurysms bleed and some develop rapidly and rupture soon thereafter. A screening procedure would be unlikely to detect rapidly growing aneurysms of this nature. In addition, physicians and patients must decide whether the morbidity and mortality rates of the treatment of aneurysms (less than 5% and 2%, respectively) are acceptable. The lifetime risk of hemorrhage for someone with only one first-degree relative who had had a subarachnoid hemorrhage is 1% by the age of 50 and 2% by the age of 70; for these patients screening is generally not recommended, but it may be worthwhile for those with two or more affected relatives or for patients with polycystic kidney disease.[1]

REFERENCES

1. Schievink WI: Intracranial aneurysms, *N Engl J Med* 336:28-40, 1997.

SYNCOPE

(See also diagnosis of seizures)

A number of elderly patients have a significant drop in blood pressure within 45 to 60 minutes after a meal. In one study of nursing home residents with a mean age of 80, 24% had a systolic pressure reduction of more than 20 mm Hg during the postprandial period. Those with a history of falls or syncope in the previous 6 months had a greater mean blood pressure loss than did patients without such a history.[1]

Mass fainting at rock concerts is common. The patients are girls between 11 and 17 years of age, and the cause seems to be a combination of fatigue, a long period of fasting (from standing in line for hours), compression by crowds, and hyperventilation as part of a panic attack.[2]

REFERENCES

1. Aronow WS, Ahn C: Postprandial hypotension in 499 elderly persons in a long-term health care facility, *J Am Geriatr Soc* 42: 930-932, 1994.
2. Lempert T, Bauer M: Mass fainting at rock concerts (letter), *N Engl J Med* 332:1721, 1995.

TOURETTE'S SYNDROME

Gilles de la Tourette's syndrome is characterized primarily by motor tics. These brief, jerky movements involve primarily the head and neck but may also affect the trunk or limbs. The tics are involuntary but usually can be voluntarily suppressed. The symptoms begin by 11 years of age in 96% of patients. Although symptoms are often lifelong, their severity often decreases at puberty. Among children the ratio of males to females is as great as 9:1, whereas among adults it is 4:1. Coprolalia is a rare complication of the disorder, occurring in less than 10% of cases.[1-3]

Although some authors group all tics together in the spectrum of Tourette's syndrome, others place transient tic disorder in a separate category. Patients with Tourette's syndrome have a high incidence of obsessive-compulsive disorder and attention deficit disorder.[3]

Transient tic disorder lasts less than 1 year.[3]

REFERENCES

1. Suchowersky O: Recognizing Tourette's syndrome, *Can J Diagn,* August 1993, 10:109-119.
2. Hyde TM, Weinberger DR: Tourette's syndrome: a model neuropsychiatric disorder, *JAMA* 273:498-501, 1995.
3. American Psychiatric Association: *Diagnostic and statistical manual of mental disorders,* ed 4, Washington, DC, 1994, The Association, pp 101-103.

TREMORS

(See also Parkinson's disease)

Both propranolol (Inderal), usually in doses of 40 to 160 mg/day, and primidone (Mysoline), usually in doses of 125 to 250 mg bid, are effective in about 70% of patients.[1] Other beta-blockers such as timolol (Blocadren) or sotalol (Sotacor) may be used instead of propranolol. If a patient does not respond to one beta-blocker, trying another is often worthwhile.

REFERENCES

1. Martin WR: Investigating the source of tremors, *Can J Diagn,* September 1993, 10:51-59.

COMMUNITY HEALTH

Topics covered in this section

PERIODIC HEALTH EXAMINATION

(See also attitudes, physician; prevention; skepticism; screening)

Three organizations in the forefront of making recommendations about the periodic health examination are the Canadian Task Force on the Periodic Health Examination (CTF),[1] the U.S. Preventive Services Task Force (USTF),[2] and the American College of Physicians (ACP).[3]

Evidence for inclusion or exclusion from the periodic health examination as determined by the Canadian Task Force on the Periodic Health Examination and the U.S. Preventive Services Task Force is classified as follows:

A. There is good evidence to include.
B. There is fair evidence to include.

C. There is poor evidence to include.
D. There is fair evidence to exclude.
E. There is good evidence to exclude.

Examples of "A" and "B" recommendations for the general population from both the Canadian Task Force on the Periodic Health Examination and the U.S. Preventive Services Task Force are smoking cessation, folic acid for women at risk of pregnancy, fluoride to prevent dental caries, mammography for women 50 to 69 years of age, and age-appropriate routine immunizations. Examples of "D" and "E" recommendations are periodic chest x-ray examination to detect lung cancer, prostate specific antigen (PSA) screening of men over 50 to detect prostate cancer, pelvic examination to detect ovarian cancer, and urine dipstick examination to detect bladder cancer. The largest category is "C" and includes items such as mammography for women 40 to 49 years of age, screening of blood or urine for non-insulin-dependent diabetes mellitus, and tonometry or funduscopy to detect glaucoma.[1,2]

REFERENCES

1. Canadian Task Force on the Periodic Health Examination: *Clinical preventive health care,* Ottawa, 1994, Canadian Communication Group—Publishing.
2. US Preventive Services Task Force: *Guide to clinical preventive services,* ed 2, Baltimore, 1996, Williams & Wilkins.
3. Eddy DM, editor: *Common screening tests,* Philadelphia, 1991, American College of Physicians.

PRACTICE PATTERNS

(See also attitudes, physician; consultations; coronary artery bypass grafting; detrimental effects of investigations; cholecystectomy; lumpectomy; performance reports; prescribing habits and the elderly; prevention; secondary prevention of myocardial infarction; radical prostatectomy)

Variations in Medical Practice

Variations in medical practice patterns are common. Several examples are discussed in the ensuing paragraphs.

Variations in local resection for breast cancer

Local resection (breast-conserving surgery) plus radiation therapy is as effective as mastectomy for node-negative breast cancer.[1-5] The main exceptions are multiple tumors or a tumor of such a nature, usually because of its size, that local removal would result in unacceptable cosmetic results.[1] Despite this, mastectomy continues to be a widely practiced procedure. The frequency with which it is performed varies considerably from one geographical region to another.[1-4] A review of more than 500 U.S. hospitals found that only 15% of women with breast cancer were treated with breast-conserving surgery.[3] The rates of local resection are higher in Canada than in the United States, but the rates vary among provinces; in British Columbia they were 44%, while in Ontario they were 68%.[2] Numerous factors are used to explain different treatment modalities in different locations, including accessibility of radiation therapy facilities, patients' preferences, and preferences of the attending surgeons. In general, university-affiliated surgeons perform more breast-conserving operations.[2,3]

Variations in invasive cardiac procedures following myocardial infarctions

An international study involving two Canadian and three U.S. centers concluded that 1 year after a myocardial infarction (MI), Canadian patients had more cardiac symptoms and worse functional status than did those in the United States. This correlated with more visits to specialists, more coronary angiographies, more coronary angioplasties, and more coronary bypass surgery in the U.S. cohort than in the Canadian cohort. The authors suggest that the more aggressive pattern of care in the United States may be responsible for a slightly better quality of life after an MI.[6]

A 1997 report of nearly a quarter of a million elderly Americans and nearly 10,000 elderly Ontario residents, all of whom had suffered an initial MI, found a slightly lower 30-day mortality rate in the American cohort but no differences in mortality between the two groups at 1 year. In this study the rates of interventions for Americans versus Canadians were angiography 35% versus 7%, percutaneous transluminal coronary angioplasty 12% versus 2%, and coronary artery bypass surgery 11% versus 1%.[7] Several other studies have failed to find any correlation between the numbers of invasive cardiac procedures performed in the management of MI and mortality rates.[8-12]

Within the United States itself the rates of invasive interventions after MI vary widely.[10,11] An enthusiasm for diagnostic testing may be an important cause of invasive cardiac procedures; positive stress tests lead to more angiograms, which in turn lead to more revascularization procedures.[12]

Variations in medical care after myocardial infarctions

Drugs of proven value after an MI, such as beta-blockers, angiotensin-coverting enzyme (ACE) inhibitors, and nitrates, are prescribed more frequently in New England than in other regions of the United States.[10]

Variations in psychiatric care

A larger proportion of the U.S. population receives outpatient psychiatric care than is the case in the province of Ontario, Canada. However, the proportion of patients with moderate to severe psychiatric illnesses in the United States who are treated as outpatients is lower than in Ontario.[13,14]

Variations in rates of radical prostatectomy

It has been estimated that in 1989 a white male from Seattle had a 6.4% chance of having a radical prostatectomy by the time he was 75, whereas the odds of this happening in Connecticut was only 1.3%.[15] This is a fivefold difference.

Community Health

Causes of variability in practice patterns

The probable reason for the marked variability in practice patterns from one region to another is that the norms of the local medical milieu have a more powerful influence on the behavior of individual physicians than does the national and international medical literature or national and international meetings. According to Greer,[16] change within a particular milieu frequently depends on a sequence of events, especially if the innovation is in some ways controversial. Often a "local innovator" enthusiastically adopts a new technology, but this in itself is not enough. A local "opinion leader" usually has to endorse and support the change, experts in the technology have to be available in the local community to teach its application, and finally a "consensus" that it is desirable has to develop among the local physicians.

Medical Specialists

In the 1990s subspecialists accounted for 70% of physicians in the United States.[17] There are suggestions that health indices and patient satisfaction are inversely related to the number of subspecialists in a country. This certainly seems to be the case for Germany and the United States, both of which have highly subspecialized medical care.[18] Cost is another issue that seems to be related to degree of specialization. A comparison of Sweden and Norway found that health indices were almost identical in the two countries, but that Sweden, which is more specialty oriented, had 14 hospital beds per 1000 population compared with Norway's 6.5 per 1000, and that Sweden spent 9.4% of its gross national product on health care versus 6.5% for Norway.[19]

Although the preceding data certainly suggest that having too many specialists is undesirable, another aspect of the issue is the quality of care administered. As yet no clear answer to that is available, but there are suggestions that in some areas of practice specialists may do a better job.[6,20-22] A Canadian-U.S. comparison of post-MI patients concludes that specialty care and aggressive interventions in the United States probably resulted in a better quality of life 1 year after the infarct,[6] another study showed that cardiologists' knowledge of several key aspects of MI management was superior to that of either general internists or family physicians,[21] and a third found that patients with MI admitted by primary care physicians had a 12% higher mortality after 1 year than those admitted by cardiologists.[22] The better outcomes in the last study correlated with more investigations, more medications, and more therapeutic procedures among the patients treated by cardiologists.[22] A cross-sectional study of patients with asthma indicated that the quality of life was better for patients treated by allergists than for those treated by general internists, pediatricians, or family physicians. In part this correlated with a greater use of steroids by patients seeing allergists.[23]

Another important aspect of the issue of specialists versus generalists is the expectations of patients. A view expressed by two U.S. residents in specialty training is that patients with knee injuries do not want to see family physicians or even general orthopedists, but rather orthopedists with subspecialty practices in arthroscopy, and that patients with earaches want to see otolaryngologists, not primary care physicians.[24]

REFERENCES

1. Starreveld A: A surgical subculture: the use of mastectomy to treat breast cancer (editorial), *Can Med Assoc J* 156:43-45, 1997.
2. Goel V, Olivotto I, Hislop TG, et al: Patterns of initial management of node-negative breast cancer in two Canadian provinces, *Can Med Assoc J* 156:25-35, 1997.
3. Johantgen ME, Coffey RM, Harris DR, et al: Treating early-stage breast cancer: hospital characteristics associated with breast-conserving surgery, *Am J Public Health* 85:1432-1434, 1995.
4. Margolese R: Surgical considerations in selecting local therapy, *J Natl Cancer Inst Monogr* 11:41-48, 1992.
5. Jacobson JA, Danforth DN, Cowan KH, et al: Ten-year results of a comparison of conservation with mastectomy in the treatment of stage I and II breast cancer, *N Engl J Med* 332:907-911, 1995.
6. Mark DB, Naylor CD, Phil D, et al: Use of medical resources and quality of life after acute myocardial infarction in Canada and the United States, *N Engl J Med* 331:1130-1135, 1994.
7. Tu JV, Pashos CL, Naylor D, et al: Use of cardiac procedures and outcomes in elderly patients with myocardial infarction in the United States and Canada, *N Engl J Med* 336:1500-1505, 1997.
8. Van de Werf F, Topol EJ, Lee KL, et al: Variations in patient management and outcomes for acute myocardial infarction in the United States and other countries: results from the GUSTO Trial, *JAMA* 273:1586-1591, 1995.
9. Every NR, Parsons LS, Hlatky M, et al (Myocardial Infarction Triage and Intervention Investigators): A comparison of thrombolytic therapy with primary coronary angioplasty for acute myocardial infarction, *N Engl J Med* 335:1253-1260, 1996.
10. Pilote L, Califf RM, Sapp S, et al: Regional variation across the United States in the management of acute myocardial infarction, *N Engl J Med* 333:565-572, 1995.
11. Guadagnoli E, Hauptman PJ, Ayanian JZ, et al: Variation in the use of cardiac procedures after acute myocardial infarction, *N Engl J Med* 333:573-578, 1995.
12. Wennberg DE, Kellett MA, Dickens JD Jr, et al: The association between local diagnostic testing intensity and invasive cardiac procedures, *JAMA* 275:1161-1164, 1996.
13. Kessler RC, Frank RG, Edlund M, et al: Differences in the use of psychiatric outpatient services between the United States and Ontario, *N Engl J Med* 336:551-557, 1997.
14. Michels R: Improving outpatient psychiatric care (editorial), *N Engl J Med* 336:578-579, 1997.
15. Lu-Yao GL, McLerran D, Wasson J, et al (Patient Outcomes Research Team): An assessment of radical prostatectomy: time trends, geographic variation, and outcomes, *JAMA* 269:2633-2636, 1993.
16. Greer AL: The state of the art versus the state of the science: the diffusion of new medical technologies into practice, *Int J Technol Assessment Health Care* 4:5-26, 1988.

17. Rivo ML, Satcher D: Improving access to health care through physician workforce reform: direction for the 21st century, *JAMA* 270:1074-1078, 1993.
18. Starfield B: Primary care and health: a cross-national comparison, *JAMA* 266:2268-2271, 1991.
19. Agdestein S, Roemer MI: Good health at a modest price: the fruit of primary care, *J Public Health Policy* 13:485-490, 1992.
20. Kassirer JP: Access to specialty care (editorial), *N Engl J Med* 331:1151-1153, 1994.
21. Ayanian JZ, Hauptman PJ, Guadagnoli E, et al: Knowledge and practices of generalist and specialist physicians regarding drug therapy for acute myocardial infarction, *N Engl J Med* 331: 1136-1142, 1994.
22. Jollis JG, DeLong ER, Peterson ED, et al: Outcome of acute myocardial infarction according to the specialty of the admitting physician, *N Engl J Med* 335:1880-1887, 1996.
23. Vollmer WM, O'Hollaren M, Ettinger KM, et al: Specialty differences in the management of asthma: a cross-sectional assessment of allergists' patients and generalists' patients in a large HMO, *Arch Intern Med* 157:1201-1208, 1997.
24. Whyte JJ, Beall DP: A physician's freedom to choose, *JAMA* 273:1303, 1995.

PREVENTION

(See also detrimental effects of investigations; informed consent; informed consent for digital rectal examination and prostate specific antigen screening for prostate cancer; methods of reporting benefits of clinical trials; screening; labeling as ill person; patient education; psychological consequences of abnormal Papanicolaou smears; wellness)

Before participating in a preventive program, patients and their physicians should be able to answer the following questions[1]:

1. Are there any proven benefits?
2. If so, how great are they?
3. Are there potential adverse effects?
4. If so, what are they, how serious are they, and how frequently do they occur?

Some preventive programs such as accident prevention, avoidance of high-risk behavior, and selection of healthy life-style choices have virtually no adverse consequences. Even if the benefits have not been proved, there seems little harm in participating in such endeavors. On the other hand, preventive programs that involve screening for disease, classification of individuals into high- or low-risk categories for certain diseases, dietary interventions, or prophylactic drug regimens often have uncertain benefits and may have significant adverse consequences.[1]

Reporting methods of the benefits of preventive programs may have a profound influence on whether preventive programs appear useful.[1] The standard reporting methods are as follows[1]:

1. Relative reduction of morbidity or mortality rates
2. Absolute reduction of morbidity or mortality rates
3. Number of patients who need to be treated to prevent one adverse event
4. Total cohort mortality rates

Reporting methods for benefits are discussed in more detail in the section on statistics under "Methods of Reporting Benefits of Clinical Trials." The essential clinical point is that relative reduction rates tend to exaggerate the benefits greatly and should never be used to make decisions about the clinical usefulness of a program.[1]

The clinical significance of the benefits of preventive programs may be misconstrued in numerous other ways, including these[2]:

1. Surrogate rather than clinically significant outcomes are used (e.g., more "small" cancers are found, rather than decreased mortality rates).
2. The risk level or disease prevalence of the population involved is not considered (e.g., lipid-lowering drugs are more effective for patients with proven coronary disease than for asymptomatic persons).
3. The interval between the intervention and the benefit is not considered (e.g., if a decrease in prostate cancer death rates is ever proved to occur as a result of PSA screening, this benefit will not be evident until 10 years after radical prostatectomy).
4. The duration of the intervention required to achieve the benefit is not considered (e.g., hormone replacement therapy must be given for several decades to prevent hip fractures).
5. One benefit may be overshadowed by another (e.g., the value of exercise in the prevention of coronary artery disease and fractures may be deemphasized by the promotion of hormone replacement therapy for the same purpose).
6. The benefits shown for one variant of a disease are inappropriately applied to another (e.g., the unwarranted assumption may be made that very tight control of NIDDM will result in decreased morbidity because fewer microvascular complications in IDDM have been proved to occur in patients subjected to intensive insulin therapy).
7. Benefits documented in clinical trials are assumed to occur in clinical practice (in many instances this is not the case because the populations are different or compliance is less stringent).
8. There is publication bias (positive results of preventive interventions are more often published than are negative results).
9. Studies showing positive results are preferentially cited (authors may cite positive studies more often than negative ones).
10. False negative results are present (if a study has inadequate power, a true beneficial result may not be shown—type II error).

All preventive screening or case-finding programs have the potential for causing harm.[3] In general, the degree of harm increases with each level of the "screening cascade." Harm is least for the initial level, which is the screening process itself, intermediate for the second level, which is the investigation

Community Health

of abnormal screening results, and greatest for the third level, which is the treatment of identified disorders.[3] The types of harm induced may be physical such as breast pain from compression during mammography or syncope from a venipuncture at level 1 of the screening cascade, urinary tract infection from prostate biopsy or perforated colon from colonoscopy at level 2, and impotence or death as a result of radical prostatectomy or the precipitation of an eating disorder as a result of dietary therapy at level 3.[3] The psychological and social harm of preventive programs may be categorized as follows[3]:

1. Anticipated discomfort or perception of adverse effects resulting from preventive interventions
2. Unpleasant interactions with health care workers
3. Time required for preventive programs
4. Excessive overall awareness of health
5. Anxiety while anticipating the results of a screening test
6. Anxiety induced by a positive screening test result
7. Distress from being labeled as "sick" or at "high risk"
8. Psychopathological effects directly induced by a therapeutic program (such as strict dieting)
9. False assurance of disease-free status as a result of a negative screening test

An important aspect of preventive screening programs is the issue of informed consent.[4] Since the benefits of such programs are often small or uncertain, and since they all place the patient at risk of harm, informed consent should be a prerequisite for participation. Unfortunately, implementing this is difficult because of physicians' lack of knowledge, patients' problems assimilating data, and lack of time for the process to unfold. Suggested ways around this are for physicians to base their recommendations, whenever possible, on evidence-based guidelines, such as those put forward by the Canadian Task Force on the Periodic Health Examination and the U.S. Preventive Services Task Force, and never to promote a preventive program on the basis of relative reduction of morbidity rates. Patient information material should be used whenever it is available in a balanced form.[4]

Once a preventive intervention is determined to be worthwhile, what are the logistics of implementing such a program in a physician's office setting? In 1994, kits for prevention based on the recommendations of the U.S. Preventive Services Task Force became available for family physicians through the American Academy of Family Practice. These "Put Prevention into Practice" (PPIP) kits contain, among other items, child and adult educational booklets for patients, a summary of recommended preventive services for physicians, pediatric and adult flow sheets, patient record alert stickers, and wall posters. McVea and associates[5] from the University of Nebraska surveyed eight midwestern practices that were interested enough in prevention to have requested these kits. They found that even though all the clinicians were enthusiastic about and reasonably knowledgeable about prevention, none of them used the kits. The reasons depended entirely on the efficiency or lack of efficiency of their office organizational systems. Those offices that did not already have an organized system could not integrate the material into their routines. On the other hand, well-organized offices already had preventive interventions integrated into their programs and had no need of the PIPP kits. A huge benefit of well-organized offices was that clinicians had time for preventive interventions even with caseloads of up to 50 patients a day. In contrast, one physician with a disorganized practice saw about 20 patients a day, was constantly rushed, and had little time for preventive interactions.

Specific aspects of prevention are covered in many sections of the text, and these can be located by looking up prevention and its many subheadings in the index.

REFERENCES

1. Marshall KG: Prevention. How much harm? How much benefit? 1. Influence of reporting methods on perception of benefits, *Can Med Assoc J* 154:1493-1499, 1996.
2. Marshall KG: Prevention. How much harm? How much benefit? 2. Ten potential pitfalls in determining the clinical significance of benefits, *Can Med Assoc J* 154:1837-1843, 1996.
3. Marshall KG: Prevention. How much harm? How much benefit? 3. Physical, psychological and social harm, *Can Med Assoc J* 155:169-176, 1996.
4. Marshall KG: Prevention. How much harm? How much benefit? 4. The ethics of informed consent for preventive screening programs, *Can Med Assoc J* 155:377-383, 1996.
5. McVea K: Crabtree BF, Medder JD, et al: An ounce of prevention? Evaluation of the "Put Prevention into Practice" program, *J Family Pract* 43:361-369, 1996.

Behavioral Changes for Prevention

Behavioral or life-style change is an essential aspect of many preventive programs, but as everyone knows, this is an extraordinarily difficult undertaking for patients and physicians. Understanding why we behave as we do facilitates approaches to change. Six stages of change have been defined by Dr. James Prochaska. By identifying and understanding them, physicians can direct their interventions toward patients' current levels with the goal of helping them move to the next level. This process takes time, and a reasonable goal is to advance from one stage to another at monthly intervals. The stages are as follows[1]:

1. Precontemplation. Patients are not prepared to change, often feel that they are unable to do so, and may rationalize this by concluding that the cons outweigh the pros. Interventions that can be used at this stage include:
   a. Fully informing patients of the risks of their current behavior (e.g., smoking, sedentary life-style)
   b. Using life events, such as the death of a friend from an illness related to the same high-risk behavior, or the unhappiness of spouses or children with the behavior as reasons for contemplating change
   c. Pointing out the benefits of change not only to themselves, but to their social environment (e.g., less risk that their children will smoke if they quit)

2. Contemplation. Patients in this stage are seriously considering changing their behavior within the next 2 to 6 months but not within the next month. Interventions that may be used here often involve suggesting short-term, limited trials of change. Giving two or three choices, such as delaying the first cigarette of the morning by 30 minutes, cutting the daily consumption by five cigarettes, or refraining from smoking for 24 hours, often gives patients a feeling of empowerment and confidence that they can move on to a more permanent program.
3. Preparation. Patients in this stage generally have a plan that they expect to implement within 1 month. Their major fear is that they may fail. Interventions include helping them formalize the details of the plan and supporting their self-confidence.
4. Action. Most of the published literature on life-style changes deals with this stage. This is the point at which nicotine patches are given or serious dieting or regular exercise begins. This phase usually takes 6 months, and relapses are frequent if patients let down their guard after just 2 or 3 months. One of the more important therapeutic interventions in this stage is frequent positive reinforcement for a job well done. As many social supports as possible should be mobilized, which includes telling a lot of people what one is trying to accomplish.
5. Maintenance. For most programs such as smoking cessation it takes at least 5 years before the risk of relapse becomes relatively low. Vigilance is required throughout the maintenance period. Continuing social supports should be mobilized.
6. Termination. Termination is a theoretical stage in which there is no risk of relapse. Some achieve it, but for most, prolonged maintenance is a more realistic goal.

REFERENCES

1. Prochaska JO: Why do we behave the way we do? *Can J Cardiol* 11(suppl A):20A-25A, 1995.

Bicycle Helmets

(See also motor vehicle accidents)

Head injuries cause 75% of bicycle-related deaths.[1,2] In one case-control study, bicycle helmets were shown to reduce the risk of head injury by 85% and the risk of brain injury by 88%[3]; in a second to reduce head injuries by 69%, brain injuries by 65%, and severe brain injuries by 74%[4]; and in a third to reduce head injuries by 63% and loss of consciousness by 86%.[5] In a Canadian study of deaths from bicycle-related injuries in Ontario between 1986 and 1991, 75% of the deaths were due to head injuries but only 4% of those killed were wearing bicycle helmets.[2] In this study 91% of deaths were the result of collisions with motor vehicles, males outnumbered females 3.5:1, and the risk of being killed was four times greater at night than during the day.[2] In Victoria, Australia, mandatory bicycle helmet use was associated with a 51% decrease in the number of cyclists killed or hospitalized with head injuries.[6] A case-control study has also shown that helmets protect against upper face and midface injuries.[7]

All types of helmets (soft shelled as well as hard shelled, although evidence suggests that the latter are better) are protective, and this applies to all age groups.[5] Children under 6 years of age do not require a different type of helmet.[5]

An argument given against mandatory use of bicycle helmets is that fewer people might bicycle and therefore fewer people would gain the health benefits of that activity.[8] Several letters to the editor published in the *British Medical Journal*[9-11] and *JAMA*[12,13] suggest that this has happened in Australian states where such laws have been enacted. In fact, the decrease in bicycle usage reported there was mainly in teenagers while adult bicycling actually increased.[6,14]

Making either individual or public health policy decisions on the basis of letters to the editor would be inappropriate. The peer-reviewed literature firmly supports the use of bicycle helmets as a protection against serious injury, and no solid evidence has been presented that mandatory helmet use decreases bicycle use.

REFERENCES

1. Friede AM, Azzara CV, Gallagher SS, et al: The epidemiology of injuries to bicycle riders, *Pediatr Clin North Am* 32:141-151, 1985.
2. Rowe BH, Rowe AM, Bota GW: Bicyclist and environmental factors associated with fatal bicycle-related trauma in Ontario, *Can Med Assoc J* 152:45-53, 1995.
3. Thompson RS, Rivara FP, Thompson DC: A case-control study of the effectiveness of bicycle safety helmets, *N Engl J Med* 320:1361-1367, 1989.
4. Thompson DC, Rivara FP, Thompson RS: Effectiveness of bicycle safety helmets in preventing head injuries: a case-control study, *JAMA* 276:1968-1973, 1996.
5. Thomas S, Acton C, Nixon J, et al: Effectiveness of bicycle helmets in preventing head injury in children: case-control study, *BMJ* 308:173-176, 1994.
6. Centers for Disease Control and Prevention: Mandatory bicycle helmet use—Victoria, Australia, *JAMA* 269(23):2967, 1993.
7. Thompson DC, Nunn ME, Thompson RS, et al: Effectiveness of bicycle safety helmets in preventing serious facial injury, *JAMA* 276:1974-1975, 1996.
8. DeMarco T: Helmet legislation could decrease cycling (letter), *Can Family Physician* 40:1703-1704, 1994.
9. Davis A: Cyclists should wear helmets: increasing the number of cyclists is more important (letter), *BMJ* 314:69, 1997.
10. Robinson DL: Cyclists should wear helmets: Australian laws making helmets compulsory deterred people from cycling (letter), *BMJ* 314:69-70, 1997.
11. Hillman M: Cyclists should wear helmets: health benefits of cycling greatly outweigh loss of life years from deaths (letter), *BMJ* 314:70, 1997.
12. Bayliss J: Do bicycle helmets protect, and should they be mandatory? (letter), *JAMA* 277:883, 1997.
13. Goldman D: Do bicycle helmets protect, and should they be mandatory? (letter), *JAMA* 277-278:883-884, 1997.

14. Thompson DC, Thompson RS: Do bicycle helmets protect, and should they be mandatory? (in reply to letters), *JAMA* 884:277-278, 1997.

Causes of Preventable Deaths in the United States

Any public health policy must be based in part on the frequency of occurrence of the disorders the policy aims to prevent. One estimate is that 19% of U.S. deaths could be prevented or delayed by cessation of smoking, 14% by exercise and diet, and 5% by abstention from excessive alcohol intake.[1]

REFERENCES

1. McGinnis JM, Foege WH: Actual causes of death in the United States, *JAMA* 270:2207-2212, 1993.

Guns

(See also adverse effects associated with low cholesterol levels; homicide; suicide)

In 1994 guns were owned by 33% of urban, 39% of suburban, and 60% of rural U.S. households, and pistols made up more than 50% of the weapons in each category. Gun ownership is highest in southern and Rocky Mountain states. More guns are owned by men than women, whites than blacks, Republicans than Democrats, and persons whose parents owned a gun than those whose parents did not.[1] According to some studies there is a threefold increase in homicides[2] and a threefold[3] to fivefold[4] increase in suicides in homes where guns are kept. Accidental shootings, which are usually self-inflicted by young men, are also a common sequel of gun ownership.[5]

Guns have not proved to be protective in cases of homicides associated with forced entry[2] and indeed are far more likely to kill a family member than an intruder.[6] According to one study, family members are 18 times more likely to be killed by firearms kept in the home than are intruders.[7] The sheer number, easy accessibility, and lethality of guns probably account for the climbing death rate from firearms in the United States. In cases of assault, guns are three times as likely to kill as knives and 23 times as likely to kill as other weapons.[8]

An analysis of the type of gun used in firearm-related homicides and suicides in Milwaukee, Wisconsin, between 1991 and 1994 found that handguns accounted for 89% of the homicides and 71% of the suicides.[9]

According to 1989 U.S. data, firearms accounted for 11% of childhood deaths, 17% of deaths among adolescents aged 15 to 19, and 41% of deaths of black males aged 15 to 19.[10] Many high school students take guns to school. A Seattle survey found that 6% of the students had brought a handgun to school at least once,[11] and in Illinois a third of students had done so.[12] A survey of predominantly Hispanic adolescents in three New York City schools found that 21% carried a weapon to school and 42% reported having had a relative or close friend who was shot.[13]

Adequate storage of guns in the home requires that they be unloaded and locked. A survey of parents of children in 29 urban, suburban, and rural pediatric practices from across the United States found that a third of families reported owning at least one gun. Of gun-owning families, 61% had at least one unlocked gun and 15% had at least one loaded gun. Only 30% kept all guns unloaded and locked.[14] An Oregon survey found that 6.2% of households with children contained loaded, unlocked firearms.[15]

REFERENCES

1. Blendon RJ, Young JT, Hemenway D: The American public and the gun control debate, *JAMA* 275:1719-1722, 1996.
2. Kellermann AL, Rivara FP, Rushforth NB, et al: Gun ownership as a risk factor for homicide in the home, *N Engl J Med* 329:1084-1091, 1993.
3. Sloan JH, Rivara FP, Reay DT, et al: Firearm regulations and rates of suicide: a comparison of two metropolitan areas, *N Engl J Med* 322:369-373, 1990.
4. Kellermann AL, Rivara FP, Somes G, et al: Suicide in the home in relation with gun ownership, *N Engl J Med* 327:467-472, 1992.
5. Sinauer N, Annest JL, Mercy JA: Unintentional, nonfatal firearm-related injuries, *JAMA* 275:1740-1743, 1996.
6. Webster DW, Chaulk CP, Teret SP, et al: Reducing firearm injuries, *Issues Sci Technol* 7:73-79. 1991.
7. Kellermann AL, Reay DT: Protection or peril? An analysis of firearm-related deaths in the home, *N Engl J Med* 314:1557-1560, 1986.
8. Saltzman LE, Mercy JA, O'Carroll PW, et al: Weapon involvement and injury outcomes in family and intimate assaults, *JAMA* 267:3043-3047, 1992.
9. Hargarten SW, Karison TA, O'Brien M, et al: Characteristics of firearms involved in fatalities, *JAMA* 275:42-45, 1996.
10. Fingerhut LA, Kleinman FC: *Firearm mortality among children and youth: advance data from Vital and Health Statistics No 178,* Hyattsville, Md, 1989, National Center for Health Statistics, US Dept of Health and Human Services pub no PHS 90-1250.
11. Callahan CM, Rivara FP: Urban high school youth and handguns: a school-based survey, *JAMA* 267:3038-3042, 1992.
12. Koop CE, Lundberg GB: Violence in America: a public health emergency; time to bite the bullet back (editorial), *JAMA* 267:3075-3076, 1992. [Published errata appear in *JAMA* 268:3074, 1992, and 271:1404, 1994.]
13. Vaughan RD, Mccarthy JF, Armstrong B, et al: Carrying and using weapons—a survey of minority junior high school students in New York City, *Am J Public Health* 86:568-572, 1996.
14. Senturia YD, Christoffel KK, Donovan M (Pediatric Practice Research Group): Gun storage patterns in US homes with children, *Arch Pediatr Adolesc Med* 150:265-269, 1996.
15. Nelson DE, Grant-Worley JA, Powell K, et al: Population estimates of household firearm storage practices and firearm carrying in Oregon, *JAMA* 275:1744-1748, 1996.

Homicide

(See also abuse; adverse effects associated with low cholesterol levels; cocaine; guns; poverty; suicide)

In the United States homicide is the eleventh leading cause of death in all age groups, the second leading cause among 15- to 24-year-olds, and the leading cause among black males aged 15 to 34. Homicides in homes are perpetrated by relatives or acquaintances in 76.7% of cases and by strangers in only 3.6% of cases. In 17.4% of cases the perpetrator is unknown. In homes 50% of killings are with guns and 25% with knives or sharp instruments. The presence of a gun in the home is an independent risk factor for homicide, along with the use of illicit drugs and a history of physical abuse.[1] Users of alcohol and illicit drugs are at increased risk of being murdered, as are nonusers of these agents who live in the same house as alcohol or drug abusers.[2]

Studies in both Atlanta, Georgia,[3] and New Orleans, Louisiana,[4] have shown that the domestic homicide rate among blacks was six times greater than among whites. However, when the white and black populations were stratified in terms of household crowding (a measure of socioeconomic status), there was no difference in the homicide rates; the underlying cause seems to be poverty.[3,4]

REFERENCES

1. Kellermann AL, Rivara FP, Rushforth NB, et al: Gun ownership as a risk factor for homicide in the home, *N Engl J Med* 329: 1084-1091, 1993.
2. Rivara FP, Mueller BA, Somes G, et al: Alcohol and illicit drug abuse and the risk of violent death in the home, *JAMA* 278:569-575, 1997.
3. Centerwall BS: Race, socioeconomic status, and domestic homicide, Atlanta, 1971-72, *Am J Public Health* 74:813-815, 1984.
4. Centerwall BS: Race, socioeconomic status, and domestic homicide, *JAMA* 273:1755-1758, 1995.

In-Line Skating

Elbow and wrist guards have been shown to decrease injuries to the elbows and wrists in in-line skaters. Data documenting the efficacy of helmets in this sport are not yet available.[1]

REFERENCES

1. Schieber RA, Branche-Dorsey CM, Ryan GW, et al: Risk factors for injuries from in-line skating and the effectiveness of safety gear, *N Engl J Med* 335:1630-1635, 1996.

Motor Vehicle Accidents

(See also alcohol; bicycle helmets; cocaine; prescriptions for elderly; whiplash injury)

Air bags

The safety and efficacy of air bags have been well documented.[1] However, a number of childhood fatalities have been reported to result from air bag deployment when the child was sitting in the front passenger seat, particularly if the child was unrestrained or in a rear-facing child safety seat.[2,3] Current recommendations are that children in rear-facing safety seats should never be in the front seat, that whenever possible children should be in the back seat, and that if the vehicle has no back seat, the front seat where the child is sitting should be pushed as far back as possible.[2,3]

Seat belts and car seats

The American Academy of Pediatrics has made a number of recommendations about infant and child car seats and the use of seat belts. Some of these are[4]:

1. No matter what the age, rear seats are safer than front seats.
2. All infants should be in a backward-facing seat strapped into the back seat until they are 1 year of age and weigh 20 lb (9 kg). Such seats should never be placed in the front passenger seat. The shoulder straps in rear-facing seats should be in the lowest slots until the child's growth places the shoulders above that slot. If because of the tilt of the car seat the infant's head flops forward, a rolled towel or newspaper should be placed under the depressed edge of the seat to raise it sufficiently that the infant's head rests against the back of the seat.
3. Children between 20 lb (9 kg) and 40 lb (18 kg) should be placed in a forward-facing child seat that is fastened into the back seat.
4. Once the child surpasses 40 lb (18 kg), a belt-positioning booster with lap and shoulder belts may be used.
5. Once the child surpasses 50 lb (23 kg), regular seating using seat belts is acceptable. Ideally the child should be in the back seat, but if he or she is in the front passenger seat, the seat should be pushed as far back as possible to avoid injury if the air bag deploys.

Head restraints

Evidence indicates that in rear-end collisions head restraints are useful.[5] The head rest should be adjusted so it reaches at least as high as the midocciput. The horizontal distance of the head rest from the occiput should be 2.5 to 10 cm.

Alcohol

In the United States, motor vehicle accidents are the leading cause of death of all ages from 1 to 34, and slightly less than half of these fatal accidents are alcohol related. The cutoff point for blood alcohol levels in determining the above statistics is $\geq$0.10 g/dl ($\geq$100 mg/dl). This level is used because in the general population the risk of a motor vehicle accident has been shown to be much greater when this level is reached than at lower blood alcohol levels.[6,7] This should not be construed as implying that lower levels are risk free because they are not. The risk begins to increase at levels of 0.02 g/dl, increases significantly at 0.05 g/dl, and increases rapidly at levels over 0.1 g/dl.[7]

Drivers 16 to 24 years of age are five times as likely to be involved in alcohol-related driving fatalities as drivers aged 35 to 64, and in many instances this increased risk occurs with very low levels of blood alcohol. The reasons are uncertain, but the "risk-taking" behavior of adolescents coupled with inexperience is thought to be the major factor. It is also probable that less alcohol is required to impair adolescents than older drivers.[8]

One study has shown that arrests for drunk driving correlate with an increased risk of death from an alcohol-related crash.[9]

Breathalyzers were developed in 1954, but small portable models did not become available until the early 1960s. One of the medicolegal problems with these devices is that they require the patient to blow into the device for a brief period. This has led to a number of court challenges in which individuals who had such conditions as asthma, chronic obstructive pulmonary disease, tracheostomy, or ankylosing spondylitis or who were experiencing severe emotional or physical distress have in some jurisdictions been considered to have reasonable excuses for not complying with police requests for breathalyzer tests.[10]

Sleep deprivation

Serious sleep deprivation is common among long-distance truck drivers, especially those who drive at night, and is responsible for numerous accidents.[11,12]

Geriatric drivers

Elderly people drive relatively few miles and tend to be law abiding. Therefore they account for a small proportion of total road accidents. On the other hand, on a per mile traveled basis the accident rate is higher than for younger individuals; by age 85 and over it is three times that of other drivers and is exceeded only by teenage drivers. Older drivers involved in accidents are more likely to be killed than are younger persons; those over 85 have the highest death rate per accident of any group.[13] Use of long-acting benzodiazepines is associated with an increased rate of motor vehicle accidents in the elderly.[14]

Motorcycles

The death rate for motorcyclists is 35 times greater than that of car occupants. Major injuries in motorcycle accidents are to the head and lower extremities. Helmets decrease fatal head injuries by 25%.[15]

REFERENCES

1. National Center for Statistics and Analysis, National Highway Traffic Safety Administration: *Traffic safety facts 1994: occupant protection,* Washington, DC, 1995, US Department of Transportation.
2. Centers for Disease Control and Prevention: Air-bag-associated fatal injuries to infants and children riding in front passenger seats—United States, *JAMA* 274:1752-1753, 1995.
3. Centers for Disease Control and Prevention: Update: fatal air bag-related injuries to children—United States, 1993-1996, *JAMA* 277:11-12, 1997.
4. Committee on Injury and Poison Prevention of the American Academy of Pediatrics: Selecting and using the most appropriate car safety seats for growing children: guidelines for counseling parents, *Pediatrics* 97:761-763, 1996.
5. Spitzer WO, Rachid S, Skovron ML, et al: Redéfinir le "whiplash" et sa prise en charge, *Médecin du Québec,* May 1995, supplement.
6. Update: Alcohol-related traffic fatalities—United States, 1982-1993, *MMWR* 43:861-867, 1994.
7. Madden C, Cole TB: Emergency intervention to break the cycle of drunken driving and recurrent injury, *Ann Emerg Med* 26:177-179, 1995.
8. Augustyn M, Simons-Morton BG: Adolescent drinking and driving: etiology and interpretation, *J Drug Educ* 25:41-59, 1995.
9. Brewer RD, Morris PD, Cole TB, et al: The risk of dying in alcohol-related automobile crashes among habitual drunk drivers, *N Engl J Med* 331:513-517, 1994.
10. Marks P: Drink driving legislation: medicine and the law, *Medico-Legal J* 63:119-127, 1995.
11. Mitler MM, Miller JC, Lipsitz JJ, et al: The sleep of long-haul truck drivers, *N Engl J Med* 337:755-761, 1997.
12. Dement WC: The perils of drowsy driving (editorial), *N Engl J Med* 337:783-784, 1997.
13. Martinez R: Older drivers and physicians (editorial), *JAMA* 274:1060, 1995.
14. Hemmelgarn B, Suissa S, Huang A, et al: Benzodiazepine use and the risk of motor vehicle crash in the elderly, *JAMA* 278: 27-31, 1997.
15. Rivara FP, Grossman DC, Cummins P: Injury prevention [First of two parts], *N Engl J Med* 337:543-548, 1997.

Poverty

(See also homicide; medical economics; unemployment)

Within developed nations, poverty correlates with increased morbidity and mortality.[1-7] For example, the chance that an adolescent male in Harlem will live to be 65 has been shown to be 37%.[5] Causes of excess mortality among the poor vary from one region to another. The poor have an excess death rate from cardiovascular disease in all regions and from cancer in most. In certain urban areas HIV infection and homicides are the leading causes of death, while in others accidents top the list.[5]

Repeated studies have shown that in developed countries increases in mortality and morbidity correlate far more with relative poverty than with absolute poverty. The probable explanation is not simply lack of adequate housing or food, but rather high-risk behaviors such as smoking, excessive eating, and excessive drug and alcohol use. Societies with less income disparity tend to have more social cohesion and lower variances in mortality and morbidity rates among income groups.[7]

Loss of social cohesiveness is in part a result of a decrease in the number of neighborhoods shared by rich and poor as the wealthy escape to more affluent districts. The poor are left to deal not only with their own economic and social problems, but also with the problems inherent in living in

Statistical Techniques

If you are like me, your eyes glaze over when you run across a term such as statistical techniques. The bad news is that when we read the medical literature, we keep seeing such terms as *p* value, confidence intervals, type I error, type II error, and inadequate power, so to make sense of it we have to learn what they mean. The good news is that Guyatt and associates[1-4] from McMaster University have published in the *Canadian Medical Association Journal* a series of simple clear articles for the statistically illiterate.

Null hypothesis

Many studies involve comparing the efficacy of one treatment with another treatment or a placebo. One way of determining if there is a statistically significant difference between treatments is for the study authors to start out with the assumption that there will be no difference. This is called the null hypothesis. If the results clearly show that one treatment is superior to the other (see below), the null hypothesis is disproved.[1]

p Value

The *p* value is a way of recording probability. A *p* value of .01 is another way of saying that chance alone would account for the observed results in 1% of cases, while a *p* value of .05 means that chance alone would account for the results in 5% of cases.[1]

Statistical significance

A study result is said to be statistically significant if the odds are that chance alone is unlikely to account for the results. By convention the boundary between statistically significant and statistically insignificant is a *p* value of .05. Any *p* value of .05 or less is statistically significant.[1]

Type I error

A type I error is falsely concluding that an observed difference is due to the intervention being studied and not to chance alone. The lower the *p* value, the less likely that a type I error is present. However, with a *p* value of .05, any observed differences in results could be explained by chance alone in 5% of cases.[1]

Type II error

A type II error is falsely concluding that no difference exists between two treatment plans (or a treatment and a placebo) when actually there is a difference. This error may occur because the study had inadequate power (see below).[1]

Power

If a study fails to disprove the null hypothesis, one reason may be that too few subjects were in the study to allow a true difference to become apparent. If this is the case, the study is said to have inadequate power and a type II error has occurred. The larger the sample, the less likelihood of inadequate power and a resulting type II error.[1]

Multiple tests

When multiple independent tests or variables are assessed at the same time in any study, the odds that one of them will show a difference with a p value $\leq .05$ by chance alone increases with the number of variables assessed. If a single variable is assessed, the odds are 5%. If six variables are assessed, the odds are 26% (or 1 in 4), and for 10 variables they are 40%.[1]

In family medicine this problem is seen most frequently when a physician makes the mistake of ordering a batch of laboratory tests for a healthy person "just to make sure everything is all right." Ordering 10 tests is very easy, and if the physician does so, close to half the patients will have falsely abnormal results.

Point estimate

If a study comparing a drug with a placebo shows that 35% of patients taking the placebo died at 1 year whereas only 30% of those taking the drug died, the difference of 5% is called the point estimate. One way of determining whether this point estimate is statistically significant is to calculate confidence intervals (see below).[2]

Confidence intervals

The likelihood that the 5% difference in mortality rate described above under "Point Estimate" is due to chance rather than the drug being tested depends largely on the number of subjects assessed. If only 10 were in each group, the result might well be due to chance; if there were 1000, it might well be the beneficial effects of the drug. This type of probability calculation can be quantified to produce confidence intervals around the point estimation. The wider the confidence intervals, the greater the chance that the observed point estimate is a result of chance, and the narrower they are, the greater the chance that the point estimate is due to the intervention applied.[2]

Methods of Reporting the Benefits of Clinical Trials

The benefits of clinical studies are usually reported in one of four ways.[5] These are relative reduction of morbidity, absolute reduction of morbidity, numbers of patients who need treatment to prevent adverse events, and total cohort mortality. The meaning of these terms and their clinical significance are discussed in the ensuing paragraphs.

Relative reduction of risk

Relative reduction of risk or mortality is the percentage reduction of morbidity or mortality in a population that is subject to an intervention compared with a control population that is not subject to the intervention.[3] A mammographic trial might report a 35% reduction in death rate from breast cancer in the mammographically screened population, or a cholesterol-lowering drug trial might report a 45% decrease in myocardial infarction rate in the treated compared with the control population. The calculations of relative risk and relative risk reductions are simple.[3,5,6] For example, a mammographic study enrolled 10,000 women in the screened group and 10,000 women in the control group. If after 5 years six women in the control group had died of breast cancer and only four in the screened group had died of this disease, these figures could be presented as percentages. In the screened group 0.04% of women died of breast cancer, while in the control group 0.06% died. The relative risk of dying of breast cancer in this study is 0.04/0.06 × 100 or 66%. Put another way, the relative risk of dying of breast cancer if a woman had mammography is two thirds that of women who did not have mammography.

Still another way of looking at the figures given above is to determine the relative risk reduction. This is simply the reciprocal of the relative risk.[3] The relative risk in the screened population is 66%, so the relative reduction of risk has to be 34%. The latter figure is the one most often quoted in studies such as this. (Although the example given here is hypothetical, a 34% relative reduction of risk is fairly representative of figures reported from actual mammographic screening programs; see discussion of mammography).

A 34% relative reduction of risk of dying of breast cancer looks impressive. However, the clinical significance of such relative risk or mortality reductions may be deceiving because they are often quite unrelated to the magnitude of the actual numbers, a trap that many of us have fallen into on more than one occasion. It is the absolute figures, as well as the numbers of patients who must be screened or treated for one beneficial event to accrue, that are important.[5,6] These methods of reporting are discussed below.

Odds ratios

Odds ratios are the bane of many family physicians, including this one. They are useful for statisticians and confusing for clinicians. The odds ratio in the example of mammographic screening given above would be calculated as follows[3]:

Death rate in screened population	4	A
Survival rate in screened population	9,996	B
Death rate in unscreened population	6	C
Survival rate in unscreened population	9,994	D
Odds Ratio (A/C) / (B/D)	(4/6) / (9,994/9,996) = 0.6667.	

In this case the odds ratio and the relative reduction of mortality are virtually identical; this is common when dealing with rare events.

Absolute risk reduction

Absolute risk reduction or absolute mortality reduction is the actual morbidity rate or death rate of the screened population subtracted from the actual morbidity rate or death rate of the control population. An example from the hypothetical mammographic screening program described in the previous section might be as follows[3,5,6]:

We have already determined that after 5 years, 4 of 10,000 women in the screened group died of breast cancer, compared with 6 of 10,000 women in the unscreened control group. Expressed as percentages, these number are 0.04% and 0.06%. The absolute risk reduction (or mortality reduction) that can be attributed to screening is 0.06 to 0.04 or 0.02%.

The salient point for patients and physicians is that the small absolute risk reduction figure is far more important clinically than is the larger relative risk reduction figure.

Numbers of patients who must be screened[3,5,6]

If a screening procedure or a therapeutic intervention is undertaken with the object of preventing adverse effects, many of the individuals screened or treated will not benefit from the intervention.[5,6] This is well illustrated in the mammography screening example discussed previously. The relative mortality reduction rate was 34%, and the absolute mortality reduction 0.02%. The latter figure means that two lives were saved by screening 10,000 women over a 5-year period or, putting it another way, 5000 women would have to be screened by mammography to save one life. Although the example given here is theoretical, the figures used are quite close to those that have actually been reported (see discussion of mammography).

Disease prevalence or severity and risk reduction

An important association exists between the severity or prevalence of a disease and the absolute risk reduction or the number of patients who must be screened or treated to prevent one adverse effect. The greater the severity or prevalence of the disease, the higher the absolute risk reduction and the fewer patients who must be treated to prevent one adverse outcome.[6,7] We must be aware of this because the relative risk reduction does not necessarily vary with prevalence rates. The following examples are an illustration: One thousand high-risk patients have a disease of such lethality that 500 of them will die within 1 year without treatment. If a treatment is available that reduces the risk of death by 50% (relative risk reduction of 50%), only 250 will die, an absolute mortality reduction of 25%. Let us compare this with 1000 low-risk patients who have a disease that will kill two of them within 1 year without treatment. If the treatment reduces the risk of death by 50% (relative risk reduction of 50%), only one will die, an absolute reduction of 0.1%. The relative reduction rate is the same in both examples, but the clinical indications for treatment probably exist only in the former. These same figures can be presented as numbers of patients who must be treated to prevent one adverse event. In the high-risk group the number is 4, while in the low-risk group it is 1000.

If all of the above sounds theoretical, a real-life example from the field of commercial aviation can be used to illustrate the huge disparity that may be found between relative and absolute risk reduction figures. Since the introduction of the jet airliner in the 1960s, major commercial aviation accidents have decreased by 94.4%.[8] This imposing number is the relative reduction figure. The absolute reduction, however, is minuscule. Before 1960 the rate of major accidents was 45 per million departures, whereas by 1994 it was 2 per million departures. The difference between 45 accidents per million departures and 2 accidents per million departures is 43 accidents per million departures or 0.0043%. The reason that the absolute figures are so low is because flying on commercial airlines was extremely safe before the 1960s, even though it is safer now.

Effect of Benefit Reporting Methods on Decision Making of Physicians and Patients

The discrepancies between relative reduction figures and absolute reduction figures or between relative reduction figures and number of patients who must be treated to prevent one adverse event are constantly influencing clinical decisions. For example, physicians are frequently asked by patients if they should take an aspirin a day to prevent heart attacks. As Smith and Egger point out, in virtually all the aspirin trials for the reduction of myocardial infarction, the relative reduction rate is about 40%.[9] Using that figure alone, physicians might be tempted to put everyone on aspirin whether or not they had evidence of vascular disease or risks for vascular disease. However, the actual numbers of patients who need to be treated for 1 year to prevent one nonfatal myocardial infarction vary tremendously. For high-risk patients, such as those who have had a previous MI, the number is 100, whereas for low-risk patients, such as healthy British physicians, it is 1000.[9] If we use actual numbers of patients who need to be treated, we might be less likely to prescribe aspirin for healthy low-risk individuals.

Several studies have examined the way physicians respond to the various methods of reporting clinical benefits for preventive programs. All of them show that interventions (such as prescribing lipid-lowering agents) are more likely to ensue when benefits are presented as relative reduction figures than when they are given as absolute reduction figures or as the number of patients who must be treated to prevent one adverse event.[10-13] Methods of reporting benefits also have a major influence on patient decisions to participate or not participate in certain preventive interventions.[14]

Physicians who are advising their patients must try to be judicious. They should always remember that the methods of reporting benefits lead to cognitive biases on the part of both physicians and patients.[5,15] They should not forget the principle stated by Rose[16] that in mass screening programs any one individual has only a very small chance of achieving any benefit and therefore this can easily be counterbalanced by a small risk.

Some aspects of statistical reports physicians need to understand are described in the following paragraphs.

Total cohort mortality rates

One of the most important pieces of information a clinician needs to know about a study is how the total mortality rates compare in the intervention group and the control group. Good examples are the cholesterol-lowering studies in patients without known cardiovascular disease. Although a number of them showed decreased cardiovascular events or even reduced cardiovascular mortality, the total mortality in the treated groups was unchanged or even increased.[5] (An exception is the study by the West of Scotland Coronary Prevention Study Group.[17])

Sensitivity of a test

Sensitivity is the percentage of test results that are positive among patients who have the disease for which one is testing.

Specificity of a test

Specificity is the percentage of test results that are negative in patients who do not have the disease for which one is testing.

Positive predictive value

The positive predictive value is the percentage of positive test results that are true positives. The positive predictive value varies directly with the prevalence of the disorder in the population being tested. If the disorder is uncommon, most test results will be false positives even if the specificity is high. For example, Westhoff and Randall[18] have calculated that if a test were developed for the detection of ovarian cancer that had a 98% specificity (only 2% of all positive tests were false positives), the most optimistic positive predictive value of the test for women 45 to 74 years of age would be 2%. This is based on the premise that approximately 2500 women would have to be screened to find one case of ovarian cancer. Such a screening test would involve considerable morbidity for many women, even if it saved a few lives. Further examples of the relationship of disease prevalence to the positive predictive value of a test can be found under "Investigations."

Surrogate outcomes

A surrogate or intermediate outcome is one that is used in a study instead of the truly desired clinical outcome.[7,19] For example, if a study on the efficacy of a lipid-lowering drug uses as an endpoint the degree by which cholesterol is lowered in the treated cohort, this is a surrogate outcome for the true endpoints, which are cardiovascular events, cardiovascular deaths, or total mortality rates. The finding of small breast cancers by mammography is a surrogate outcome for a decreased death rate from breast cancer. In a study of the diagnosis and control of gestational diabetes, the incidence of large babies is a surrogate for neonatal or maternal morbidity and mortality. No guarantee can be provided that surrogate outcomes will eventually translate into the desired clinical outcomes.[7,19]

REFERENCES

1. Guyatt G, Jaeschke R, Heddle N, et al: Basic statistics for clinicians. 1. Hypothesis testing, *Can Med Assoc J* 152:27-32, 1995.
2. Guyatt G, Jaeschke R, Heddle N, et al: Basic statistics for clinicians. 2. Interpreting study results: confidence intervals, *Can Med Assoc J* 152:169-173, 1995.
3. Jaeschke R, Guyatt G, Shannon H, et al: Basic statistics for clinicians. 3. Assessing the effects of treatment: measures of association, *Can Med Assoc J* 152:351-357, 1995.
4. Guyatt G, Walter S, Shannon H, et al: Basic statistics for clinicians. 4. Correlation and regression, *Can Med Assoc J* 152:497-504, 1995.
5. Marshall KG: Prevention. How much harm? How much benefit? 1. Influence of reporting methods on perception of benefits, *Can Med Assoc J* 154:1493-1499, 1996.
6. Laupacis A, Sackett DL, Roberts RS: An assessment of clinically useful measures of the consequences of treatment, *N Engl J Med* 318:1728-1733, 1988.
7. Marshall KG: Prevention. How much harm? How much benefit? 2. Ten potential pitfalls in determining the clinical significance of benefits, *Can Med Assoc J* 154:1837-1843, 1996.
8. Phelan P: Cultivating safety: cultural differences in the cockpit must be ironed out, if air safety is to continue to improve, *Flight International* 24:22-24, 1994.
9. Smith GD, Egger M: Who benefits from medical interventions? (editorial), *BMJ* 308:72-74, 1994.
10. Forrow L, Taylor WC, Arnold RM: Absolutely relative: how research results are summarized can affect treatment decisions, *Am J Med* 92:121-124, 1992.
11. Naylor CD, Chen E, Strauss B: Measured enthusiasm: does the method of reporting trial results alter perceptions of therapeutic effectiveness? *Ann Intern Med* 117:916-921, 1992.
12. Bobbio M, Demichelis B, Giustetto G: Completeness of reporting trial results: effect on physicians' willingness to prescribe, *Lancet* 343:1209-1211, 1994.
13. Bucher HC, Weinbacher M, Gyr K: Influence of method of reporting study results on decision of physicians to prescribe drugs to lower cholesterol concentration, *BMJ* 309:761-764, 1994.
14. Hux JE, Naylor CD: Communicating the benefits of chronic preventive therapy: does the format of efficacy data determine patients' acceptance of treatment? *Med Decision Making* 15:152-157, 1995.
15. Hux JE, Naylor CD: In the eye of the beholder (editorial), *Arch Intern Med* 155:2277-2280, 1995.
16. Rose G: Sick individuals and sick populations, *Int J Epidemiol* 14:32-38, 1985.
17. Shepherd J, Cobbe SM, Ford I, et al: Prevention of coronary heart disease with pravastatin in men with hypercholesterolemia, *N Engl J Med* 333:1301-1307, 1995.
18. Westhoff C, Randall MC: Ovarian cancer screening: potential effect on mortality, *Am J Obstet Gynecol* 165:502-505, 1991.
19. Skrabanek P, McCormick J: *Follies and fallacies in medicine,* Glasgow, 1989, Tarragon Press.

DENTISTRY

(See also hormone replacement therapy for the reduction of long-term morbidity and mortality)

Topics covered in this section

NOMENCLATURE

Dentists have different ways of identifying specific teeth. A common approach in the United States is to use a numerical system for naming the 32 adult teeth and an alphabetical system for the 20 primary teeth. For adult teeth number 1 is the upper right third molar (wisdom tooth) and from there the numbers move across the upper teeth so that the upper left third molar is 16. Number 17 is the lower left third molar, and the counting then moves across the lower teeth toward the right so that the right lower third molar is 32. For the primary teeth "A" is the upper right second molar, "J" the upper left second molar, "K" the lower left second molar, and "T" the lower right second molar.[1]

An international system that is used in many parts of Canada and the rest of the world divides the adult mouth into four equal quadrants, each containing eight teeth. Each quadrant has a number:

Right upper	1
Left upper	2
Left lower	3
Right lower	4

Within each quadrant, each tooth is also given a number, so that the medial incisor is 1 and the third molar 8. By use of a double number, the first to name the quadrant and the second the tooth, each tooth can be precisely identified. Thus 2-3 is the left upper canine and 4-8 is the right lower third molar or wisdom tooth.

In the international system the quadrants of a child's mouth are labeled 5 to 8:

Right upper	5
Left upper	6
Left lower	7
Right lower	8

As in the adult, each baby tooth within a quadrant is specifically identified, but with a letter rather than a number. The medial incisor is A, the lateral incisor B, the canine C, the first molar D, and the second molar E. Thus 6-C is the left upper canine and 8-E is the right lower second molar.

REFERENCES

1. Clark MM, Album MM, Lloyd RW: Preventive dentistry and the family physician, *Am Fam Physician* 53:619-626, 1996.

ANTIBIOTIC PROPHYLAXIS

Endocarditis Prophylaxis

In 1990 the American Heart Association (AHA) drew up guidelines for the prevention of bacterial endocarditis. The AHA advised using prophylactic antibiotics for all dental interventions that cause bleeding except for the bleeding produced by injection of a local anesthetic.[1] This covered a wide variety of procedures, many of which, such as fillings, crowns, and root canals, are not associated with significant bacteremia.[2] Antibiotics were to be given both 1 hour before the procedure and 6 hours afterward. Standard protocols for adults were[1]:

Amoxicillin	3 g 1 hour before the procedure; 1.5 g 6 hours later *or*
Erythromycin	1 g 2 hours before the procedure; 500 mg 6 hours later *or*
Clindamycin	300 mg po 1 hour before the procedure; 150 mg 6 hours later

In 1997 the AHA revised its guidelines for the prevention of endocarditis.[3] The new guidelines state that the only persons requiring prophylaxis are those at high or moderate risk of endocarditis—patients with prosthetic heart valves, a past history of endocarditis, congenital heart disease (except for isolated secundum atrial septal defect), acquired valvular disease, and hypertrophic cardiomyopathy. Patients with mitral valve prolapse usually need antibiotics only if they have a regurgitant murmur.[3] The specific dental procedures for which prophylaxis is recommended include extractions, dental implant placement, periodontal surgery, and scaling or cleaning associated with bleeding. Antibiotic prophylaxis is not recommended for most local anesthetics, fillings, crowns, or root canals provided the latter do not extend beyond the apex of the tooth. However, if unexpected bleeding is encountered during one of these procedures, antibiotic prophylaxis may be given if the medication is taken no later than 4 hours after the intervention.[3]

Two major antibiotic regimens are recommended by the new guidelines[3]:

Amoxicillin	2 g po 1 hour before the procedure (children 50 mg/kg) *or*
Clindamycin	600 mg po 1 hour before the procedure (children 20 mg/kg)

The dose of amoxicillin has been decreased from 3 to 2 g, and postprocedure antibiotics are no longer considered necessary because of their long duration of action and the short period of bacteremia. Clindamycin has replaced erythromycin as the drug of choice for patients unable to take amoxicillin, but other alternatives are cephalexin 2 g (children 50 mg/kg) or azithromycin or clarithromycin 500 mg (children 15 mg/kg), all taken po 1 hour before the procedure.[3]

An interesting note is that the revised guidelines of the American Heart Association closely approximated those published in the *Lancet* in 1990 by a British working party on endocarditis.[4]

When prescribing prophylactic antibiotics, practitioners should inform patients that in the vast majority of cases bacterial endocarditis of oral origin is caused by poor oral hygiene, not dental procedures.[2,3] Therefore receiving regular dental care is particularly important, and patients should not avoid going to the dentist because they do not want to take antibiotics.

All guidelines for endocarditis prophylaxis are based on expert opinion because no prospective randomized controlled trials have shown that antibacterial prophylaxis for dental procedures is effective.[3,5] Indirect evidence suggests that it is, but even if this is so, only a small proportion of cases (4% to 19%) are related to procedures for which prophylaxis is recommended.[5] A study in the Netherlands has estimated that only 6% of cases of endocarditis could be prevented if 100% of patients requiring prophylactic antibiotics received them.[6,7]

REFERENCES

1. Dajani AS, Bisno AL, Chung KF, et al: Prevention of bacterial endocarditis: recommendations by the American Heart Association, *JAMA* 264:2919-2922, 1990.
2. Wahl MJ: Myths of dental-induced endocarditis, *Arch Intern Med* 154:137-144, 1994.
3. Dajani AS, Taubert KA, Wilson W, et al: Prevention of bacterial endocarditis: recommendations by the American Heart Association, *JAMA* 277:1794-1801, 1997.
4. Simmons NA, Cawson RA, Eykyn SJ, et al: Antibiotic prophylaxis of infective endocarditis: recommendations from the Endocarditis Working Party of the British Society for Antimicrobial Chemotherapy, *Lancet* 335:88-89, 1990.
5. Durack DT: Prevention of infective endocarditis, *N Engl J Med* 332:38-44, 1995.
6. van der Meer JTM, van Wijk W, Thompson J, et al: Efficacy of antibiotic prophylaxis for prevention of native-valve endocarditis, *Lancet* 339:135-139, 1992.
7. van der Meer JTM, Thompson J, Valkenburg HA, et al: Epidemiology of bacterial endocarditis in the Netherlands. II. Antecedent procedures and use of prophylaxis, *Arch Intern Med* 152:1869-1873, 1992.

Prosthetic Joint Infection Prophylaxis

Whether or not patients with prosthetic joints should receive prophylactic antibiotics for dental treatments is controversial. There have been no randomized trials dealing with this issue, so recommendations are based on expert opinion.[1,2] The Working Party of the British Society for Antimicrobial Chemotherapy recommends against antibiotic prophylaxis because infections of prosthetic joints are rarely caused by oral streptococci and because infections of prosthetic joints have rarely been reported to follow dental work.[3] For the same reasons the American Dental Association and the American Academy of Oral Medicine do not recommend antibiotic prophylaxis.[2] However, even though a majority of American orthopedic surgeons do not believe that a relationship exists between dental procedures and prosthetic joint infections, most recommend antibiotic prophylaxis, usually with a cephalosporin.[4] One British author suggests that this tendency to recommend prophylaxis for dental surgery by American surgeons may reflect a fear of litigation in the United States.[1]

REFERENCES

1. Uyemura MC: Antibiotic prophylaxis for medical and dental procedures: a look at AHA guidelines and controversial issues, *Postgrad Med* 98:137-140, 147, 151-152, 1995.
2. Averns HL, Kerry R: Role of prophylactic antibiotics in the prevention of late infection of prosthetic joints: results of a questionnaire and review of the literature, *Br J Rheumatol* 34:380-382, 1995.
3. Working Party of the British Society for Antimicrobial Therapy: Case against antibiotic prophylaxis for dental treatment of patients with joint prostheses, *Lancet* 339:301, 1992.
4. Little JW: Antibiotic prophylaxis for prevention of bacterial endocarditis and infections of major joint prostheses, *Curr Opin Dent* 2:93-101, 1992.

AVULSED TOOTH

An avulsed tooth that is reimplanted within 30 minutes will survive in 90% of cases. After 30 minutes the success rate decreases by about 1% per minute. The avulsed tooth should be held by the crown, rinsed off in water (with a plug in the sink so that it is not lost down the drain), and reimplanted. The patient can hold it in place by biting gently on it through an overlying piece of gauze until he or she sees a dentist. If unable to replace the tooth in the socket, the physician should rinse it and have it transported to the dentist in milk or water. Primary teeth need not be reimplanted.[1]

REFERENCES

1. Clark MM, Album MM, Lloyd RW: Medical care of the dental patient, *Am Fam Physician* 52:1126-1132, 1995.

DENTAL ABSCESS

A dental abscess can often be diagnosed by percussing the suspected tooth to see if this elicits pain. The emergency treatment of dental abscesses is penicillin plus analgesics.[1]

REFERENCES

1. Clark MM, Album MM, Lloyd RW: Medical care of the dental patient, *Am Fam Physician* 52:1126-1132, 1995.

FLUORIDES

For some time the amount of fluoride children should receive and the ages at which it should be administered have been controversial issues. Because a significant amount of fluoride is present in toothpaste, mouthwash, and even soft drinks and juices reconstituted with fluoridated water, many young children receive their daily fluoride requirements in this fashion even if their drinking water is not fluoridated. There is fear that excessive supplementation could lead to fluorosis.[1] There are varying degrees of fluorosis; most cases in North America are so mild that the alterations in the enamel are visible only to experts and therefore do not produce detrimental esthetic effects.[2,3]

The optimal fluoridation levels of the water supply should be 0.6 or 0.7 to 1.2 ppm.[2-5] If the levels are below that, supplementation is indicated. The recommended doses and age at onset of supplementation vary according to both the fluoride level of the water supply and the viewpoints of the issuing organizations.[1-4] The trend has been to initiate fluoride supplementation later in life (2 to 3 years) and to give lower doses than were previously the case. This is done not only to prevent fluorosis, but also because the traditional view that fluorides had to be incorporated into the tooth enamel before tooth eruption is false and therefore administration of the agent can be delayed until after tooth eruption.[2,3] Thus the American Academy of Pediatrics advises no supplementation before the age of 6 months regardless of the concentration of fluorides in the water and from 6 months to 3 years recommends 0.25 mg/day only if the water supply fluorides are less than 0.3 ppm.[5] The Canadian Dental Association goes even further and recommends no supplementation before the age of 3 years regardless of the fluoride concentration of the water.[2,3] Whether or not fluoride supplements are given, young children should brush their teeth twice daily under adult supervision using only a pea-sized amount of (fluoridated) toothpaste, and they should be taught to spit it out, not swallow it.[1-3]

The Canadian Task Force on the Periodic Health Examination updated its evaluation of dental caries in 1995.[6] It gave "A" recommendations for fluoridation of the water supply, the use of fluoride dentifrices, daily fluoride supplementation when the water is not fluoridated, and annual or biannual professional application of topical fluorides. The latter is effective but costly and is therefore not recommended for the general populace. The U.S. Preventive Services Task Force also gives an "A" recommendation to fluoride supplementation if the fluoride concentration in the water supply is inadequate.[7]

REFERENCES

1. Raves J: MDS call for more study before endorsing dentists' new recommendations on fluoride, *Can Med Assoc J* 149:1820-1822, 1993.
2. Clark DC: Appropriate uses of fluorides for children: guidelines from the Canadian Workshop on the Evaluation of Current Rec-

ommendations Concerning Fluorides, *Can Med Assoc J* 149: 1787-1793, 1993.
3. Clark DC: Appropriate use of fluorides in the 1990s, *J Can Dent Assoc* 59:272-279, 1993.
4. Jakush J: New fluoride schedule adopted, *ADA News* 25:12, 14, 1994.
5. American Academy of Pediatrics Committee on Nutrition: Fluoride supplementation for children: interim policy recommendations, *Pediatrics* 95:777, 1995.
6. Lewis DW, Ismail AI (Canadian Task Force on the Periodic Health Examination): Periodic health examination, 1995 update. 2. Prevention of dental caries, *Can Med Assoc J* 152:836-846, 1995.
7. US Preventive Services Task Force: *Guide to clinical preventive services,* ed 2, Baltimore, 1996, Williams & Wilkins, pp 711-721.

PAIN

Nonsteroidal antiinflammatory drugs are, in general, the analgesics of choice for dental pain.[1]

REFERENCES

1. Seymour RA, Walton JG: Analgesic efficacy in dental pain, *Br Dent J* 153:291-298, 1982.

DERMATOLOGY

(See also keloids; pruritus ani)

Topics covered in this section

ACNE VULGARIS

(See also selective progestins)

About 80% of the population suffers from some degree of acne between the ages of 11 and 30. Acne develops earlier in girls than boys but affects boys more frequently and more severely.[1,2]

Pathogenesis

The basic pathogenetic factors in acne are an increased desquamation of epithelial cells, which block the follicular orifices, and an increased production of sebum. Sebum accumulating behind the obstruction favors the growth of *Propionibacterium acnes,* which is a normal commensal within the pilosebaceous units. *P. acnes* secretes lipolytic enzymes, leading to the release of free fatty acids, as well as secreting chemotactic factors that attract neutrophils. The hydrolytic enzymes of the neutrophils damage the follicular wall, and these as well as the free fatty acids are released into the tissues, causing inflammation.[1,2]

Clinical Manifestations

A whitehead or closed comedone is caused by accumulation of sebum behind a plugged pilosebaceous follicle. Continued distention leads to a partial protrusion from the follicular opening, which has the clinical appearance of an opened comedone or blackhead. The black color of a blackhead is due to melanin and oxidized lipids, not dirt. Once the sebaceous contents rupture into the dermis, the pattern becomes one of inflammatory acne with papule, and in more severe cases nodule or "cyst," formation. Acne usually develops at puberty when androgens stimulate the sebaceous follicles. Premenstrual flares of acne are common because the follicular orifices become more obstructed at that time of the cycle.[1,2]

Specific etiological factors

Endocrine disorders with excess androgen production such as polycystic ovary syndrome and Cushing's syndrome can cause acne. Medications known to be associated with acne include corticosteroids, androgens, certain oral contraceptives containing antiestrogenic progestins, phenytoin, barbiturates, lithium, isoniazid, cyclosporine, iodides, and bromides. Oil-based cosmetics and occupational exposure to oils are other known precipitants of acne.[1]

Principles of Acne Vulgaris Therapy

Diet has no influence on acne. Vigorous scrubbing of the affected areas may aggravate rather than ameliorate the situation.[2] Gentle washing (20 minutes before the application of topical medications) is all that is required.[1,2]

Use of cosmetics, especially oil-based cosmetics and moisturizers, should be avoided. If the patient insists on using cosmetics, they should be water based.[1]

Gels are more potent than creams. Gels are best for oily skin or for hot, humid climates, while creams are best for sensitive skins and for cold, dry climates.[1,2] Topical therapy should be started at low doses for short periods. Some drying, erythema, and scaling are to be expected. If they are not excessive, the duration of application is increased to 8 to 12 hours. The concentrations of topical medications may be increased, if necessary, at 4- to 8-week intervals.[1,2] A therapeutic response to any treatment modality may take 2 months.[1,2]

Most of the pharmacological agents target one or more of three pathogenetic mechanisms of acne production—excessive sebum production (estrogens, isotretinoin, spironolactone); abnormal desquamation of epithelial cells (isotretinoin, tretinoin, adapalene, azelaic acid, benzoyl peroxide); or *P. acnes* (antibiotics, benzoyl peroxide, azelaic acid).[2]

Blackheads may be removed with a comedone extractor, and whiteheads with a no. 25 needle. Comedone extraction hastens the resolution of the disorder.[1]

Sequence of therapeutic regimens

For noninflammatory acne the initial regimen of choice is tretinoin (Retin-A) or adapalene (Differin). These drugs decrease the adhesiveness of follicular epithelial cells and increase cell turnover. By doing this they inhibit the formation of comedones and hasten the expulsion of those already formed. Treatment should start with once daily low doses and increase gradually. Adapalene is as effective as tretinoin but causes less irritation.[3] For patients with both comedonal and papulopustular acne a combination of tretinoin and a topical antibiotic such as erythromycin (Stievamycin) or tretinoin and a systemic antibiotic should be given.[2]

For mild papulopustular acne, benzoyl peroxide (Panoxyl, Desquam-X, Dermoxyl, Loroxide), a topical antibiotic such as erythromycin (Staticin), clindamycin (Cleocin T, Dalacin T), or a combination of erythromycin and benzoyl peroxide (Benzamycin) is the agent of first choice.[2] Benzoyl peroxide not only is a potent antibacterial agent that inhibits *P. acnes*, but also has mild comedolytic and exfoliant properties. If both tretinoin and benzoyl peroxide are used, one should be applied in the morning and the other in the evening. If a combination of tretinoin and 10% benzoyl peroxide is not effective or not tolerated, a topical antibiotic may be substituted for benzoyl peroxide. The topical antibiotic should not be applied at the same time as the tretinoin unless it is in a commercial formulation such as Stievamycin that combines tretinoin and erythromycin. If tretinoin plus a topical antibiotic is ineffective, the patient requires oral antibiotics.[1] The oral antibiotics of choice are doxycycline (Vibra-Tabs) or minocycline (Minocin) in daily doses of 50 to 200 mg, or trimethoprim-sulfamethoxazole (Septra, Bactrim) as one regular tablet daily or bid or one double-strength tablet daily. Alternatives, which are probably less effective, are tetracycline and erythromycin. In general, the dose should not be reduced for 2 to 4 months.[2] Although concomitant use of antibiotics and oral contraceptives has been commonly believed to decrease the efficacy of the contraceptives, there is no good evidence supporting this claim in terms of the usual antibiotics for treating acne.[4]

In cases of moderate or severe inflammatory acne the initial treatment should include oral antibiotics.[1,2] A new topical antibacterial agent with some effect on comedogenesis is azelaic acid (Azelex).[2]

Isotretinoin (Accutane) is an oral retinoid that is effective for widespread, severe, nodular cystic lesions. It is teratogenic, so proof that the patient is not pregnant and is using effective measures to prevent conception is essential before starting it. The usual treatment regimen is 4 to 5 months at a dosage of 0.1 to 1 mg/kg/day.

For women, spironolactone (Aldactone) in daily doses of 25 to 200 mg or oral contraceptives may help control acne. Third-generation oral contraceptives containing "selective" progestins such as desogestrel (Marvelon, Ortho-Cept) or norgestimate (Cyclen, Tri-Cyclen) are often recommended for this purpose because they are thought to have few androgenic side effects. It may take 2 to 4 months for beneficial effects to be observed, and relapses occur frequently if the agents are discontinued.[2]

REFERENCES

1. Nguyen QH, Kim YA, Schwartz RA: Management of acne vulgaris, *Am Fam Physician* 50:89-96, 1994.
2. Leyden JJ: Therapy for acne vulgaris, *N Engl J Med* 336:1156-1162, 1997.
3. Adapalene for acne, *Med Lett* 39:19-20, 1997.
4. Rasmussen JE: The effect of antibiotics on the efficacy of oral contraceptives, *Arch Dermatol* 125:1562-1564, 1989.

ALOPECIA

The growth of hair follicles is cyclical. Normally 85% to 90% of scalp hair is in the anagen phase, the period of active hair growth. This is followed by the catagen or involutional phase, which lasts about 6 weeks. The final stage is the telogen phase, which lasts 2 to 4 months and terminates with the hair falling out. On average about 100 scalp hairs are lost daily.[1]

A common cause of diffuse hair loss is telogen effluvium. This is hair loss resulting from psychological, physiological, or pathological stress. The disorder usually declares itself 2 to 4 months after the precipitating event, and up to 50% of hair may be lost. Specific causes include childbirth; surgery and anesthesia; crash dieting; infections; hypothyroidism; ingestion of a variety of drugs, including antidepressants, lithium, beta-blockers, angiotensin-converting enzyme (ACE) inhibitors, and anticoagulants; and discontinuation of oral contraceptives. Hair regrows in 2 to 3 months if the precipitating event is no longer present.[1]

Other causes of hair loss are trichotillomania, in which hairs are broken off in the region of the alopecia, and traction alopecia. In alopecia areata, "exclamation point" hairs appear around the periphery of the bald spots.[1]

A medical treatment for male pattern baldness is minoxidil (Rogaine). Only 20% to 40% of men using this treatment have noticeable improvement. The drug, which is sold as a 2% solution, should be applied bid to the dry scalp for 6 to 12 months to determine whether it will be effective. Continuation of therapy for an indefinite period is required to maintain hair growth. Minoxidil is more effective if the area involved is on the vertex than temporal and is less than 10 cm in diameter, as well as if the alopecia is of less than 10 years' duration.[1]

Female androgenetic alopecia is common in women and is manifested as diffuse hair loss in the temporoparietal region and a more than usually apparent central part. The frontal hairline is usually maintained in women. Treatment of this condition in women with 2% minoxidil has resulted in minimal hair growth in about half of them and moderate hair growth in 13%.[2]

The currently favored surgical treatment of male pattern baldness is the use of autografts taken from the occipital region and transplanted to the frontal and vertex balding areas. Multiple minigrafts (four to six hairs) or micrografts (one or two hairs) are used. The process works because the hair follicles in the occipital area tend not to be sensitive to androgens and to retain this characteristic when transplanted.[3]

REFERENCES

1. Nielsen TA, Reichel M: Alopecia: diagnosis and management, *Am Fam Physician* 51:1513-1522, 1995.
2. De Villez RL, Jacobs JP, Szpunar CA, et al: Androgenetic alopecia in the female: treatment with 2% topical minoxidil solution, *Arch Dermatol* 130:303-307, 1994.
3. Taylor EK: Management of male pattern baldness, *Can J CME* 7(11):107-113, 1995.

CONTACT DERMATITIS

A common cause of contact dermatitis from earrings, watches, or eyeglass frames is nickel allergy. One method of preventing the contact is to coat the offending object with clear nail polish and let it dry. Repeat applications every 2 to 8 weeks are usually required.[1]

REFERENCES

1. Gore BQ: For nickel allergy, *Patient Care Can* 7(3):22, 1996.

FOLLICULITIS

Patients with recurrent staphylococcal skin infections tend to reinfect themselves through nasal carriage of the organism. In one study a monthly 5-day course of mupirocin (Bactroban) ointment applied to the nose over a 1-year period resulted in fewer recurrent skin infections than were seen in the placebo control group.[1]

REFERENCES

1. Raz R, Miron D, Colodner R, et al: A 1-year trial of nasal mupirocin in the prevention of recurrent staphylococcal nasal colonization and skin infection, *Arch Intern Med* 156:1109-1112, 1996.

HIRSUTISM

More than 95% of cases of hirsutism are idiopathic or secondary to polycystic ovary syndrome.[1] Other causes include late-onset congenital adrenal hyperplasia, Cushing's syndrome, testosterone-secreting tumors, starvation, anorexia nervosa, obesity (sometimes), and drugs (progestins in some oral contraceptive pills, danazol, phenytoin, minoxidil).[1-3]

Source of Androgens

The ovary produces testosterone, androstenedione, and dehydroepiandrosterone (DHEA). The adrenal gland produces these, as well as the sulfated form of DHEA (DHEA-S). Testosterone is 99% bound to sex hormone–binding globulin, and only the free portion is biologically active. In some women sex hormone–binding globulin is decreased in association with obesity, and in them hirsutism is related to weight gain.[2,3]

Investigations

The main purpose of investigating patients with hirsutism is to rule out ominous causes of hirsutism. Investigations are usually not indicated if the clinical picture is one associated with a benign cause of hirsutism. These patients are usually between the ages of 15 and 25, have had hirsutism for more than a year (not a rapid new onset), and have no evidence of virilization. Investigations are required in the small group of women who do not have this clinical pattern. In particular, investigations should be carried out if the onset of hirsutism is rapid, if there are signs of virilism (frontal balding, voice deepening, increased muscle mass, clitoromegaly), or if Cushing's syndrome is suspected.[1]

It is not important clinically to distinguish among idiopathic hirsutism, polycystic ovarian syndrome, and late-onset congenital adrenal hyperplasia, all of which may be associated with mild elevations of testosterone level (usually less than twice the normal value). When indicated, initial investigations should include the following[1,2]:

1. Total testosterone. Levels greater than twice the normal value suggest tumor.[2]
2. Dehydroepiandrosterone sulfate (DHEA-S). Levels greater than twice the normal value suggest tumor.[2]
3. 17-Hydroxyprogesterone. Blood for this assay should be drawn in the early morning. The level is usually significantly elevated in patients with the more common and innocuous forms of congenital adrenal hyperplasia.[1]
4. Dexamethasone suppression test if Cushing's syndrome is suspected. This test is performed by giving 1 mg dexamethasone po at 11 PM and measuring the serum cortisol level by 9 AM the next day.

Treatment of Benign Forms of Hirsutism

Methods of treating benign forms of hirsutism include weight loss (if obese), electrolysis, birth control pills, and spironolactone (Aldactone). If birth control pills are chosen, they should have a low level of androgenic progestin, as is the case in the third-generation oral contraceptives containing desogestrel or norgestimate. The usual dosage of spironolactone is 50 to 100 mg/day or even 200 mg/day in 2 divided doses. This drug may cause hyperkalemia. Other methods that have been used for treating hirsutism are androgen-suppressing drugs such as flutamide (Euflex) and finasteride (Proscar).[2]

REFERENCES

1. McKennal TJ: Screening for sinister causes of hirsutism (editorial), *N Engl J Med* 331:1015-1016, 1994.
2. Kalve E, Klein J: Evaluation of women with hirsutism, *Am Fam Physician* 54:117-124, 1996.
3. Conway GS, Jacobs HS: Hirsutism: treatable and usually caused by the polycystic ovary syndrome (editorial), *BMJ* 301:619-620, 1996.

HYPERHIDROSIS PALMARIS

A solution of aluminum chloride hexahidride 20% (Drysol) may be used to treat sweaty palms. The usual regimen is to apply to the palms qhs for 3 nights and to wear polyethylene gloves all night. The maintenance regimen is the same program once or twice a week.[1]

REFERENCES

1. Hurley HF: Questions and answers, *JAMA* 259:3325, 1988.

MELANOMA

Certain types of nevi are risk factors for melanoma. Multiple small nondysplastic nevi are associated with a slight increase in risk, but the presence of 10 or more dysplastic nevi increases the risk 12 fold. Dysplastic nevi are flat, vary in color, and have a diameter greater than 5 mm, irregular poorly defined borders, and an asymmetrical appearance.[1]

REFERENCES

1. Tucker MA, Halpern A, Holly EA, et al: Clinically recognized dysplastic nevi: a central risk factor for cutaneous melanoma, *JAMA* 277:1439-1444, 1997.

PEDICULOSIS PUBIS AND PEDICULOSIS CAPITIS

Transmission of head lice is usually by direct contact (head to head) and rarely if ever through fomites.[1] A 1% solution of permethrin (Nix Creme Rinse) is the pharmacological treatment of choice for pediculosis pubis and capitis.[2-4] After the area is shampooed, rinsed, and dried, the permethrin solution is applied in sufficient quantities to saturate the area and is left in place for 10 minutes before being rinsed off with water. One systematic review concluded that evidence is insufficient to justify the use of lindane (Kwellada).[4] Unfortunately, there is evidence that some lice have become resistant to permethrin.[5] Although a single treatment is sufficient to kill both the nits and the adult lice, many experts recommend a second treatment 7 to 10 days later as insurance.[1] The policy of some schools that children must be free of nits before returning is not based on scientific evidence and should be discouraged. However, if the school insists on this policy, nits can be removed by applying a damp towel to the scalp for 30 to 60 minutes (or by applying a mixture of equal parts water and white vinegar to the scalp, which is then covered with a damp towel soaked in the same material for 15 minutes), followed by combing with a fine-toothed comb.[1]

Pesticides are not always needed to control pediculosis capitis. An alternative is to wash the hair with ordinary shampoo and then add conditioner. Immediately afterward, while the hair is still wet, it is combed thoroughly with a fine-toothed comb. The procedure is repeated every 3 or 4 days for a total of four shampoos and combings over a 2-week period. Wetting the hair slows down the lice, and conditioner makes the hair slippery so they have difficulty gripping the shafts. Thus the initial combing removes all adult and nymphal lice. Subsequent shampooing and combing remove further nymphal lice that have hatched from the nits (incubation period of 7 to 10 days) before they mature, mate, and lay still more eggs.[6]

REFERENCES

1. Infectious Diseases and Immunization Committee of the Canadian Paediatric Society: Head lice infestations: a persistent itchy "pest," *Paediatr Child Health* 1:237-240, 1996.
2. Drugs for sexually transmitted diseases, *Med Lett* 37:117-122, 1995.
3. Drugs for parasitic infections, *Med Lett* 37:99-108, 1995.
4. Vander Stichele RH, Dezeure EM, Bogaert MG: Systematic review of clinical efficacy of topical treatments for head lice, *BMJ* 311:604-608, 1995.
5. Mumcuoglu CY, Hemingway J, Miller J, et al: Permethrin resistance in the head louse *Pediculus capitis* from Israel, *Me Vet Entomol* 9:427-432, 1995.
6. Ibarra J, Hall DM: Head lice in schoolchildren, *Arch Dis Child* 75:471-473, 1996.

PHYTOPHOTODERMATITIS

Limes and lemons may be a cause of phytophotodermatitis. Erythema, vesicles, or bullae occur hours to days after contact with the fruit and may take weeks or months to resolve.[1]

REFERENCES

1. Goskowicz MO, Friedlander SF, Eichenfield LF: Endemic "lime" disease phytophotodermatitis in San Diego County, *Pediatrics* 93:828-830, 1994.

PORT-WINE STAINS

Vascular skin lesions, including port-wine stains, can often be treated effectively by lasers, but the recurrence rate is high.[1]

REFERENCES

1. Cosmetic surgery with lasers, *Med Lett* 39:10-11, 1997.

PSORIASIS

(See also psoriatic arthritis; topical steroids)

The common form of psoriasis is plaque psoriasis. Other variants include guttate, pustular, and arthritic psoriasis. Unless otherwise specified, this section deals with plaque psoriasis.[1,2] Psoriasis affects between 1% and 3% of all individuals. The two peak ages of onset are the late teens to early twenties and the late fifties to early sixties. The natural history is one of exacerbations and remissions. Factors known to exacerbate psoriasis are trauma to the skin (physical, sunburn, or infection), psychological stress, and certain drugs. Drug classes to avoid prescribing, if possible, for patients with psoriasis are beta-blockers, ACE inhibitors, indomethacin, lithium, and antimalarials.[1]

A variety of treatment options are available for the control of psoriasis. Avoidance of precipitating factors is common to all of them. If lesions are sparse and do not bother the patient, no treatment is needed. If less than 20% of the body is involved, topical agents are often effective, but if more than 20% is involved, systemic therapy may be required from the onset.[1,2]

Topical agents commonly used in North America include emollients that hydrate and soften the scaly surface of lesions, medium- or high-potency topical steroids, and an analogue of vitamin D, calcipotriene, which is also called calcipotriol (Dovonex). Emollients are not especially effective but have virtually no adverse effects. Steroids usually are very effective initially, but in time they become less effective. Calcipotriene is reasonably effective, being equivalent to moderate-potency steroids, but it may be irritating.[1,2] Other effective topical agents are coal tar preparations and anthralin. Both are usually combined with ultraviolet B phototherapy. Anthralin stains the skin and clothes.[1]

Systemic therapies and phototherapies are usually administered by or in conjunction with a dermatologist. They include ultraviolet B phototherapy combined with topical tars or anthralin, ultraviolet A phototherapy combined with the photosensitizing drug methoxsalen, methotrexate, and in some cases cyclosporine.[1]

REFERENCES

1. Greaves MW, Weinstein GD: Treatment of psoriasis, *N Engl J Med* 332:581-588, 1995.
2. Phillips TJ: Current treatment options in psoriasis, *Hosp Pract (Office Edition)* 31:155-157, 161-64, 166, 1996.

ROSACEA

Acne rosacea has four classic phases. These are[1,2]:

1. Facial flushing
2. Persistent erythema with telangiectasias
3. Inflammatory lesions (papules, pustules, nodules)
4. Rhinophyma

Factors that aggravate acne rosacea include exposure to heat or cold, exposure to sunlight, and ingestion of alcohol and hot spicy foods. Avoidance of these precipitants is required for all patients.[1] Standard drug therapy is oral antibiotics, and these are particularly effective in the papular and pustular phase of the disease. First-line therapy is tetracycline (Achromycin) or tetracycline derivatives such as minocycline (Minocin) and doxycycline (Vibramycin). A suggested initial dosage of tetracycline is 1 g/day in divided doses for 2 to 3 weeks followed by 0.5 g/day for another 2 to 3 weeks. If a good response is not obtained, second-line drugs such as sulfamethoxazole-trimethoprim (Septra, Bactrim) or oral metronidazole (Flagyl) may be used.[2]

Topical 0.75% metronidazole cream or gel may be used alone for the treatment of acne rosacea, but improvement takes longer and is usually not as great as that seen with oral antibiotics. However, metronidazole is useful in maintaining remissions that have been achieved with oral antibiotics.[2]

REFERENCES

1. Thiboutot DM: Acne rosacea, *Am Fam Physician* 50:1691-1697, 1994.
2. Wilkin JK: Rosacea: pathophysiology and treatment (editorial), *Arch Dermatol* 130:359-362, 1994.

SCABIES

Permethrin 5% (Nix Dermal Cream) is the treatment of choice for scabies.[1] The usual way to apply it is to wash and dry the skin and rub in the cream from head (except scalp) to toe over all parts of the body; 30 g will do for the average adult. It should be washed off after 12 to 14 hours. A single treatment is usually effective, but itch may persist for a significant period and does not mean treatment failure. All sexual contacts and close family members should be treated at the same time. All clothes and bedclothes used in the 48 hours before treatment should be washed. Nix Dermal Cream is the agent of choice for scabies, whereas Nix Cerme Rinse is used for pediculosis capitis and pubis. For children under age 2 years, 10% precipitated sulfur in petrolatum should be used. It should be left in place for 24 hours and the treatment repeated in 24 hours or 1 week.

REFERENCES

1. Drugs for sexually transmitted diseases, *Med Lett* 37:117-122, 1995.

SCALP LOTIONS, STEROID

Some of the steroid-containing scalp lotions that are available are betamethasone valerate 0.1% (Valisone, Betnovate), betamethasone dipropionate 0.05% plus salicylic acid (Diprosalic), and clobetasol-17-propionate 0.05% (Temovate, Dermovate).

SCALP SHAMPOOS, MEDICATED

The usual way of using medicated scalp shampoos is to shake thoroughly, rub well into the scalp, leave for 4 minutes, and then rinse off. Some of the medicated scalp shampoos that are available are salicylic acid shampoo (Ionil, Sebcur), salicylic acid–tar shampoo (Ionil T, Sebcur/T), salicylic acid–sulfur shampoo (Sebulex), and salicylic acid–sulfur–tar shampoo (Sebutone).

SEABATHER'S ERUPTION

(See also swimmer's itch)

Seabather's eruption or sea lice is a pruritic dermatitis occurring mainly on areas of the body covered by the bathing suit in ocean swimmers. The eruption develops 3 to 30 minutes after swimming. The condition is usually found in Florida and the Caribbean but has been reported as far north as Long Island. The probable cause is the planula larvae of *Edwardsiella lineata,* a sea anemone. It has also been considered to be due to the larvae of the thimble jellyfish *(Linuche unguiculata).*[1] Treatment is antihistamines and topical steroids.

REFERENCES

1. Tomchik RS, Russell MT, Szmant AM, et al: Clinical perspectives on seabather's eruption, also known as "sea lice," *JAMA* 269:1669-1672, 1993.

SUN DAMAGE

(See also wrinkles and skin aging)

Solar radiation in the ultraviolet B (UVB) spectrum (290 to 320 nm) is a major cause of sunburn, chronic skin injury including aging, and skin cancers. Ultraviolet B is blocked by window glass. Ultraviolet A (UVA) (320 to 400 nm) causes polymorphous light eruption and most photosensitivity reactions to drugs. It also contributes to chronic skin damage or photoaging, skin cancer, and to a lesser extent sunburn.[1-4] Photoaging, especially wrinkling, and skin cancer are more prevalent in smokers than nonsmokers with equal exposure to ultraviolet rays.[4]

Clouds give little protection against ultraviolet radiation, since they allow approximately 80% of it to be transmitted. Snow and beaches reflect almost all of this radiation, and immersion in water filters out only about 50%. Maximum exposure to ultraviolet radiation occurs between the hours of 10 AM and 3 PM. Aside from staying indoors, clothing and especially hats are probably the most effective protection against sun damage. However, wet clothes, loosely woven fabrics, and nylon stockings allow about 20% to 30% of ultraviolet rays to pass through to the skin.[1-3]

Traditionally, sunscreens have protected against UVB only. This is no longer acceptable. Although UVA is only about 1/1000 as potent in producing skin erythema as UVB, between 10 to 100 times as much UVA reaches the earth's surface as UVB. Furthermore, UVA penetrates more deeply in the dermis and is a major contributor to photoaging and tumor promotion. Sunscreens should protect against both UVA and UVB, and indeed most of them now do; patients should be advised to buy only those stating on the labels that both UVA and UVB are screened. Although it is generally accepted that the sun protective factor (SPF) must be at least 15,[2,3] evidence suggests that an SPF of 30 is more efficient in protecting against markers of radiation-induced DNA damage.[3] However, the degree of improved protection may be minimal; a sunscreen with an SPF of 30 blocks out only 3% more UVB than one with an SPF of 15.[5]

Sunscreens are an essential adjunct to the primary prevention of photoaging and skin cancers. However, they will not work if they are used merely as a method of staying in the sun longer[6]; tanning of any degree is a sign of sun damage.[2,3] Sunscreens are also valuable for patients who have already sustained the ravages of ultraviolet radiation, since they facilitate the repair of photoaging.[4]

Various formulations of sunscreens are available. The most frequently used are lotions or creams, but for those exposed to dust, such as farmers, ranchers, and construction workers, gels may be better because the dirt will not stick to them as readily. Children sometimes prefer sprays. Some sunscreens are specifically formulated to be waterproof or water resistant, and these should be used by those going swimming.[3] Ideally sunscreens should be applied liberally half an hour before exposure and reapplied after swimming or perspiring, as well as every 2 to 3 hours on a regular basis.[2] Even waterproof or very water-resistant preparations have a duration of action limited to about 80 minutes,[7] so lovers of the water should come out at least every hour for a reapplication of sunscreen.

REFERENCES

1. Shade UVAGuard, *Med Lett* 35:53-54, 1993.
2. Guercio-Hauer C: Photodamage, photoaging and photoprotection of the skin, *Am Fam Physician* 50:327-332, 1994.
3. Wentzell JM: Sunscreens: the ounce of prevention, *Am Fam Physician* 53:1713-1733, 1996.
4. Gilchrest BA: A review of skin ageing and its medical therapy, *Br J Dermatol* 135:867-875, 1996.
5. Trouton KJ, Mills CJ: A place in the shade: reducing the risks of UV exposure, *Can Med Assoc J* 157:175-176, 1997.
6. McGregor JM, Young AR: Sunscreens, suntans, and skin cancer—sunscreens should not be seen as a safe way to prolong sun exposure, *BMJ* 312:1621-1622, 1996.
7. Farmer KC, Naylor MF: Sun exposure, sunscreens, and skin cancer prevention: a year-round concern, *Ann Pharmacother* 30:662-673, 1996.

SWIMMER'S ITCH

(See also seabather's eruption)

Swimmer's itch is caused by the penetration into the skin of the larval or cercarial form of an animal schistosome. (The usual natural cycle is duck-snail-duck.) Since humans are not the definitive host, the cercariae die after penetrating the skin and cause a delayed hypersensitivity reaction.

The person often has a brief period of skin stinging when first exposed to the cercaria and perhaps a transient macular or urticarial rash. This is followed by a latent period of 1 to 14 days before the development of the maculopapular-vesicular rash, which is usually seen over body areas not protected by clothing. Resolution begins in a few days and is complete within 2 weeks. Treatment is symptomatic and includes antihistamines, topical antipruritics, and in severe cases corticosteroids.[1,2]

Most cases of swimmer's itch come from exposure in fresh water. The cercariae are most abundant in warm, shallow water.[1,2] Elimination of snails from the water eliminates swimmer's itch.

REFERENCES

1. Mulvihill CA, Burnett JW: Swimmer's itch: a cercarial dermatitis, *Cutis* 46:211-213, 1990.
2. Chapman A, Ekelund C, Tominaga J: Rash and pruritus after a camping trip, *Pediatr Infect Dis J* 12:966, 968-969, 1993.

TATTOOS

Tattoos can often be treated effectively with lasers.[1]

REFERENCES

1. Cosmetic surgery with lasers, *Med Lett* 39:10-11, 1997.

TOPICAL STEROIDS

One of the most useful ways of classifying topical steroids is by potency. The standard classification puts the most potent drugs in group I and the least potent in group VII. Selected products are listed this way in Table 23. You will note that this table lists only creams. The same concentration of drug in a different vehicle such as an ointment might be more potent. The same drug (e.g., triamcinolone) in different concentrations would also have different potencies. It would take a large table indeed to cover all drugs, all doses, and all formulations. These can be found in standard textbooks of dermatology. Topical steroids should be applied as a thin film. In general, only the mildest steroids should be used on the face, axillae, or genitals.

Table 23 Selected Topical Steroid Creams

Generic names	Selected trade names
Group I	
Betamethasone dipropionate/propylene glycol 0.05%	Diprolene
Clobetasol 17-propionate 0.05%	Dermovate, Temovate
Group II	
Desoximetasone 0.25%	Topicort
Fluocinonide 0.05%	Lidex Regular
Halcinonide 0.1%	Halog-E
Group III	
Triamcinolone acetonide 0.5%	Aristocort "C"oncentrate
Group IV	
Amcinonide 0.1%	Cyclocort
Fluocinolone acetonide 0.2%	Synalar HP
Halcinonide 0.025%	Halog
Group V	
Betamethasone-17-valerate 0.1%	Betnovate, Celestoderm-V, Valisone
Fluocinolone acetonide 0.025%	Synalar Regular
Hydrocortisone 0.2%	Westcort
Triamcinolone acetonide 0.1%	Aristocort "R"egular, Kenalog
Group VI	
Desonide 0.05%	Tridesilon
Triamcinolone acetonide 0.025%	Aristocort "D"ilute
Group VII	
Hydrocortisone 1%	Hytone, Synacort, Cortate
Methylprednisolone 0.25%	Medrol

TINEA

Tinea pedis has generally been treated topically with one of the imidazoles such as clotrimazole (Lotrimin, Mycelex, Canesten), miconazole (Micatin, Monistat), or ketoconazole (Nizoral). Some of the more recently introduced allylamines, such as terbinafine (Lamisil) or Naftifine (Naftin), and the benzylamine butenafine (Penederm) appear to be more potent, at least in vitro.[1]

Like tinea pedis, tinea versicolor is traditionally managed with topical antifungal agents applied once or twice a day for 2 to 4 weeks,[2] or alternatively by the application of a 2.5% selenium sulfide solution (Selsun) for 10 minutes a day for 7 days or for 24 hours once a week for 4 weeks. In extensive or recurrent cases a single oral dose of 400 mg of fluconazole (Diflucan) may be effective.[3] In some recurrent cases prophylaxis with the oral agent once monthly may be indicated.[4]

Fungal infections are only one cause of dystrophic nails, so it is important to obtain culture results or positive potassium hydroxide smears before initiating oral treatment for onychomycosis. The best specimens are obtained from the more proximal portions of the nail.[5] Onychomycosis cannot be cured by topical treatment,[5,6] but it can sometimes be controlled with the use of topical lotions.[6] Definitive treatment is with oral agents.[5,6] In one study the mycological cure rate for 250 mg of terbinafine (Lamisil) daily for 12 weeks was 81% while that for itraconazole (Sporanox) 200 mg daily for 12 weeks was 63%.[7] Part of the reason for the efficacy of the newer oral agents such as terbinafine (Lamisil), itraconazole (Sporanox), and fluconazole (Diflucan) in curing onychomycosis is that these agents bind to nail keratin and persist in the nails for several weeks after oral therapy is discontinued.[5] Because of this an alternative to daily oral therapy is pulse therapy. Reports of using this technique for onychomycosis of the toenails with itraconazole (Sporanox) found that 200 mg of the drug given bid 1 week a month for two to four cycles was as effective as continuous therapy with daily doses of 100 to 200 mg/day for 3 to 4 months.[8,9]

REFERENCES

1. Topical butenafine for tinea pedis, *Med Lett* 39:63-64, 1997.
2. Kovacs SO, Hruza LL: Superficial fungal infections: getting rid of lesions that don't want to go away, *Postgrad Med* 98:61-75, 1995.
3. Faergemann J: Treatment of pityriasis versicolor with a single dose of fluconazole, *Acta Derm Venereol* 72:74-75, 1992.
4. Faergemann J: Pityriasis versicolor, *Semin Dermatol* 12:276-279, 1993.
5. Gupta AK, Shear NH: Onychomycosis: going for cure, *Can Fam Physician* 43:299-305, 1997.
6. Bergus GR, Johnson JS: Superficial tineal infections, *Am Fam Physician* 48:259-268, 1993.
7. Brautigam M, Nolting S, Schopf RE, et al (Seventh Lamisil German Onychomycosis Study Group): Randomised double blind comparison of terbinafine and itraconazole for treatment of toenail tinea infection, *BMJ* 311:919-922, 1995.
8. De Doncker PRG, Scher RK, Baran RL, et al: Itraconazole therapy is effective for pedal onychomycosis caused by some nondermatophyte molds and in mixed infection with dermatophytes and molds: a multicenter study with 36 patients, *J Am Acad Dermatol* 36(2 Part 1):173-177, 1997.
9. Havu V, Brandt H, Heikkila H, et al: A double-blind, randomized study comparing itraconazole pulse therapy with continuous dosing for the treatment of toe-nail onychomycosis, *Br J Dermatol* 136:230-234, 1997.

ULCERS, DERMAL

(See also venous ulcers)

Staging of skin ulcers is as follows[1]:

Stage 1	Nonblanchable erythema of the intact skin
Stage 2	Partial thickness loss involving the epidermis or dermis or both; presents clinically as an abrasion, blister, or shallow crater
Stage 3	Full-thickness loss extending into the subcutaneous tissue, but not through the underlying fascia
Stage 4	Full-thickness loss extending to muscle, bone tendons, joint capsule, and so on

Occlusive dressings

The modern treatment of skin ulcers often involves the use of occlusive dressings, and a confusingly large number of these are on the market. Occlusive dressings not only protect the area, but also maintain a moist wound surface that facilitates autolytic debridement and the formation of granulation tissue and increases the rate of reepithelialization. Pain is relieved, and the degree of scarring diminished. Although bacterial colonization takes place in this milieu, the rate of clinical infections is actually less than in wounds treated with gauze or other conventional dressings. Occlusive dressings should not be used if the lesion is clearly infected.[1,2]

Occlusive dressings can be applied only if the surrounding skin is intact and healthy. The dressings should be large enough to give a 2.5-cm or 1-inch margin around the borders. They should be changed when they leak or look as if they are going to leak, or at least once a week. Patients wearing occlusive dressings can bathe or shower with them on. The dressings come in various sizes and shapes, so that the physician can keep a list handy to prescribe the specific size required or can tell the pharmacist the size and shape of the ulcer and let him or her dispense the appropriate product.

The following are some occlusive dressings and wound fillers that family physicians may use reasonably frequently[1,2]:

1. Transparent polymer films (e.g., Tegaderm Transparent Dressing, Duoderm Extra Thin Dressings and Border Dressings, Opsite Wound Dressing). These are generally used to cover first- and second-degree ulcers. They are impermeable to water and nonabsorbent, so serous fluid may accumulate. This is not in itself harmful, but if enough accumulates, it may break the seal and leak out.
2. Hydrocolloid dressings (e.g., Tegasorb Ulcer Dressing, Duoderm CGF [Controlled Gel Formulation] Dressings, IntraSite Wound Dressing). These dressings are used for third- and fourth-degree ulcers. They are self-adhering and contain gelling agents. Before application the wound should be cleaned with normal saline. When the dressing is removed, a viscous gel remains in the ulcer, but it can be easily removed by saline irrigations (not hydrogen peroxide or other antiseptic solutions).
3. Calcium alginate dressings (e.g., Kaltostat Wound Dressing, Algoderm calcium alginate wound packing, Sorbsan). Alginates are seaweed-derived polysaccharides that are useful for packing large exuding cavities because they are highly absorbent. Only half of the cavity should be gently packed because these products expand.[1]
4. Hydrocolloid pastes and polyurethane foam (e.g., Cutinova Cavity, Duoderm Hydroactive Paste or Hydroactive Granules, Allevyn Hydrophilic Polymer Foam Dressing, LYOfoam). These absorbent agents, like calcium alginate dressings, are used for large exuding cavities. Only about half the wound cavity should be gently packed.

REFERENCES

1. Findlay D: Practical management of pressure ulcers, *Am Fam Physician* 54:1519-1528, 1996.
2. Helfman T, Ovington L, Falanga V: Occlusive dressings and wound healing, *Clin Dermatol* 12:121-127, 1994.

URTICARIA AND ANGIOEDEMA

(See also anaphylactic reactions to insect stings; antihistamines)

Urticaria and angioedema are said to affect 15% to 25% of the population at least once in a lifetime. Among patients with these disorders, 40% have urticaria alone, 10% angioedema alone, and 50% a combination of the two. Urticaria involves swelling of the superficial dermal tissues, whereas angioedema is located in the deep dermal, subcutaneous, or submucosal tissues. The swelling of angioedema is usually found in the extremities, eyelids, and lips, but it may involve the gastrointestinal tract or the respiratory tract. In the latter instance respiratory obstruction is a real possibility.

Patients with angioedema usually complain of burning or tingling rather than itching. Individual lesions of both urticaria and angioedema come on rapidly, usually resolve in 2 to 4 hours, and rarely last more than 24 hours.[1]

Common causes of acute urticaria are Hymenoptera insect stings; foods such as nuts, chocolate, shellfish, eggs, and milk; viral infections including hepatitis B; and drugs, especially antibiotics.[1] In several reported cases angioedema has developed months or even years after a patient started taking ACE inhibitors.[2-4] In one case the patient continued taking his enalapril because the initial episode of angioedema resolved, but it recurred several days later.[4]

Chronic urticaria is defined as the presence of widespread wheals daily or almost daily for at least 6 weeks. In about 75% of cases no etiological factor is found,[1,5] and about half of these patients will be symptom free after 1 year.[1] Physical urticarias such as cold, solar, pressure, and cholinergic (brought on by exercise or hot shower) should be considered in the differential diagnosis. The most important condition to be ruled out is urticarial vasculitis. Urticarial vasculitis is associated with connective tissue diseases such as lupus and Sjögren's syndrome. In this condition the individual wheals last more than 24 hours, and often purpura and sometimes skin pigmentation are seen. Fever, arthralgia, nephritis, and abdominal pain may also be present. The diagnosis can be made with a skin biopsy. A rare condition causing recurrent episodes of urticaria or angioedema is deficiency of C1 esterase inhibitor. It is diagnosed by finding a low C4 complement level.[1,5]

In one small U.S. study, patients with acute-onset urticaria, regardless of cause, had better itch control if given a 4-day course of prednisone 20 mg in addition to hydroxyzine (Atarax) 25 mg q4-8h prn compared with those given only hydroxyzine.[6]

Patients with chronic urticaria should avoid taking ACE inhibitors, aspirin, and other nonsteroidal antiinflammatory drugs.[5] For patients who fail to respond to H_1-receptor antagonists alone, the addition of an H_2 antagonist such as cimetidine or ranitidine may result in the control of symptoms.[7,8] The antidepressant doxepin (Sinequan) has significant H_1 antihistaminic activity and may be used in doses of 25 to 50 mg hs.[5]

REFERENCES

1. Kulp-Shorten CL, Callen J: Urticaria, angioedema, and rheumatologic disease: rheumatic disease, *Clin North Am* 22:95-115, 1996.
2. Jain M, Armstrong RP, Hall J: Predisposition to and late onset of upper airway obstruction following angiotensin-converting enzyme inhibitor therapy, *Chest* 102:871-874, 1992.
3. Forslund T, Tohmo H, Weckström G, et al: Angio-oedema induced by enalapril, *J Intern Med* 238:179-181, 1995.
4. Shionoiri H, Takasaki I, Hirawa N, et al: A case report of angioedema during long-term (66 months) angiotensin converting enzyme inhibition therapy with enalapril, *Jpn Circ J* 60:166-170, 1996.
5. Greaves MW: Chronic urticaria, *N Engl J Med* 332:1767-1772, 1995.
6. Pollack CV, Romano TJ: Outpatient management of acute urticaria—role of prednisone, *Ann Emerg Med* 26:547-551, 1995.
7. Paul E, Bödecker RH: Treatment of chronic urticaria with terfenadine and ranitidine: a randomized double-blind study in 45 patients, *Eur J Clin Pharmacol* 31:277-280, 1986.
8. Bleehen SS, Thomas SE, Greaves MW, et al: Cimetidine and chlorpheniramine in the treatment of chronic idiopathic urticaria: a multi-centre randomized double-blind study, *Br J Dermatol* 117:81-88, 1987.

WARTS

Between 5% and 10% of children and young adults have warts, which are lesions caused by the human papillomavirus.[1] The peak age is 12 to 16 years.[2] About 70% of warts resolve spontaneously within 2 years (most within 1 year), but because new lesions develop in a number of patients, only about 50% of patients are lesion free after 2 years if left untreated.[3]

Treatment of warts is not very effective, as indicated by the fact that the American Academy of Dermatology lists at least 23 therapeutic options.[4] Since many of the lesions resolve spontaneously, no treatment is the preferred choice in many instances.[2,3] Specific indications for treatment include symptomatic warts, lesions that are disfiguring or disabling, large numbers of lesions, and an immunocompromised host.[4]

Topical treatments, which are usually accomplished with cantharidin (Cantharone) or salicylic acid, are as effective as more invasive therapies such as cryotherapy, laser treatment, or cautery.[1,3] The main disadvantage of topical treatments is that they often require considerable time until complete resolution is achieved.

One of the frequently used topical agents is cantharidin, which is an extract of the blister beetle or "Spanish fly." The method of using cantharidin is as follows: Apply the liquid to the wart, allow to dry, and cover with nonporous tape for 24 hours. After 24 hours replace the tape with a loose bandage such as a Band-Aid. After 2 weeks reassess and remove necrotic tissue. One treatment is usually effective for hand and body warts, but a second application may be given if necessary. Two or more treatments at 2-week intervals are usually required for plantar warts.

If salicylic compounds are used, the lesion should be soaked in water or a shampoo solution for 5 minutes before application. It should be rinsed and dried, and any debris should be mechanically removed from the lesion. The liquid should be applied to the lesion, with care not to include surrounding normal skin. Treatments should be repeated every 24 to 48 hours until the skin lines can be seen over the base of the lesion. Examples of the many available products are salicylic acid 17% (Compound W gel), salicylic acid 20% (Compound W liquid), salicylic acid 30% (Compound W plus), salicylic acid 16.7%–lactic acid 16.7% (Duofilm liquid), and salicylic acid 27% (Duoforte 27). Salicylic acid compounds specifically formulated for plantar warts include 40% salicylic acid disks and plasters (Carnation Callous and Corn Caps, Clear Away Plantar Wart Remover, Scholl Corn Removers), and salicylic acid 25%, lactic acid 10%, and formalin 5% (Duoplant). Disks or plaster should be purchased or cut to fit the lesion exactly so that normal surrounding skin is not affected. The plaster should then be applied and covered with waterproof tape, and treatments should be repeated every 48 hours. Once skin lines can be seen across the base of the lesion, treatment can be stopped. Total duration of treatment varies but may be up to 12 weeks. Liquid salicylic acid products such as Duoplant may be applied to the wart and covered with a waterproof bandage.

Cryotherapy may require repeat treatments every 2 to 3 weeks until the lesions resolve. With cryotherapy a single freeze-thaw cycle lasting 5 to 30 seconds with white margins extending 1 to 3 mm beyond the lesion is usually adequate. Laser treatments probably offer no significant advantages over other therapeutic modalities.[3]

As indicated previously, in addition to watchful waiting or "benign neglect" and invasive therapies, numerous other therapeutic modalities have been reported, although many of these are anecdotal. There are reports that "magic" such as transferring the virus to a coin is effective for some children.[3] High-dose cimetidine (Tagamet) over a 3-month period has been reported to be effective for adults[5] and children[6] with multiple recalcitrant warts. Response to treatment may not be seen for 4 to 6 weeks.[6] The adult regimen is 30 to 40 mg/kg/day in 3 divided doses for 3 months with a maximum daily dose of 3.5 g,[5] and that for children is 25 to 40 mg/kg/day in 3 or 4 divided doses.[6] In adults the treatment was found to be particularly efficacious for patients with plantar warts.[5] Cimetidine is thought to modulate the immune system. Immersing the affected area in a water bath at 45° C (113° F) for 30 minutes three times a week has been reported to be effective in immunocompromised patients with HIV who had widespread warts refractory to usual treatment modalities.[7] There are also anecdotal reports that recurrent applications of heat may be effective for plantar warts in nonimmunocompromised persons. The feet are soaked in hot water for 15 minutes once a week for 6 weeks.[8]

REFERENCES

1. Sterling J: Treating the troublesome wart, *Practitioner* 239:44-47, 1995.
2. Siegfried EC: Warts on children: an approach to therapy, *Pediatr Ann* 25:79-90, 1996.
3. Landow K: Nongenital warts: when is treatment warranted? *Postgrad Med* 99:245-249, 1996.
4. Committee on Guidelines of Care: Guidelines of care for warts: human papillomavirus, *J Am Acad Dermatol* 32:98-103, 1995.
5. Glass AT, Solomon BA: Cimetidine therapy for recalcitrant warts in adults, *Arch Dermatol* 132:680-682, 1996.
6. Orlow SJ, Paller A: Cimetidine therapy for multiple viral warts in children, *J Am Acad Dermatol* 28:794-796, 1993.
7. Kang S, Fitzpatrick TB: Debilitating verruca vulgaris in a patient infected with the human immunodeficiency virus: dramatic improvement with hyperthermia therapy, *Arch Dermatol* 130:294-296, 1994.
8. Larimore WL, Hartman JR: Family physician's notebook: diary from a week in practice, *Am Fam Physician* 47:1589-1590, 1993.

WRINKLES AND SKIN AGING

(See also sun damage)

Sun exposure and smoking are major risk factors for skin aging. Clinically aging skin is characterized by blotchy pigmentation, wrinkles, and in some cases actinic keratoses and skin cancer (see sun damage).[1]

A formulation of tretinoin (Renova) is available as a 0.05% cream for the treatment of facial wrinkles and mottled hyperpigmentation. For wrinkles it is applied lightly over the entire face once daily at bedtime. According to the manufacturer 6 months may be necessary for full effects to occur.

REFERENCES

1. Farmer KC, Naylor MF: Sun exposure, sunscreens, and skin cancer prevention: a year-round concern, *Ann Pharmacother* 30: 662-673, 1996.

EXERCISE

(See also bed rest; congestive heart failure; coronary artery disease; hypertension; cerebrovascular accidents; colon cancer; geriatrics; medical management of intermittent claudication; menopause; osteoarthritis; insulin-dependent diabetes mellitus; non-insulin-dependent diabetes mellitus; osteoporosis; obesity; secondary prevention of myocardial infarction)

Topics covered in this section

EPIDEMIOLOGY

An analysis of self-reported leisure time physical activity in the United States in 1991 indicated that 58.1% of adults participated in no physical activity or did so only on an irregular basis.[1] Another U.S. study found that 22% of adults over the age of 20 reported no leisure time physical activity. The rates were higher for the subgroups of Mexican Americans, black women, and the elderly.[2]

REFERENCES

1. Centers for Disease Control and Prevention: Prevalence of sedentary lifestyle, *MMWR* 42:576-579, 1993.
2. Crespo CJ, Keteyian SJ, Heath GW, et al: Leisure-time physical activity among US adults: results from the Third National Health and Nutrition Examination Survey, *Arch Intern Med* 156:93-98, 1996.

AEROBIC EXERCISE EQUIVALENCIES

(See also nutrition)

The energy consumed by aerobic exercise depends on the individual's weight and the type of exercise. Compared with brisk walking (7.5 kph or 4.5 mph), swimming at 20 yards (or meters) per minute consumes one third less energy, bicycling at 21 kph or 13 mph one third more, and cross-country skiing or jogging at 13 kph or 8 mph a little more than twice as much.[1]

A study from Wisconsin measured energy expenditure in healthy volunteers at given ratings of perceived exertion for six indoor exercise machines (Airdyne, cross-country skiing simulator, cycle ergometer, rowing ergometer, stair stepper, and treadmill). The most energy was expended with the treadmill and the least with the Airdyne and cycle.[2]

REFERENCES

1. *Consumer Reports,* July 1993, 58(7):421.
2. Zeni AI, Hoffman MD, Clifford PS: Energy expenditure with indoor exercise machines, *JAMA* 275:1424-1427, 1996.

BENEFITS OF EXERCISE

Overview and All-Cause Mortality

(See also breast cancer risk factors; exercise as a protection against anxiety and depression; exercise as a protection against colon cancer; medical management of intermittent claudication; exercise and congestive heart failure; exercise as a protection against coronary artery disease; exercise and hypertension; exercise as a protection against non-insulin-dependent diabetes mellitus; exercise and osteoarthritis; exercise as a protection against osteoporosis; exercise as a protection against stroke; exercise in the elderly; risk of exercise; life-style changes for disease prevention in menopausal women)

Proven and reputed benefits of exercise include a decreased risk of all-cause mortality,[1-3] coronary artery disease,[1-3] hypertension,[4] non-insulin-dependent diabetes mellitus,[5] strokes,[6] osteoporosis,[7,8] colon cancer,[9] and breast cancer.[10] Exercise increases mobility in the very elderly,[11] improves the functioning of patients with osteoarthritis of the knees,[12] is beneficial for depression,[13] anxiety,[14] and chronic fatigue syndrome,[15] and may decrease the incidence of serious gastrointestinal hemorrhages in the elderly.[16] It is the cornerstone of the medical management of intermittent claudication,[17] and it has been shown to improve insomnia in the elderly.[18] Recent evidence shows that moderate exercise (a daily brisk walk of 30 to 60 minutes or the equivalent) significantly decreases the all-cause mortality rate.[1-3,19-22] Smokers who participate in vigorous exercise also have decreased mortality rates.[23]

Two important papers on the beneficial effects of exercise have been published by Blair and associates.[1,2] In the first paper the authors measured physical fitness in 9777 men by treadmill testing on two occasions at mean intervals of 4.9 years. On the basis of the initial tests the men were divided into quintiles of fitness. Those in the lowest quintile were labeled unfit and all others fit. The results showed that men who were unfit at both assessments had the highest total and cardiovascular mortality, those who were fit at both assessments had the lowest, and those who were unfit at the first and fit at the second assessment fell between.[1] The second paper recorded the results of similar studies on 25,341 men and 7080 women. Results were similar, and in both sexes the most fit had the lowest all-cause and cardiovascular mortality.[2] Furthermore, these beneficial results were seen in individuals with a variety of other risk factors such as smoking, hypertension, hyperlipidemia, and obesity, even if no change occurred in smoking habits, blood pressure levels, cholesterol levels, or weight.[2]

Evidence that an increase in physical activity reduces mortality has been well documented in the Harvard Alumni Study.[19-21] The degree of benefit correlated with the total increase in energy expenditure per week.[20] The most recent report from the Harvard Alumni Study concluded that vigorous activities, but not nonvigorous activities, were associated with longevity.[21] It is important to realize that the term "vigorous" included not only running or jogging, swimming laps, playing tennis, or shoveling snow, but also brisk walking.[21] The Iowa Women's Health Study documented decreased mortality in postmenopausal women participating in moderate activity.[3]

It is difficult to quantitate exercise in the general population and to correlate it with mortality statistics. However, one assessment that attempted to do this came to the conclusion that poor dietary habits and sedentary life-style combined accounted for 14% of deaths in the United States, and smoking accounted for 19%.

REFERENCES

1. Blair SN, Kohl HW III, Barlow CE, et al: Changes in physical fitness and all-cause mortality: a prospective study of healthy and unhealthy men, *JAMA* 273:1093-1098, 1995.
2. Blair SN, Kampert JB, Kohl HW III, et al: Influences of cardiorespiratory fitness and other precursors on cardiovascular disease and all-cause mortality in men and women, *JAMA* 276:205-210, 1996.
3. Kushi LH, Fee RM, Folsom AR, et al: Physical activity and mortality in postmenopausal women, *JAMA* 277:1287-1292, 1997.
4. Kokkinos PF, Narayan P, Colleran JA, et al: Effects of regular exercise on blood pressure and left ventricular hypertrophy in African-American men with severe hypertension, *N Engl J Med* 333:1462-1467, 1995.
5. Helmrich SP, Ragland DR, Leung RW, et al: Physical activity and reduced occurrence of non-insulin-dependent diabetes mellitus, *N Engl J Med* 325:147-152, 1991.

6. Shinton R, Sagar G: Lifelong exercise and stroke, *BMJ* 307: 231-234, 1993.
7. Dalsky GP, Stocke KS, Ehsani AA, et al: Weight-bearing exercise training and lumbar bone mineral content in postmenopausal women, *Ann Intern Med* 108:824-828, 1988.
8. Grisso JA, Kelsey JL, Strom BL, et al: Risk factors for hip fracture in black women, *N Engl J Med* 330:1555-1559, 1994.
9. Lee I, Paffenbarger RS, Hsieh C: Physical activity and risk of developing colorectal cancer among college alumni, *J Natl Cancer Inst* 83:1324-1329, 1991.
10. Thune I, Brenn T, Lund E, Gaard M: Physical activity and the risk of breast cancer, *N Engl J Med* 336:1269-1275, 1997.
11. Fiatarone MA, O'Neill EF, Ryan ND, et al: Exercise training and nutritional supplementation for physical frailty in very elderly people, *N Engl J Med* 330:1769-1775, 1994.
12. Ettinger WH Jr, Burns R, Messier S, et al: A randomized trial comparing aerobic exercise and resistance exercise with a health education program in older adults with knee osteoarthritis: the Fitness, Arthritis, and Senior Trial (FAST), *JAMA* 277: 25-31, 1997.
13. Taylor CB, Sallis JF, Needle R: The relationship of physical activity and exercise to mental health, *Public Health Rep* 100: 195-201, 1995.
14. Petruzello SJ, Landers DM, Hatfield BD, et al: A meta-analysis on the anxiety-reducing effects of acute and chronic exercise, *Sports Med* 11:143-182, 1991.
15. Fulcher KY, White PD: Randomised controlled trial of graded exercise in patients with the chronic fatigue syndrome, *BMJ* 314:1647-1652, 1997.
16. Pahor M, Guralnik JM, Salive ME, et al: Physical activity and risk of severe gastrointestinal hemorrhage in older persons, *JAMA* 272:595-599, 1994.
17. Gardner AW, Poehlman ET: Exercise rehabilitation programs for the treatment of claudication pain: a meta-analysis, *JAMA* 274:975-980, 1995.
18. King AC, Oman RF, Brassington GS, et al: Moderate-intensity exercise and self-rated quality of sleep in older adults: a randomized controlled trial, *JAMA* 277:32-37, 1997.
19. Paffenbarger RS Jr, Hyde RT, Wing AL, et al: The association of changes in physical-activity level and other life-style characteristics with mortality among men, *N Engl J Med* 328:538-545, 1993.
20. Paffenbarger RS Jr, Kampert JB, Lee I-M, et al: Changes in physical activity and other lifeway patterns influencing longevity, *Med Sci Sports Exerc* 26:857-865, 1994.
21. Lee I-M, Chung-Cheng H, Paffenbarger RS Jr: Exercise intensity and longevity in men: the Harvard Alumni Health Study, *JAMA* 273:1179-1184, 1995.
22. McGinnis JM, Foege WH: Actual causes of death in the United States, *JAMA* 270:2207-2211, 1993.
23. Hedblad B, Ogren M, Isacsson S-O, et al: Reduced cardiovascular mortality risk in male smokers who are physically active: results from a 25-year follow-up of the Prospective Population Study Men Born in 1914, *Arch Intern Med* 157:893-899, 1997.

Exercise as a Protection Against Coronary Artery Disease

(See also exercise as a protection against anxiety and depression; exercise as a protection against colon cancer; exercise as a protection against non-insulin-dependent diabetes mellitus; exercise as a protection against osteoporosis; exercise and congestive heart failure; exercise as a protection against stroke; exercise in the elderly; female athletes; hormone replacement therapy; life-style changes for disease prevention in menopausal women; overview of exercise benefits; risk of exercise)

Protection against coronary artery disease is probably the most important health gain from exercise programs. Numerous studies have demonstrated this benefit in the prevention of both first-time events[1-5] and recurrences of myocardial infarction (MI).[6] Powell and associates[1] critically reviewed the English language literature on the subject and determined that the better the quality of a study, the more likely that it showed a beneficial effect of exercise on the risk of coronary artery disease. They concluded that the increase in relative risk of coronary artery disease in sedentary persons was of equal magnitude to that caused by hypertension, smoking, or hypercholesterolemia. Results of the Harvard Alumni Study gave similar results; the quantitative benefit of exercise in reducing coronary artery mortality was as great as avoiding obesity, achieving good blood pressure control, or stopping smoking.[3]

A question of great clinical importance is the quantity of exercise that is necessary to produce a cardioprotective effect. An encouraging finding in recent years is that moderate exercise appears to be as or almost as beneficial as intense exercise in protecting against cardiovascular events.[4,5,7-9] Another important finding in this area is that brief bouts of exercise are as beneficial as more prolonged exercise periods, provided the total amount of exercise is sufficient (30 minutes day).[10]

Relatively few studies have evaluated the cardioprotective effects of exercise in women; those that have been done showed a significant decrease in the risk of coronary events.[5,8,11] Even fewer studies have evaluated the effect of exercise in smokers; a Swedish prospective study found that vigorous physical activity decreased cardiovascular mortality in smokers by almost 40%.[12]

Some theoretical ways in which exercise may protect against coronary artery disease are through lowering cholesterol levels, raising high-density lipoprotein levels, reducing weight, improving glucose tolerance, lowering blood pressure, increasing fibrinolysis, and enhancing myocardial electrical stability.[1]

REFERENCES

1. Powell KE, Thompson PD, Caspersen CJ, et al: Physical activity and the incidence of coronary heart disease, *Annu Rev Public Health* 8:253-287, 1987.
2. Morris JN, Clayton DG, Everitt MG, et al: Exercise in leisure time: coronary attack rate and death rates, *Br Heart J* 63:325-334, 1990.

3. Paffenbarger RS Jr, Hyde RT, Wing AL, et al: The association of changes in physical-activity level and other lifestyle characteristics with mortality among men, *N Engl J Med* 328:538-545, 1993.
4. Lakka TA, Venalainen JM, Rauremaa R, et al: Relation of leisure-time physical activity and cardiorespiratory fitness to the risk of acute myocardial infarction in men, *N Engl J Med* 330:1549-1554, 1994.
5. Kushi LH, Fee RM, Folsom AR, et al: Physical activity and mortality in postmenopausal women, *JAMA* 277:1287-1292, 1997.
6. Oldridge NB, Guyatt GH, Fischer ME, et al: Cardiac rehabilitation after myocardial infarction: combined experience of randomized clinical trials, *JAMA* 260:945-950, 1988.
7. Blair SN, Kohl HW III, Barlow CE, et al: Changes in physical fitness and all-cause mortality: a prospective study of healthy and unhealthy men, *JAMA* 273:1093-1098, 1995.
8. LaCroix AZ, Leveille SG, Hecht JA, et al: Does walking decrease the risk of cardiovascular disease hospitalizations and death in older adults? *J Am Geriatr Soc* 44:113-120, 1996.
9. Blair SN: Dose of exercise and health benefits (editorial), *Arch Intern Med* 157:153-154, 1997.
10. Pate RR, Pratt M, Blair SN, et al: Physical activity and public health: a recommendation from the Centers for Disease Control and Prevention and the American College of Sports Medicine, *JAMA* 273:402-407, 1995.
11. Rich-Edwards JW, Manson JE, Hennekens C, et al: The primary prevention of coronary heart disease in women, *N Engl J Med* 332:1758-1766, 1995.
12. Hedblad B, Ogren M, Isacsson S-O, et al: Reduced cardiovascular mortality risk in male smokers who are physically active: results from a 25-year follow-up of the Prospective Population Study Men Born in 1914, *Arch Intern Med* 157:893-899, 1997.

Exercise as a Protection Against Stroke

(See also exercise as a protection against anxiety and depression; exercise as a protection against colon cancer; exercise as a protection against coronary artery disease; exercise and congestive heart failure; exercise as a protection against non-insulin-dependent diabetes mellitus; exercise as a protection against osteoporosis; exercise in the elderly; overview of exercise benefits; risk of exercise)

In one British study, moderate physical activity such as frequent walking was associated with a decreased incidence of stroke and heart attacks in middle-aged men.[1] In another study a history of vigorous exercise at ages 15 to 25 and a history of recent walking or vigorous exercise appeared to protect against stroke.[2]

REFERENCES

1. Wannamethee Gl, Shaper AG: Physical activity and stroke in British middle-aged men, *BMJ* 304:597-601, 1992.
2. Shinton R, Sagar G: Lifelong exercise and stroke, *BMJ* 307:231-234, 1993.

Exercise as a Protection Against Non-Insulin-Dependent Diabetes Mellitus

(See also exercise as a protection against anxiety and depression; exercise as a protection against colon cancer; exercise and congestive heart failure; exercise as a protection against coronary artery disease; exercise as a protection against osteoporosis; exercise as a protection against stroke; exercise in the elderly; overview of exercise benefits; risk of exercise)

A follow-up study of male alumni from the University of Pennsylvania found a significant protective effect of exercise against the development of non-insulin-dependent diabetes.[1] The incidence was much lower in the most physically active compared with the least active, and a significant difference remained even after correction for obesity. The greatest protection was noted for men at highest risk for the disease (because of obesity, hypertension, and a family history of diabetes).[1] Similar results have been reported in a study of Finnish men.[2] Aside from decreasing the level of obesity, the mechanism of protection is probably an increased insulin sensitivity induced by the exercise.[3]

REFERENCES

1. Helmrich SP, Ragland DR, Leung RW, et al: Physical activity and reduced occurrence of non-insulin-dependent diabetes mellitus, *N Engl J Med* 325:147-152, 1991.
2. Lynch J, Helmrich SP, Lakka TA, et al: Moderately intense physical activities and high levels of cardiorespiratory fitness reduce the risk of non-insulin-dependent diabetes mellitus in middle-aged men, *Arch Intern Med* 156:1307-1314, 1996.
3. Horton ES: Exercise and decreased risk of NIDDM (editorial), *N Engl J Med* 325:196-198, 1991.

Exercise as a Protection Against Osteoporosis

(See also exercise as a protection against anxiety and depression; exercise as a protection against colon cancer; exercise and congestive heart failure; exercise as a protection against coronary artery disease; exercise as a protection against non-insulin-dependent diabetes mellitus; exercise as a protection against stroke; exercise in the elderly; osteoporosis; overview of exercise benefits; risk of exercise)

Although the relationship between exercise and osteoporosis has been well studied, this does not seem to be the case with major fractures. For example, a review of the various risk factors for hip fracture assessed many variables, including body weight, smoking, alcohol intake, thiazide use, and estrogen replacement therapy, but did not evaluate or even refer to exercise in the discussion of literature on the subject.[1]

The amount of physical activity in childhood seems to correlate directly with the adult bone density.[2] In addition, a number of reports indicate that exercise decreases the rate of bone density loss in postmenopausal women. This is discussed more fully under "Osteoporosis."

REFERENCES

1. Grisso JA, Kelsey JL, Strom BL, et al: Risk factors for hip fracture in black women, *N Engl J Med* 330:1555-1559, 1994.
2. McCulloch RG, Bailey DA, Houston S, et al: Effects of physical activity, dietary calcium intake and selected lifestyle factors on bone density in young women, *Can Med Assoc J* 142:221-227, 1990.

Exercise as a Protection Against Colon Cancer

(See also exercise as a protection against anxiety and depression; exercise as a protection against coronary artery disease; exercise and congestive heart failure; exercise as a protection against non-insulin-dependent diabetes mellitus; exercise as a protection against stroke; exercise in the elderly; overview of exercise benefits; risk of exercise)

A few studies have suggested that physical inactivity is associated with an increased risk of colon cancer.[1-4] A Swedish study covering a 14-year follow-up period found that the relative risk of colon cancer in the least physically active group was 3.6 times that of the most physically active group.[1] Rates of rectal cancer were unaffected. The Health Professionals Follow-up Study found that the colon cancer risk for men in the highest quintile of leisure time physical activity was 0.53 that of those in the lowest quintile.[4] A possible explanation of this finding is that exercise decreases intestinal transit time and so diminishes exposure of the colonic mucosa to fecal carcinogens.

REFERENCES

1. Gerhardsson M, Floderus B, Norell SE: Physical activity and colon cancer risk, *Int J Epidemiol* 17:743-746, 1988.
2. Powell GE, Caspersen CJ, Hoplan JP, et al: Physical activity and chronic diseases, *Am J Clin Nutr* 49:999-1006, 1989.
3. Lee I, Paffenbarger RS, Hsieh C: Physical activity and risk of developing colorectal cancer among college alumni, *J Natl Cancer Inst* 83:1324-1329, 1991.
4. Giovannucci E, Ascherio A, Rimm EB, et al: Physical activity, obesity, and risk for colon cancer and adenoma in men, *Ann Intern Med* 122:327-334, 1995.

Exercise as a Protection Against Anxiety and Depression

(See also exercise as a protection against anxiety and depression; exercise as a protection against colon cancer; exercise as a protection against coronary artery disease; exercise as a protection against non-insulin-dependent diabetes mellitus; exercise as a protection against stroke; exercise in the elderly; overview of exercise benefits; risk of exercise)

Evidence supports the role of exercise as a protective factor against or therapeutic agent for anxiety and depression.[1-4]

REFERENCES

1. King AC, Taylor CB, Haskell WL, et al: Influence of regular aerobic exercise on psychological health, *Health Psychol* 8:305-324, 1989.
2. Taylor CB, Sallis JF, Needle R: The relationship of physical activity and exercise to mental health, *Public Health Rep* 100:195-201, 1995.
3. Martinsen EW: Physical activity and depression: clinical experience, *Acta Psychiatr Scand* 377(suppl):23-27, 1994.
4. Byrne A, Byrne DG: The effect of exercise on depression, anxiety and other mood states: a review, *J Psychosom Res* 37:565-574, 1993.

Exercise in the Elderly

(See also exercise as a protection against anxiety and depression; exercise as a protection against colon cancer; exercise and congestive heart failure; exercise as a protection against coronary artery disease; exercise as a protection against non-insulin-dependent diabetes mellitus; exercise as a protection against stroke; overview of exercise benefits; risk of exercise)

A number of studies have shown that mild to moderate endurance exercise in the elderly is beneficial.[1-3]

A study from the Hebrew Rehabilitation Center for the Aged in Roslindale, Massachusetts, has demonstrated a dramatic effect of resistance exercises in improving the mobility of the very elderly.[4] The patients who were evaluated were all residents of a nursing home. All were over 70 years of age, 38% were over 90 years of age, and the mean age was 87. The resisted exercise group underwent a regimen of high-intensity progressive resistance training of the hip and knee extensors lasting 45 minutes three times a week for 10 weeks. Muscle strength and mass increased significantly, but more important, the exercise intervention increased the habitual gait velocity, improved the ability to climb stairs, and produced an overall growth in physical activity. A liquid nutritional supplement did not improve the performance of either the exercising group or the nonexercising control group. The authors postulated that the failure of some other studies to show benefits in nursing home residents given endurance training[5,6] (in contrast to resistance training) was because the patients had insufficient muscle strength to benefit from it.

For the ambulatory elderly, Shephard[7] recommends endurance exercises plus 8 to 10 repetitions or resistance exercises twice a week for each set of major muscle groups. The degree of resistance should be enough to induce slight fatigue by the tenth repetition. The goal of such exercises is to maintain lean muscle mass.

A 1994 study of elderly patients in various U.S. communities found that the relative risk of severe gastrointestinal hemorrhage in elderly patients with a mean age of 77 was 0.7 for those who exercised at least three times per week compared with the nonexercising control group.[8] Exercise was defined as walking, gardening, or "doing vigorous physical activity" three times a week or more. One theoretical explanation is that exercise decreases ischemia in the splanchnic circulation.

REFERENCES

1. Blair SN, Kohl HW, Paffenberger RS Jr, et al: Physical fitness and all-cause mortality: a prospective study of healthy men and women, *JAMA* 262:2395-2401, 1989.

2. Powell KE, Thompson PD, Caspersen CJ, et al: Physical activity and the incidence of coronary heart disease, *Annu Rev Public Health* 8:253-287, 1987.
3. Guralnik JM, Kaplan GA: Predictors of healthy aging: prospective evidence from the Alameda County Study, *Am J Public Health* 79:703-708, 1989.
4. Fiatarone MA, O'Neill EF, Ryan ND, et al: Exercise training and nutritional supplementation for physical frailty in very elderly people, *N Engl J Med* 330:1769-1775, 1994.
5. Blankfort-Doyle W, Waxman H, Coughey K: An exercise program for nursing home residents. In Ostrow AC, ed: *Aging and motor behavior,* Indianapolis, 1989, Benchmark Press, pp 201-206.
6. Waters R, Yakura J: Energy expenditure of normal and abnormal ambulation. In Smidt GL, ed: *Gait in rehabilitation,* New York, 1990, Churchill Livingston, pp 65-96.
7. Shephard RJ: Physical activity, fitness and cardiovascular health: a brief counselling guide for older patients, *Can Med Assoc J* 151:557-561, 1994.
8. Pahor M, Guralnik JM, Salive ME, et al: Physical activity and risk of severe gastrointestinal hemorrhage in older persons, *JAMA* 272:595-599, 1994.

RISKS OF EXERCISE

(See also cardiac arrest; cardiopulmonary resuscitation; diarrhea and hematochezia in runners; exercise as a protection against anxiety and depression; exercise as a protection against colon cancer; exercise and congestive heart failure; exercise as a protection against coronary artery disease; exercise as a protection against non-insulin-dependent diabetes mellitus; exercise as a protection against stroke; exercise-induced hematuria; female athletes; overview of exercise benefits; preparticipation medical examinations; urinalysis-blood)

Exercise entails a number of risks, the most common of which are probably musculoskeletal problems. These are most likely to occur with high-intensity exercise.[1] Other important adverse effects in women come about when weight loss from the exercise is of such a degree as to induce amenorrhea. This is associated with osteoporosis and an increased risk of infertility.[1] Cultural pressures on women athletes may also foster eating disorders and the so-called female athlete triad of an eating disorder, amenorrhea, and osteoporosis.[2]

The relative risk of sudden death is two to three times greater during the exercise period but is decreased by 50% for the remaining 23 hours of the day. The relative risk of MI during vigorous exercise (6 METS [metabolic equivalents of oxygen consumption]) is increased in sedentary individuals but not in physically active ones.[3-5]

About 5% of MIs are associated with heavy exercise. The mechanism is uncertain. Platelets are activated with exercise in sedentary individuals but not in those who are regularly physically active. Regular exercise increases the endogenous fibrinolytic system.[3-5]

Acute exertional rhabdomyolysis is caused by damage to skeletal muscle with the release of myoglobin and other cellular constituents into the circulation. In severe cases there may be intravascular coagulation, renal failure, and even death. Mild to moderately severe cases may result in hyperkalemia, hypernatremia, hyperphosphatemia, hypocalcemia (from deposition of calcium in necrotic muscle), and lactic acidosis. The condition should be suspected when the patient has a significant overuse syndrome involving pain and often swelling of muscles. Particular risk factors are high ambient temperature, high humidity, and inadequate fluid intake; the untrained exerciser is probably at greater risk than the trained athlete. A urine dipstick test will be positive for blood, but no red blood cells will be seen. Usually the serum creatine kinase level is markedly elevated. Fluid replacement is the cornerstone of treatment.[6]

REFERENCES

1. Manson JE, Lee I-M: Exercise for women—how much pain for optimal gain? (editorial), *N Engl J Med* 334:1325-1327, 1996.
2. Nattiv A, Agostini R, Drinkwater B, et al: The female athlete triad: the inter-relatedness of disordered eating, amenorrhea, and osteoporosis, *Clin Sports Med* 13:405-418, 1994.
3. Mittleman MA, Maclure M, Tofler GH, et al: Triggering of acute myocardial infarction by heavy physical exertion—protection against triggering by regular exertion: determinants of Myocardial Infarction Onset Study Investigators, *N Engl J Med* 329: 1677-1683, 1993.
4. Willich SN, Lewis M, Löwel H, et al: Physical exertion as a trigger of acute myocardial infarction: triggers and mechanisms of Myocardial Infarction Study Group, *N Engl J Med* 329:1684-1690, 1993.
5. Curfman G: Is exercise beneficial—or hazardous—to your heart? (editorial), *N Engl J Med* 329:730-731, 1993.
6. Line RL, Rust GS: Acute exertional rhabdomyolysis, *Am Fam Physician* 52:502-506, 1995.

EXERCISE GUIDELINES

Traditional Exercise Prescriptions

The traditional exercise prescription is aimed at developing cardiovascular fitness and, as discussed previously, is probably unnecessary for producing a cardioprotective effect. Traditional programs have aimed to increase the pulse rate to the following levels:

Healthy individuals	70%-85% of 220–Age
Cardiovascular-compromised individuals	50%-70% of 220–Age

The overall traditional exercise prescription is outlined below:

Frequency	3-5 times a week
Intensity	220–Age etc. (see above)
Time	40-60 minutes
Type	Aerobic

Exercise Prescription Recommendations of U.S. Expert Panels

Some of the major recommendations of the 1996 NIH Consensus Conference on exercise are as follows[1]:

1. Children and adults should attempt to accumulate 30 minutes of moderate-intensity exercise on most and preferably all days of the week.

2. Several brief bouts of moderate activity are beneficial.
3. Types of exercise that are classified as moderate activity include many occupational functions or activities of daily living, as well as leisure time activity: brisk walking, cycling, swimming, home repair, and yard work.
4. Persons already meeting these recommendations may gain further benefits through more exercise.
5. Exercise reduces all-cause mortality and cardiovascular mortality in patients with known cardiovascular disease. Patients with these conditions should participate in appropriately prescribed and supervised exercise training programs.

The preceding recommendations differ from many previous ones in that they are based on these principles: moderate exercise is effective in promoting health, and exercise does not have to be done in block periods to be beneficial; intermittent short bouts of exercise are also efficacious.[2]

The 1996 U.S. Surgeon General's Report on Physical Activity and Health recommends moderate exercise such as brisk walking or raking leaves for 30 minutes a day, running 1.5 miles (2.5 km) in 20 minutes every day, swimming laps for 20 minutes a day, or playing basketball for 15 to 20 minutes a day. Additional exercise will lead to added health benefits.[3] Other ways of obtaining moderate exercise are walking up stairs rather than taking elevators, walking short distances instead of driving, pedaling a stationary bicycle while watching television, and housework or dancing at an intensity equivalent to brisk walking.[2]

In a Glasgow study a sign was placed beside the escalator in an underground station saying, "Stay Healthy, Save Time, Use the Stairs." Before the sign was posted, 8% of persons used the stairs. During the 3 weeks the sign was posted, stair use increased to an average of 21%. Twelve weeks after removal of the poster fewer people used the stairs but the rate was still higher than baseline. Both at baseline and after the placard was posted, twice as many men as women used the stairs.[4]

REFERENCES

1. Physical activity and cardiovascular health: NIH Consensus Development Panel on Physical Activity and Cardiovascular Health, *JAMA* 276:241-246, 1996.
2. Pate RR, Pratt M, Blair SN, et al: Physical activity and public health. a recommendation from the Centers for Disease Control and Prevention and the American College of Sports Medicine, *JAMA* 273:402-407, 1995.
3. Centers for Disease Control and Prevention: Surgeon General's report on physical activity and health, *JAMA* 276:522, 1996.
4. Blamey A, Mutrie N, Aitchison T: Health promotion by encouraged use of stairs, *BMJ* 311:289-290, 1995.

GASTROINTESTINAL SYSTEM

Topics covered in this section

ANAL AND ANORECTAL DISORDERS

Anal Fissures

Ninety percent of anal fissures are found in the posterior midline, and almost all the others are located in the anterior midline.[1,2] If fissures are detected in other locations, underlying diseases such as Crohn's disease should be suspected.[1]

Conservative treatment is successful in most patients and consists of maneuvers to relieve spasm of the anal sphincter and avoid hard bulky stools. Stool management consists of bulking agents such as fruits and vegetables and psyllium (Metamucil) with plenty of water.[1-3] Warm baths, 1% hydrocortisone ointment,[1-3] and if necessary 5% lidocaine applied to the anus just before bowel movements[3] are generally effective.

A prospective randomized placebo-controlled trial has shown that nitroglycerin (glyceryl trinitrate) ointment dramatically increases the healing rate of persistent anal fissures. In one study a 0.2% glyceryl trinitrate ointment was applied to the fissure twice a day for 4 to 6 weeks. A few patients had mild headaches. The drug is believed to relax the anal sphincter muscle. If prescribing this ointment, the physician should be sure to underline the dosage of 0.2%, since the concentration of nitroglycerin ointment used for angina is generally 2.0%.[4] Similar results were previously reported in a small group of patients using a 0.5% nitroglycerin ointment. Pain was relieved within 3 to 4 minutes, especially the pain that followed bowel movements, and the relief lasted for 4 to 6 hours. The major adverse effect was headaches.[5]

If conservative treatment fails, surgery is probably indicated. The procedure of choice is a lateral internal sphincterotomy with the goal of breaking the cycle of internal sphincter spasm.[1-3] Digital stretching of the anal sphincter no longer has a role.[1,2]

Hemorrhoids

Hemorrhoids may be external or internal. External hemorrhoids lie distal to the dentate line and are covered by skin; internal hemorrhoids are proximal to the dentate line and are covered by mucosa.[1]

External hemorrhoids become symptomatic when they become thrombosed. Pain peaks in 48 to 72 hours and then gradually resolves. If the patient has intense pain and is seen within 72 hours, incision and evacuation of the thrombus or excision of the lesion with overlying skin may be performed.[1,2] The usual conservative treatment consists of warm baths, increased fiber, and fluids.[2] An alternative may be the application of a 0.5% or 0.2% nitroglycerin ointment to the anus and distal anal canal. In a series of five patients a 0.5% ointment produced marked immediate pain relief, probably through relief of sphincter spasm.[5]

Four categories of internal hemorrhoids have been established. Grade I internal hemorrhoids are small and do not prolapse; grade II hemorrhoids prolapse with bowel movement but return spontaneously; grade III hemorrhoids prolapse but can be replaced manually; grade IV hemorrhoids prolapse and cannot be replaced manually. Internal hemorrhoids usually lie in the right anterior, right posterior, and left lateral positions.[1,2]

Anemia from rectal bleeding secondary to internal hemorrhoids is well documented. Among 43 patients with this condition reported from the Mayo Clinic, the mean hemoglobin concentration was 9.4 g/dl (94 g/L). Eighty-four percent of the patients gave a history of blood squirting from the anus or the passage of clots. Six of the 43 had coagulation defects.[6]

Conservative management of internal hemorrhoids is the initial treatment of choice for grade I to III lesions. This consists of avoiding straining at stool, increasing dietary fiber in the form of fruit, vegetables, and fiber products such as psyllium, and maintaining a high fluid intake (six to eight glasses of caffeine-free fluid per day).[2] Interventional options include rubber band ligation, infrared photocoagulation, and injection sclerotherapy. Hemorrhoidectomy is indicated for grade IV lesions and for other cases that do not respond to less invasive procedures.[1,2]

Proctalgia Fugax

Proctalgia fugax is characterized by infrequent episodes of severe perianal pain. These episodes usually last only a few minutes and are sometimes relieved by defecation. In some patients the episodes are precipitated by orgasm. Proctalgia fugax is a disorder of adults and affects both sexes. No serious underlying diseases are associated with this condition, and when patients give a typical history, no investigations are required. Because the pain is brief and infrequent, there is generally no specific treatment, although digital dilatation of the anus by the patient has been reported to give relief, presumably by relaxing the sphincter.[7,8] There are anecdotal reports that clonidine (Catapres) 0.15 mg bid or diltiazem (Cardizem) 80 mg bid is effective for very severe cases.[7]

Pruritus Ani

Pruritus ani has been estimated to occur in about 5% of the population, and men are four times more likely to be affected than women.[1] Most cases of pruritus ani are primary, but in some instances the condition is secondary to other benign or malignant anorectal or systemic disorders, including pinworms, hemorrhoids, fissures, fistulas, chronic dermatoses, diabetes, rectal carcinomas, Paget's disease, and Bowen's disease.[1-3,9] In children the most common cause is pinworms.[2] A thorough workup for secondary causes is indicated if suggested by the initial history or physical examination or if the patient fails to respond to treatment within a month or so.[2,3]

A variety of foods are said to cause or aggravate pruritus ani. Coffee seems to be high on the list of responsible agents; others are said to be tea, colas, beer, chocolate, tomatoes, and milk.[1-3,9] As far as I know, no good controlled studies have been published supporting these claims.

Treatment of primary pruritus ani consists of eliminating aggravating nutrients and potentially irritating local agents such as scented soaps and over-the-counter medications. If the area is acutely inflamed and weeping, warm baths may be helpful. Good perianal hygiene is important. After bowel movements or when washing, the perianal area may be gently cleansed and then dried by blotting with cotton balls or, even better, with the use of a hair dryer. Rubbing and scrubbing of the area should be avoided.[1,2] Although failure to clean the perianal region adequately after bowel movements may aggravate pruritus ani, excessive cleansing is equally detrimental.[2] As the condition improves, corn starch may be applied to keep the area dry; absorbent pads and loose undergarments also help in keeping moisture down.[1,2] In some cases a short course of 1% hydrocortisone cream hastens symptomatic relief.[1]

REFERENCES

1. Fazio VW, Tjandra JJ: The management of perianal diseases, *Adv Surg* 29:59-78, 1996.
2. Nagle D, Rolandelli RH: Primary care office management of perianal and anal disease, *Primary Care* 23:609-620, 1996.
3. Mazier WP: Hemorrhoids, fissures, and pruritus ani, *Surg Clin North Am* 74:1277-1292, 1994.
4. Lund JN, Armitage NC, Scholefield JH: Use of glyceryl trinitrate ointment in the treatment of anal fissure, *Br J Surg* 83:776-777, 1996.
5. Gorfine SR: Treatment of benign anal disease with topical nitroglycerin, *Dis Colon Rectum* 38:453-456, 1995.
6. Kluiber RM, Wolff BG: Evaluation of anemia caused by hemorrhoidal bleeding, *Dis Colon Rectum* 37:1006-1007, 1994.
7. Nidorf DM, Jamison ER: Proctalgia fugax, *Am Fam Physician* 52:2238-2240, 1995.
8. Rockefeller R: Digital dilatation for relief of proctalgia fugax (letter), *Am Fam Physician* 54:72, 1996.
9. Daniel GL, Longo WE, Vernava AM 3d: Pruritus ani: causes and concerns, *Dis Colon Rectum* 37:670-674, 1994.

BILIARY SYSTEM

Cholecystectomy

Clear indications for cholecystectomy are acute cholecystitis and gallstone-associated pancreatitis. The presence of asymptomatic gallstones is not an indication for surgery because the incidence of biliary pain in such circumstances is only 1% to 2% per year and decreases over time; serious sequelae are 10 times less frequent in asymptomatic cases. A more difficult decision is whether a patient who has had one episode of biliary colic needs surgery. In 30% no more episodes of pain occur, but the overall risk of recurrent pain is 30% to 50% per year for a few years.[1]

The pain of gallbladder disease must be differentiated from other causes of abdominal pain. Biliary colic tends to be infrequent, episodic, and intense. Short or fleeting pain or continuous pain is usually not due to gallstones.[1]

Advantages of laparoscopic cholecystectomy are better cosmetic results and a more rapid return to work or full activity. In one study the mean time to full recovery was 2 weeks for the laparoscopic procedures versus 8 weeks for the open procedure.[2] A concern about laparoscopic cholecystectomy is that the rate of injury to the common bile duct, although low (up to 0.5%), is higher than that with open cholecystectomy (0.1% to 0.2%). This higher rate might result from a learning curve among surgeons who are adopting the procedure.[1]

Postcholecystectomy diarrhea develops in about 18% of patients subjected to cholecystectomy.[2] Some cases may be due to bile acid malabsorption,[3,4] but for others the cause is uncertain.[4] The efficacy of cholestyramine in controlling diarrhea is variously reported as "dramatic"[3] to useful for only a minority of patients.[4]

REFERENCES

1. Ransohoff DF, McSherry CK: Why are cholecystectomy rates increasing? (editorial), *JAMA* 273:1621-1622, 1995.
2. Vander Velpen GC, Shimi SM, Cuschieri A: Outcome after cholecystectomy for symptomatic gall stone disease and effect of surgical access: laparoscopic versus open approach, *Gut* 34:1448-1451, 1993.
3. Arlow FL, Dekovich AA, Priest RJ, et al: Bile acid–mediated postcholecystectomy diarrhea, *Arch Intern Med* 147:1327-1332, 1987.
4. Fromm H, Tunuguntla AK, Malavolti M, et al: Absence of significant role of bile acids in diarrhea of a heterogeneous group of postcholecystectomy patients, *Dig Dis Sci* 32:33-44, 1987.

Endoscopic Retrograde Cholangiopancreatography and Sphincterotomy

Endoscopic retrograde cholangiopancreatography (ERCP) is often combined with sphincterotomy. In one multicenter study the most common indications for sphincterotomy were common bile duct stones and the placement of biliary stents for malignant obstruction. The overall complication rate in this series was just under 10%. Pancreatitis was the most common sequela, followed by hemorrhage and cholangitis. Complications were greater when the sphincterotomy was performed by endoscopists who did so rarely and in patients being treated for "suspected dysfunction of the sphincter of Oddi."[1]

Dysfunction of the sphincter of Oddi is largely an American disorder; in other parts of the world patients with similar symptoms are usually considered to have irritable bowel disease. Dysfunction of the sphincter of Oddi is an ill-defined condition in which the major symptoms are abdominal pain and occasionally transient elevations of liver enzyme levels. It is most frequently diagnosed in middle-aged women who have had previous cholecystectomies. Sphincterotomy relieves symptoms in less than 75% of cases and with a complication rate of over 20%.[2]

REFERENCES

1. Freeman ML, Nelson DB, Sherman S, et al: Complications of endoscopic biliary sphincterotomy, *N Engl J Med* 335:909-918, 1996.
2. Huibregtse K: Complications of endoscopic sphincterotomy and their prevention (editorial), *N Engl J Med* 335:961-963, 1996.

CELIAC DISEASE

Celiac disease is often diagnosed in childhood or in the third or fourth decade. Patients may have minimal or no gastrointestinal symptoms. Presenting findings may be weight loss, bone pain from fractures, or unexplained hypocalcemia, anemia, or folate deficiency. Patients with celiac disease have an increased incidence of autoimmune thyroiditis.[1]

REFERENCES

1. Shaker JL, Brickner RC, Findling JW, et al: Hypocalcemia and skeletal disease as presenting features of celiac disease, *Arch Intern Med* 157:1013-1016, 1997.

COLON

(See also inflammatory bowel disease; irritable bowel disease)

Colon Cancer

(See also gastrointestinal bleeding and iron deficiency anemia)

Epidemiology

About 15% of newly diagnosed cancers in both men and women occur in the colon and rectum. Colorectal cancer is the second most common cancer in the United States and has the second highest mortality rate. The incidence increases progressively with age; in North America the lifetime risk of having the disease is estimated to be 6% and the lifetime risk of dying of the disease is about 2.6%.[1] The median age at diagnosis is 70, and only 4% of cases occur in persons under 50.

The distribution of cancers within the colon has changed over the past few decades so that more lesions are now found on the right side and fewer on the left side. At present about one fourth of the cancers are in the proximal colon and a little over half in the sigmoid colon and rectum.[2] Another way of putting this is that at least half of all colonic polyps and cancers are within 60 cm of the anus and so are at least theoretically within reach of the long flexible sigmoidoscope.[3]

Risk factors.[4-13] The risk of colon cancer for untreated persons with the familial polyposis syndrome is 100%.

The relative risk of colon cancer is generally considered to be two to three times greater in persons with a first-degree relative who has had the disease. A recent prospective study of U.S. health professionals found an overall increased relative risk of 1.72 for those who had a father, mother, or sibling with the disease compared with those who had no such family history, and this risk increased to 2.75 for persons with two or more first-degree relatives who had the disease. The relative risk was much higher for individuals under the age of 45 (5.37) and was negligible for those 60 years of age or more.[4]

The relative risk of colon cancer for siblings and parents of patients with adenomatous polyps is 1.78. This risk is particularly great if the polyps were diagnosed in patients under the age of 60.[5]

The risk of colon cancer is increased in those who have a history of large adenomatous colonic polyps or colon cancer.[1]

Women in whom breast, ovarian, or endometrial cancer has previously been diagnosed are at increased risk.[1]

Ulcerative colitis and to a lesser extent Crohn's disease are risk factors. In the case of ulcerative colitis the risk is greatest if the patient has had extensive colonic involvement for over 7 years. The risk is greater with right-sided colonic involvement, and there is virtually no increased risk if the disease is limited to the sigmoid colon and rectum.[6]

Cigarette smoking is a risk factor for colorectal adenomas and carcinomas. The risk increases with the number of cigarettes smoked and the duration of smoking. The induction period for cancer development is very long, on the order of 35 years.[7,8]

Epidemiological evidence points to a correlation between diets high in red meat and saturated fats and low in fiber and colorectal cancer. This association has also been shown for colorectal adenomas.[9]

Sedentary life-style and obesity increase the risk of colorectal cancer, whereas leisure time physical activity decreases the risk.[10]

A number of case-control[11] and prospective[12,13] studies have shown a protective effect of hormone replacement therapy against the development of colon cancer. Possibly this is mediated through alterations of bile acids by estrogens.[11]

The overall mortality rate for cancer of the large bowel is 50%. The rate depends on the stage of the cancer. For stage I disease (Dukes' stages A and B-1) in which invasion is limited to the muscularis propria without nodal involvement, the cure rate is 90%. For stage II (Dukes' stage B-2) in which there is invasion through the muscularis to the serosa but no nodal involvement, the cure rate is 75%. For stage III disease (Dukes' stage C), in which the disease has metastasized to the regional nodes, the cure rate is 35%.[14]

REFERENCES

1. US Preventive Services Task Force: *Guide to clinical preventive services,* ed 2, Baltimore, 1996, Williams & Wilkins, pp 89-103.
2. Kelvin FM, Gaglinte DDT, Stephens BA: Colorectal carcinoma detected initially with barium enema examination: site distribution and implications, *Radiology* 169:649-651, 1988.
3. Lieberman D, Smith F: Screening asymptomatic subjects for colon malignancy with colonoscopy, *Am J Gastroenterol* 86:946-951, 1991.
4. Fuchs CS, Giovannucci EL, Colditz GA, et al: A prospective study of family history and the risk of colorectal cancer, *N Engl J Med* 331:1169-1174, 1994.
5. Winawer SJ, Zauber AG, Gerdes H, et al: Risk of colorectal cancer in the families of patients with adenomatous polyps, *N Engl J Med* 334:82-87, 1996.
6. Donald JJ, Burhenne HJ: Colorectal cancer: can we lower the death rate in the 1990s? *Can Fam Physician* 39:107-114, 1993.
7. Giovannucci E, Rimm EB, Stampfer MF, et al: A prospective study of cigarette smoking and risk of colorectal adenoma and colorectal cancer in U.S. men, *J Natl Cancer Inst* 86:183-191, 1994.
8. Giovannucci I, Colditz GA, Stampfer MJ, et al: A prospective study of cigarette smoking and risk of colorectal adenoma and colorectal cancer in U.S. women, *J Natl Cancer Inst* 86:162-164, 1994.
9. Giovannucci E, Stampfer MJ, Colditz G, et al: Relationship of diet to risk of colorectal adenoma in men, *J Natl Cancer Inst* 84:91-98, 1992.
10. Giovannucci E, Ascherio A, Rimm EB, et al: Physical activity, obesity, and risk for colon cancer and adenoma in men, *Ann Intern Med* 122:327-334, 1995.
11. Newcomb PA, Storer BE: Postmenopausal hormone use and risk of large-bowel cancer, *J Natl Cancer Inst* 87:1067-1071, 1995.
12. Grodstein F, Martinez ME, Giovannucci EL, et al: Postmenopausal hormone use and colorectal cancer in the Nurses' Health Study, *Am J Epidemiol* 143(suppl):S63, 1996.
13. Calle EE, Miracle-McMahill HL, Thun MJ, et al: Estrogen replacement therapy and risk of fatal colon cancer in a prospective cohort of postmenopausal women, *J Natl Cancer Inst* 87:517-523, 1995.
14. Moertel CG: Chemotherapy for colorectal cancer, *N Engl J Med* 330:1136-1142, 1994.

Primary prevention of colon cancer

(See also exercise)

Diet. Two major dietary factors that have been thought to affect the risk of colon cancer are fiber and fat. Evidence suggests that altering diet might slightly alter risk, but at this time the evidence is insufficient to justify major efforts to change dietary habits for this reason alone. It would seem that a high-fiber diet that includes fruits and vegetables[1] or high-fiber grains[2] would be beneficial. That fat might be a significant factor in colon cancer is suggested by a prospective study of the Nurses' Health Study cohort. It was found that the relative risk of colon cancer in women who ate beef, pork, or lamb as a main dish every day was 2.49 that of women who ate these foods less than once a month. Fish and chicken were associated with a decreased risk.[3]

Exercise. Some preliminary evidence suggests that the incidence of colon cancer may be lower in those who exercise. This is discussed more fully in the section on exercise.

Nonsteroidal antiinflammatory drugs. Several prospective studies involving men and women have shown a significant decrease in the incidence[4-7] and mortality[6] of colon cancer in persons taking 325 mg of aspirin at least four to six times a week; this benefit may not become obvious until 10 years has elapsed.[7] Two studies failed to show such a relationship,[8,9] although one involved only 5 years of follow-up.[9] Aspirin and other nonsteroidal antiinflammatory drugs (NSAIDs) reduce the incidence of adenomas in humans, and various NSAIDs inhibit carcinogenesis in the colon of experimental animals.[6] One editorialist's recommendation is that patients at elevated risk of colon cancer take an aspirin a day; such patients are those with a past history of colonic adenoma or cancer, with a family history of colorectal cancer or adenoma, with inflammatory bowel disease, or with breast, ovarian, or endometrial cancer.[10]

Hormone replacement therapy. A case-control study of 694 women receiving hormone replacement therapy and 1622 control subjects found a significantly decreased risk of colon cancer among recent hormone users.[11]

REFERENCES

1. Willett W: The search for the causes of breast and colon cancer, *Nature* 338:389-394, 1989.
2. Boffetta P, Garfinkel L, Heath CW Jr: Risk factors for fatal colon cancer in a large prospective study, *J Natl Cancer Inst* 84: 1491-1500, 1992.
3. Willett WC, Stampfer MJ, Colditz GA, et al: Relation of meat, fat, and fiber intake to the risk of colon cancer in a prospective study among women, *N Engl J Med* 1323:1664-1672, 1990.
4. Schreinemachers DM, Everson RB: Aspirin use and lung, colon, and breast cancer incidence in a prospective study, *Epidemiology* 5:138-146, 1994.
5. Giovannucci I, Rimm EB, Stampfer MJ, et al: Aspirin use and the risk for colorectal cancer and adenoma in male health professionals, *Ann Intern Med* 121:241-246, 1994.
6. Thun MJ, Namboodiri MM, Heath CW Jr: Aspirin use and risk of fatal cancer, *Cancer Res* 53:1322-1327, 1993.
7. Giovannucci E, Egan KM, Hunter DJ, et al: Aspirin and the risk of colorectal cancer in women, *N Engl J Med* 333:609-614, 1995.
8. Pagannini-Hill A, Chao A, Ross RK, et al: Aspirin use and chronic diseases: a cohort study of the elderly, *BMJ* 229:1247-1250, 1989.
9. Gann PH, Manson JE, Glynn RJ, et al: Low-dose aspirin and incidence of colorectal tumors in a randomized trial, *J Natl Cancer Inst* 85:1220-1224, 1993.
10. Marcus AJ: Aspirin prophylaxis against colorectal cancer (editorial), *N Engl J Med* 333:656-657, 1995.
11. Newcomb PA, Storer BE: Postmenopausal hormone use and risk of large-bowel cancer, *J Natl Cancer Inst* 87:1067-1071, 1995.

Secondary prevention of colon cancer

(See also positive predictive value; relative risk reduction; prevention; informed consent)

Fecal occult blood screening. In a study by Mandel and associates[1] from the University of Minnesota, mortality from colon cancer was decreased by a relative rate of 33% over 13 years by annual Hemoccult testing of six specimens obtained from three different stool samples. This relative mortality reduction rate of 33% translates into an absolute mortality reduction rate of 3:1000 or 0.3%. In another arm of the study, Hemoccult testing was performed only every second year, and in this group no decrease in colon cancer mortality was detected. Total mortality was not reduced in either of the screened groups. The positive predictive value of the Hemoccult testing for cancer was 2.2%, but for cancer and polyps combined it was 30%.

Over the 13-year study period 12,246 colonoscopies were performed at the University of Minnesota on the total trial population of approximately 30,000 patients.[1] Among the 15,000 patients in the annual Hemoccult testing group, 4,500 had colonoscopies,[2] and some critics have suggested that this high rate of colonoscopy may in itself have accounted for the decreased cancer mortality.[3] Among all the colonoscopies performed, there were four perforations requiring surgery and 11 episodes of serious bleeding, three of which required surgery.[1]

Two large prospective studies of fecal occult blood screening were published in the *Lancet* in 1996, one from Great Britain[4] and one from Denmark.[5] Both screened patients only every 2 years, and both showed a small but significant decline in colon cancer–related mortality (but not total cohort mortality) in the screened cohort. In the British study the 15% relative reduction in colon cancer deaths over 8 years of follow-up meant that screening 1000 patients led to one fewer colon cancer death,[4] while in the Danish study the 18% relative reduction of colon cancer deaths over 10 years of follow-up meant that screening 1000 patients led to almost two fewer colon cancer deaths.[5] Both these studies are notable in that only about 4% of the screened cohort had full colonoscopies. In both studies the positive predictive value of a positive stool occult blood test for cancer was between 9% and 17%, whereas for adenomas it was between 20% and 45%.[4,5]

The Canadian Task Force on the Periodic Health Examination gives fecal occult blood testing a "C" recommendation,[6] while the U.S. Preventive Services Task Force gives annual fecal occult blood testing (or sigmoidoscopy, time interval not specified) a "B" recommendation.[7] In 1997 guidelines for screening for colorectal cancer were issued by a multidisciplinary expert panel administered by the American Gastroenterological Association under the auspices of the Agency for Health Care Policy and Research. These guidelines were endorsed by a number of other organizations, including the American Cancer Society. They recommend that average-risk men and women 50 years and over undergo screening. Although the only screening programs that have been proved by randomized controlled studies to decrease colon cancer mortality are those that used fecal occult blood testing, the new guidelines offer several screening options to be selected by individual patients and their physicians. These are annual fecal occult blood testing, flexible sigmoidoscopy every 5 years, flexible sigmoidoscopy plus fecal occult blood testing, barium enema every 5 to 10 years, and full colonoscopy every 10 years.[8]

As in so many screening programs, even when benefit has been proved, as seems likely in the case of screening stool for occult blood, the benefit is gained by only a small number of persons undergoing the test. Is it worth it? That is up to the individual patient, who needs to know the pros and cons and give a thoughtful informed consent (see discussion of informed consent and prevention).

Colonoscopy and sigmoidoscopy screening. No prospective randomized controlled trials have been published to show that screening sigmoidoscopy or colonoscopy decreases colon cancer mortality. However, case-control studies suggest a protective effect from sigmoidoscopy. Selby and coworkers[9] from the Kaiser Permanente Program in Oakland, California, studied a group of patients who died of colon cancer and compared them with a series of matched control subjects without colon cancer. When cancers within reach of the sigmoidoscope were evaluated, 8.8% of the cancer patients had had one or more previous rigid sigmoidoscopies compared with 24.2% of the control group. In contrast, when cancers above the reach of the sigmoidoscope were assessed, the rates of previous sigmoidoscopies were equal in the cancer cases and the controls. The protective effect of sigmoidoscopy was apparent even when it had been performed as long as 10 years previously.

Another study suggesting a protective effect of sigmoidoscopy was that of Atkin and associates[10] in Great Britain, who found that removal of tubular adenomas at sigmoidoscopy was associated with a low rate of cancer at follow-up. Similar results were reported from a case-controlled Veterans Administration study in the United States; the odds ratio of mortality for patients who had a diagnostic procedure of the large bowel was 0.41 compared with control subjects who had not had such procedures. This protective effect was most marked if tissue had been removed.[11]

If flexible sigmoidoscopy or colonoscopy is to be used as a screening method for the detection of colon cancer, the complication rates for these interventions must be known. Unfortunately, the literature on the subject is scanty.[12] Major complications are perforation, major hemorrhage, and death. Both perforation and hemorrhage are more common if a polypectomy is performed during the endoscopy. In 1996 Waye, Kahn, and Auerbach[12] analyzed the combined complication rates of the few prospective studies of colonoscopy complications reported between 1987 and 1994. The perforation rate was 1:2,222, the rate of significant hemorrhage was 1:81 if a polypectomy had been performed and 1:1352 if it had not, and the mortality rate was 1:16,745. These rates were lower than those reported in previous decades, and the authors attributed this to improved physician training and better instruments. They cautioned, however, that reports from centers with extensive experience in endoscopy may not reflect the experience of the broader medical community, since complication rates are known to be higher for inexperienced compared with experienced operators.[12] A rare but serious complication of colonoscopy is the nosocomial transmission of hepatitis C infection from inadequate cleaning of the colonoscope.[13]

Waye, Kahn, and Auerbach[12] were unable to find any randomized prospective trials reporting the complications of flexible sigmoidoscopy. Cohen and associates[14] quoted a perforation rate of 1:8795, and a 1996 Swedish report recorded a rate of 1:716.[15] The authors of the latter study explained their high rate by the initial inexperience of the endoscopists.[15] A survey of British gastroenterologists reported a perforation rate of 1:16,810 for flexible fiberoptic sigmoidoscopy and 1:65,763 for rigid sigmoidoscopy. Significant bleeding rates were 1:16,810 for flexible sigmoidoscopy and 1:9394 for rigid sigmoidoscopy.[16]

Considering these data, what recommendations should a family physician make to patients about screening for colon cancer by sigmoidoscopy or colonoscopy? As stated previously, the American Gastroenterological Association strongly recommends colorectal cancer screening for all average-risk adults 50 years or older but does not favor one particular modality.[8] On the other hand, the Canadian Task Force on the Periodic Health Examination found insufficient evidence to recommend sigmoidoscopic screening ("C" recommendation) of asymptomatic individuals over the age of 40 who were not at high risk.[6] This recommendation also applies to individuals with only one or two relatives with colon cancer. However, the Canadian Task Force on the Periodic Health Examination does recommend colonoscopy for the rare cancer family syndrome (uterine, stomach, breast, ovarian, and colorectal).[6] The U.S. Preventive Services Task Force gives a "B" recommendation to screening all persons over 50 years of age by annual fecal occult blood testing or sigmoidoscopy or both. It does not specify the frequency of sigmoidoscopy.[7] This is probably because little information dealing with that topic is available. One 1996 study reported on the follow-up of complete colonoscopy in 154 patients who had negative complete colonoscopies 5 years previously. No patient had cancer, and only one had an adenoma larger than 1 cm.[17]

Both Selby[18] and Atkin[19] have suggested that a cost-effective screening program for colon cancer might be to perform a single flexible sigmoidoscopy between the ages of 55 and 60 with follow-up colonoscopy if high-risk polyps are found. Another approach, for which no substantiating evidence has yet appeared, would be to screen only high-risk patients such as those with a strong family history.[20] Even though the benefit of such a policy for decreasing colon cancer death rates is as yet unproved, the worried relatives of patients with colon cancer may derive considerable psychological benefit.[20]

Strong evidence suggests that screening by flexible fiberoptic sigmoidoscopy may decrease the incidence and mortality of colon cancer, but whether these probable benefits outweigh the adverse effects remains in question. In weighing these issues, both physicians and patients should be aware that the published complication rates of sigmoidoscopy and colonoscopy are mostly from centers with considerable experience in the use of these instruments. The odds are that complication rates are higher for practitioners who only occasionally perform these procedures; as far as I have been able to determine, such statistics are not currently available. Physicians and patients should also realize that if such screening is undertaken, the value, if any, of repeat screening in negative cases and the time intervals at which it should be performed are unknown.

Barium enema screening. Although no definitive studies have shown a decrease in colorectal mortality associated with double-contrast barium enema screening, the American Gastroenterological Association recommends this procedure every 5 to 10 years as an alternative to fecal occult blood or endoscopy screening (see previous discussion).[8] The rationale is that any procedure that can detect polyps and so allow their removal should prevent colorectal cancer.

REFERENCES

1. Mandel JS, Bond JH, Church TR, et al: Reducing mortality from colorectal cancer by screening for fecal occult blood, *N Engl J Med* 328:1365-1371, 1993.
2. Mandel JS, Church TR, Ederer F: Screening for colorectal cancer (letter), *N Engl J Med* 329:1353-1354, 1993.
3. Ahlquist DA, Moertel CG, McGill DB: Screening for colorectal cancer (letter), *N Engl J Med* 329:1351, 1993.
4. Hardcastle JD, Chamberlain JO, Robinson MH, et al: Randomised controlled trial of faecal-occult-blood screening for colorectal cancer, *Lancet* 348:1472-1477, 1996.
5. Kronborg O, Fenger C, Olsen J, et al: Randomised study of screening for colorectal cancer with faecal-occult-blood test, *Lancet* 348:1467-1471, 1996.
6. Canadian Task Force on the Periodic Health Examination: *Clinical preventive health care,* Ottawa, 1994, Canadian Communication Group—Publishing, pp 798-809.
7. US Preventive Services Task Force: *Guide to clinical preventive services,* ed 2, Baltimore, 1996, Williams & Wilkins, pp 89-103.
8. Winawer SJ, Fletcher RH, Miller L, et al: Colorectal cancer screening and surveillance: clinical guidelines, evidence and rationale, *Gastroenterology* 112:594-642, 1997.
9. Selby JV, Friedman GD, Quesenberry CP Jr, et al: A case-control study of screening sigmoidoscopy and mortality from colorectal cancer, *N Engl J Med* 326:653-657, 1992.
10. Atkin WS, Morson BC, Cuzick J: Long-term risk of colorectal cancer after excision of rectosigmoid adenomas, *N Engl J Med* 326:658-662, 1992.
11. Mueller AD, Sonnenberg A: Protection by endoscopy against death from colorectal cancer: a case-control study among veterans, *Arch Intern Med* 155:1741-1748, 1995.
12. Waye JD, Kahn O, Auerbach ME: Complications of colonoscopy and flexible sigmoidoscopy, *Gastrointest Endosc Clin North Am* 6:343-374, 1996.
13. Bronowicki J-P, Venard V, Botté C, et al: Patient-to-patient transmission of hepatitis C virus during colonoscopy, *N Engl J Med* 337:237-240, 1997.
14. Cohen LB, Basuk PM, Waye JD: *Practical flexible sigmoidoscopy,* New York, 1995, Igaku-Shoin, pp 117-125.
15. Kewenter J, Brevinge H: Endoscopic and surgical complications of work-up in screening for colorectal cancer, *Dis Colon Rectum* 39:676-680, 1996.
16. Robinson RJ, Stone M, Mayberry JF: Sigmoidoscopy and rectal biopsy—a survey of current UK practice, *Eur J Gastroenterol Hepatol* 8:149-151, 1996.
17. Rex DK, Cummings OW, Helper DJ, et al: 5-Year incidence of adenomas after negative colonoscopy in asymptomatic average-risk persons, *Gastroenterology* 111:1178-1181, 1996.
18. Selby JV: Screening sigmoidoscopy for colorectal cancer (commentary), *Lancet* 341:728-729, 1993.
19. Atkin WS, Cuzick J, Northover JMA, et al: Prevention of colorectal cancer by once-only sigmoidoscopy, *Lancet* 341:736-740, 1993.
20. Mulcahy HE, Farthing MJ, O'Donoghue DP: Screening for asymptomatic colorectal cancer, *BMJ* 314:285-291, 1997.

Colonoscopy versus barium enema for investigation of suspected colon cancer

(See also secondary prevention of colon cancer)

If clinical findings indicate that a patient may have colon cancer, the major investigative techniques of choice are colonoscopy and barium enema. Fecal occult blood testing in this context has little or no value, since further investigation is required whether or not it is positive.

A complete colonoscopy and a well-performed barium enema are excellent means of detecting cancers and polyps. A double-contrast barium enema is thought to give a greater yield for polyps smaller than 1 cm than does a single-contrast study, but for polyps larger than that they are equally effective.[1] Both barium enema and colonoscopy detect a few cases that were missed by the other. One review of the radiological literature found that colorectal cancer was detected by barium enema in 90% to 99% of cases.[2] In general, rigid sigmoidoscopy detects about 25% of colonic polyps and flexible 60-cm fiberoptic sigmoidoscopy detects 50% to 60%.[3]

One clear advantage of colonoscopy is that a biopsy can be performed at once if a cancer is detected, or a polyp, if seen, can be removed during the procedure. Another advantage, according to one survey, is that patients prefer colonoscopy to a double-contrast barium enema, probably because of the sedating and analgesic medications given with the former.[4]

An important factor influencing the choice of any investigative procedure is the complication rates. For a barium enema the perforation rate is 1:10,000 and the mortality rate is 1:50,000.[3] For a full colonoscopy these numbers are higher (see discussion of secondary prevention of colon cancer).

REFERENCES

1. Donald JJ, Burhenne HJ: Colorectal cancer: can we lower the death rate in the 1990s? *Can Fam Physician* 39:107-114, 1993.
2. Levine R, Tenner S, Fromm H: Prevention and early detection of colorectal cancer, *Am Fam Physician* 45:663-668, 1992.
3. Gelfand DW, Ott DJ: The economic implications of radiologic screening for colonic cancer, *Am J Roentgenol* 156:939-943, 1991.
4. Van Ness MM, Chobanian SJ, Winters C Jr, et al: A study of patient acceptance of double-contrast barium enema and colonoscopy: which procedure is preferred by patients? *Arch Intern Med* 147:2175-2176, 1987.

Therapy for colorectal cancer

(See also follow-up of cancer patients who have had curative treatments)

Adjuvant chemotherapy. A combination of fluorouracil and levamisole has been shown to decrease the rate of recurrence of stage III colon cancer by 40% and the death rate by 33%.[1,2] A slight decrease in the recurrence rate has been shown for stage II disease. Fluorouracil plus high-dose folinic acid has also proved effective.[3] Unfortunately, no adjuvant therapy has been found for rectal cancer.

Adjuvant radiation therapy. A randomized prospective study from Sweden compared surgery alone to preoperative radiation plus surgery for resectable rectal carcinoma. After 5 years the local recurrence rate in those who did not receive radiation therapy was 27% compared with 11% in those who received irradiation. The overall 5-year survival was 48% in the surgery-only group and 58% in the surgery plus radiation therapy group.[4]

REFERENCES

1. Moertel CG: Chemotherapy for colorectal cancer, *N Engl J Med* 330:1136-1142, 1994.
2. Goertel CG, Fleming TR, Macdonald JS, et al: Fluorouracil plus levamisole as effective adjuvant therapy after resection of stage III colon carcinoma: a final report, *Ann Intern Med* 122:321-326, 1995.
3. Labianca R, Marsoni S, Pancera G, et al: Efficacy of adjuvant fluorouracil and folinic acid in colon cancer, *Lancet* 345:939-944, 1995.
4. Swedish Rectal Cancer Trial: Improved survival with preoperative radiotherapy in resectable rectal cancer, *N Engl J Med* 336: 980-987, 1997.

Familial polyposis

Presymptomatic diagnosis of adenomatous familial polyposis is possible in the majority of cases by a blood test involving molecular genetic diagnosis.[1]

REFERENCES

1. Powell SM, Petersen GM, Krush AJ, et al: Molecular diagnosis of familial adenomatous polyposis, *N Engl J Med* 329:1982-1987, 1993.

CONSTIPATION

(See also pain, chronic)

Normally persons have between three bowel movements a day and three bowel movements a week.[1] A working definition accepted by many experts in the field is the "Rome criteria." Constipation according to these criteria is the presence of two or more of the following for at least 3 months[2]:

1. Two or fewer bowel movements a week
2. Stool weight of less than 35 g/day
3. Hard lumpy stool on more than 25% of occasions
4. Straining on more than 25% of occasions
5. Sensation of incomplete evacuation on more than 25% of occasions

Management of Constipation in the Community

Once organic disease is ruled out, most cases of true constipation may be managed at home by exercise, good hydration, and fiber. Constipated patients should be started on regular supplements of bran or psyllium (Metamucil, Prodiem), beginning with 1 tbsp/day and working up as rapidly as possible to 3 tbsp/day. Each dose should be accompanied or followed by 8 ounces of water or other fluid. If this does not resolve the problem, the patient should be given an osmotic laxative, such as lactulose (Lactulax) 30 to 60 ml hs or magnesium hydroxide (Milk of Magnesia) 15 to 30 ml hs. Use of other types of laxatives, including mineral oil, those that cause intestinal secretion (docusate [Colace, Regulex]), and stimulant laxatives (sennosides [Senokot], bisacodyl [Dulcolax], glycerin suppositories), should be avoided because they may lead to the laxative abuse syndrome. An important behavioral aspect of the treatment plan is instructing the patient to sit on the toilet for 15 to 20 minutes after breakfast without any distractions and to avoid straining during this time.[1]

Laxatives in Palliative Care

The discussion on the uses of laxatives in this section applies primarily to immobilized patients and those receiving narcotics. Stool softeners and peristaltic stimulants take 6 to 9 hours to work, so they should be given at bedtime. The two should be given together because using only a stool softener may cause soft stool to accumulate in the rectum. Suppositories work within the hour, so they should be given half an hour before breakfast or supper.[3] The suppositories should be pushed against rectal mucosa, not into stool. They should also should be inserted with the "base" and not the pointed end first.[4]

Gastrointestinal System

The following sequence of therapeutic interventions for constipation is one author's guideline for palliative care.[3] Missing here is the osmotic laxative lactulose (Lactulax). In doses of 15 to 60 ml/day it is usually very effective.

1. Encourage fluids, fiber, and exercise.
2. Use one of these: standardized sennosides (Senokot) 1 to 2 tablets hs plus docusate sodium (Colace, Regulex) 100 mg bid; *or* bisacodyl (Dulcolax) 5 to 15 mg po hs plus docusate sodium (Colace, Regulex) 100 mg bid; *or* magnesium hydroxide (Milk of Magnesia) 15 to 30 ml hs plus docusate sodium (Colace, Regulex) 100 mg bid.
3. Increase docusate sodium (Colace, Regulex) to 200 to 300 mg bid and double the dose of one of the other three laxatives.
4. Add one glycerin suppository and one bisacodyl (Dulcolax) suppository before breakfast.
5. Prescribe a phosphate enema (Fleet enema).
6. Prescribe an oil enema if the stool is hard or a saline enema if the stool is soft.
7. Disimpact the bowel.

REFERENCES

1. Camilleri M, Thompson WG, Fleshman JW, et al: Clinical management of intractable constipation, *Ann Intern Med* 121:520-528, 1994.
2. Thompson WG, Creed F, Drossman DA, et al: Functional bowel disease and functional abdominal pain, *Gastroenterol Int* 5:75-91, 1992.
3. Van Tilburg EG: Constipation: a frequent iatrogenic complication in cancer patients receiving narcotics, *Can Fam Physician* 36:967-970, 1990.
4. Larimore WL, Hartman JR, Shupe TB: Diary from a week in practice, *Am Fam Physician* 50:1673-1674, 1994.

DIARRHEA

(See also cryptosporidiosis; cyclosporiasis; diarrhea and hematochezia in runners; food poisoning; giardiasis; travelers' diarrhea)

Infectious Diarrhea

Many bacterial, viral, and parasitic organisms may cause diarrhea, and some of these are listed in Table 24. Toxins such as ciguatoxin and tetrodotoxin that cause diarrhea are discussed under "Food Poisoning."

Mild to moderate community-acquired acute infectious diarrhea can be treated in adults with the antimotility agent loperamide (Imodium) 4 mg stat and 2 mg after each loose stool to a maximum of 16 mg/day. Severe diarrhea and some cases of moderate diarrhea require the addition of a quinolone antibiotic such as ciprofloxacin 500 mg bid for 2 to 5 days.[1]

Table 24 Selected Infectious Diseases Causing Diarrhea

Bacterial	Viral	Parasitic
Salmonella	Rotaviruses	*Giardia lamblia*
Shigella	Norwalk viruses	*Entamoeba histolytica*
Campylobacter	Adenoviruses	*Cyclospora cayetanensis*
Yersinia	Astroviruses	Cryptosporidiosis
Enterotoxigenic *Escherichia coli*		
Enteroinvasive *E. coli*		
Verotoxin-producing *E. coli* (hamburger disease; hemorrhagic colitis)		
Clostridium difficile		
Clostridium perfringens		
Vibrio cholerae		
Vibrio parahaemolyticus		

Chronic Diarrhea

Chronic diarrhea is defined as persistent diarrhea lasting more than 4 weeks. Before being placed into this category, a patient should be on a lactose-free diet for several days, since lactase deficiency may be a result of an infectious agent and cause persistence of symptoms after the organism itself has been eradicated.[2]

Excluding irritable bowel disease, lactase deficiency, and diarrhea in HIV-positive patients, the following are the most common causes of chronic diarrhea, in order of frequency as seen by gastroenterologists[2]:

1. Infections (giardiasis, amebiasis, *Clostridium difficile,* cyclosporiasis)
2. Inflammatory bowel disease
3. Steatorrhea (greasy or bulky stools difficult to flush, bad odor, oil in toilet bowel requiring brush for removal, weight loss)
4. Medications (e.g., antibiotics, antihypertensives, magnesium-containing antacids), foods (ethanol, caffeine), sweeteners (sorbitol in gum or mints, fructose in corn syrup)
5. Previous gastrointestinal surgery
6. Endocrine (Addison's disease, diabetes mellitus, hyperthyroidism, hypothyroidism)
7. Laxative abuse (often concealed by patient or parent)
8. Ischemic bowel disease
9. Radiation enteritis or colitis
10. Colon cancer
11. Idiopathic (functional)

Screening tests for celiac disease are serum and red blood cell folate levels, which are almost always low in persons with untreated celiac disease.[3]

Symptomatic Therapy for Diarrhea

Loperamide (Imodium) and diphenoxylate (Lomotil) are the drugs most frequently used for the symptomatic control of diarrhea. The usual dose of loperamide is 4 mg (2 tablets) initially and then 2 mg after each subsequent loose stool. Maximum is 16 mg (8 tablets) per day. The usual dose of diphenoxylate is 5 mg (2 tablets) initially and then 2.5 to 5 mg tid or qid. Cholestyramine (Questran) is also an effective symptomatic treatment for many cases of chronic diarrhea. The usual dose is 2 to 4 g (a half to a full packet) one to six times a day.

REFERENCES

1. Gorbach SL: Treating diarrhoea (editorial), *BMJ* 314:1776-1777, 1997.
2. Donowitz, Kokke FT, Saidi R: Evaluation of patients with chronic diarrhea, *N Engl J Med* 332:725-729, 1995.
3. Ballinger AB, Cevallos AM, Clark ML: Patients with chronic diarrhea (letter), *N Engl J Med* 333:257, 1995.

HEMATOCHEZIA

(See also colon cancer; gastrointestinal bleeding and anemia; diarrhea and hematochezia in runners; hemorrhoids)

In a British community study 24% of respondents to a questionnaire reported at least one episode of rectal bleeding in their lifetimes, and 19% had had such bleeding within the past 12 months. Only 41% of those who had ever had rectal bleeding sought medical advice.[1] Data like these suggest that most of these incidents were innocuous. That this might not be the case is indicated by a study of U.S. veterans (almost all male and 80% over the age of 40). They were specifically asked about a history of rectal bleeding and, if it had occurred in the past 3 months, were given a complete examination of the colon. Colon cancer was detected in 6.5%, polyps in 13%, and inflammatory bowel disease in 4.5%. The character of the bleeding (e.g., frequency of bleeding, on the toilet paper, mixed with stool) did not distinguish innocuous from severe disease. The only two clinical features that correlated with a diagnosis of cancer were age and duration of bleeding of less than 2 months.[2]

Occult blood in the stools has been found in 20% of marathon runners immediately after the race. Frank blood in stools occurs in about 6% of such runners.[3]

REFERENCES

1. Crosland A, Jones R: Rectal bleeding—prevalence and consultation behaviour, *BMJ* 311:486-488, 1995.
2. Helfand M, Marton KI, Zimmer-Gembeck MJ, et al: History of visible rectal bleeding in a primary care population: initial assessment and 10-year follow-up, *JAMA* 277:44-48, 1997.
3. McCabe ME 3d, Peura DA, Kadakia SC, et al: Gastrointestinal blood loss associated with running a marathon, *Dig Dis Sci* 31:1229-1232, 1986.

ESOPHAGUS

(See also cough; esophageal candidiasis; peptic ulcer disease)

Achalasia

Patients with achalasia have an approximately 16-fold increased risk for esophageal cancer. However, there is no evidence that endoscopic surveillance improves the prognosis. One study concluded that 406 endoscopies would be needed to detect one cancer in men and 2220 endoscopies to detect one cancer in women.[1] Injection of botulinum toxin into the lower esophageal sphincter gives excellent immediate results in most patients with achalasia, and this benefit is sustained at 6 months in about half the patients.[2]

Dysphagia

Dysphagia may be esophageal or oropharyngeal. If a patient has trouble getting the food bolus out of the mouth or has nasal regurgitation, choking, or coughing on swallowing it is likely to be oropharyngeal, whereas a definite feeling of sticking in the retrosternum indicates esophageal dysphagia. The initial symptom of organic strictures is difficulty swallowing solids, whereas motor disorders such as may be associated with cerebrovascular accidents, amyotrophic lateral sclerosis, myasthenia gravis, or other neurological conditions may produce episodic difficulty in swallowing both liquids and solids from the beginning. Idiopathic oropharyngeal neuromuscular dysphagia is common in the elderly, and many such persons never seek medical help for the condition.[3]

Adenocarcinoma of the Esophagus

The incidence of adenocarcinoma of the esophagus has been increasing dramatically in the Western world over the past two decades. Most such tumors have regional lymph node involvement at the time of diagnosis, and the 5-year survival rate from surgical resection is less than 10%. One study found that preoperative radiation therapy and chemotherapy increased the 3-year survival rate for resectable tumors from 6% to 32%.[4]

Gastroesophageal Reflux Disease and Barrett's Esophagus

Reflux is a result of transient relaxation of the lower esophageal sphincter and not of a low resting sphincter pressure. If an associated hiatus hernia is present, gastric reflux is more likely to occur during the periods of sphincter relaxation.[5]

Coronary artery disease is often an important part of the differential diagnosis of gastroesophageal reflux disease (GERD). According to one study this condition can be ruled out with reasonable certainty if symptoms are controlled by omeprazole (Prilosec, Losec) 40 mg bid for 7 days (omeprazole test). Lower doses of omeprazole and ranitidine are not effective for this purpose.[6]

A number of reports suggest that reflux at times induces "acid laryngitis," which manifests itself as persistent cough, hoarseness, and a continual need to clear the throat. The existence of this entity is controversial. Believers treat the patients with omeprazole (Losec, Prilosec) for 2 months,[5] but no randomized controlled studies have been published documenting benefit from this therapy.[7] Other reports suggest that reflux may have a role in causing bronchoconstriction (asthma) and pulmonary fibrosis. As with "acid laryngitis" this connection is controversial. If it does exist, actual aspiration may not be the pathogenetic mechanism; more likely it is a reflex lowering of the threshold for bronchoconstriction by acidification of the esophageal mucosa. Those who believe in this syndrome give the patients a trial of omeprazole (Losec, Prilosec) for 2 months,[5] but as in the case of "acid laryngitis" no controlled studies have shown the benefits of this regimen.[7]

The initial treatment of symptomatic esophageal reflux involves life-style changes and over-the-counter medications. Most cases can be successfully controlled by these measures,[7] which include the following:

1. Avoiding bedtime snacks
2. Avoiding foods that relax the lower esophageal sphincter, such as fats, whole milk, chocolate, orange juice, tomatoes, carminatives (peppermint), and ethanol
3. Discontinuing smoking
4. Raising the head of the bed by at least 14 cm
5. Taking alginic acids such as Gaviscon Heart Burn Relief Formula (there are Gaviscon products without alginic acid) or Gastrocote. The usual dose is 2 to 4 tablets well chewed tid or qid.

Aside from the alginic acid products mentioned, medications of various classes have been used for treating reflux.[7] For many patients antacids are effective. Initial treatment with an H_2-blocker such as cimetidine (Tagamet) 800 mg bid or ranitidine (Zantac) 150 mg bid may be tried for 8 weeks. If this is unsuccessful, omeprazole (Losec, Prilosec) 20 to 40 mg/day or lansoprazole (Prevacid) 30 mg/day is usually effective. Once control is achieved, maintenance therapy is continued with the lowest possible dose of the effective drug.

Prokinetic agents are another option for esophageal reflux. Metoclopramide (Maxeran) in doses of 5 to 10 mg tid or qid is minimally effective as a single agent, but cisapride (Prepulsid), which is usually given as 5 to 10 mg tid ac or qid ac and hs, seems to be more effective.[8] Cisapride is about as effective as an H_2-blocker and so may be used for mild esophagitis.[7] It has also been reported to have a synergistic effect with H_2-blockers.[7,8]

For some patients relapses are frequent. In one 12-month study of maintenance therapy after initial treatment with omeprazole the relapse rate was lower in patients taking omeprazole 20 mg/day or omeprazole 20 mg/day plus cisapride 10 mg tid than in those taking ranitidine 150 mg/day, cisapride 10 mg tid, or ranitidine 150 mg tid plus cisapride 10 mg tid.[9] As an editorial accompanying the report points out, only a minority of patients require such rigorous therapy.[10]

A condition that may be associated with GERD is Barrett's esophagus. This is defined as the presence of columnar (not gastric) mucosa extending 3 cm or more proximal to the gastroesophageal junction. The condition is important because affected patients have an increased risk for adenocarcinoma of the lower esophagus.[11,12] The male/female ratio of Barrett's esophagus is 4:1, and it is much more common in whites than blacks. Among patients with GERD the incidence of Barrett's esophagus is much higher in those with persistent symptoms over more than 5 years, dysphagia, esophageal stricture, severe esophagitis, or esophageal ulceration. From the viewpoint of the family physician, patients with severe or persistent GERD are the ones who usually need referral for endoscopy to determine whether they have Barrett's esophagus.[11] Patients with proven Barrett's esophagus require regular endoscopic monitoring.[11,12]

Esophageal Varices

Beta-blockers and sclerotherapy have been used to decrease the incidence of recurrent bleeding from esophageal varices.[13] A metaanalysis of these two therapeutic modalities found the rate of rebleeding to be less with sclerotherapy but survival to be the same.[14] Even after successful sclerotherapy the rate of rebleeding is as high as 50%, and complications of the procedure such as esophageal ulcerations and strictures are common.[13] In a Spanish study the rate of rebleeding in patients treated with a combination of nadolol (Corgard) and an oral isosorbide mononitrate (Imdur) was significantly less than in control subjects treated with sclerotherapy, and complications were fewer.[13]

Beta-blockers lower by about 50% the risk of an initial variceal bleeding episode in patients with cirrhosis and portal hypertension. In an Italian study the addition of isosorbide mononitrate (Imdur) to nadolol (Corgard) further decreased the risk.[15]

Patients with portal hypertension and esophageal bleeding who do not respond to other therapeutic modalities may be treated by creating a shunt between the portal and hepatic veins. This is done by interventional radiologists who introduce a catheter through the jugular vein and pass it through the liver into the portal vein. The procedure is called a transjugular intrahepatic portosystemic shunt (TIPS).[16]

REFERENCES

1. Sandler RS, Nyrén O, Ekbom A, et al: The risk of esophageal cancer in patients with achalasia: a population-based study, *JAMA* 274:1359-1362, 1995.
2. Pasricha PJ, Ravich WJ, Hendrix TR, et al: Intrasphincteric botulinum toxin for the treatment of achalasia, *N Engl J Med* 332:774-778, 1995.
3. Paterson WG: Dysphagia in the elderly, *Can Fam Physician* 42:925-932, 1996.
4. Walsh TN, Noonan N, Hollywood D, et al: A comparison of multimodal therapy and surgery for esophageal adenocarcinoma, *N Engl J Med* 335:462-467, 1996.
5. Pope CE II: Acid-reflux disorders, *N Engl J Med* 331:656-660, 1994.
6. Schindlbeck NE, Klauser AG, Voderholzer WA, et al: Empiric therapy for gastroesophageal reflux disease, *Arch Intern Med* 155:1808-1812, 1995.
7. Kahrilas PJ: Gastroesophageal reflux disease, *JAMA* 276:983-988, 1996.
8. Cisapride for nocturnal heartburn, *Med Lett* 36:11-12, 1994.
9. Vigneri S, Termini R, Leandro G, et al: A comparison of five maintenance therapies for reflux esophagitis, *N Engl J Med* 333:1106-1110, 1995.
10. Tytgat GN: Long-term therapy for reflux esophagitis (editorial), *N Engl J Med* 333:1148-1150, 1995.

11. Drewitz DJ, Sampliner RE, Garewal HS: The incidence of adenocarcinoma in Barrett's esophagus—a prospective study of 170 patients followed 4.8 years, *Am J Gastroenterol* 92:212-215, 1997.
12. Crooks GW, Lichtenstein GR: Clinical implications of Barrett's esophagus, *Arch Intern Med* 156:2174-2180, 1996.
13. Villanueva C, Balanzó J, Novella MT, et al: Nadolol plus isosorbide mononitrate compared with sclerotherapy for the prevention of variceal rebleeding, *N Engl J Med* 334:1624-1629, 1996.
14. D'Amico G, Pagliaro L, Bosch J: The treatment of portal hypertension: a meta-analytic review, *Hepatology* 22:332-354, 1995.
15. Merkel C, Marin R, Enzo E, et al: Randomised trial of nadolol alone or with isosorbide mononitrate for primary prophylaxis of variceal bleeding in cirrhosis: Gruppo-Triveneto per L'ipertesione portale (GTIP), *Lancet* 348:1677-1681, 1996.
16. Miller-Catchpole R: Transjugular intrahepatic portosystemic shunt (TIPS): diagnostic and therapeutic technology assessment (DATTA), *JAMA* 273:1824-1830, 1995.

FLATUS

Alpha-galactosidase (Beano) is available as an over-the-counter liquid preparation. Its mode of action is to hydrolyze undigestible complex sugars (oligosaccharides) of certain vegetables into their digestible monosaccharides and disaccharides. Most cruciferous vegetables and most legumes have a high content of undigestible sugars. Examples are beans, chickpeas, peas, lentils, brussels sprouts, cabbage, broccoli, carrots, corn, leeks, squash, onions, parsnips, oats, and wheat.

In a study from San Diego, volunteers took 8 drops of Beano or 8 drops of placebo before a meal of meatless chili consisting of navy, pinto, and kidney beans. Beano decreased the numbers of farts.[1] No solid evidence has been presented that simethicone relieves the discomfort of "gas."[2]

REFERENCES

1. Ganiats TG, Norcross WA, Halverson AL, et al: Does Beano prevent gas—a double-blind crossover study of oral alpha-galactosidase to treat dietary oligosaccharide intolerance, *J Fam Pract* 39:441-445, 1994.
2. Simethicone for gastrointestinal gas, *Med Lett* 38:57-58, 1996.

INFLAMMATORY BOWEL DISEASE

(See also biliary cirrhosis; colon; diarrhea; beneficial effects of smoking; psoriatic arthritis)

Crohn's Disease

Relapses of Crohn's disease are more frequent in smokers than nonsmokers.[1] Relapse rates are significantly decreased in patients maintained with 5-aminosalicylic acid or mesalazine (Asacol, Mesasal, Pentasa, Salofalk),[2] enteric-coated fish oil (it has antiinflammatory properties),[3] and, in the case of patients who have had ileal resections, metronidazole (Flagyl).[4] Methotrexate at a dose of 25 mg/week intramuscularly has been effective in the management of chronically active Crohn's disease requiring steroid therapy.[5] Azathioprine and 6-mercaptopurine are also effective in treating active disease and maintaining remissions.[6]

Ulcerative Colitis

Ulcerative colitis is found three to four times as frequently in whites as in other races. Both sexes are equally affected. About 5% of patients have severe disease manifested as fulminating hemorrhagic colitis, toxic megacolon, or severe diffuse colitis. Ulcerative colitis is more common in nonsmokers than in smokers. The onset of the disease often correlates with discontinuing smoking, and smoking may control the symptoms of the disease. These apparently beneficial effects are not seen in Crohn's disease.[7]

A complication of long-term ulcerative colitis is colon cancer; this association is most marked in patients with pancolitis. The risk begins to develop 10 to 15 years after the diagnosis, and for patients with widespread disease the risk approaches 30% 35 years after the original diagnosis. If the disease began before the age of 15, the risk after 35 years is close to 50%. The risk in patients with only left-sided colitis is considerably less.[8,9]

Mild and moderate cases of ulcerative colitis may be managed on an outpatient basis. Standard therapy consists of oral medications and medicated enemas. Therapy usually begins with relatively low doses of oral medications such as mesalazine (Asacol, Mesasal, Pentasa, Salofalk) or olsalazine (Dipentum), with increases to full therapeutic doses at a rate tolerable for the patient. Enemas are used for disease of the distal colon or rectum. They are usually given hs for 3 weeks. The patient is instructed to try to retain the enema all night. Some of the newer steroid enemas such as tixocortol (Rectovalone) are not readily absorbed and do not suppress the pituitary-adrenal axis.[10] Short-term, randomized, double-blind studies of patients with ulcerative colitis have demonstrated symptom reduction with the use of nicotine patches,[11,12] but at the cost of significant side effects.[2] The use of nicotine patches to help maintain remission in ulcerative colitis has not shown any benefit.[13]

Extraintestinal Manifestations of Inflammatory Bowel Disease

Peripheral arthritis, involving primarily the hips and ankles, and ankylosing spondylitis are fairly common complications of inflammatory bowel disease. Ocular manifestations are also common and include episcleritis and uveitis.[14] Sclerosing cholangitis is a rare complication of inflammatory bowel disease. Some patients are asymptomatic, but others have fatigue and pruritus. Levels of aspartate aminotransferase (AST or SGOT) and alanine aminotransferase (ALT or SGPT) may be normal or elevated, whereas alkaline phosphatase and gamma-glutamyl transferase levels are markedly elevated.[15]

REFERENCES

1. Duffy LC, Zielezny MA, Marshall JR, et al: Cigarette smoking and risk of clinical relapse in patients with Crohn's disease, *Am J Prevent Med* 6:161-166, 1990.
2. Messori A, Brignola C, Trallori G, et al: Effectiveness of 5-aminosalicylic acid for maintaining remission in patients

with Crohn's disease: a meta-analysis, *Am J Gastroenterol* 89:692-698, 1994.
3. Belluzzi A, Brignola C, Campieri M, et al: Effect of an enteric-coated fish-oil preparation on relapses in Crohn's disease, *N Engl J Med* 334:1557-1560, 1996.
4. Rutgeerts P, Hiele M, Geboes K, et al: Controlled trial of metronidazole treatment for prevention of Crohn's recurrence after ileal resection, *Gastroenterology* 108:1935-1938, 1995.
5. Feagan BG, Rochon J, Fedorak RN, et al: Methotrexate for the treatment of Crohn's disease, *N Engl J Med* 332:292-297, 1995.
6. Pearson DC, May GR, Fick GH, et al: Azathioprine and 6-mercaptopurine in Crohn disease: a meta-analysis, *Ann Intern Med* 122:132-142, 1995.
7. Hanauer SB: Nicotine for colitis—the smoke has not yet cleared (editorial), *N Engl J Med* 330:856-857, 1994.
8. Lennard-Jones JE, Melville DM, Morson BC, et al: Precancer and cancer in extensive ulcerative colitis: findings among 401 patients over 22 years, *Gut* 31:800-806, 1990.
9. Ekbom A, Helmick C, Zack M, et al: Ulcerative colitis and colorectal cancer: a population-based study, *N Engl J Med* 323: 1228-1233, 1990.
10. Hanauer SB: Inflammatory bowel disease, *N Engl J Med* 334: 841-848, 1996.
11. Pullan RD, Rhodes J, Ganesh S, et al: Transdermal nicotine for active ulcerative colitis, *N Engl J Med* 330:811-815, 1994.
12. Sandborn WJ, Tremaine WJ, Offord KP, et al: Transdermal nicotine for mildly to moderately active ulcerative colitis, *Ann Intern Med* 126:364-371, 1997.
13. Thomas GAO, Mani V, Williams GT, et al: Transdermal nicotine as maintenance therapy for ulcerative colitis, *N Engl J Med* 332:988-992, 1995.
14. Hastings GE, Wever RJ: Inflammatory bowel disease. I. Clinical features and diagnosis, *Am Fam Physician* 47:598-608, 1993.
15. Buckley SE, Dipalma JA: Recognizing primary biliary cirrhosis and primary sclerosing cholangitis, *Am Fam Physician* 53: 195-200, 1996.

IRRITABLE BOWEL SYNDROME

(See also lactase deficiency)

Irritable bowel disease is common, affecting an estimated 15% of the adult population. Many patients do not seek medical attention, but the disorder is probably the single most common reason for referral to a gastroenterologist. The long-term prognosis is excellent.[1] A number of cases appear to be precipitated by an episode of acute bacterial gastroenteritis.[2] Symptoms of irritable bowel syndrome resemble those of lactase deficiency; the latter should always be considered in the differential diagnosis of irritable bowel syndrome.[3]

For a clinical diagnosis of irritable bowel syndrome the patient must have had at least 3 months of continuous or recurrent symptoms of abdominal pain or discomfort that is relieved with defecation and is associated with a change in the frequency or consistency of the stool. In addition, two or more of the following symptoms must occur on at least 25% of occasions or days[4]:

1. Altered stool frequency
2. Altered stool form (lumpy and hard or loose and watery)
3. Altered stool passage (straining, urgency, or feeling of incomplete evacuation)
4. Passage of mucus
5. Bloating or feeling of abdominal distention

There is no proof that any specific treatment is effective for irritable bowel syndrome[5]; a good physician-patient relationship is important.[1] Traditional therapeutic regimens are based on symptom control.[4] Constipation is managed with fiber, such as ½ to 1 cup of bran per day or ½ to 1 tbsp psyllium (Metamucil, Prodiem) one to four times a day taken with plenty of fluids, or with prokinetic agents, such as cisapride (Prepulsid) 5 to 10 mg tid. Pain may be treated with antispasmodics, such as dicyclomine (Bentyl, Bentylol) 10 to 20 mg tid or qid, hyoscine butylbromide (Buscopan) 10 mg tid or qid, or trimebutine (Modulon) 200 mg tid, or with smooth muscle relaxants, such as the calcium channel blocker pinaverium bromide (Dicetel) 50 mg tid with meals. Antidiarrheal agents include loperamide (Imodium) 2 to 4 mg tid or qid prn, diphenoxylate-atropine (Lomotil) 2.5 to 5 mg tid or qid prn, or cholestyramine (Questran) 2 to 4 g bid to qid.

REFERENCES

1. Owens DM, Nelson DK, Talley NJ: The irritable bowel syndrome: long-term prognosis and the physician-patient interaction, *Ann Intern Med* 122:107-112, 1995.
2. Neal KR, Hebden J, Spiller R: Prevalence of gastrointestinal symptoms six months after bacterial gastroenteritis and risk factors for development of the irritable bowel syndrome: postal survey of patients, *BMJ* 324:779-782, 1997.
3. Tolliver BA, Gerrerea JL, DiPalma JA: Evaluation of patients who meet clinical criteria for irritable bowel syndrome, *Am J Gastroenterol* 89:176-178, 1994.
4. Thompson WG: Irritable bowel syndrome: strategy for the family physician, *Can Fam Physician* 40:307-316, 1994.
5. Klein KB: Controlled treatment trials in the irritable bowel syndrome: a critique, *Gastroenterology* 95:232-241, 1988.

LACTASE DEFICIENCY

(See also irritable bowel syndrome)

Within Europe the incidence of lactose intolerance is lowest in Scandinavia and Northwest Europe (3% to 8%) and highest in the southeastern regions (70% in southern Italy and Turkey). The incidence in black Africa is high except among cattle-raising nomads. In Southeast Asia the incidence is almost 100%.[1]

Lactase levels in the small intestine normally fall with increasing age. The levels in a 1-year-old are about 25% to 50% of those in a newborn. Levels continue to fall thereafter in populations subject to lactase deficiency, so that between the ages of 2 and 20 the levels in these groups reach only about 10% of the neonatal levels. This process continues into old age, particularly in blacks.[2]

The major symptoms of lactase deficiency are abdominal pain, diarrhea, bloating, borborygmi, and flatulence. These symptoms are similar to those in patients with irritable bowel syndrome, and numerous reports have found an increased incidence of lactase deficiency in patients with irritable bowel syndrome. In fact, in one study about half the patients meeting the criteria for irritable bowel syndrome were lactase deficient.[3] Lactase deficiency is probably responsible for a number of cases of recurrent abdominal pain in children.[4]

Not all patients who claim to be milk intolerant are as intolerant as they think. A double-blind study of lactose-intolerant patients who claimed they had symptoms even if they added milk to coffee found that they were able to tolerate 240 ml of milk a day taken in the morning with breakfast.[5]

The standard investigation for lactose deficiency is the breath hydrogen test. According to Thompson and co-workers[6] a cheaper and equally effective method is to have the patient abstain from all milk products for 1 week and then drink a quart of milk. If significant symptoms result, the test is positive.

A simple treatment for lactase deficiency is the avoidance of milk and milk products containing lactose. Aged cheese does not contain lactose because it is destroyed during the fermentation process. However, processed cheeses such as cream cheese, cottage cheese, and ricotta cheese do contain lactose and should be avoided. The adverse effect of limiting dairy products may be an inadequate calcium intake, so supplementary calcium should often be prescribed. An alternative to avoiding milk products is to have the patients buy milk that has had lactase added, add lactase enzyme (Lactaid) to ordinary milk, or take lactase enzymes before ingesting dairy products. Lactase enzyme is supplied as a liquid in dropper bottles and as tablets. The usual dose is ½ to 3 tablets just before the ingestion of lactose-containing milk products or 5 to 15 drops added to each liter or quart of refrigerated milk 24 hours before its use. Five drops of lactase will hydrolyze 70% of the lactose in 1 liter of milk in 24 hours at refrigerator temperature; 15 drops in a liter of milk will hydrolyze 99% of the lactose. The reaction is much faster at room temperature.

There is evidence that lactose-intolerant individuals can adapt to some extent if given gradually increasing amounts of lactose.[7]

REFERENCES

1. Gudmand-Hoyer E: The clinical significance of disaccharide maldigestion, *Am J Clin Nutr* 59(suppl 3):S735-S741, 1994.
2. Rao DR, Bello H, Warren AP, et al: Prevalence of lactose maldigestion: influence and interaction of age, race, and sex, *Dig Dis Sci* 39:1519-1524, 1994.
3. Tolliver BA, Gerrerea JL, DiPalma JA: Evaluation of patients who meet clinical criteria for irritable bowel syndrome, *Am J Gastroenterol* 89:176-178, 1994.
4. Gudmand-Hoyer E: The clinical significance of disaccharide maldigestion, *Am J Clin Nutr* 59(suppl 3):S735-S741, 1994.
5. Suarez FL, Savaiano DA, Levitt MD: A comparison of symptoms after the consumption of milk or lactose-hydrolyzed milk by people with self-reported severe lactose intolerance, *N Engl J Med* 333:1-4, 1995.
6. Thompson WG, Drossman DA, Whitehead WE: Approaching IBS with confidence, *Patient Care Can* 31:51-66, 1993.
7. Johnson AO, Semenya JG, Buchowski MS, et al: Adaptation of lactose maldigesters to continued milk intakes, *Am J Clin Nutr* 58:879-881, 1993.

LIVER

Alcoholic Hepatitis

(See also alcohol)

The spectrum of illness in patients with alcoholic hepatitis varies from mild nonspecific symptoms (fatigue, anorexia, and weight loss) through liver failure with jaundice, ascites, and hepatic encephalopathy. Alcoholic hepatitis is generally limited to persons who drink 80 g or more of ethanol per day. This is more than eight 12-ounce beers, 1 liter (one and a half bottles) of 12% wine, or one-half pint of 80-proof whiskey.[1]

Patients may have anemia with macrocytosis, leukocytosis (white blood cell count usually more than 15,000/mm^3, but 8% have leukopenia), elevated prothrombin time, elevated bilirubin level, and mild elevation of liver enzyme levels. Usually the AST (or SGOT) level is less than five times normal. The ALT (or SGPT) level is usually less than half the AST. An AST/ALT ratio greater than 2 virtually establishes the diagnosis of alcoholic hepatitis (about 60% of cases). In more than 90% of cases of alcoholic hepatitis the AST is greater than the ALT level.[1]

REFERENCES

1. Woods SE, Hitchcock M, Meyer A: Alcoholic hepatitis, *Am Fam Physician* 47:1171-1178, 1993.

Ascites

Ascites is usually treated with a potassium-sparing diuretic and a loop diuretic. A frequent combination is spironolactone and furosemide.[1] One regimen is to start with spironolactone (Aldactone) 100 mg po and furosemide (Lasix) 40 mg po with all pills given at once in the morning. If weight does not decrease in 2 to 3 days, both drug doses should be doubled (200 mg and 80 mg, respectively). The maximum dose is 400 mg of spironolactone and 160 mg of furosemide. Amiloride (Midamor) may be used instead of spironolactone, starting with 10 mg qam and increasing to a maximum of 40 mg/day. Amiloride has a faster action and does not cause painful gynecomastia.[1]

REFERENCES

1. Runyon BA: Care of patients with ascites, *N Engl J Med* 330:337-342, 1994.

Biliary Cirrhosis

(See also connective tissue diseases; hypothyroidism; inflammatory bowel disease)

Ninety-five percent of patients with biliary cirrhosis are women, and most are middle aged. The usual clinical presentation is pruritus and fatigue, although many asymptomatic cases are detected when an unexpectedly elevated alkaline phosphatase level is discovered during biochemical screening procedures. AST and ALT concentrations may be normal or only slightly elevated, whereas alkaline phosphatase and GGT levels are markedly elevated. Most patients are found to have increased levels of antimitochondrial antibodies, and low titers of smooth muscle and antinuclear antibodies are common.[1,2] Serum lipid levels are often strikingly elevated, with total cholesterol levels as high as 1000 mg/dl (26 mmol/L). However, patients are not at increased risk of cardiovascular disease, probably because of a marked elevation of HDL cholesterol levels.[2]

The median survival is between 10 and 16 years for asymptomatic patients and 7 years for symptomatic patients. Although symptoms develop after 2 to 4 years in most asymptomatic patients, approximately a third remain symptom free for many years. The most common symptom is pruritus, which can usually be controlled with cholestyramine (Questran) 4 g po tid.[2]

An association has been reported between biliary cirrhosis and immunological disorders such as lupus, rheumatoid arthritis, scleroderma, CREST syndrome (calcinosis, Raynaud's phenomenon, esophageal involvement, sclerodactyly, and telangiectasia), Sjögren's syndrome, and thyroiditis.[1,2] About one fifth of the patients are hypothyroid.[2]

REFERENCES

1. Buckley SE, Dipalma JA: Recognizing primary biliary cirrhosis and primary sclerosing cholangitis, *Am Fam Physician* 53:195-200, 1996.
2. Kaplan MM: Primary biliary cirrhosis, *N Engl J Med* 335:1570-1580, 1996.

Table 25 Hepatitis Terminology

Liver Enzymes	
ALT (SGPT)	Alanine aminotransferase
AST (SGOT)	Aspartate aminotransferase
Hepatitis A	
HAV	Hepatitis A virus
IgM anti-HAV	Acute hepatitis A infection
IgG anti-HAV	Previous hepatitis A infection
Hepatitis B	
HBV	Hepatitis B virus
HBsAg	Hepatitis B surface antigen; elevated in acute infections and in the carrier state
Anti-HBs	Anti-hepatitis B surface antigen; develops 1-3 months after recovery from acute infection
HBcAg	Hepatitis B core antigen
IgM anti-HBc	Positive in the window phase of acute hepatitis B when HBsAg has declined but anti-HBs has not yet developed
HBeAg	Hepatitis B e antigen; present during acute hepatitis B infection and in chronic hepatitis B
Anti-HBe	Develops after acute infection; not usually tested
HBIG	Hepatitis B immune globulin
Hepatitis C	
HCV	Hepatitis C virus
Anti-HCV	May not develop until 3 months after infection
Hepatitis D	
HDV	Hepatitis D virus; occurs only in patients who are carriers of HBsAg
Anti-HDV	Order only for patients who are HBsAg positive and have clinical symptoms of acute hepatitis
Hepatitis E	
HEV	Hepatitis E virus; clinical picture similar to hepatitis A; uncommon in developed countries

Hepatitis

(See also alcoholic hepatitis; biliary cirrhosis; hemochromatosis; immunization schedules for children; transfusions; vaccines)

The common forms of viral hepatitis seen in family medicine, hepatitis A, B, and C, are discussed below. Rare causes of hepatitis that should be ruled out when investigating for the cause of chronic hepatitis are hemochromatosis, alpha$_1$-antitrypsin deficiency, and primary biliary cirrhosis.

Terminology and clinical correlations of laboratory tests used in investigating hepatitis

A discussion of viral hepatitis requires a knowledge of several terms and abbreviations (Table 25).[1]

Hepatitis A

About 20% of patients with hepatitis A have a brief relapse after initial improvement. Fulminant hepatitis occurs in 0.1% of patients with this disease. The diagnosis of acute infection may be confirmed by elevated titers of IgM anti-HAV. Gamma globulin 0.02 ml/kg is effective for the prophylaxis of family member contacts if given within 8 days of exposure.[2]

Travelers from industrialized countries to developing nations are at risk of acquiring hepatitis A even if they are staying in luxury hotels. The overall risk if unprotected by passive or active immunization is estimated to be 3 to 6 per 1000 travelers per month with the risk increasing to 20 per 1000 per month among those eating and drinking under poor hygienic conditions. Less than 20% of persons from industrialized countries born after 1945 have acquired natural immunity.[2,3]

For travelers, passive immunization with immune globulin (human) is effective for 3 to 5 months in 85% to 90% of cases. Active immunization with a two-dose series of inactivated HAV vaccine (Havrix, Vaqta) is available. Hepatitis A vaccination is effective, and immunity is estimated to persist for 7 to 10 years or more.[2,3] Patients at risk of exposure to hepatitis A within 4 weeks of vaccination may be given immune globulin at the same time as they are vaccinated, but in a different body site.[4] The usual adult dose of immune globulin is 2 ml for travel of less than 3 months and 5 ml for travel of 3 to 5 months. For postexposure prophylaxis of household or sexual contacts the dose of immune globulin is 0.02 mg/kg given as soon as possible and no later than 2 weeks after exposure.[5]

Hepatitis B

Five percent of Canadians are anti-HBs positive and 0.5% are HBsAg positive. In Canada less than 3% of reported cases of acute infection are in children.[6] In adults about half the patients who acquire hepatitis B are asymptomatic, one fourth have jaundice, and one fourth have nonspecific symptoms. Complete cure occurs in 90% of cases, and the carrier state develops in about 10%. In a quarter of this 10%, cirrhosis, chronic hepatitis, or liver cancer will develop. Hepatocellular cancer is most likely to develop in patients whose liver biopsies show severe chronic active hepatitis, cirrhosis, or both.[7]

In patients with acute hepatitis B, detectable HBsAg usually develops about 3 weeks before the onset of clinical symptoms. HBsAg declines over the next few weeks as the patient recovers, and shortly thereafter anti-HBs develops. A "window phase" may occur in the recovery stage of hepatitis B when neither HBsAg nor anti-HBs is present; at that time tests for IgM anti-HBc are usually positive.[1]

A patient with clinical hepatitis who has anti-HBs does not have acute hepatitis B. HBeAg is present during acute hepatitis B infection and in chronic hepatitis B. If a patient from an endemic area has elevated liver enzyme levels and is HBsAg and HBeAg positive, he or she probably has chronic hepatitis.[1]

A person is defined as a chronic carrier of hepatitis B if two samples of sera taken 6 months apart are both HBsAg positive or if a single serum sample is HBsAg positive and anti-HBc negative. The risk of development of the carrier state depends on the age of the patient at the time of infection. Specific risks are infants 90% to 95%, children under 5 25% to 50%, and adults 6% to 10%.[8]

Immunization against hepatitis B. See immunization schedules for children and vaccines.

Treatment of chronic hepatitis B. Interferon alpha (interferon alfa-2a [Roferon-A] or interferon alfa-2b [Intron A]) has been used for the treatment of chronic active hepatitis B. The drug is given subcutaneously either as 5 million units daily or 10 million units three times a week. The usual indications for treatment are elevations of the serum aminotransferase level and chronic hepatitis on liver biopsy. A course of 4 to 6 months gives a remission rate of about 33%. Acute reactions to interferon are flulike symptoms; chronic side effects include fatigue, myalgias, mood changes, and bone marrow suppression.[9] Interferon alfa-n1 (Wellferon) may also be used to treat chronic hepatitis B.

Hepatitis C

Before the discovery and implementation of anti-HCV in blood banks in 1989, hepatitis developed in approximately 3% to 4% of transfusion recipients.[10] Hepatitis C was responsible for 90% of these transfusion-related cases of non-A, non-B hepatitis. Another form of non-A, non-B hepatitis was known to be enterically transmitted, and it is now clear that most of those cases were due to hepatitis E.[10] Recognized risk factors for hepatitis C are intravenous drug use, transfusions, and living in an endemic area. In the United States more than 35% of cases occur without known risk factors and are labeled as sporadic.

Transmission of infection by close physical contact or through sexual relations may occur but is rare. For example, a 10- to 15-year follow-up of husbands of hepatitis C–positive women in Germany showed no evidence of transmission; in the same study only 1.3% of the children developed antibodies to hepatitis C.[11] However, evidence that heterosexual transmission does occur is beginning to accumulate.[12-14]

Perinatal transmission of hepatitis C also occurs rarely.[15,16] In one Italian study of pregnant women who were anti-HCV positive, none of the babies became infected unless the mother was also HIV positive; in that circumstance a third of the babies became infected with HCV.[16]

The presence of hepatitis C viremia can now be determined by detecting hepatitis C RNA through polymerase chain reaction methods. A systematic review of studies of hepatitis C transmission found that the risk of transmission is extremely low if the polymerase chain reaction is negative. This may be important in advising patients about sexual practices (whether to use condoms) and risks of transmitting the disease through pregnancy. When the polymerase chain reaction is positive, the risk of transmission from occupational exposure (needle sticks) and pregnancy is about 6%, whereas the risk with blood transfusions is around 80%.[17]

The incubation period of hepatitis C is 40 to 90 days, and the acute clinical illness is usually mild. Only 25% of patients have jaundice. Anti-HCV may not develop until 3 months after the onset of infection. Chronic hepatitis is a common complication of the disease. Chronic hepatitis develops in an estimated 50% of patients with posttransfusion hepatitis C, and in 20% of these cirrhosis occurs. Hepatocellular carcinoma is an important complication that is most likely to develop in patients whose liver biopsies show severe chronic active hepatitis, cirrhosis, or both.[7]

Treatment of chronic hepatitis C. Interferon alpha (interferon alfa-2a [Roferon-A] or interferon alfa-2b [Intron A]) has been used for the treatment of chronic active hepatitis C. Indications for therapy are elevated serum aminotransferase enzymes and chronic hepatitis on liver biopsy. The currently recommended treatment is 3 million units of interferon subcutaneously three times a week for 6 to 12 months. Response ceases in many patients once the drug is stopped; the overall sustained response rate is 15% to 25%.[10] However, in a study from Japan, interferon-alfa given to patients with hepatitis C and cirrhosis protected most of them from hepatocellular carcinoma.[18] Adverse effects of interferon are as described for hepatitis B (see discussion of treatment of chronic hepatitis B) but are less severe because the dose is lower.[18]

REFERENCES

1. Friedman G, Sherker AH: The ABCs of hepatitis, *Can J Diagn,* March, 13:85-97, 1996.
2. Steffen R, Kane MA, Shapiro CN, et al: Epidemiology and prevention of hepatitis A in travelers, *JAMA* 272:885-889, 1994.

3. Furesz J, Scheifele DW, Palkonyay L: Safety and effectiveness of the new inactivated hepatitis A virus vaccine, *Can Med Assoc J* 152:343-348, 1995.
4. Public health: hepatitis A, *Can Med Assoc J* 156:545, 1997.
5. *Canadian immunization guide,* ed 4, Ottawa, 1993, Minister of Supply and Services Canada.
6. From the CCDR: report of the Hepatitis B Working Group, *Can Med Assoc J* 151:1294-1297, 1994.
7. Curley SA, Izzo F, Gallipoli A, et al: Identification and screening of 416 patients with chronic hepatitis at high risk to develop hepatocellular cancer, *Ann Surg* 222:375-380, 1995.
8. Mahoney FJ, Burkholder BT, Matson CC: Prevention of hepatitis B virus infection, *Am Fam Physician* 866:865-872, 1993.
9. Hoofnagle JH, Bisceglie AM: The treatment of chronic viral hepatitis, *N Engl J Med* 336:347-356, 1997.
10. A-Kader HH, Balistreri WF: Hepatitis C virus: implications to pediatric practice, *Pediatr Infect Dis J* 12:853-867, 1993.
11. Meisel H, Reip A, Faltus B, et al: Transmission of hepatitis C virus to children and husbands by women infected with contaminated anti-D immunoglobulin, *Lancet* 345:1209-1211, 1995.
12. Thomas DL, Zenilman JM, Alter HJ, et al: Sexual transmission of hepatitis C virus among patients attending sexually transmitted diseases clinics in Baltimore—an analysis of 309 sex partnerships, *J Infect Dis* 171:768-775, 1995.
13. Piazza M, Sagliocca L, Tosone G, et al: Sexual transmission of the hepatitis C virus and efficacy of prophylaxis with intramuscular immune serum globulin, *Arch Intern Med* 157:1537-1544, 1997.
14. Kao JH, Hwang YT, Chen PJ, et al: Transmission of hepatitis C virus between spouses—the important role of exposure duration, *Am J Gastroenterol* 91:2087-2090, 1996.
15. Nakashima K, Ikematsu H, Hayashi J, et al: Intrafamilial transmission of hepatitis C virus among the population of an endemic area of Japan, *JAMA* 274:1459-1461, 1995.
16. Zanetti AR, Tanzi E, Paccagnini S, et al (Lombardy Study Group on Vertical HCV Transmission): Mother-to-infant transmission of hepatitis C virus, *Lancet* 345:1122-1123, 1995.
17. Dore GJ, Kaldor JM, McCaughan GW: Systematic review of role of polymerase chain reaction in defining infectiousness among people infected with hepatitis C virus, *BMJ* 315:333-337, 1997.
18. Nishiguchi S, Kuroki T, Nakatani S, et al: Randomised trial of effects of interferon-alpha on incidence of hepatocellular carcinoma in chronic active hepatitis C with cirrhosis, *Lancet* 346: 1051-1055, 1995.

PANCREAS

Pancreatic Cancer

Diabetic patients who have had the disease for at least 5 years have double the risk of pancreatic carcinoma compared with nondiabetic control subjects.[1] Current smokers have a 2.5-fold increase in the relative risk for this malignancy.[2] Overall, 80% of patients with pancreatic cancer are dead within a year of diagnosis.[3] A multicenter study of 100 U.S. veterans' hospitals found that the operative mortality for the Whipple procedure was 8%. Patients who underwent the surgery for pancreatic cancer had a mean survival of 15 months and a projected 5-year survival of 9%.[4]

REFERENCES

1. Everhart J, Wright D: Diabetes mellitus as a risk factor for pancreatic cancer: a meta-analysis, *JAMA* 273:1605-1609, 1995.
2. Fuchs CS, Colditz GA, Stampfer MJ, et al: A prospective study of cigarette smoking and the risk of pancreatic cancer, *Arch Intern Med* 156:2255-2260, 1996.
3. Taylor WF, Everhart JE: Pancreatic cancer. In Everhart JE, ed: *Digestive diseases in the United States: epidemiology and impact,* Washington, DC, 1994, US Dept of Health and Human Services, Public Health Service, National Institutes of Health, National Institute of Diabetes and Digestive and Kidney Diseases, NIH Pub No 94-1447, pp 247-270.
4. Wade TP, Elghazzawy AG, Virgo KS, et al: The Whipple resection for cancer in US Department of Veterans Affairs hospitals, *Ann Surg* 221:241-248, 1995.

STOMACH AND DUODENUM

Nonsteroidal Antiinflammatory Drug Gastropathy

(See also absolute risk reduction; nonsteroidal antiinflammatory drugs; nonpharmacological treatment of hypertension; numbers of patients who need to be screened or treated; relative risk reduction; osteoarthritis)

NSAIDs are associated not only with peptic ulcers and their complications, but also with a small bowel enteropathy that may cause loss of blood and protein.[1] No solid evidence has been offered that any of the "traditional" NSAIDs are more likely to induce gastropathy than others. One meta-analysis of studies comparing a number of these drugs concluded that ibuprofen (Motrin, Advil) and diclofenac (Voltaren) were the least likely to cause major gastrointestinal complications, that ketoprofen (Orudis, Oruvail, Actron) and piroxicam (Feldene) were the most likely to do so, and that aspirin, sulindac (Clinoril), naproxen (Naprosyn), and indomethacin (Indocid, Indocin) were intermediate in this respect. However, it was clear that ibuprofen was used in low doses, and the lower rates of gastropathy noted with this drug and some of the others were probably related to dosage rather than the characteristics of the drugs themselves.[2]

Several short-term studies have shown fewer adverse gastrointestinal and renal effects from two newer NSAIDs, etodolac (Ultradol, Lodine) and nabumetone (Relafen). The theoretical basis is that these two agents inhibit cyclooxygenase 2 (COX-2) to a greater extent than cyclooxygenase 1 (COX-1). COX-1 normally facilitates the production of protective prostaglandins in the stomach and kidneys, whereas COX-2 is found in joints and aggravates inflammation.[1]

NSAIDs are associated with many adverse gastrointestinal effects, including peptic ulcer and its complications, small and large bowel bleeding, perforation, esophageal strictures, and small intestine inflammation. The most important risk factors for NSAID gastropathy appear to be old age, history of previous peptic ulcer disease, high-dose NSAIDs, and concomitant administration of corticosteroids.[1,3,4] Other risk factors are hypertension, congestive heart failure, renal failure, hepatic failure, and volume depletion.[1]

A controversial issue is whether misoprostol (Cytotec) is beneficial to patients taking NSAIDs. The drug can certainly decrease the incidence of gastric erosions (so-called NSAID gastropathy) or even ulcers defined as a mucosal defect of 0.5 cm or greater as detected by gastroscopy.[5] (The distinction between "erosion" and "ulcer" is controversial.) Whether this has clinical significance is unknown. Definitive evidence that misoprostol has any protective effect with respect to clinically significant gastrointestinal bleeding, perforation, hospitalization, or subjective dyspepsia was reported for the first time in 1995.[6] A multicenter, randomized, double-blind, placebo-controlled study of patients with rheumatoid arthritis who were taking NSAIDs continually found that after 6 months there was a 40% relative reduction in major upper gastrointestinal complications in the patients receiving 200 μg of misoprostol qid.[6] The absolute reduction rate was 0.4%, or put another way, 250 patients taking NSAIDs would have to be treated with misoprostol for 6 months to prevent one major upper gastrointestinal event.

Should patients taking NSAIDs be given misoprostol (Cytotec)? If the risk of major upper gastrointestinal events continued at the same rate in subsequent months as in the first 6 months of the study quoted above,[6] the argument for using misoprostol becomes more persuasive. Additional risk factors for adverse events in this study were age, a history of peptic ulcer or gastrointestinal bleeding, and cardiovascular disease; patients with all of these risks had a 9% complication rate by the end of 6 months. Treating at least high-risk patients seems reasonable. On the other hand, the risk of a major gastrointestinal complication among patients who were taking NSAIDs (without misoprostol) continually for 6 months and had none of the previous risk factors was only 0.4% in the above study.[6] There does not seem to be much logic to prescribing misoprostol for low-risk patients on short-term NSAID regimens.[7] A Canadian consensus panel recommends avoiding the use of NSAIDs if possible, but if they must be given to high-risk patients, using the lowest possible dose, adding misoprostol (Cytotec), and considering use of a weak cyclooxygenase 1 inhibitor (COX-1) such as etodolac (Ultradol, Lodine) or nabumetone (Relafen).[1]

The H_2-blocker famotidine (Pepcid) in doses of 40 mg bid over a 2-year period has been shown to decrease the incidence of endoscopically identified duodenal and gastric ulcers (defined as excavated mucosal breaks greater than 3 mm in diameter) in patients taking NSAIDs.[8] Whether this would significantly decrease the clinical complications of ulcer disease has not been determined.[7]

A related issue is whether NSAIDs are the drugs of choice for osteoarthritis. Degenerative arthritis or osteoarthritis is probably the most common reason for prescribing NSAIDs for elderly people,[9] and it is done with alacrity, since 60% of persons who use NSAIDs in the United States are 60 years or older,[10] while 27% of persons in Alberta, Canada, over the age of 65 received at least one NSAID prescription during a 6-month study period.[11] Yet the evidence that NSAIDs are any better than acetaminophen, weight loss, or exercise programs for the control of osteoarthritis symptoms is tenuous at best.[12-15] An obvious way of decreasing the gastrointestinal complications of NSAIDs is to avoid using them for osteoarthritis.

The standard dose of misoprostol is 200 μg qid; a 1995 endoscopic study found that 200 μg of misoprostol bid or tid was effective in reducing the incidence of endoscopically detectable duodenal and gastric ulcers in patients taking NSAIDs and that these dosages were much better tolerated than the qid doses.[16]

REFERENCES

1. Tannenbaum H, Davis P, Russell AS, et al (Canadian NSAID Consensus Participants): An evidence-based approach to prescribing NSAIDs in musculoskeletal disease: a Canadian consensus, *Can Med Assoc J* 155:77-88, 1996.
2. Henry D, Lim LL-Y, Rodriguez LA, et al: Variability in risk of gastrointestinal complications with individual non-steroidal anti-inflammatory drugs: results of a collaborative meta-analysis, *BMJ* 312:1563-1566, 1996.
3. Griffin MR, Piper JM, Daugherty JR, et al: Nonsteroidal anti-inflammatory drug use and increased risk for peptic ulcer disease in elderly persons, *Ann Intern Med* 114:257-263, 1991.
4. Gabriel SE, Jaakkimainene L, Bambardier C: Risk for serious gastrointestinal complications related to use of nonsteroidal anti-inflammatory drugs: a meta-analysis, *Ann Intern Med* 115: 787-796, 1991.
5. Graham DY, White RH, Moreland LW: Duodenal and gastric ulcer prevention with misoprostol in arthritis patients taking NSAIDs, *Ann Intern Med* 119:257-262, 1993.
6. Silverstein FE, Graham DY, Senior JR, et al: Misoprostol reduces serious gastrointestinal complications in patients with rheumatoid arthritis receiving nonsteroidal anti-inflammatory drugs—a randomized, double-blind, placebo-controlled trial, *Ann Intern Med* 123:241-249, 1995.
7. Levine JS: Misoprostol and nonsteroidal anti-inflammatory drugs: a tale of effects, outcomes, and costs (editorial), *Ann Intern Med* 123:309-310, 1995.
8. Taha AS, Hudson N, Hawkey CJ, et al: Famotidine for the prevention of gastric and duodenal ulcers caused by nonsteroidal antiinflammatory drugs, *N Engl J Med* 334:1435-1439, 1996.
9. Murray MD, Brater DC: NSAIDs, *Clin Geriatr Med* 6:365-441, 1990.
10. Gurwitz JH, Avorn J: The ambiguous relation between aging and adverse drug reactions, *Ann Intern Med* 114:956-966, 1991.
11. Hogan DB, Campbell NRC, Crutcher R, et al: Prescription of nonsteroidal anti-inflammatory drugs for elderly people in Alberta, *Can Med Assoc J* 151:315-322, 1994.
12. Dieppe PA, Frankel SJ, Toth B: Is research into the treatment of osteoarthritis with NSAID misdirected? *Lancet* 341:353-354, 1993.
13. Bradley JD, Brandt KD, Katz BP, et al: Comparison of an anti-inflammatory dose of ibuprofen, an analgesic dose of ibuprofen and acetaminophen in the treatment of patients with osteoarthritis of the knee, *N Engl J Med* 325:87-91, 1991.

Gastrointestinal System

14. Kovar PA, Allegrante JP, MacKenzie CR, et al: Supervised fitness walking in patients with osteoarthritis of the knee, *Ann Intern Med* 116:529-534, 1992.
15. Felson DT, Zhang Y, Anthony JM, et al: Weight loss reduces the risk for symptomatic knee osteoarthritis in women: the Framingham Study, *Ann Intern Med* 116:535-539, 1992.
16. Raskin JB, White RH, Jackson JE, et al: Misoprostol dosage in the prevention of nonsteroidal anti-inflammatory drug-induced gastric and duodenal ulcers—a comparison of three regimens, *Ann Intern Med* 123:344-350, 1995.

Peptic Ulcer

(See also nonsteroidal antiinflammatory drug gastropathy; stomach cancer)

Differentiation from nonulcer dyspepsia

A major issue in clinical practice is distinguishing peptic ulcer from nonulcer dyspepsia. Should patients with symptoms of uncomplicated peptic ulcer disease have a barium swallow or endoscopy, or should they be treated with H_2-blockers on clinical grounds only? Thompson makes a cogent case for investigation[1]:

1. At least half of patients with "ulcer symptoms" do not have an ulcer; they have nonulcer dyspepsia.
2. Both nonulcer dyspepsia and peptic ulcer are recurrent diseases, so a definitive diagnosis is desirable.
3. H_2-blockers are no more effective in treating nonulcer dyspepsia than placebo (the placebo effect is about 30%).
4. Peptic ulcer is an infectious disease and should be treated with antibiotics.
5. Studies of patients with nonulcer dyspepsia have shown that those who underwent endoscopy had a decrease in physician visits and drug use compared with those who did not have endoscopy.

A British group screened patients with dyspepsia for "sinister" symptoms, NSAID use, and *Helicobacter pylori*. Those who were positive in any of these areas underwent endoscopy, and the rest (37%) did not. The investigators then compared drug use in the nonendoscopy patients with a cohort of patients who had endoscopy but in whom no abnormalities were detected. The patients who underwent endoscopy used more medications than those who did not, which is the contrary of the studies quoted previously by Thompson.[2]

The issue is more complex in the United States where the costs of endoscopy are high; in that situation it may be more cost effective to treat patients empirically and order endoscopy only for nonresponders.[3]

Bleeding peptic ulcers

Bleeding peptic ulcers account for 50% of upper gastrointestinal hemorrhages. In 80% of cases the bleeding stops spontaneously and recovery is uneventful. Rebleeding, when it occurs, usually takes place within the first 3 days. NSAIDs appear to be a major risk factor not only for the development of peptic ulcers, but also for bleeding from peptic ulcers (see later discussion).[4] The concomitant use of steroids and NSAIDs is associated with a 10-fold increased risk of upper gastrointestinal hemorrhage.[5]

The appearance of an ulcer as seen at gastroscopy helps determine the prognosis, and in patients with uncontrolled bleeding, hemostasis can often be achieved through gastroscopic procedures.[4] Intensive therapy with H_2-blockers has not been effective in controlling acute upper intestinal bleeding, but in India a trial of omeprazole (Losec, Prilosec) 40 mg po bid for 5 days for endoscopically documented bleeding peptic ulcers showed a significant decrease in requirements for transfusion or surgery. No endoscopic therapeutic interventions were attempted in this study.[6] Whether these results could be duplicated in North America or Western Europe is unknown. At present, endoscopic treatment is the first-line therapy for active bleeding from peptic ulcers, but proton pump inhibitors may be a useful adjunct to this procedure or an alternative for patients who are unable to be receive it.[7]

Once a patient has stopped bleeding and is in a stable condition, medical treatment is aimed at healing the ulcer and preventing recurrences of the ulcer and bleeding. If possible, NSAIDs should be discontinued. If the patient is positive for *H. pylori* (as are about 75% of patients with bleeding peptic ulcers), the organisms should be eradicated (see later discussion). Healing is facilitated by omeprazole 20 mg/day for 6 to 8 weeks or by an H_2-receptor antagonist for 2 to 3 months.[4]

Helicobacter pylori infection

Excluding patients taking NSAIDs, more than 80% of those with gastric ulcers and more than 90% of those with duodenal ulcers are infected with *H. pylori*. However, ulcers develop in only 15% to 20% of those infected with the organism. The ulcer recurrence rate is markedly decreased in patients treated for *H. pylori*.[8,9]

H. pylori infection is recognized as a cause of gastric and duodenal ulcers, as well as gastric carcinoma,[8-10] but whether it is related to nonulcer dyspepsia is uncertain.[9] An interesting observation is that the incidence of gastric cancer is decreased in patients with a history of duodenal ulcer.[11] The probable explanation is that *H. pylori* acquired in early childhood (as occurs frequently in developing countries) leads to atrophic gastritis, which is both a predisposing factor for malignancy and, because of decreased acid secretion, a defense against duodenal ulcer formation. When the infection is acquired later in life, atrophic gastritis is less likely to develop and so acid secretion is not inhibited.[10]

Diagnostic procedures for *H. pylori* include gastric biopsies, breath urea tests, and serological tests.[8,9] Serological findings remain positive after eradication of the organisms and cannot be used to measure the efficacy of therapy; breath urea tests and gastric biopsies may be used for this purpose, but the indications for doing so are few.[8]

Treatment of *H. pylori* infections leads to faster healing of ulcers and a marked reduction in the relapse rate.[9,10] Since

Gastrointestinal System

95% of duodenal ulcers that are not NSAID related are associated with *H. pylori* infection, a reasonable approach is to treat all such patients with antimicrobial therapy without testing for the presence of the organism.[8,9,12] Whether treating patients with *H. pylori* but no evidence of peptic ulcers will prevent gastric carcinoma is unknown, but on the basis of current knowledge it seems a reasonable option.[13]

Because *H. pylori* is difficult to eradicate, two or more antibiotics should be used. The adjunct use of a proton pump inhibitor such as omeprazole (Prilosec, Losec) or lansoprazole (Prevacid), which have some in vitro inhibitory effects against the organism, augments the efficacy of the antibiotics.[9] Most studies to date have used omeprazole 20 mg bid, but new data suggest that other proton pump inhibitors such as lansoprazole (Prevacid) 30 mg bid or pantoprazole (Pantoloc) 40 mg bid are equally effective.[9] Acquired resistance to metronidazole (Flagyl) and clarithromycin (Biaxin) is common if these drugs are used as single agents. Resistance to amoxicillin, tetracycline, and bismuth has not been reported.[12]

A variety of treatments for *H. pylori* have been used, and some of these are listed below.[9,13] Cure rates with any of these regimens are on the order of 85% to 90%.[9,12,14] Doxycycline may not be substituted for tetracycline, or ampicillin for amoxicillin.[8] Most of the studies of bismuth have been with bismuth subcitrate, which is not available in North America; probably bismuth subsalicylate (Pepto-Bismol), which is the standard form in North America, is equally effective.[14] The current trend is to use amoxicillin or clarithromycin (Biaxin) plus metronidazole plus omeprazole (treatment protocols no. 3 and no. 4 as listed below),[14] but the least expensive treatment is bismuth-metronidazole-tetracycline (protocol no. 1 below).[9]

1. Bismuth subsalicylate (Pepto-Bismol) 2 tablets (262 mg each) qid for 7 to 14 days *plus* metronidazole (Flagyl) 250 mg qid for 7 to 14 days *plus* tetracycline 500 mg qid for 7 to 14 days[9]
2. Amoxicillin 1 g bid for 7 days *plus* clarithromycin (Biaxin) 500 mg bid for 7 days *plus* omeprazole 20 mg bid for 7 days[9]
3. Amoxicillin 1 g bid with meals for 7 days *plus* metronidazole (Flagyl) 500 mg bid with meals for 7 days *plus* omeprazole (Prilosec, Losec) with a loading dose of 20 mg tid on the day before beginning antibiotics followed by 20 mg bid before meals for 7 days[13]
4. Clarithromycin (Biaxin) 250 mg[9] to 500 mg[13] bid with meals for 7 days *plus* metronidazole (Flagyl) 500 mg bid[9,13] with meals for 7 days *plus* omeprazole (Prilosec, Losec) with a loading dose of 20 mg tid on the day before beginning of the antibiotic regimen[13] followed by 20 mg bid before meals for 7 days[9,13]

Specific ulcer medications

Traditional medications used for the treatment of peptic ulcers are listed in Table 26.

Table 26 Peptic Ulcer Medications

Drug	Usual doses
H_2-Blockers	
Cimetidine (Tagamet)	800 mg qhs or 600 mg bid
Famotidine (Pepcid)	40 mg qhs
Nizatidine (Axid)	300 mg qhs
Ranitidine (Zantac)	300 mg qhs or 150 mg bid
Proton Pump Inhibitors	
Lansoprazole (Prevacid)	15 mg qam
Omeprazole (Losec, Prilosec)	20 mg qam
Pantoprazole (Pantoloc)	40 mg qam
Prostaglandins	
Misoprostol (Cytotec)	200 µg qid or 400 µg bid
Cytoprotectives	
Sucralfate (Sulcrate)	1-2 g qid ac and hs

REFERENCES

1. Thompson WG: Dyspepsia: is a trial of therapy appropriate? *Can Med Assoc J* 153:293-299, 1995.
2. Patel P, Khulusi S, Mendall MA, et al: Prospective screening of dyspeptic patients by *Helicobacter pylori* serology, *Lancet* 18 (346):1315-1318, 1995.
3. Fendrick AM, Chkernew ME, Hirth RA, Bloom B: Alternative management strategies for patients with suspected peptic ulcer disease, *Ann Intern Med* 123:260-268, 1995.
4. Laine L, Peterson WL: Bleeding peptic ulcer, *N Engl J Med* 331:717-727, 1994.
5. Piper JM, Ray WA, Daugherty JR, et al: Corticosteroid use and peptic ulcer disease: role of nonsteroidal anti-inflammatory drugs, *Ann Intern Med* 114:735-740, 1991.
6. Khuroo MS, Yattoo GN, Javid G, et al: A comparison of omeprazole and placebo for bleeding peptic ulcer, *N Engl J Med* 336:1054-1058, 1997.
7. Saltzman JR, Zawacki JK: Therapy for bleeding peptic ulcers (editorial), *N Engl J Med* 336:1091-1093, 1997.
8. Walsh JH, Peterson WL: The treatment of *Helicobacter pylori* infection in the management of peptic ulcer disease, *N Engl J Med* 333:984-991, 1995.
9. Veldhuyzen van Zanten SJ, Sherman PM, Hunt RH: *Helicobacter pylori:* new developments and treatments, *Can Med Assoc J* 156:1565-1574, 1997.
10. Parsonnet J: *Helicobacter pylori* in the stomach—a paradox unmasked (editorial), *N Engl J Med* 335:278-280, 1996.
11. Hansson L-E, Nyrén O, Hsing AW, et al: The risk of stomach cancer in patients with gastric or duodenal ulcer disease, *N Engl J Med* 335:242-249, 1996.
12. Shafran SD: *Helicobacter pylori* and duodenal ulcer: guilty as charged, *Can J Infect Dis* 5:257-258, 1994.
13. Axon A, Forman D: *Helicobacter* gastroduodenitis: a serious infectious disease: antibiotic treatment may prevent deaths in the decades ahead (editorial), *BMJ* 314:1430-1431, 1997.
14. Soll AH: Medical treatment of peptic ulcer disease: practice guidelines, *JAMA* 275:622-629, 1996.

Stomach Cancer

(See also *Helicobacter pylori*)

In the 1930s gastric carcinoma was the leading cause of cancer death in North America among men and the third leading cause among women; since then the incidence has dropped dramatically in that part of the world but continues to be high in Japan, China, South America, and Eastern Europe. A correlation exists between the incidence of gastric carcinoma and the prevalence of *H. pylori* infection. Surgery is the treatment of choice. The 5-year survival of stage I tumor that has not invaded the muscularis, spread to nodes, or metastasized is 50% to 60% in North America, but stage I accounts for less than 10% of North American cases; the 5-year survival for stage II (invasion of muscularis propria but no serosal involvement) is 30%, and stages III and IV have much lower survival rates. Overall survival is better in Japan, probably because screening has led to detection of earlier stage lesions. Chemotherapy and radiation therapy offer relatively little for this form of cancer.[1]

REFERENCES

1. Fuchs CS, Mayer RJ: Gastric carcinoma, *N Engl J Med* 333:32-41, 1995.

GERIATRICS

(See also bacteriuria and pyuria in the elderly; dementia; elderly abuse; exercise; falls; hypertension in the elderly; motor vehicle accidents; nonsteroidal antiinflammatory drugs; nonsteroidal antiinflammatory drugs in the treatment of osteoarthritis; practice patterns; prescribing habits; pseudohypertension; osteoporosis)

Topics covered in this section

Epidemiology
Delirium
Exercise
Falls
Isolation
Prescriptions for the Elderly
Retirement

EPIDEMIOLOGY

Persons who are 85 or older are often labeled as the "oldest old." Among this group half of the men are living with their wives (most wives are younger than their husbands), whereas only 10% of women are living with their husbands (most of their husbands are dead). About half have impaired hearing, and a third have some degree of dementia. In the United States 25% of women over the age of 84 and 15% of men of similar age live in nursing homes.[1]

The average life expectancy of 80-year-old U.S. women is 9.1 years, while for 80-year-old U.S. men it is 7 years.[2] Among 85-year-olds in the United States the life expectancy is 6.4 years for women and 5.2 years for men.[1]

DELIRIUM

Five important precipitating factors for delirium in elderly hospitalized patients are malnutrition, physical restraints, bladder catheterization, more than three medications added, and any iatrogenic event.[3]

EXERCISE

Resisted exercises of the knee and hip extensors in the very elderly have been shown to increase mobility in nursing home residents.[4] Exercise emphasizing balance decreases the risk of falls in the elderly.[5]

FALLS

Falls in the elderly often result in fractures, and fracture rates are higher in patients whose physicians are known to prescribe a lot of medications.[6] The risk is particularly high if the patient is taking a benzodiazepine.[7] The risk of falls is reduced by exercise programs emphasizing balance and by home assessments that lead to modification of risk factors.[5]

ISOLATION

The risk that a person living alone will become helpless from an illness or die without help increases with age. The highest risk group is men over the age of 85 who are living alone. The longer the interval between the onset of helplessness and being found, the higher the mortality rate.[8] Suggested solutions are frequent checking on such individuals[8,9] and use of electronic alert devices.[9]

PRESCRIPTIONS FOR THE ELDERLY

Inappropriate prescription of drugs for the elderly is rampant. A study by Tamblyn and associates[10] determined that over a 1-year period about one third of elderly Quebec residents received prescriptions for benzodiazepines to be taken for more than 30 consecutive days. A similar survey in British Columbia found that over a 1-year period 17% of noninstitutionalized persons over the age of 65 received at least one prescription for benzodiazepines while 4% of elderly patients received a prescription for 20 mg of diazepam or its equivalent to be taken daily for more than 2 months.[11] A U.S. report found that 60% of individuals in the United States who use nonsteroidal antiinflammatory drugs (NSAIDs) are 60 years of age or older,[12] and in Alberta 27% of persons over the age of 65 received at least one NSAID prescription during a 6-month study period.[13] A Canadian study of the prescribing habits of New Brunswick physicians treating elderly patients showed that high prescribers had more practice days, saw more patients per day, billed more per patient, and billed on average 30% more than did low prescribers. On average, high prescribers ordered 45% more prescriptions than did low prescribers.[14] Similar results have been found in Great Britain.[15]

A follow-up of the New Brunswick general practitioner study quoted previously found that morbidity, hip fracture rates, and mortality rates were higher among patients of high-prescribing physicians than among those of low prescribers.[6] The chances of sustaining a hip fracture in elderly patients taking benzodiazepines was found to be increased in a study from the Netherlands. The risk was particularly marked with short-acting benzodiazepines, sudden dose increases, higher doses, and use of more than one benzodiazepine.[7]

The number of potentially inappropriate drug combinations that are prescribed to elderly patients increases with the number of prescribing physicians seen by the patients.[16]

RETIREMENT

According to Finnish studies, retirement is not associated with a deterioration of physical health and in many instances mental health improves.[17,18]

REFERENCES

1. Campion EW: The oldest old (editorial), *N Engl J Med* 30: 1819-1820, 1994.
2. Manton KG, Vaupel JW: Survival after the age of 80 in the United States, Sweden, France, England, and Japan, *N Engl J Med* 333:1232-1235, 1995.
3. Inouye SK, Charpentier PA: Precipitating factors for delirium in hospitalized elderly persons: predictive model and interrelationship with baseline vulnerability, *JAMA* 275:852-857, 1996.
4. Fiatarone MA, O'Neill EF, Ryan ND, et al: Exercise training and nutritional supplementation for physical frailty in very elderly people, *N Engl J Med* 330:1769-1775, 1994.
5. NHS Centre for Reviews and Dissemination and Nuffield Institute for Health: Preventing falls and subsequent injury in older people, *Eff Health Care* 2:1-16, 1996.
6. Davidson W, Molloy DW, Bédard M: Physician characteristics and prescribing for elderly people in New Brunswick: relation to patient outcomes, *Can Med Assoc J* 152:1227-1234, 1995.
7. Herings RM, Stricker BH, de Boer A, et al: Benzodiazepines and the risk of falling leading to femur fractures, *Arch Intern Med* 155:1801-1807, 1995.
8. Gurley RJ, Lum N, Sande M, et al: Persons found in their homes helpless or dead, *N Engl J Med* 334:1710-1716, 1996.
9. Campion EW: Home alone, and in danger (editorial), *N Engl J Med* 334:1738-1739, 1996.
10. Tamblyn RM, McLeod PJ, Abrahamowicz M, et al: Questionable prescribing for elderly patients in Quebec, *Can Med Assoc J* 150:1801-1809, 1994.
11. Thomson M, Smith WA: Prescribing benzodiazepines for noninstitutionalized elderly, *Can Fam Physician* 41:792-798, 1995.
12. Gurwitz JH, Avorn J: The ambiguous relation between aging and adverse drug reactions, *Ann Intern Med* 114:956-966, 1991.
13. Hogan DB, Campbell NRC, Crutcher R, et al: Prescription of nonsteroidal anti-inflammatory drugs for elderly people in Alberta, *Can Med Assoc J* 151:315-322, 1994.
14. Davidson W, Molloy W, Somers G, et al: Relation between physician characteristics and prescribing for elderly people in New Brunswick, *Can Med Assoc J* 150:917-921, 1994.
15. Wilson AD: Consultation length: general practitioners' attitudes and practices, *BMJ* 290:1322-1324, 1985.
16. Tamblyn RM, McLeod PJ, Abrahamowicz M, et al: Do too many cooks spoil the broth? Multiple physician involvement in medical management of elderly patients and potentially inappropriate drug combinations, *Can Med Assoc J* 154:1177-1184, 1996.
17. Joukamaa M, Saarijarvi S, Salokangas RK: The TURVA project: retirement and adaptation in old age, *Ztschrft Gerontol* 26: 170-175, 1993.
18. Salokangas RK, Joukamaa M: Physical and mental health changes in retirement age, *Psychother Psychosom* 55:100-107, 1991.

GYNECOLOGY

Topics covered in this section

Abortion
Amenorrhea
Cervix
Circumcision, Female
Contraception
Dysfunctional Uterine Bleeding
Ectopic Pregnancy
Endometrium
Human Papillomavirus
Infertility, Female
Menopause
Ovaries
Pelvic Inflammatory Disease
Premenstrual Dysphoric Disorder
Vaginismus
Vaginitis and Vulvitis

ABORTION

(See also antenatal care for physicians who do not practice obstetrics; breast cancer risk factors; ectopic pregnancy; postcoital contraception)

Risk of Breast Cancer

Claims have been made that induced abortions are associated with an increased risk of breast cancer.[1] This is almost certainly untrue (see discussion of breast cancer risk factors).[2]

Mifepristone

A drug that has been used in many parts of the world for inducing abortion is RU 486, or mifepristone. It appears to be effective, particularly when given in combination with an intravaginal instillation of prostaglandins.[3,4] In one study of pregnant women who had amenorrhea for 63 days or less, all patients were given 600 mg of mifepristone po and 48 hours later four 200-µg tablets of misoprostol (Cytotec) either po or by deep vaginal insertion. Of the study group, 95% of those who took the misoprostol vaginally and 87% of those who took it orally had a complete abortion without the need for surgical intervention.[4] Mifepristone can also be used for postcoital contraception (see discussion of postcoital contraception). In 1997 the French manufacturer of mifepristone bowed to pressure from antiabortionists in the United States and stopped production of the drug.[5]

Methotrexate Plus Misoprostol

Methotrexate is known to be cytotoxic to trophoblast and is used in the treatment of trophoblastic neoplasms and ectopic pregnancies; misoprostol (Cytotec) is a prostaglandin E_1 analogue.[6] A study from San Francisco compared the efficacy of methotrexate plus misoprostol and misoprostol alone in inducing therapeutic abortions in women whose pregnancies were of 56 days' duration or less. The first group was given a single intramuscular injection of methotrexate at a dose of 50 mg/m^2 of body surface followed 3 days later by 800 µg of misoprostol given by the vaginal route. If abortion did not occur, the misoprostol dose was repeated 24 hours later. The second group was given misoprostol alone in the same fashion as the first group. Complete abortion occurred in 90% of the combined methotrexate-misoprostol group and in 47% of the misoprostol only group. Another 27% of the misoprostol only group had incomplete abortions.[7] A previous smaller trial led the authors to conclude that oral misoprostol was not as effective in inducing abortion as intravaginal misoprostol.[6]

In a New York study of 171 women, successful abortion was achieved in 86% with a single intramuscular dose of methotrexate 50 mg/m^2 followed in 5 to 7 days by the vaginal insertion of 800 µg of misoprostol. The 25 women who did not have an abortion with this protocol were given a second intravaginal dose of misoprostol; 18 aborted and 7 required suction curettage. Since misoprostol is not available in commercial form as vaginal suppositories, half the women were treated with four 200-µg suppositories made up by a pharmacist and the other half were treated with the intravaginal insertion of four 200-µg oral tablets held in place by a vaginal tampon.[8] An almost identical protocol at another center had equally good results; side effects were nausea (70%), diarrhea (46%), and vomiting (23%).[9] Misoprostol is a common illicit method of inducing abortions in Brazil.[10]

Coffee

In a case-controlled study the rate of spontaneous abortion was increased in women who drank 3 or more cups of coffee daily before pregnancy, as well as in those who had 1½ to 3 cups a day during pregnancy. Each cup was estimated to contain 107 mg caffeine.[11]

Grief and Depression

Grief reactions among women who have had spontaneous abortions may be as intense as that which follows a neonatal death.[12-14] The male partners of women who abort may also suffer from grief reactions.[15] Spontaneous abortion is a a risk factor for major depression, especially in women who are childless or who have a past history of depressive illness. In a case-controlled study the incidence of depression in the first 6 months after a spontaneous abortion was 11% compared with 4.3% among control subjects over the same period.[16]

REFERENCES

1. Brind J, Chichilli VM, Severs WB, et al: Induced abortion as an independent risk factor for breast cancer: a comprehensive review and meta-analysis, *J Epidemiol Community Health* 50:481-496, 1996.
2. Melbye M, Wohlfahrt J, Olsen J, et al: Induced abortion and the risk of breast cancer, *N Engl J Med* 336:81-85, 1997.
3. World Health Organisation Task Force on Post-Ovulatory Methods of Fertility Regulation: Termination of pregnancy with reduced doses of mifepristone, *BMJ* 307:684, 1993.
4. El-Refaey H, Rajasekar D, Abdalla M, et al: Induction of abortion with mifepristone (RU 486) and oral or vaginal misoprostol, *N Engl J Med* 332:983-987, 1995.
5. Dorozynski A: Boycott threat forces French company to abandon RU 486, *BMJ* 314:1150, 1997.
6. Creinin MD, Darney PD: Methotrexate and misoprostol for early abortion, *Contraception* 48:339-348, 1993.
7. Creinin MD, Vittinghoff E: Methotrexate and misoprostol vs misoprostol alone for early abortion: a randomized controlled trial, *JAMA* 19:1190-1195, 1994.
8. Hausknecht RU: Methotrexate and misoprostol to terminate early pregnancy, *N Engl J Med* 333:537-540, 1995.
9. Schaff EA, Eisinger SH, Franks P, et al: Combined methotrexate and misoprostol for early induced abortion, *Arch Fam Med* 4:774-779, 1995.
10. Coelho HL, Teixeira AC, Santos AP, et al: Misoprostol and illegal abortion in Fortaleza, Brazil, *Lancet* 341:1261-1263, 1993.
11. Infante-Rivard C, Fernandez A, Gauthier R, et al: Foetal loss associated with caffeine intake before and during pregnancy, *JAMA* 270:2940-2943, 1993.
12. Cecil R, Leslie JC: Early miscarriage: preliminary results from a study in Northern Ireland, *J Reprod Infant Psychol* 15:347-352, 1993.
13. Lasker JN, Toedter LJ: Acute versus chronic grief: the case for pregnancy loss, *Am J Orthopsychiatry* 61:510-522, 1991.
14. Prettyman RJ, Cordle CJ, Cook GD: A three-month follow-up of psychological morbidity after early miscarriage, *Br J Med Psychol* 66:363-372, 1993.
15. Johnson MP, Puddifoot JE: The grief response in the partners of women who miscarry, *Br J Med Psychol* 69:313-327, 1996.
16. Neugebauer R, Kline J, Shrout P, et al: Major depressive disorder in the 6 months after miscarriage, *JAMA* 277:383-388, 1997.

AMENORRHEA

(See also anorexia nervosa; female athletes)

Amenorrhea is divided into primary and secondary forms.[1] Primary amenorrhea is rare and is defined as the absence of vaginal bleeding in a 14-year-old with no secondary sexual characteristics or in a 16-year-old with normal secondary sexual development. Primary amenorrhea in a woman with normal breast development but absence of pubic and axillary hair may be due to an androgen insensitivity syndrome (testicular feminization). Secondary amenorrhea is the absence of menstruation for 6 months in women who previously had normal periods or for 12 months in those who previously had oligomenorrhea. The overall prevalence rate of secondary amenorrhea is 1% to 3%, but the rate is 3% to 5% among college students, 5% to 60% among competitive athletes, and 19% to 44% among ballet dancers.[1]

The most frequent cause of secondary amenorrhea is pregnancy, and it must always be ruled out before any further investigations are undertaken. Home pregnancy tests have neither the sensitivity nor the specificity to be reliable for this purpose.[2] The following are other important causes of secondary amenorrhea[1,3]:

1. Hypothalamic dysfunction brought about by psychological stress
2. Anorexia nervosa
3. Strenuous exercise
4. Weight loss
5. Drugs such as oral contraceptives, antipsychotics, tricyclic antidepressants, and calcium channel blockers
6. Pituitary tumors, many of which are prolactinomas
7. Thyroid disorders
8. Premature ovarian failure
9. Hyperandrogenic disorders such as polycystic ovarian syndrome, adrenal hyperplasia, and Cushing's syndrome[1]

The essential elements in the initial evaluation of a patient with secondary amenorrhea are as follows[1,3]:

1. History. Drugs, exercise, weight loss, psychological stress, galactorrhea, thyroid disease, gynecological surgery, hot flashes, and androgenic symptoms such as hirsutism, acne, frontal balding, and lowering of the voice
2. Physical examination. Signs of thyroid disease, galactorrhea, androgen excess, or genital tract abnormalities
3. Laboratory investigations. Pregnancy test, thyroid-stimulating hormone, prolactin; if the patient is hypoestrogenic, follicle-stimulating hormone (FSH) and luteinizing hormone; testosterone is not needed unless the patient shows clinical evidence of androgen excess

If the prolactin level is elevated above 100 ng/ml (100 μg/L)—normal maximum is 20—a careful neurological examination and imaging of the sella turcica are indicated.[1]

The estrogen status of a nonpregnant amenorrheic woman may be evaluated by performing a progesterone challenge test.[1,3] The patient is given 10 mg of medroxyprogesterone acetate (Provera) orally for 5 days.[3] The test is positive if any vaginal bleeding occurs within 2 to 7 days of completion of the drug course. A failure to bleed indicates inadequate estrogen stimulation, an unresponsive endometrium, or outflow tract obstruction such as Asherman's syndrome (intrauterine adhesions).[1] In most young women who fail to bleed, the underlying disorder is hypothalamic amenorrhea caused by psychological stress, excessive exercise, or excessive weight loss. In this condition the FSH level is normal or low (with primary ovarian failure it would be high).[3]

If an amenorrheic woman is hypoestrogenic, she is at high risk for osteoporosis. If the amenorrhea persists for more than 6 months, she probably requires hormone replacement therapy. The potency of estrogen in the standard postmenopausal replacement dose of 0.625 mg of conjugated equine estrogen (Premarin) is only one fifth that of 30 to 50 μg of ethinyl estradiol, which is the estrogenic component of most of the low-dose birth control pills. A small prospective randomized controlled trial of amenorrheic young women found that over a 12-month period birth control pills containing 35 μg of ethinyl estradiol increased lumbar spine density and total body bone mineral compared with control subjects receiving placebo and medroxyprogesterone.[4]

REFERENCES

1. Kiningham RB, Apgar BS, Schwenk TL: Evaluation of amenorrhea, *Am Fam Physician* 53:1185-1194, 1996.
2. Bastian LA, Piscitelli JT: Is this patient pregnant? Can you reliably rule in or rule out early pregnancy by clinical examination? *JAMA* 278:586-589, 1997.
3. Davis A: A 21-year-old woman with menstrual irregularity, *JAMA* 277:1308-1314, 1997.
4. Hergenroeder AC, O'Brian Smith E, Shypailo R, et al: Bone mineral changes in young women with hypothalamic amenorrhea treated with oral contraceptives, medroxyprogesterone, or placebo over 12 months, *Am J Obstet Gynecol* 176:1017-1025, 1997.

CERVIX

Cervical Cancer

(See also *Chlamydia*; human papillomavirus; prevention; screening; *Trichomonas vaginalis*)

Epidemiology

Risk factors for cervical cancer are early onset of sexual intercourse, multiple partners, a partner who has had multiple partners, and smoking. A number of varieties of human papillomavirus (HPV), such as types 16, 18, 31, 33, and 35, are associated with cervical intraepithelial neoplasia (CIN) II and III and invasive cancer, whereas other types such as 6 and 11 are associated with condylomata acuminata and not neoplasia (see discussion of human papillomavirus).[1]

Techniques of obtaining Papanicolaou smears

A metaanalysis of randomized and quasirandomized studies of various sampling devices used for obtaining cervical cytology specimens found no differences in the yields of abnormal results between the Ayre spatula, the Cytobrush, and the cotton swab when each was used alone. However, better results were obtained with the extended tip spatula, the cervix brush, or a combination of any spatula plus the Cytobrush or cotton swab.[2]

Guidelines for cervical cytology screening

Canadian recommendations for cervical cytology screening as reported by Miller and associates[3] are as follows:

1. An initial smear should be obtained from any woman over the age of 18 who has had sexual intercourse.
2. A second smear should be obtained 1 year after the initial smear.
3. If the first two smears are satisfactory and normal, further screening should be conducted every 3 years until age 69.
4. The above recommendations are applicable to all women between the ages of 18 and 69 regardless of risk classification.
5. Women over age 69 who have had at least two satisfactory normal smears within the past 9 years and who have never had biopsy-confirmed severe dysplasia or carcinoma in situ do not require any further routine smears.
6. Women entering a screening program at age 67 or older should have two satisfactory smears at least 6 months apart; those over age 69 can be dropped from the program if the smears show no epithelial abnormality.
7. Women who have never had sexual intercourse do not need to be screened, nor do women who have had a hysterectomy for a benign condition and whose previous smears have been normal.

The Canadian Task Force on the Periodic Health Examination has accepted Miller's recommendations and given them a "B" recommendation. This group's only caveat was that high-risk women may need screening more frequently than every 3 years.[4] The U.S. Preventive Services Task Force has advised that women have regular Papanicolaou (Pap) smears ("A" recommendation) beginning at the onset of sexual activity with repeat examinations at least every 3 years ("B" recommendation). According to their guidelines, women who have had a hysterectomy for benign disease do not need to be screened.[5] The U.S. Preventive Services Task Force found insufficient evidence for establishing 65 as the upper age limit of screening, although it accepted as reasonable the discontinuation of screening if the patient has had regular negative smears in the past.[5]

If a patient has had a hysterectomy for cervical dysplasia or carcinoma in situ, she should have follow-up vaginal vault smears at regular intervals. If the hysterectomy was for benign disease, there is no need to perform routine pelvic examinations or vaginal Pap smears.[5-7] Despite the evidence that Pap smears in women who have had hysterectomies for benign disease are not beneficial, the 1995 Guidelines of the American College of Obstetricians and Gynecologists recommends that they be done.[8]

Classification of Papanicolaou smears

Several classifications for abnormal Pap smears have been developed. One of the common ones uses the terminology cervical intraepithelial neoplasia (CIN). CIN grade 1 is the equivalent of mild dysplasia, CIN grade 2 of moderate dysplasia, and CIN grade 3 of severe dysplasia or carcinoma in situ. The newer Bethesda System, which is achieving widespread use in the United States, has three categories: atypical squamous cells of undetermined significance (ASCUS); low-grade squamous intraepithelial lesions (LSIL), which is equivalent to CIN grade 1; and high-grade squamous intraepithelial lesions (HSIL), which is equivalent to CIN grades 2 and 3.[9,10]

Discrepancies often occur between the degree of cytological abnormalities reported and the underlying histological lesions. Between 17.5% and 40% of smear reports are said to underestimate the severity of the lesion.[11] Conversely up to 75% of patients with smears reported as ASCUS are normal histologically, and in most cases these cytological abnormalities revert to normal spontaneously over the next few months.[9,12,13] When the Pap smear result is LSIL, two thirds to three fourths of the cases revert to normal spontaneously, in most cases because of regression of the underlying histological abnormalities. For these reasons follow-up cytological studies in 4 to 6 months, rather than immediate colposcopy, are recommended by many for low-grade abnormal cytology reports.[12,13]

The traditional view has been that a Pap smear was adequate only if endocervical or metaplastic cells were present on the smear, indicating that the transition zone (squamocolumnar junction) had been sampled. In a review of nearly 19,000 Pap smears, no increased incidence of subsequent cytological abnormalities was found in women whose original smears failed to show endocervical or metaplastic cells.[14] Thus recall of a patient for repeat smears in cases in which endocervical or metaplastic cells are absent is unnecessary if the patient has no past history of abnormal cytology and there is no clinical suspicion of cervical abnormalities.[12]

Incidence of abnormal smears

The percentage of abnormal smears is generally reported as between 5% and 10%,[15] and only about 5% of these show high-grade atypia.[15,16] It is generally agreed that less than 5% of smears using the Bethesda System should be reported as ASCUS,[12,13] but unfortunately in some centers up to 30% of smears are placed in this category.[9]

In a study from Bristol, England, the rate of mild to moderate dyskaryosis (dysplasia) and borderline changes increased markedly over the last decade, while the rate of severe dyskaryosis remained stable. In the latest screening round, 10% of young women were found to have some degree of abnormality and the rate of abnormalities for the entire population was 6.8%; 2.5% were referred for colposcopy. Although a true rise in CIN may account for the increased rate of abnormal smears, the authors believe that a

Gynecology 129

more likely explanation is a tendency to overdiagnose cases to avoid litigation.[17]

Inflammation detected by Papanicolaou smears

A study from the University of Washington in Seattle correlated cytology reports of "dense inflammation" and genital tract findings on examination, as well as cultures for *Neisseria gonorrhoeae, Chlamydia trachomatis,* herpes simplex virus, and *Trichomonas vaginalis*. Two cohorts were studied, women in a sexually transmitted disease (STD) clinic and university students. Dense inflammation was found in 33% of the women attending the STD clinic and in 19% of the students. Among the patients with STDs, half of the smears showing dense inflammation were associated with *N. gonorrhoeae, C. trachomatis,* herpes simplex, or trichomoniasis, whereas in the student group only 10% were associated with positive cultures, which were almost always *C. trachomatis*. In both cohorts many women with dense inflammation had negative cultures but cervical ectopy on examination. Inflammation on the smears also correlated with cervical mucopus.[18]

My interpretation of the above results is that in regard to infections, a report of dense inflammation requires no specific action if the patient is in a low-risk group for STDs. If she is in a high-risk group, guidelines suggest that cultures for STDs should already have been obtained.[19,20] If they have not, she should be recalled and this should be done. If the cytopathologist's report suggests that the inflammation is of such a degree that the epithelial cells are obscured and cannot be interpreted, the smear is unsatisfactory and should be repeated.

The presence of trichomonads may be noted in cytological reports. In asymptomatic women 20% to 30% of such findings are falsely positive.[21]

Psychological consequences of abnormal Papanicolaou smears

Raffle and associates[17] point out that the death rate for cervical cancer in Britain is about 10 per million women in their twenties and 40 per million women in their thirties. Since 10% of women were declared at risk on the basis of cytological findings, large numbers of women who would never have cancer were subject to persistent anxiety about cancer, the effect of treatment on their ability to bear children, and in some cases their ability to obtain life insurance.

Patients' responses to learning that they had abnormal smears have been documented by Posner and Vessey.[22] The women used such words as shocked, devastated, stunned, and petrified to describe their reactions.

Campion and associates[23] found that women had a statistically significant decrease in sexual functioning 6 months after they received a diagnosis of CIN compared with control subjects who did not have CIN. Specifically, they had decreased spontaneous interest in sex, decreased frequency of intercourse, less arousal, fewer orgasms, more dyspareunia, and more negative feelings about sex. The authors postulated that this may be related to the widespread knowledge that CIN is an STD. Patients may be angry at their partners, fear that continued sexual intercourse could be harmful, or, in a more encompassing way, have a diminished sense of worth and body image. Posner and Vessey[24] reported that 43% of women referred to a colposcopy clinic experienced psychosexual disturbances as a result of the diagnosis and this was still present 6 to 9 months later in 14% of the women.

Management of abnormal Papanicolaou smears

Experts generally agree that patients whose cervical cytological examination shows severe atypia (CIN II or III, severe dysplasia or dyskaryosis, carcinoma in situ, or invasive carcinoma) require immediate colposcopic evaluation.[3,12] Greater controversy exists about the management of lesser degrees of atypia (mild dysplasia, CIN I, low-grade intraepithelial lesion). Studies indicate that a high percentage of women with such reports will subsequently have normal smears without any therapeutic interventions[25,26] and that even among those subjected to immediate colposcopy, one third will have no abnormal histological findings.[27] Current evidence is that only a few low-grade lesions progress, and when they do, the rate of progression is slow.[28] In many cases lesions regress.[29] Because of this biological behavior, cases of mild atypia can be managed without immediate colposcopy but with careful follow-up cytological smears.[3,12,30] Both the National Cancer Institute in the United States[12] and a Canadian expert panel[3] state that acceptable management of mild atypias is to repeat the Pap smear at 6-month intervals. If this results in three normal smears, the patient may revert to the normal screening interval. If any smear shows high-grade atypia, or if abnormalities persist for 24 months, the patient should be referred for colposcopy.[3,12]

Standard treatment methods for lesions detected by colposcopy have been electrocautery, cryosurgery, and laser surgery. The most modern technique is loop electrosurgical excision (LEEP).

Invasive cervical cancer

Very early "microinvasive" cancer is usually treated with hysterectomy or in some cases cone biopsy. For more extensive but potentially curable disease, radical hysterectomy or radiation therapy gives equal results.[1] One complication of radiation therapy is vaginal stenosis, which may prevent sexual intercourse.[1]

REFERENCES

1. Cannistra SA, Niloff DIM: Cancer of the uterine cervix, *N Engl J Med* 334:1030-1038, 1996.
2. Buntinx F, Brouwers M: Relation between sampling device and detection of abnormality in cervical smears: a meta-analysis of randomised and quasi-randomised studies, *BMJ* 313:1285-1290, 1996.
3. Miller AB, Anderson G, Brisson J, et al: Report of a National Workshop on Screening for Cancer of the Cervix, *Can Med Assoc J* 145:1301-1325, 1991.

4. Canadian Task Force on the Periodic Health Examination: *Canadian guide to clinical preventive health care,* Ottawa, 1994, Canada Communication Group—Publishing, pp 882-889.
5. *Report of the U.S. Preventive Services Task Force: guide to clinical preventive services,* ed 2, Baltimore, 1996, Williams & Wilkins, pp 105-117.
6. Piscitelli JT, Bastian LA, Wilkes A, et al: Cytologic screening after hysterectomy for benign disease, *Am J Obstet Gynecol* 173:424-430, 1995.
7. Pearce KF, Haefner HK, Sarwar SF, et al: Cytopathological findings on vaginal Papanicolaou smears after hysterectomy for benign gynecologic disease, *N Engl J Med* 335:1559-1562, 1996.
8. *ACOG committee opinion: recommendations on frequency of Pap test screening,* no 152, Chicago, 1995, American College of Obstetricians and Gynecologists.
9. Zuber TJ: The minimally abnormal Pap smear: a conservative approach (editorial), *Am Fam Physician* 53:1042-1057, 1996.
10. The revised Bethesda system for reporting cervical/vaginal cytologic diagnoses: report of the 1991 Bethesda workshop, *J Reprod Med* 37:383-386, 1992.
11. Ferris DG: ASCUS and LSIL Pap smear results: triage considerations (editorial), *Am Fam Physician* 53:1057-1066, 1996.
12. Kurman RJ, Henson DE, Herbst AL, et al: Interim guidelines for management of abnormal cervical cytology: the 1992 National Cancer Institute Workshop, *JAMA* 271:1866-1869, 1994.
13. *Cervical cytology: evaluation and management of abnormalities,* ACOG Tech Bull No 183, Washington, DC, 1993, American College of Obstetricians and Gynecologists, pp 1-8.
14. Kivlahan C, Ingram E: Papanicolaou smears without endocervical cells: are they inadequate? *Acta Cytol* 30:258-260, 1986.
15. Nuovo GJ: *Cytopathology of the lower female genital tract: an integrated approach,* Baltimore, 1994, Williams & Wilkins.
16. Sadeghi SB, Hsieh EW, Gunn SW: Prevalence of cervical intraepithelial neoplasia in sexually active teenagers and young adults, *Am J Obstet Gynecol* 148:726-729, 1984.
17. Raffle AE, Alden B, Mackenzie EFD: Detection rates for abnormal cervical smears: what are we screening for? *Lancet* 345:1469-1473, 1995.
18. Eckert LO, Koutsky LA, Kiviat NB, et al: The inflammatory Papanicolaou smear—what does it mean? *Obstet Gynecol* 86: 360-366, 1995.
19. Davies HD, Wang EE (Canadian Task Force on the Periodic Health Examination): Periodic health examination, 1996 update. 2. Screening for chlamydial infections, *Can Med Assoc J* 154:1631-1644, 1996.
20. US Preventive Services Task Force: *Guide to clinical preventive services,* ed 2, Baltimore, 1996, Williams & Wilkins, pp 325-334.
21. Weinberger MW, Harger JH: Accuracy of the Papanicolaou smear in the diagnosis of asymptomatic infection with *Trichomonas vaginalis*, *Obstet Gynecol* 82:425-429, 1993.
22. Posner T, Vessey M: *Prevention of cervical cancer: the patient's view,* London, 1988, King's Fund Publishing Office, pp 45-73.
23. Campion MJ, Brown JR, McCance DJ, et al: Psychosexual trauma of an abnormal cervical smear, *Br J Obstet Gynaecol* 95:175-181, 1988.
24. Posner T, Vessey M: Psychosexual trauma of an abnormal cervical smear (letter), *Br J Obstet Gynaecol* 95:729, 1988.
25. Jones MH, Jenkins D, Cuzick J, et al: Mild cervical dyskaryosis: safety of cytological surveillance, *Lancet* 339:1440-1443, 1992.
26. Kirby AJ, Speigelhalter DJ, Day NE, et al: Conservative treatment of mild/moderate cervical dyskaryosis: long-term outcomes, *Lancet* 339:828-831, 1992.
27. Nuovo J, Kreiter L: Frequency of nondiagnostic findings on colposcopy: implications for management, *J Am Board Family Pract* 6:209-214, 1993.
28. Nasiell M, Nasiell K, Vaclavinkova V: Natural history of CIN with particular emphasis on the biologic behaviour of CIN II (moderate dysplasia). In Bender HG, Beck L, eds: *Cancer of the uterine cervix*, New York, 1985, Fischer, pp 81-90.
29. Montz FJ, Monk BJ, Fowler JM, Nguyen L: Natural history of the minimally abnormal Papanicolaou smear, *Obstet Gynecol* 80:385-388, 1992.
30. Nuovo J, Melnikow J, Paliescheskey M: Management of patients with atypical and low-grade Pap smear abnormalities, *Am Fam Physician* 52:2243-2250, 1995.

Cervicitis

An infectious cervicitis should be suspected if the endocervical mucus is yellow and contains more than 10 white blood cells per high-power field.[1-3]

REFERENCES

1. Megran DW: Treat PID effectively in four simple steps, *Patient Care Can* 6:16-26, 1995.
2. Romanowski B: Pelvic inflammatory disease: current approaches, *Can Fam Physician* 39:346-349, 1993.
3. Newkirk GR: Pelvic inflammatory disease: a contemporary approach, *Am Fam Physician* 53:1127-1135, 1996.

CIRCUMCISION, FEMALE

Female circumcision is practiced almost exclusively in Africa and among immigrants from Africa. Depending on the area, the prevalence rate varies from 5% to 99%. Female circumcision is practiced not only by those who espouse indigenous African religions, but also by Christians, Muslims, and Jews. It is a custom that involves all socioeconomic groups.[1]

Circumcision is usually performed by lay operators without the use of anesthesia on girls between the ages of 4 and 10. The procedure may involve removal of the clitoris alone ("Sunna circumcision") or the clitoris along with some of the labia minora, or it may involve clitorectomy plus removal of the labia minora plus incisions on the labia majora that are stitched together for near-occlusion of the vaginal orifice (infibulation).[1]

REFERENCES

1. Toubia N: Female circumcision as a public health issue, *N Engl J Med* 331:712-716, 1994.

CONTRACEPTION

Comparative Efficacy of Various Contraceptive Methods

Contraceptive efficacy can be calculated on the basis of theoretical effectiveness and real-use effectiveness. The typical pregnancy rate in 1 year when no contraception is used is 85%. This compares with 1-year pregnancy rates of less than 3% with the use of combined and progestin only oral contraceptives, progesterone T or copper T intrauterine devices, levonorgestrel subdermal implants (Norplant), and medroxyprogesterone acetate (Depo-Provera) injections. Mechanical barrier methods with or without spermicides have 1-year rates ranging from about 12% for the male condom to about 20% for the female condom, diaphragm, and cervical cap. Spermicide alone and the rhythm method also have rates of around 20%. For some methods theoretical effectiveness is much better than are typical use rates. For example, the theoretical effectiveness of the condom alone is 3%, and that of diaphragm plus spermicide is 6%.[1,2] Figures given for efficacy are generally derived from studies of young women. The efficacy of all modes is better in older women, partly because of decreasing fertility and partly because of a lower frequency of intercourse.[3]

REFERENCES

1. US Public Health Service: Counseling to prevent unintended pregnancy, *Am Fam Physician* 50:971-974, 1994.
2. Choice of contraceptives, *Med Lett* 37:9-12, 1995.
3. Reid R: Which contraceptive methods are suitable for the older women? *J SOGC* 15:933-944, 1993.

Natural Family Planning Methods

Basal body temperature

A slight drop in temperature indicates ovulation. Proof of ovulation is a subsequent persistent rise of 0.2° to 0.5° C over 3 days.

Billings or ovulation method

Days on which a woman is considered infertile are during the menstrual period, the subsequent days when the vagina is dry, and the interval beginning 4 days after the onset of spinnbarkeit (see below) and lasting until the next menstrual period. The time of relative fertility is the days when vaginal secretions are wet and the first 4 days of spinnbarkeit. Spinnbarkeit is the phenomenon whereby the cervical mucus has become sufficiently sticky to allow it to be stretched out between thumb and fingers like an egg white. Samples of cervical mucus are obtained by placing the fingers in the lower vagina; touching the cervix is not necessary. Spinnbarkeit occurs 24 hours before the luteinizing hormone surge and 48 hours before ovulation.[1]

Symptothermal method

The symptothermal method combines the Billings method and basal body temperature measurements.[1]

REFERENCES

1. Geerling JH: Natural family planning, *Am Fam Physician* 52:1749-1756, 1995.

Barrier Contraceptives

Condoms

Regular condom use decreases the transmission of all sexually transmitted diseases, including HIV. Aside from noncompliance, condom failures are usually due to breakage or slippage, and both of these events are more common among inexperienced users. Breakage is more likely if condoms are stored in hot humid environment, exposed to light, or used with oil-based lubricants. The storage problem is particularly acute in developing countries.[1] In a small survey of male college students in Georgia, one third of the men who experienced a condom breakage failed to inform their partners of this event.[2]

Diaphragms

The diaphragm may be inserted up to 6 hours before intercourse. It should be left in place for 6 hours after intercourse. For repeated intercourse, contraceptive jelly should be placed in the vagina before each episode without removal of the diaphragm.

There have been reports that diaphragms are effective without use of a spermicide.[3] In a nonrandomized trial of this method, 110 women were instructed to wear "fit-free" (60-mm) diaphragms continuously, removing them only once a day for washing, but not within 6 hours of intercourse. The accidental pregnancy rate was 24.1% after 12 months.[3] Another study compared diaphragm plus spermicide to diaphragm alone. The pregnancy rates were lower with the diaphragm plus spermicide. Although the difference was not statistically significant, the authors point out this may have been because the study lacked sufficient power to prove a difference.[4]

The role of diaphragms in preventing STDs, especially HIV infection, is controversial. When compared directly with condoms, they are less effective, but evidence suggests that they provide some protection. Since their use is controlled by women, they may prevent more infections than condoms, which many men refuse to use.[1,5]

Female condoms

In an open study of the female condom as the only method of contraception for couples in monogamous relationships, the pregnancy rates after 6 months were 12.4% among U.S. users and 22.2% among Latin American users.[6] The female condom would probably be an effective method of lowering the incidence of HIV transmission.[6,7]

REFERENCES

1. Faúndes A, Elias C, Coggins C: Spermicides and barrier contraception, *Curr Opin Obstet Gynecol* 6:552-558, 1994.
2. Warner DL, Boles J, Goldsmith J: Disclosure of condom breakage to sexual partners (letter), *JAMA* 278:291-292, 1997.
3. Smith C, Farr G, Feldblum PJ, Spence A: Effectiveness of the non-spermicidal fit-free diaphragm, *Contraception* 51:289-291, 1995.

4. Bounds W, Guillebaud J, Dominik R, et al: The diaphragm with and without spermicide: a randomized, comparative efficacy trial, *J Reprod Med* 40:764-774, 1995.
5. Stein ZA: More on women and the prevention of HIV infection (editorial), *Am J Public Health* 85:1485-1488, 1995.
6. Farr G, Gabelnick H, Sturgen K, et al: Contraceptive efficacy and acceptability of the female condom, *Am J Public Health* 84: 1960-1964, 1994.
7. Trussell J, Sturgen K, Strickler J, et al: Comparative contraceptive efficacy of the female condom and other barrier methods, *Fam Plann Perspect* 26:66-72, 1994.

Spermicidal Contraceptives

On the market are numerous spermicidal contraceptives, which come in the form of foams, creams, or gels applied with an applicator or of sponges or ovules inserted with a finger. The active agent in most is nonoxynol-9. The general recommendation for foams and creams is that the products be inserted no more than an hour before intercourse and that if intercourse is to be repeated, further applications are required. Manufacturers of some of the newer products such as Advantage Gel claim that it can be applied up to 24 hours before intercourse, with further applications if intercourse is to be repeated. Sponges or ovules should be inserted at least 15 minutes before intercourse and remain in place for a maximum period of 12 hours to decrease the risk of toxic shock syndrome. They should not be removed until 6 hours after intercourse. Instructions for individual products should be followed. Whether nonoxynol-9 has a protective effect against HIV infection is uncertain.[1]

REFERENCES

1. Faúndes A, Elias C, Coggins C: Spermicides and barrier contraception, *Curr Opin Obstet Gynecol* 6:552-558, 1994.

Intrauterine Devices

IUDs are an effective method of contraception. The risk of pelvic inflammatory disease (PID) is not increased in women who do not have a sexually transmitted disease and who are in a monogamous relationship. The devices may be inserted at any time during the menstrual cycle if the patient is known not to be pregnant. If a second-generation copper T is used, it is effective for at least 5 years. The TCu-380A has been approved by the FDA for 10 years of use.[1]

REFERENCES

1. IUDs—an update, *Popul Rep Series B* 6:1-35, 1995.

Oral Contraceptives

(See also dysfunctional uterine bleeding; thrombophlebitis)

Benefits

Aside from contraception, the use of oral contraceptive pills has a number of reputed advantages. These include control of dysfunctional uterine bleeding,[1,2] relief of hot flushes in perimenopausal women,[3] and reduced incidence of endometrial cancer,[4] ovarian cancer,[5] PID,[6] ectopic pregnancy,[7] iron deficiency anemias,[7] dysmenorrhea,[7] functional ovarian cysts,[7] benign breast disease,[7] and possibly osteoporosis.[8]

Adverse effects

Mild adverse effects are well known and not discussed here.

Cardiovascular effects. A number of studies in the 1960s and 1970s showed an increased incidence of ischemic strokes and subarachnoid hemorrhages in women who used oral contraceptives. This was particularly marked if the women were smokers and over the age of 35.[9] However, other long-term investigations, such as the Nurses' Health Study, did not confirm these findings.[10,11] Because of concern about the cardiovascular complications of oral contraceptives during that era, both the FDA in the United States and the Health Protection Branch of Health and Welfare Canada recommended that oral contraceptive pills be stopped at 35 years of age.

Only a few studies of the cardiovascular complications of oral contraceptives have been published since the advent of low-dose estrogen birth control pills. One case-controlled study using mailed questionnaires and including cerebral hemorrhage in the group with "stroke" found that the risk from low-dose oral contraceptives was significantly less than the risk from high-dose contraceptives,[12] and another study found no increased risk of stroke in a healthy cohort of users of low-dose oral contraceptives.[13] Furthermore, an evaluation of the risks of contraceptives should include the risks associated with pregnancy in the control groups. For example, the annual mortality rates for oral contraceptive users aged 35 to 39 has been calculated as 4.5:100,000 for nonsmokers and 13.4:100,000 for smokers. In contrast the mortality rate for women in this age group using no contraceptive methods is 20.8:100,000 per year.[3] As a result of such evidence, official recommendations have changed in both Canada and the United States. Oral contraceptive use by nonsmoking women is now considered safe until the time of menopause. However, smokers should discontinue oral contraceptives at the age of 35 and substitute another form of contraception.

Third-generation oral contraceptives containing desogestrel (Marvelon, Ortho-Cept) or gestodene (none marketed in North America) have been reported to increase the risk of venous thromboembolic disease compared with second-generation oral contraceptives.[14-16] The relative risk is twice as high for users of these third-generation products, while the absolute increase is about 16 cases per 100,000 women-years.[14,16] The risk of death from thromboembolic events is much lower; according to one estimate it is 5 per 1 million per year for non-pill users, 14 per million per year for users of second-generation products, and 20 per million per year for users of third-generation products.[17]

An estimated 5% of the white population carries factor V Leiden. The risk of venous thrombosis in carriers who do not take oral contraceptives is 5.7:10,000 women-years, whereas for carriers taking oral contraceptives it is 28.5:10,000 women years. Is this sufficient reason to screen all women for factor V Leiden before prescribing the birth control pill? Vandenbroucke and associates[18] claim that it is not, for the following reasons: even though the relative risk of thrombophlebitis is increased in factor V Leiden carriers, the absolute risk is small; the major serious complication of thrombophlebitis is fatal pulmonary embolism, and this is rare; and screening all women who want contraception for factor V Leiden and denying the pill to those who were positive would deprive 5% of women of an effective method of contraception (about 20,000 women per year would be denied oral contraceptives to save one life per year). An additional consideration is that screening of this nature would be expensive. The authors suggest that a more practical solution is to screen patients carefully for a personal or family history of thrombotic events.

An evaluation of the risks of thromboembolism associated with oral contraceptives must take into account that any increased risk is relative to nonusers of the pill. If comparison were made to pregnant patients, all oral contraceptive pill users would have a lower incidence of thromboembolism.

Breast cancer. The risk of breast cancer is slightly increased among current pill users.[19,20] For example, a 1994 update of the Nurses' Health Study, which was begun in 1976, found no increase in breast cancer in women who had used oral contraceptives before 1976 but who were not using them at the beginning of the study; in contrast, women who were current users of the pill in 1976 had a 1.63 increase in the relative risk of dying of breast cancer within 12 years.[19] However, the overall total mortality and the total cancer mortality were not increased, in part because the ovarian cancer incidence was decreased. A 1996 systematic review of 54 case-controlled studies found that the odds ratio for development of breast cancer among current users of the pill was 1.24 whereas for women who had stopped the pill 1 to 4 years before it was 1.16. No increase in risk was found for women who had stopped the pill 10 years before.[20]

Adenocarcinoma of cervix. In a case-controlled study from Los Angeles an association between oral contraceptive use and adenocarcinoma of the cervix was noted.[1] The relative risk for women who had ever used the pill was 2.1 and for users taking the pill for 12 or more years it was 4.4. However, since the incidence of adenocarcinoma of the cervix is very low (2 to 4:100,000 women per year), the absolute increase was minuscule.[21]

Total mortality

There is no increase in mortality in women who have ever used oral contraceptives compared with women who have not, nor is there evidence that prolonged use of oral contraceptives increases mortality.[19]

Selection of product

Low-dose oral contraceptives containing estrogens and progestins are divided into three main classes: fixed dose products, phasic products, and "selective" progestins (third-generation oral contraceptives).

In theory, selective progestins and triphasics have fewer androgenic side effects. A number of the currently available oral contraceptives are listed in Table 27.

No firm rules govern selection of a pill. All the low-estrogen pills are safe and effective. Patients with large, tender breasts or heavy bleeding and clots may benefit from a low-estrogen, full-progestin pill such as Ortho 1/35. Patients prone to acne, oily skin, hirsutism, and mood swings or premenstrual tension might benefit from selective progestin pills or triphasics.

Starting day

Different starting days may be used. Common ones are the first day of the cycle, the fifth day of the cycle, the first Sunday after the beginning of the cycle, or anytime during the first 6 days of the cycle. The last is acceptable for all products. If the starting day is after the fifth day of the cycle, contraceptive reliability is uncertain until 7 daily consecutive tablets have been taken. For double assurance in this circumstance, an alternative form of contraception should be used during the first 7 days of taking the pill. Pills should be taken at the same time each day.

Table 27 Selected Oral Contraceptive Pills

Composition	Trade names
Fixed Dose Products	
Norethindrone 0.5 mg plus ethinyl estradiol 35 μg	Brevicon 0.5/35 Ortho 0.5/35 Synphasic 0.5/35
Norethindrone 1 mg plus ethinyl estradiol 35 μg	Brevicon 1/35 Ortho 1/35 Synphasic 1/35
Levonorgestrel 150 μg plus ethinyl estradiol 30 μg	Levlen Min-Ovral Nordette
Levonorgestrel 250 μg plus ethinyl estradiol 50 μg	Ovral
Norgestrel 300 μg plus ethinyl estradiol 30 μg	Lo/Ovral
Triphasic Products	
Norethindrone in variable concentrations plus ethinyl estradiol 35 μg	Ortho 777
Levonorgestrel in variable concentrations plus ethinyl estradiol 32 μg	Tri-Levlen Triphasil Triquilar
"Selective" Progestins (Monophasic and Triphasic)	
Norgestimate 0.25 mg plus ethinyl estradiol 35 μg	Cyclen
Norgestimate in variable levels plus ethinyl estradiol 35 μg	Tri-Cyclen
Desogestrel 0.15 mg and ethinyl estradiol 30 μg	Desogen Marvelon Ortho-Cept

Missed pills

The protocol for missed pills varies with the number of pills missed and the time in the cycle when they were missed.

If one pill is missed at any time in the cycle, the missed pill should be taken as soon as it is remembered.

If two pills are missed during the first 2 weeks of the cycle, one should be taken as soon as it is remembered, as well as the regular pill for that day. The next day, two pills should be taken, one in the morning and one in the evening. Backup contraception should be used for the next 7 days.

If two pills are missed during the third week of the cycle and the patient is not on a Sunday start, she should begin a new package of pills immediately and use backup contraception for 7 days. If on a Sunday start, she should take one pill daily until the following Sunday, at which time another package should be started whether or not the menses has commenced. Backup contraception should be used until completion of the first 7 days of the new cycle.

If three or more pills are missed at any time in the cycle and the patient is not on a Sunday start, she should start a new package of pills immediately and use backup contraception for 7 days. If on a Sunday start, the patient should take one pill daily until the following Sunday, at which time another package should be started whether or not the menses has commenced. Backup contraception should be used until completion of the first 7 days of the new cycle.

Discontinuing the pill in perimenopausal women

If a nonsmoking perimenopausal woman is taking an oral contraceptive pill on a regular basis, how does the physician know when menopause has occurred so that the birth control pill may be discontinued and hormone replacement therapy started (assuming the latter is clinically indicated)? Haney[1] suggests simply stopping oral contraceptives arbitrarily at age 51 or 52. If periods do not resume within 3 months, or if vasomotor symptoms develop, menopause has occurred and hormone replacement therapy may be started if indicated. If menses does recur, the physician can either wait for menopause to occur or restart oral contraceptives for another year. Steinberg[22] goes one step further and suggests simply stopping oral contraceptives at age 50 and switching to hormone replacement therapy immediately. Another alternative is to measure FSH levels at yearly intervals toward the end of a pill-free week. Levels of 40 U/ml or higher suggest menopause. However, false-negatives occur because in some women the birth control pills prolong the inhibition of gonadotropins.

REFERENCES

1. Haney AF: Hormonal needs of the perimenopausal woman, *J SOGC* 15:1-8, 1993.
2. Farrell SA: Contraception in the perimenopause, *J SOGC* 16 (suppl):1-7, 1994.
3. Reid R: Which contraceptive methods are suitable for the older women? *J SOGC* 15:933-944, 1993.
4. Jick SS, Walker AM, Jick A: Oral contraceptives and endometrial cancer, *Obstet Gynecol* 82:931-935, 1993.
5. Cancer and Steroid Hormone Study of the Centers for Disease Control and the National Institute of Child Health and Human Development: The reduction in risk of ovarian cancer associated with oral contraceptive use, *N Engl J Med* 316:650-655, 1987.
6. Rulbin GL, Ory HW, Layde PL: Oral contraceptives and pelvic inflammatory disease, *Am J Obstet Gynecol* 144:630-635, 1982.
7. Peterson HB, Lee NC: The health effects of oral contraceptives: misperceptions, controversies and continuing good news, *Clin Obstet Gynecol* 32:339-355, 1989.
8. Kleerekoper M, Brienza RS, Schultz LR, et al (Henry Ford Hospital Osteoporosis Cooperative Research Group): Oral contraceptive use may protect against low bone mass, *Arch Intern Med* 151:1971-1976, 1991.
9. Longstreth WT: Oral contraceptives and stroke, *Stroke* 15:747-750, 1984.
10. Stampfer MJ, Willet WC, Colditz GA, et al: A prospective study of past use of oral contraceptive agents and risk of cardiovascular diseases, *N Engl J Med* 319:1313-1317, 1988.
11. Stampfer MJ, Willet WC, Colditz GA, et al: Past use of oral contraceptives and cardiovascular disease: a meta-analysis in the context of the Nurses' Health Study, *Am J Obstet Gynecol* 163:285-291, 1990.
12. Lidegaard O: Oral contraception and risk of a cerebral thromboembolic attack: results of a case-control study, *BMJ* 306: 956-963, 1993.
13. Petitti DB, Sidney S, Bernstein A, et al: Stroke in users of low-dose oral contraceptives, *N Engl J Med* 335:8-15, 1996.
14. Jick H, Jick SS, Gurewich V, et al: Risk of idiopathic cardiovascular death and nonfatal venous thromboembolism in women using oral contraceptives with differing progestogen components, *Lancet* 346:1589-1593, 1995.
15. World Health Organization Collaborative Study of Cardiovascular Disease and Steroid Hormone Contraception: effect of different progestogens in low oestrogen oral contraceptives on venous thromboembolic disease, *Lancet* 346:1582-1588, 1995.
16. Weiss N: Third-generation oral contraceptives: how risky? (editorial), *Lancet* 346:1570, 1995.
17. Spitzer WO, Lewis MA, Heinemann LA, et al (Transnational Research Group on Oral Contraceptives and the Health of Young Women): Third generation oral contraceptives and risk of venous thromboembolic disorders: an international case-control study, *BMJ* 312:83-88, 1996.
18. Vandenbroucke JP, van der Meer FJ, Helmerhorst FM, et al: Factor V Leiden: should we screen oral contraceptive users and pregnant women? *BMJ* 313:1127-1130, 1996.
19. Colditz GA (Nurses' Health Study Research Group): Oral contraceptive use and mortality during 12 years of follow-up: the Nurses' Health Study, *Ann Intern Med* 120:821-826, 1994.
20. Collaborative Group on Hormonal Factors in Breast Cancer: Breast cancer and hormonal contraceptives: collaborative reanalysis of individual data on 53,297 women with and 100,239 women without breast cancer from 54 epidemiological studies, *Lancet* 347:1713-1727, 1996.
21. Ursin G, Peters RK, Henderson BE, et al: Oral contraceptive use and adenocarcinoma of cervix, *Lancet* 344:1390-1394, 1994.
22. Steinberg WM: Benefits of perimenopausal contraception: HRT when? *Patient Care Can* 7(6):8-10, 1996.

Postcoital Contraception

(See also mifepristone)

The usual method of using the "morning after pill" is the Yuzpe regimen consisting of 100 μg of ethinyl estradiol and 500 mg of levonorgestrel (two Ovral pills) repeated in 12 hours. Standard guidelines state that this must be started within 72 hours of intercourse; the failure rate is 2.5%.[1] This hormonal intervention is thought to prevent endometrial implantation.[2] Fifty percent of women have nausea, and 25% vomit[1]; dimenhydrinate (Gravol, Dramamine) or some other antiemetic, as well as extra Ovral pills, should be prescribed in case the original ones are regurgitated.

Lower dose contraceptive pills may also be used. A prescription of eight tablets containing the active ingredients (four initially and four in 12 hours) of any of the following brands is acceptable: Levlen, Lo/Ovral (Min-Ovral), Nordette, Tri-Levlen, or Triphasil.[2]

A review of nine published studies of the Yuzpe regimen found a high success rate that was unrelated to whether the pills were started immediately or 1, 2, or 3 days after intercourse. In view of this the authors suggest that the regimen might be effective even 4 or 5 days after intercourse.[2]

Mifepristone (RU 486) as a single dose of 600 mg has been shown in Britain to be effective and to cause less nausea and vomiting than the Yuzpe regimen.[3,4] Insertion of a copper IUD within 5 days of intercourse is also effective.[1]

REFERENCES

1. After the morning after and the morning after that (editorial), *Lancet* 345:1381-1382, 1995.
2. Trussell J, Ellertson C, Rodriguez G: The Yuzpe regimen of emergency contraception: how long after the morning after? *Obstet Gynecol* 88:150-154, 1996.
3. Webb AM, Russell J, Elstein M: Comparison of the Yuzpe regimen, danazol, and mifepristone (RU 486) in oral postcoital contraception, *BMJ* 305:927-931, 1992.
4. Glasier A, Thong KJ, Dewar M, et al: Mifepristone (RU 486) compared with high-dose estrogen and progetogen for emergency postcoital contraception, *N Engl J Med* 327:1041-1044, 1992.

Progestin Only Contraceptives

Levonorgestrel implants

Levonorgestrel under the trade name Norplant is available for subcutaneous implantation.[1] The capsules are made of flexible Silastic and contain 36 mg of levonorgestrel. Contraception is achieved by the subcutaneous insertion of six capsules. The efficacy of this form of contraception is high and lasts for 5 years. The most common side effect is menstrual irregularities.[1,2]

Progestin only oral contraceptives

Progestin tablets containing 350 μg of norethindrone include Nor-QD and Micronor. This form of contraception is indicated when estrogen compounds may be contraindicated such as in smokers over the age of 35, breast-feeding women, and those with hypertension or breast cancer.[1]

Medroxyprogesterone Acetate Injections

Medroxyprogesterone acetate (Depo-Provera) for intramuscular use is available in the United States and Canada. The recommended dosage for contraception is 150 mg every 3 months injected deeply into the deltoid or gluteal muscle. Pregnancy must be ruled out, so the drug is often given only during the first 5 days of a normal menstrual period.

REFERENCES

1. Choice of contraceptives, *Med Lett* 37:9-12, 1995.
2. Baird DT, Glasier AF: Hormonal contraception, *N Engl J Med* 328:1543-1550, 1993.

Sterilization

(See also vasectomy; vasovasostomy)

Tubal sterilization

On a worldwide basis the most common form of contraception is tubal sterilization. The overall reported incidence of poststerilization regret is low but varies widely from one country to another and from one region to another within the same country. Important risk factors for regret include young age and tubal sterilization at the time of the puerperium.[1,2] Most studies of the efficacy of tubal sterilization at the time of the puerperium have found that the pregnancy rate is slightly greater than in patients who have interval tubal sterilization.[1]

REFERENCES

1. Chi IC, Petta CA, McPheeters M: A review of safety, efficacy, pros and cons, and issues of puerperal tubal sterilization—an update, *Adv Contraception* 11:187-206, 1995.
2. Chi IC, Jones DB: Incidence, risk factors, and prevention of poststerilization regret in women: an updated international review from an epidemiological perspective, *Obstet Gynecol Surv* 49:722-732, 1994.

DYSFUNCTIONAL UTERINE BLEEDING

(See also carcinoma of the endometrium; oral contraceptives)

Dysfunctional uterine bleeding (DUB) may be defined as anovulatory estrogen withdrawal bleeding that is not due to an anatomical cause such as leiomyomas of the uterus, endometrial cancer, or endometrial polyps.[1] It is common during the perimenopause (usually ages 40 to 50) and results in many surgical interventions. Hysterectomies are performed in 19% of North American women, and 40% of these are because of dysfunctional uterine bleeding.[2]

The traditional medical treatment of dysfunctional uterine bleeding has been the administration of progestins such as Provera 10 mg for 10 to 14 days every month or two. This does not alter gonadotropin secretion or prevent ovulation and pregnancy. Another traditional method has been to start cyclical hormone replacement therapy.[1]

At present the usual medical treatment for dysfunctional uterine bleeding in nonsmoking women is a low-dose estrogen (≤50 μg) oral contraceptive pill (many physicians would opt for a pill containing 35 μg or less of estrogen). For nonsmoking perimenopausal women this is effective and safe and may be used right up to the time of the menopause.[1,2] How to determine the advent of the menopause in perimenopausal women taking the pill is discussed above in the section on oral contraceptives. If the main problem is menorrhagia, an alternative treatment is the use of NSAIDs such as mefenamic acid (Ponstan) 500 mg tid or naproxen sodium (Anaprox DS) 550 mg bid during the time of bleeding. These agents decrease the loss of blood.[3]

When medical treatment of severe menorrhagia is unsuccessful, the standard surgical option has been hysterectomy. An often effective alternative is endometrial resection or ablation. This may or may not result in amenorrhea, but in one study with a 5-year follow-up period the procedure averted hysterectomy in 90% of patients.[4]

Some of the accepted methods of controlling the bleeding of severe dysfunctional uterine bleeding quickly are to give medroxyprogesterone acetate (Provera) 10 mg po daily for 5 to 7 days or four low-dose birth control pills daily for 5 to 7 days. Both of these regimens are followed by withdrawal bleeding. The oral contraceptives may cause nausea, so antiemetics should be prescribed.

REFERENCES

1. Haney AF: Hormonal needs of the perimenopausal woman, *J SOGC* 15:1-8, 1993.
2. Farrell SA: Contraception in the perimenopause, *J SOGC* 16 (suppl):1-7, 1994.
3. Rosenfeld J: Treatment of menorrhagia due to dysfunctional uterine bleeding, *Am Fam Physician* 53:165-172, 1996.
4. O'Connor H, Magos A: Endometrial resection for the treatment of menorrhagia, *N Engl J Med* 335:151-156, 1996.

ECTOPIC PREGNANCY

(See also abortion)

A single intramuscular dose of methotrexate proved to be a successful treatment for 86% of women with unruptured ectopic pregnancies that were 3.5 cm or less in maximum diameter as determined by transvaginal ultrasonography. The dose used was 50 mg/mm^3.[1]

Use of abdominal ultrasound alone permits diagnosis of about 10% of ectopic pregnancies and vaginal ultrasound about 25% of such cases. The diagnosis of ectopic pregnancy is facilitated by combining quantitative beta-human choriogonadotropin levels and abdominal or vaginal ultrasonography. With conventional abdominal ultrasonography the "discriminatory zone" (level at which a normal intrauterine pregnancy should be detected) is 6500 IU, whereas for vaginal ultrasound it is 2800 IU; 50% of normal intrauterine sacs can be detected at levels of 1000 IU.[2]

Women of childbearing age complaining of abdominal pain or vaginal bleeding who were seen in the emergency room of Boston City Hospital were evaluated according to the following protocol. All patients had a quantitative radioimmunoassay for beta-human choriogonadotropin. If it was positive and they were clinically determined to be in the first trimester (439 cases), they were enrolled in the study. All patients then underwent an abdominal or transvaginal ultrasound (all those who had an indeterminate abdominal ultrasound had a transvaginal ultrasound). Of the 439 women, 56 or 13% eventually proved to have an ectopic pregnancy. Among these 56 patients the diagnosis of ectopic pregnancy was considered highly suggestive or definitive by ultrasonography in 34 (61%) whereas in the remaining 22 (39%) the ultrasound results were indeterminate. From another perspective, about 20% to 25% of the pregnant patients with indeterminate ultrasound results had an ectopic pregnancy. Other important findings in this study were that 9% of the patients with ectopic pregnancies had no pain and one third of patients had no adnexal tenderness on examination. In other words, ectopic pregnancy cannot be ruled out on the basis of absence of abnormalities in the history or physical examination.[3]

Although ectopic pregnancy is a rare event, it does occur in women who have had previous tubal sterilization procedures.[4]

REFERENCES

1. Glock JL, Johnson JV, Brumsted JR: Efficacy and safety of single-dose systemic methotrexate in the treatment of ectopic pregnancy, *Fertil Steril* 62:716-721, 1994.
2. De Cherney AH: Case Records of the Massachusetts General Hospital: Case 3-1996, *N Engl J Med* 334:255-260, 1996.
3. Kaplan BC, Dart RG, Moskos M, et al: Ectopic pregnancy: prospective study with improved diagnostic accuracy, *Ann Emerg Med* 28:10-17, 1996.
4. Peterson HB, Xia Z, Hughes JM, et al (US Collaborative Review of Sterilization Working Group): The risk of ectopic pregnancy after tubal sterilization, *N Engl J Med* 336:762-767, 1997.

ENDOMETRIUM

(See also dysfunctional uterine bleeding; tamoxifen)

Endometrial Carcinoma

Endometrial carcinoma is primarily a disease of elderly women, although 25% of cases occur premenopausally and 5% of cases are reported in women under the age of 40. Major risk factors are obesity, diabetes, and unopposed estrogen therapy. Some increased risk is also associated with tamoxifen therapy, nulliparity, and menopause occurring after the age of 52. Smoking and combined oral contraceptives decrease the risk. Smoking probably accomplishes this feat by inactivating estrogen.[1,2] The four main stages of endometrial carcinoma are as follows[1]:

Stage I	Limited to endometrium or myometrium
Stage II	Spread to cervix
Stage III	Spread to serosa, peritoneum, regional lymph nodes, or pelvic organs
Stage IV	Distant metastases or invasion of bladder or rectal mucosa

The prognosis varies with the stage. The 5-year survival rate is 72% for stage I (almost 100% for stage IA, which is carcinoma limited to the endometrium), 56% for stage II, 32% for stage III, and 11% for stage IV. Most cases are stage I. Diagnosis is traditionally made by dilatation and curettage, but office endometrial sampling has been reported to have a high degree of sensitivity.[3,4] One suggested approach to ruling out endometrial cancer in women with abnormal vaginal bleeding is to perform endometrial aspiration biopsies on all women with this problem. If cancer is found, referral for definitive therapy is automatic. If samples fail to show malignancy, a trial of hormone therapy is reasonable for a premenopausal woman (see discussion of dysfunctional uterine bleeding), whereas a postmenopausal woman should have further investigations such as dilatation and curettage or hysteroscopy.[1]

REFERENCES

1. von Gruenigen VE, Karlen JR: Carcinoma of the endometrium, *Am Fam Physician* 51:1531-1536, 1995.
2. Rose P: Endometrial carcinoma, *N Engl J Med* 335:640-649, 1996.
3. Stovall TG, Photopulos GJ, Poston WM, et al: Pipelle endometrial sampling in patients with known endometrial carcinoma, *Obstet Gynecol* 77:954-956, 1991.
4. Stovall TG, Ling FW, Morgan PL: A prospective, randomized comparison of the Pipelle endometrial sampling device with the Novak curette, *Am J Obstet Gynecol* 165:1287-1290, 1991.

HUMAN PAPILLOMAVIRUS

(See also cervical cancer)

Human papillomavirus can be found in close to 50% of normal cervixes in sexually active women when highly sensitive techniques such as the polymerase chain reaction are used.[1]

About 60 subtypes of human papillomavirus have been identified. Subtypes 6 and 11 and most of the 40s group are associated with condylomata acuminata and, with the possible exception of the rare nonmetastasizing verrucous carcinomas of the genital tract, these are nononcogenic. Women with condylomata acuminata are not at increased risk for cervical intraepithelial neoplasia.[2] Subtypes 16 and 18 and some of the 30s, 50s, and 60s groups are associated with intraepithelial neoplasia and are thought to be oncogenic. There is no evidence that identifying these strains and instituting some form of treatment will alter morbidity or mortality.[3]

The Canadian Task Force on the Periodic Health Examination has evaluated the value of screening for human papillomavirus and concluded that it should not be done ("D" recommendation).[3] The U.S. Preventive Services Task Force gives screening for human papillomavirus a "C" recommendation but adds that "recommendations against such screening can be made on other grounds, including poor specificity and costs."[4]

A number of treatment modalities are available for condylomata acuminata. One of the newer ones is the application three times a week of 5% imiquimod (Aldara) cream. Resolution of the lesions takes 1 to 3 months.

REFERENCES

1. Bauer HM, Ting Y, Greer CE, et al: Genital human papillomavirus infection in female university students as determined by a PCR-based method, *JAMA* 265:472-477, 1991.
2. Evans BA, Bond RA, MacRae KD: A colposcopic case-control study of cervical squamous intraepithelial lesions in women with anogenital warts, *Genitourinary Med* 68:300-304, 1992.
3. Johnson K (Canadian Task Force on the Periodic Health Examination): Periodic health examination, 1995 update. 1. Screening for human papillomavirus infection in asymptomatic women, *Can Med Assoc J* 152:483-493, 1995.
4. US Preventive Services Task Force: *Guide to clinical preventive services,* ed 2, Baltimore, 1996, Williams & Wilkins, pp 105-117.

INFERTILITY, FEMALE

(See also infertility, male)

Infertility is defined as inability to conceive after 1 year of adequately timed unprotected intercourse. The incidence in developed countries is 10% to 15%. Numerous investigations may be done for cases of infertility; some of the basic ones that can be ordered by the family physician are a complete blood count, measurement of thyroid-stimulating hormone (TSH) and prolactin, semen analysis, and basal body temperature charts for three cycles.[1]

A study of the timing of intercourse and pregnancy among 221 healthy women (no fertility problems) from North Carolina who wanted to become pregnant found that pregnancy occurred only if intercourse took place during a 6-day period that ended at the time of ovulation. Intercourse on the day of ovulation resulted in pregnancy in one third of cases, whereas intercourse 6 days before ovulation led to pregnancy in only 8% of cases. No evidence was found that the timing of intercourse in relation to ovulation affected the sex of the baby or the survival of the pregnancy or that frequent intercourse decreased fertility (even though closely spaced ejaculations have been shown to decrease motile sperm counts).[2]

A 1985 study reported that smoking decreases fertility by about 15% to 20% and that this phenomenon is dose dependent.[3] Other studies have found a similar correlation but attributed it to confounding covariants.[4]

There is some evidence that laparoscopic ablation or resection of mild or minimal endometriosis increases pregnancy rates in infertile women.[5]

In vitro fertilization is an expensive, time-consuming, uncomfortable, painful, and psychologically traumatic procedure. The success rate is about 25%.[6] When infertility is related to sperm dysfunction in the male, intracytoplasmic sperm injection of the ovum is used in many centers. To date no increase has been seen in the incidence of congenital anomalies in children born as a result of this procedure.[7]

REFERENCES

1. Trantham P: The infertile couple, *Am Fam Physician* 54:1001-1010, 1996.
2. Wilcox AJ, Weinberg CR, Baird DD: Timing of sexual intercourse in relation to ovulation: effects on the probability of

conception, survival of the pregnancy, and sex of the baby, *N Engl J Med* 333:1517-1521, 1995.
3. Howe G, Westhoff C, Vessey M, Yeates D: Effects of age, cigarette smoking and other factors on fertility: findings in a large prospective study, *BMJ* 290:1967-1970, 1985.
4. deMouzan J, Spira A, Schwartz D: A prospective study of the relation between smoking and fertility, *Int J Epidemiol* 17:378-384, 1988.
5. Marcoux S, Maheux, Bérubé S (Canadian Collaborative Group on Endometriosis): Laparoscopic surgery in infertile women with minimal or mild endometriosis, *N Engl J Med* 337:217-222, 1997.
6. McCall M: Pursuing conception: a physician's experience with in-vitro fertilization, *Can Med Assoc J* 154:1075-1079, 1996.
7. Palermo GD, Colombero LT, Schattman GL, et al: Evolution of pregnancies and initial follow-up of newborns delivered after intracytoplasmic sperm injection, *JAMA* 276:1893-1897, 1996.

MENOPAUSE

(See also exercise; dysfunctional uterine bleeding; osteoporosis; oral contraceptives)

In the latter years of a woman's reproductive life the frequency of cyclical ovulation declines and the frequency of anovulatory cycles increases. This phenomenon is sometimes called the climacteric and occurs during the perimenopause, which usually covers the fifth decade of a woman's life.[1]

One of the major issues concerning menopause in the 1990s has been hormone replacement therapy. This is dealt with in several sections below. Although the evidence is clear that hormone replacement therapy has substantial benefits, physicians should be aware that the widespread enthusiasm for its use has trivialized, or at least deemphasized, life-style methods of disease prevention such as exercise and discontinuation of smoking in postmenopausal women. From the evidence available, smoking cessation and exercise may save as many lives as hormone replacement therapy; this is discussed in more detail below in the section "Life-Style Changes for Disease Prevention in Menopausal Women."

REFERENCES

1. Haney AF: Hormonal needs of the perimenopausal woman, *J SOGC* 15:1-8, 1993.

Hormone Replacement Therapy—Benefits

(See also consensus conferences; hormone replacement therapy—adverse effects; informed consent; methods of reporting benefits of clinical trials; osteoporosis; prophylaxis of recurrent urinary tract infections; sleep disturbances)

The major reasons for giving hormone replacement therapy are to prevent or control vasomotor symptoms and genital atrophy and to control long-term morbidity from cardiovascular disease and osteoporosis. Additional benefits may be a decrease in sleep disturbances, mood disorders, and cognitive decline and an improvement in libido.

Control of vasomotor symptoms

One of the initial symptoms of estrogen deficiency is hot flashes or vasomotor symptoms. These occur in 75% of postmenopausal women and persist for longer than 5 years in 25% of them. In a few women the symptoms are lifelong. Only about 30% of women seek medical help for these symptoms.[1] The standard treatment for hot flashes is estrogen replacement therapy; the choice of regimens is discussed below. Such therapy is effective, resulting in an 85% reduction in vasomotor hot flushes.[2] The beneficial effect may not be noted in the first 2 to 3 weeks, but the effect may persist for weeks after the estrogen is discontinued.[2]

If women are unable to take estrogens, hot flashes may often be controlled by megestrol acetate (Megace) 20 mg bid[3] or sometimes by clonidine (Catapres, Dixarit) 0.025 mg, 2 tablets bid.[4]

Control of vulvar and vaginal atrophy

Aside from hot flashes, a common problem of postmenopausal women is vulvar and vaginal atrophy, which often manifests itself subjectively as a feeling of vaginal dryness, vulvar itch, decreased lubrication during sexual arousal, and dyspareunia. In addition, atrophy of the urethra and base of the bladder may lead to urinary urgency and frequency and perhaps even to urethral stenosis. These symptoms are caused by estrogen deficiency and are usually relieved by estrogen hormonal replacement therapy.[1,5] If a woman already receiving estrogen replacement therapy still experiences vaginal dryness, she may use a topical estrogen cream such as vaginal Premarin cream 2 to 4 g intravaginally or applied to the vulva as necessary. Since Premarin cream is absorbed systemically, she should not use oral or transdermal estrogens on the days she uses the estrogen cream.

Control of sleep disturbances

Hot flashes may cause sleep disturbances that in turn may lead to impaired mood. A trial of estrogen replacement therapy would do no harm in this circumstance, and in one short-term study of estrogen patches without the addition of progestins it seemed to work.[6]

Control of dysphoria

Whether dysphoria is a true menopausal symptom and whether estrogen treatment improves either the mood or the quality of life is unclear. Some reports suggest that unopposed estrogens may have such a positive effect[6,7] but that it is dampened by the addition of progestins.[7] A 1996 review of 46 primary research papers on the relationship of menopause to depression concluded that evidence of a causal association is insufficient.[8]

Control of decreased libido

A number of reports have suggested that androgen plus estrogen replacement therapy is effective for women with decreased libido.[5] In Canada, replacement androgen is available only as an injectable testosterone-estradiol combination, Climacteron, which is given as 1 ml intramuscularly every 4 to 8 weeks.

Prevention of coronary artery disease

If lives are to be saved by hormone replacement therapy, the major mechanism will be through a decreased incidence of coronary artery disease. This is because the cumulative risk of death for women between the ages of 50 to 94 is 31% from coronary artery disease and only 3% each from breast cancer and hip fractures.[9] A decreased relative risk of cardiovascular disease of about 40% to 50% in women who have used, or are using, estrogens[10-13] has been shown in many studies, one of the best known of which is the Nurses' Health Study.[10,11,13] Among current estrogen users the coronary disease rate was about half of that of never users. Women who had previously taken estrogens but were no longer doing so had only a slight benefit compared with never users.[10,11,13] Similar beneficial results were reported in a group of women who had taken hormone replacement therapy for a mean of 17.1 years. The age-adjusted relative risk for all-cause mortality in hormone users versus nonusers was 0.54, while that for coronary artery disease was 0.40.[12] Unfortunately, there is an important caveat to this rosy picture. Further analysis of the Nurses' Health Study has shown that mortality benefits from the prevention of cardiovascular disease are attenuated after 10 years of hormone use, primarily because of an increased mortality from breast cancer. The overall benefit of hormone replacement therapy was most marked for women with risk factors for coronary artery disease and was least for those with no risk factors (see discussion of adverse effects of hormone replacement therapy).[13] Thus it might be wise to recommend hormone replacement therapy on the basis of individual risk factors and to limit the period for which it is prescribed.[14]

There was concern in the past that the addition of progestogens to estrogens in hormone replacement therapy would attenuate the beneficial effects of the estrogens. This has proved not to be the case.[11,13,15] The cardioprotective effects of the transdermal estrogen patches have not yet been proved; very large doses are required to lower LDL cholesterol.[1]

The mechanisms by which estrogens exert their beneficial effects on vascular disease have not been fully worked out. The effect has long been thought to be secondary to improvements in lipid profiles, but another explanation is that estrogens increase fibrinolytic activity.[16] The Postmenopausal Estrogen/Progestin Interventions (PEPI) Trial measured various surrogate outcomes in women taking combined estrogen-progestin products. HDL levels were increased, and LDL and fibrinogen levels were decreased. Little effect was seen on blood pressure or insulin measurements.[17]

Prevention of strokes

Conflicting reports have been published on the effects of hormone replacement therapy on strokes. Some studies have shown a decreased incidence,[18,19] whereas others have not found a significant effect.[11]

Prevention of osteoporosis and fractures

Estrogens have been shown to decrease the rate of development of osteoporosis, and they probably decrease the fracture rate.[20] However, to achieve this end, they must be started shortly after menopause and continued indefinitely.[21,22] Since the death rate from breast cancer is significantly increased after 10 years of hormone replacement therapy (see discussion of adverse effects of hormone replacement therapy), other modalities of decreasing the risk of osteoporosis should be considered. These include exercise, avoidance of smoking and excessive alcohol intake, and calcium and vitamin D supplementation. The role of these interventions, as well as hormone replacement therapy, is discussed in more detail under "Osteoporosis."

Prevention of tooth loss

Hormone replacement therapy may help to prevent tooth loss and the need for dentures, presumably by decreasing the degree of osteoporosis in the alveolar bone of the jaw.[23]

Preservation of cognitive functioning

A possible but as yet unproved benefit of estrogen replacement therapy is improved cognitive functioning. A few studies have demonstrated better scores in some aspects of cognitive testing, such as word or proper name recall, in postmenopausal women receiving estrogen supplementation compared with control subjects not taking estrogens.[24-26] Since Alzheimer's disease develops in three times as many men as women, an intriguing hypothesis is that estrogens protect women from the disease; this has some support from both a California and a New York study. The California study found a higher incidence of Alzheimer's disease in women who did not take hormone replacement therapy compared with women who did.[27,28] The longer the drug was taken, the greater the protection.[28] The New York study reported that elderly women who had taken postmenopausal hormones had a reduced risk of Alzheimer's disease, and if it did develop, this occurred at a later age.[29]

Diminished risk of colon cancer

Several epidemiological studies have reported a decreased incidence of colon cancer in women taking hormone replacement therapy.[30-32]

REFERENCES

1. Belchetz PE: Hormonal treatment of postmenopausal women, *N Engl J Med* 330:1062-1071, 1994.
2. Haas S, Walsh B, Evans S, et al: The effect of transdermal estradiol on hormone and metabolic dynamics over a six-week period, *Obstet Gynecol* 71:671-676, 1988.
3. Loprinzi CL, Michalak JC, Quella SK, et al: Megestrol acetate for the prevention of hot flashes, *N Engl J Med* 331:347-352, 1994.

4. Goldberg RM, Loprinzi CL, O'Fallon JR, et al: Transdermal clonidine for ameliorating tamoxifen-induced hot flashes, *J Clin Oncol* 12:155-158, 1994.
5. Walling M, Andersen BL, Johnson SR: Hormonal replacement therapy for postmenopausal women: a review of sexual outcomes and related gynecologic effects, *Arch Sex Behav* 19:119-137, 1990.
6. Wiklund I, Karlberg J, Mattison L-Å: Quality of life of postmenopausal women on a regimen of transdermal estradiol therapy: a double-blind placebo-controlled study, *Am J Obstet Gynecol* 168:824-830, 1993.
7. Sherwin BB: The impact of different doses of estrogen and progestin on mood and sexual behavior in postmenopausal women, *J Clin Endocrin Metab* 72:336-343, 1991.
8. Nicol-Smith L: Causality, menopause, and depression: a critical review of the literature, *BMJ* 313:1229-1232, 1996.
9. Cummings SR, Black DM, Rubin SM, et al: Lifetime risks of hip, Colles', or vertebral fracture and coronary heart disease among white postmenopausal women, *Arch Intern Med* 149: 2445-2448, 1989.
10. Stampfer MJ, Colditz GA, Willett WC, et al: Postmenopausal estrogen therapy and cardiovascular disease: ten-year follow-up from the Nurses' Health Study, *N Engl J Med* 325:756-762, 1991.
11. Grodstein F, Stampfer MJ, Manson JE, et al: Postmenopausal estrogen and progestin use and the risk of cardiovascular disease, *N Engl J Med* 335:453-461, 1996.
12. Ettinger B, Friedman GD, Bush T, et al: Reduced mortality associated with long-term postmenopausal estrogen therapy, *Obstet Gynecol* 87:6-12, 1996.
13. Grodstein F, Stampfer MJ, Colditz A, et al: Postmenopausal hormone therapy and mortality, *N Engl J Med* 336:1769-1775, 1997.
14. Brinton LA, Schairer C: Postmenopausal hormone-replacement therapy—time for a reappraisal? (editorial), *N Engl J Med* 336:1821-1822, 1997.
15. Psaty BM, Heckbert SR, Atkins D, et al: The risk of myocardial infarction associated with the combined use of estrogens and progestins in postmenopausal women, *Arch Intern Med* 154: 1333-1339, 1994.
16. Kwang KK, Mincemoyer R, Bui M, et al: Effects of hormone-replacement therapy on fibrinolysis in postmenopausal women, *N Engl J Med* 336:683-690, 1997.
17. Writing Group for the PEPI Trial: Effects of estrogen or estrogen/progestin regimens on heart disease risk factors in postmenopausal women: the Postmenopausal Estrogen/Progestin Interventions (PEPI) Trial, *JAMA* 273:199-208, 1995.
18. Finucane FF, Madans JH, Bush TL, et al: Decreased risk of stroke among postmenopausal hormone users, *Arch Intern Med* 153:73-79, 1993.
19. Falkeborn M, Persson I, Terent A, et al: Hormone replacement therapy and the risk of stroke: follow-up of a population-based cohort in Sweden, *Arch Intern Med* 153:1201-1209, 1993.
20. Riggs BL, Melton LJ: The prevention and treatment of osteoporosis, *N Engl J Med* 327:620-627, 1992.
21. Cauley JA, Seeley DG, Ensrud K, et al (Study of Osteoporotic Fractures Research Group): Estrogen replacement therapy and fractures in older women, *Ann Intern Med* 122:9-16, 1995.
22. Ettinger B, Grady D: The waning effect of postmenopausal estrogen therapy on osteoporosis, *N Engl J Med* 329:1192-1193, 1993.
23. Paganini-Hill A: The benefits of estrogen replacement therapy on oral health, *Arch Intern Med* 155:2325-2329, 1995.
24. Phillips S, Sherwin BB: Effects of estrogen on memory function in surgically menopausal women, *Psychoneuroendocrinology* 17:497-504, 1992.
25. Kampen DL, Sherwin BB: Estrogen use and verbal memory in healthy postmenopausal women, *Obstet Gynecol* 83:979-983, 1994.
26. Robinson D, Friedman L, Marcus R, et al: Estrogen replacement therapy and memory in older women, *J Am Geriatr Soc* 42:919-922, 1994.
27. Henderson VW, Paganini-Hill A, Emanuel CK, et al: Estrogen replacement therapy in older women: comparisons between Alzheimer's disease cases and nondemented control subjects, *Arch Neurol* 51:896-900, 1994.
28. Paganini-Hill A, Henderson VW: Estrogen replacement therapy and risk of Alzheimer disease, *Arch Intern Med* 156:2213-2217, 1996.
29. Tang MX, Jacobs D, Stern Y, et al: Effect of oestrogen during menopause on risk and age at onset of Alzheimer's disease, *Lancet* 348:429-432, 1996.
30. Newcomb PA, Storer BE: Postmenopausal hormone use and risk of large-bowel cancer, *J Natl Cancer Inst* 87:1067-1071, 1995.
31. Grodstein F, Martinez ME, Giovannucci EL, et al: Postmenopausal hormone use and colorectal cancer in the Nurses' Health Study, *Am J Epidemiol* 143(suppl):S63, 1996.
32. Calle EE, Miracle-McMahill HL, Thun MJ, et al: Estrogen replacement therapy and risk of fatal colon cancer in a prospective cohort of postmenopausal women, *J Natl Cancer Inst* 87: 517-523, 1995.

Hormone Replacement Therapy—Adverse Effects

(See also hormone replacement therapy—benefits; informed consent; thrombophlebitis)

Endometrial cancer

Routine endometrial biopsies to rule out endometrial carcinoma before starting hormone replacement therapy are unnecessary for asymptomatic women. Endometrial biopsies performed on 2964 asymptomatic women before initiation of hormone replacement detected only two cases of occult adenocarcinoma.[1]

Breast cancer

Until 1995 the existence of an association between hormone replacement therapy and breast cancer was controversial. Large numbers of articles had been published on the subject, some concluding that the risk was significant and others that it was virtually nil.[2-5] Metaanalyses of many of these studies did not prove helpful. Two of the most frequently quoted came to opposite conclusions.[6,7]

The publication in 1995 of the Nurses' Health Study made it clear that hormone replacement therapy of more than 5 years' duration is a risk factor for breast cancer. Women who were currently taking hormones and had been doing so for more than 5 years had a relative risk of acquiring breast cancer of 1.46. This risk was even greater in older women; those aged 60 to 64 who had been taking hormones for at least 5 years had a relative risk of 1.7. This study also found that progestogens had no protective effect on the incidence of breast cancer. Mortality rate from breast cancer was also increased by a relative rate of 1.45 among women who had used hormone replacement for more than 5 years.[8] Although this study did not give absolute figures, some were given by the authors in response to a letter to the editor. They calculated that the risk that a 60-year-old woman would have breast cancer if she never had hormone replacement therapy was 1.8%; if she was taking hormones and had done so for at least 5 years, her risk was 3%.[9] Ettinger and colleagues[10] found that the relative risk of death from breast cancer in long-term hormone users was 1.89 compared with nonusers. However, this detrimental effect was far outweighed by the decreased cardiovascular mortality of the hormone users (see "Hormone Replacement Therapy—Benefits").[10] An evaluation of mortality in the Nurses' Health Study has shown a relative increase in breast cancer mortality of 43% among women taking hormones for more than 10 years. As a result the overall mortality benefit, which depends on a decrease in cardiovascular disease, was seriously attenuated. The risk of breast cancer is sufficiently great with long-term hormone replacement therapy that serious consideration should be given to prescribing it for only a limited period.[12]

At this time it seems unlikely that the risk of breast cancer is increased in women who take hormone replacement therapy for 5 years or less, a view supported by the Canadian Task Force on the Periodic Health Examination[13] and the U.S. Preventive Services Task Force.[14] This knowledge should allow both patients and physicians to feel more comfortable about short-term hormonal replacement therapy for such symptoms as hot flashes. If long-term therapy is being considered, both physicians and patients must be aware of the increased absolute risk of breast cancer with this therapy as well as the decrease in morbidity and mortality from cardiovascular disease.

Hormone replacement therapy in breast cancer survivors

Most authorities consider estrogen replacement therapy to be contraindicated in women who have had breast cancer, although this is a debatable point, particularly in women who have had local resections of small tumors.[15] A 1994 review of the literature on the subject did not uncover any studies documenting adverse effects of giving estrogen replacement therapy to postmenopausal women who had had breast cancer.[16] The authors suggest mounting a randomized control study to try to resolve this issue.

One alternative method of controlling hot flashes in women who have had breast cancer is the use of a progestogen. A short-term 1994 study using low-dose (20 mg bid) megestrol acetate (Megace) in women who had had breast cancer (and in men who had had orchiectomies) found that the control of hot flashes was equal to that reported for estrogen use. As with estrogens, the beneficial effect was often delayed for a few weeks but persisted for weeks after the drug was withdrawn. In this study no significant side effects were found except for a paradoxical increase in flushing in the first few days of treatment. Long-term adverse effects have not been determined. At the doses used, appetite was not stimulated.[17]

Another method of attempting to control hot flashes is the use of clonidine (Catapres, Dixarit) 0.025 mg, 2 tablets bid. Overall, this drug has not proved very effective.[18]

Thromboembolism

Two case-controlled studies published in 1996 found that the relative risk of thromboembolic disorders in women taking hormone replacement therapy was about three times greater than among nonusers.[19,20] However, the absolute rate was very low. The authors of one of these studies estimated that the number of excess cases of thromboembolic disorders in hormone users was 1:5000 users per year.[19]

REFERENCES

1. Korhonen MO, Symons JP, Hyde BM, et al: Histologic classification and pathologic findings for endometrial biopsy specimens obtained from 2964 perimenopausal and postmenopausal women undergoing screening for continuous hormones as replacement therapy (Chart 2 Study), *Am J Obstet Gynecol* 176:377-380, 1997.
2. Delva MD: Hormone replacement therapy: risks, benefits, and costs, *Can Fam Physician* 39:2149-2154, 1993.
3. Belchetz PE: Hormonal treatment of postmenopausal women, *N Engl J Med* 330:1062-1067, 1994.
4. Kaufman DW, Palmer JR, de Mouzon J, et al: Estrogen replacement therapy and the risk of breast cancer: results from the case-control surveillance study, *Am J Epidemiol* 134:1375-1385, 1991.
5. Bergkvist L, Adami H-O, Persson I, et al: The risk of breast cancer after estrogen and estrogen-progestin replacement, *N Engl J Med* 321:293-297, 1989.
6. Steinberg KK, Thacker SB, Smith SJ, et al: A meta-analysis of the effect of estrogen replacement therapy on the risk of breast cancer, *JAMA* 265:1985-1990, 1991.
7. Dupont W, Page DL: Menopausal estrogen replacement therapy and breast cancer, *Arch Intern Med* 151:67-72, 1991.
8. Colditz GA, Hankinson SE, Hunter DJ, et al: The use of estrogens and progestins and the risk of breast cancer in postmenopausal women, *N Engl J Med* 332:1589-1593, 1995.
9. Colditz GA, Willett WC, Speizer FE: Breast cancer and hormone-replacement therapy (letter), *N Engl J Med* 333:1357-1358, 1995.
10. Ettinger B, Friedman GD, Bush T, et al: Reduced mortality associated with long-term postmenopausal estrogen therapy, *Obstet Gynecol* 87:6-12, 1996.
11. Grodstein F, Stampfer MJ, Colditz A, et al: Postmenopausal hormone therapy and mortality, *N Engl J Med* 336:1769-1775, 1997.
12. Brinton LA, Schairer C: Postmenopausal hormone-replacement therapy—time for a reappraisal? (editorial), *N Engl J Med* 336:1821-1822, 1997.

13. Canadian Task Force on the Periodic Health Examination: *Canadian guide to clinical preventive health care,* Ottawa, 1994, Canada Communication Group—Publishing, p 623.
14. US Preventive Services Task Force: *Guide to clinical preventive services*, ed 2, Baltimore, 1996, Williams & Wilkins, pp 829-843.
15. Marchant DJ: Estrogen-replacement therapy after breast cancer: risks versus benefits, *Cancer* 71(suppl):2169-2176, 1993.
16. Cobleigh MA, Berris RF, Bush T, et al: Estrogen replacement therapy in breast cancer survivors: a time for change, *JAMA* 272:540-545, 1994.
17. Loprinzi CL, Michalak JC, Quella SK, et al: Megestrol acetate for the prevention of hot flashes, *N Engl J Med* 331:347-352, 1994.
18. Goldberg RM, Loprinzi CL, O'Fallon JR, et al: Transdermal clonidine for ameliorating tamoxifen-induced hot flashes, *J Clin Oncol* 12:155-158, 1994.
19. Daly E, Vessey MP, Hawkins MN, et al: Risk of venous thromboembolism in users of hormone replacement therapy, *Lancet* 348:977-980, 1996.
20. Jick H, Derby LE, Myers MW, et al: Risk of hospital admission for idiopathic venous thromboembolism among users of postmenopausal oestrogens, *Lancet* 348:981-983, 1996.

Guidelines for Hormone Replacement Therapy

One method of trying to make sense of the complex issue of hormone replacement therapy is to try to balance advantages and disadvantages through a decision analysis. This was done in 1994 by Gorsky and associates.[1] They calculated that if a cohort of 10,000 50-year-old women took unopposed estrogens for 25 years, 642 lives would be saved; the cohort would have 567 fewer cardiovascular deaths (48% relative reduction rate) and 75 fewer deaths following hip fractures (49% relative reduction rate). However, there would be an excess of 39 breast cancer deaths (21% relative increase). According to these calculations, taking hormones for 25 years would prevent 16 times more deaths from heart disease and hip fractures than would be caused by the increased incidence of breast cancer.[1]

A thoughtful review of the pros and cons of estrogen replacement therapy was published in 1992 by Grady and associates.[2] These workers concluded that hormone replacement therapy should probably be recommended for women who have had a hysterectomy and those with, or at high risk of, coronary heart disease.

Although some organizations such as the Society of Obstetricians and Gynecologists of Canada (SOGC) strongly support the use of hormone replacement therapy for almost all postmenopausal women,[3] most evidence-based guidelines take a somewhat less interventionist position. Neither the Canadian Task Force on the Periodic Health Examination[4] nor the U.S. Preventive Services Task Force[5] has given a blanket recommendation for postmenopausal hormonal replacement therapy. Rather, they both give a "B" recommendation to the idea that all women should be counseled concerning the benefits and possible risks of estrogen replacement therapy.

An aspect of hormone replacement therapy that is rarely discussed is the possibility that the current emphasis on this mode of prevention may lead to a deemphasis of other preventive modalities, such as exercise, that may be just as useful.[6] This is discussed further under "Life-Style Changes for Disease Prevention in Menopausal Women."

REFERENCES

1. Gorsky RD, Koplan JP, Peterson HB, et al: Relative risks and benefits of long-term estrogen replacement therapy: a decision analysis, *Obstet Gynecol* 83:161-166, 1994.
2. Grady D, Rubin SM, Petitti DB, et al: Hormone therapy to prevent disease and prolong life in postmenopausal women, *Ann Intern Med* 117:1016-1037, 1992.
3. Canadian Menopause Consensus Conference, *J SOGC* 16:4-40, 1994.
4. Canadian Task Force on the Periodic Health Examination: *Canadian guide to clinical preventive health care,* Ottawa, 1994, Canada Communication Group—Publishing, pp 619-631.
5. US Preventive Services Task Force: *Guide to clinical preventive services,* ed 2, Baltimore, 1996, Williams & Wilkins, pp 829-843.
6. Marshall KG: Prevention. How much harm? How much benefit? 2. Ten potential pitfalls in determining the clinical significance of benefits, *Can Med Assoc J* 154:1837-1843, 1996.

Methods of Prescribing Hormone Replacement

Hormone replacement therapy can be administered in several ways. Most of the examples given below use conjugated estrogens (Premarin) or estrogen patches containing estradiol (Estraderm, Vivelle, Climara) plus medroxyprogesterone acetate (Provera) simply because these are the most frequently used drugs in practice. Progestogens are required only for women who have an intact uterus. Another option is to give regular combined estrogen-androgen injections, as well as cyclical progestogen if the patient has an intact uterus. Some of the methods of giving combined estrogens and progestins are as follows.

Continuous estrogen and continuous progestogen

Premarin 0.625 mg po is taken daily, or Estraderm 50 is applied twice a week, and in addition Provera 2.5 mg is given daily. This protocol is followed continuously throughout the year. Spotting or bleeding is frequent in the first 6 months. In one trial 27% of women receiving continuous 5 mg Provera and 39% of women receiving continuous 2.5 mg Provera had breakthrough bleeding.[1] After 6 to 12 months of this type of regimen, many women become completely amenorrheic, which is said to increase compliance with this therapeutic modality.[2] A metaanalysis of 42 studies of combined continuous estrogen-progestin use found that after 6 months of therapy 75% or more of women were amenorrheic.[3] A formulation containing conjugated estrogens 0.625 plus medroxyprogesterone acetate 2.5 mg (Prempro) is available in the United States for this form of treatment.

Continuous estrogen and cyclical progestogen

The standard method of using a continuous estrogen and cyclical progestogen combination is to take Premarin 0.625 mg po daily or to apply Estraderm 50 twice a week throughout the year. Provera 5 or 10 mg is taken for the first or last 10 to 14 days of each calendar month or of each 28-day cycle. The progestin withdrawal will lead to bleeding in most women. A product available in the United States is a package containing 14 tablets of 0.625 mg of conjugated estrogens, to be taken during the first 14 days, and 14 tablets of 0.625 mg of conjugated estrogens plus medroxyprogesterone acetate 5 mg, to be taken on days 15 to 28 (Premphase). In Canada patches containing both estrogen in the form of estradiol and progestin as norethindrone (Estragest) are available and can be applied twice a week for 2 weeks every month rather than using oral Provera. A monthly supply containing four Estraderm patches and four Estragest patches comes in a single package under the trade name Estracomb.

Cyclical estrogen and cyclical progestogen

Premarin 0.625 mg po is taken daily or Estraderm 50 is applied twice a week from days 1 to 25 of each month, and in addition, medroxyprogesterone acetate (Provera) 5 or 10 mg is taken daily from days 14 or 16 to 25 of each month. With cyclical estrogen and cyclical progestin about 80% of women have regular withdrawal bleeding. In addition, a number of women have a recurrence of hot flashes and perhaps sleep disturbances during the period of hormonal withdrawal at the end of the month.[1]

Table 28 Selected Medications for Hormonal Replacement

Generic names	Selected trade names
Estrogens	
Conjugated estrogens	Premarin, CES, Congest, Premarin vaginal cream
Estradiol-17 β skin patch	Estraderm, Vivelle, Climara
Estropipate	Ogen
Ethinyl estradiol	Estinyl
Dienestrol vaginal cream	Ortho Dienestrol
Estrogens Plus Progestins	
Conjugated estrogens plus medroxyprogesterone tablets	Prempro, Premphase
Estradiol plus norethindrone skin patch	Estragest
Estrogens Plus Androgens	
Testosterone plus estradiol	Climacteron (for intramuscular use)
Progesterone Derivatives	
Medroxyprogesterone acetate	Provera
Progesterone, micronized	Prometrium
Megestrol acetate	Megace
Other	
Clonidine	Dixarit

Estrogen-androgen injections and cyclical progestogen

Testosterone plus estradiol (Climacteron) is given as a 1-ml intramuscular injection deep in the gluteus muscles once every 4 to 8 weeks. If the woman has an intact uterus, Provera 5 to 10 mg should be given on days 12 to 25 of the cycle counting the day of injection as day 1.

Table 28 lists generic and selected trade names of some of the available agents used for hormonal replacement. Methods of prescribing most of them are discussed in the text.

REFERENCES

1. Archer Df, Pickar JH, Bottiglioni F: Bleeding patterns in postmenopausal women taking continuous combined or sequential regimens of conjugated estrogens with medroxyprogesterone acetate, *Obstet Gynecol* 83:686-692, 1994.
2. Rosenfeld J: Update on continuous estrogen-progestin replacement therapy, *Am Fam Physician* 50:1519-1523, 1994.
3. Udoff L, Langenberg P, Adashi EY: Combined continuous hormone replacement therapy—a critical review, *Obstet Gynecol* 86:306-316, 1995.

Life-Style Changes for Disease Prevention in Menopausal Women

(See also alcohol; exercise; osteoporosis; smoking)

Although current estrogen replacement therapy undoubtedly decreases the incidence of cardiovascular disease and osteoporosis in postmenopausal women, an equally important question is what other modalities of prevention are effective. Stopping smoking is one of the most important measures that can be taken. Another is increasing physical activity. The few studies that have specifically addressed the relationship between exercise and cardiac disease in women have shown that physical activity has a protective effect against coronary artery disease (see discussion of exercise).[1-3] For example, buried in a paper by Henderson and associates titled "Estrogen Replacement Therapy and Protection from Acute Myocardial Infarction" are the data that women who exercised for 1 hour or more daily reduced their risk of myocardial infarction by a relative rate of about 50% compared with their sedentary sisters.[1] This is as good as, or better than, the protection afforded by estrogens according to most reports. A look at the absolute figures in Henderson's paper is even more revealing. The myocardial infarction rate in sedentary women who did not use estrogen was 6.6:1000, while the rate for exercising women who did not use estrogen was 2.6:1000, a decrease of 4:1000. In contrast, nonexercising women who took estrogens had an infarction rate of 3.8:1000; the estrogen worked, but the quantitative change was not as great as with exercise alone. When estrogens were given to exercising women the infarct rate declined further, but only by 0.8:1000, leading to an infarct rate of 1.8:1000.

Exercise alone, exercise plus calcium supplementation, or exercise plus hormone replacement therapy has been shown to decrease bone loss in postmenopausal women,[4-12] and exercise correlates with a decreased incidence of hip fractures.[13-15] These issues are discussed more fully under "Osteoporosis."

Moderate alcohol intake has been shown to reduce cardiovascular mortality in both men and women.[16]

REFERENCES

1. Henderson BE, Paganini-Hill A, Ross RK: Estrogen replacement therapy and protection from acute myocardial infarction, *Am J Obstet Gynecol* 159:312-317, 1988.
2. Rich-Edwards JW, Manson JE, Hennekens C, et al: The primary prevention of coronary heart disease in women, *N Engl J Med* 332:1758-1766, 1995.
3. Kushi LH, Fee RM, Folsom AR, et al: Physical activity and mortality in postmenopausal women, *JAMA* 277:1287-1292, 1997.
4. Reid IR, Ames RW, Evans MC, et al: Effect of calcium supplementation on bone loss in postmenopausal women, *N Engl J Med* 328:460-464, 1993.
5. Reid IR, Ames RW, Evans MC, et al: Long-term effects of calcium supplementation on bone loss and fractures in postmenopausal women: a randomized controlled trial, *Am J Med* 98:331-335, 1995.
6. Dawson-Hughes B, Dallal GE, Krall EA, et al: Controlled trial of the effect of calcium supplementation on bone density in postmenopausal women, *N Engl J Med* 323:878-883, 1990.
7. Aloia JF, Vaswani A, Yeh JK, et al: Calcium supplementation with and without hormone replacement therapy to prevent postmenopausal bone loss, *Ann Intern Med* 120:97-103, 1994.
8. Prince RL, Smith M, Kick IM, et al: Prevention of postmenopausal osteoporosis: a comparative study of exercise, calcium supplementation, and hormone-replacement therapy, *N Engl J Med* 325:1189-1195, 1991.
9. Pocock NA, Eisman JA, Yeates MG, et al: Physical fitness is a major determinant of femoral neck and lumbar spine bone mineral density, *J Clin Invest* 78:618-621, 1986.
10. Simkin A, Ayalon J, Leichter I: Increased trabecular bone density due to bone-loading exercises in postmenopausal osteoporotic women, *Calcif Tissue Int* 40:59-63, 1987.
11. Dalsky GP, Stocke KS, Ehsani AA, et al: Weight-bearing exercise training and lumbar bone mineral content in postmenopausal women, *Ann Intern Med* 108:824-828, 1988.
12. Nelson ME, Fiatarone MA, Morganti CM, et al: Effects of high-intensity strength training on multiple risk factors for osteoporotic fractures: a randomized controlled trial, *JAMA* 272: 1909-1914, 1994.
13. Perez Cano R, Galan Galan F, Dilsen G: Risk factors for hip fracture in Spanish and Turkish women, Bone 14(suppl 1):S69-S72, 1993.
14. Jaglal SB, Kreiger N, Darlington G: Past and recent physical activity and risk of hip fracture, *Am J Epidemiol* 138:107-118, 1993.
15. Paganini-Hill A, Chao A, Ross RK, et al: Exercise and other factors in the prevention of hip fracture: the Leisure World study, *Epidemiology* 2:16-25, 1991.
16. Ashley MF, Room R, Rankin F, et al: Moderate drinking and health: report of an international symposium, *Can Med Assoc J* 151:809-828, 1994.

OVARIES

(See also positive predictive value; prevention; screening)

Ovarian Cancer

Epidemiology

Ovarian cancer is the fifth most common malignancy among women in the United States and is the leading cause of death from gynecological cancers. The overall lifetime risk of acquiring the disease is calculated as 1 in 70 if the patient has no relatives with ovarian cancer.[1,2] Ovarian cancer is predominantly a disease of postmenopausal women in the sixth decade. In 70% of patients the disease is advanced at diagnosis. The most important risk factor is a family history, especially if two or more first-degree relatives are affected. If a woman has one first-degree relative with ovarian cancer, her lifetime risk of the disease is estimated to be about 4% to 5%, and if she has two or more affected relatives with the disease (but does not have a hereditary ovarian cancer syndrome), her lifetime risk is about 5% to 7%.[1,2] Other risk factors are nulliparity and first birth after age 35. However, no evident risk factors are found in most women with the disease. Factors providing some protection are use of oral contraceptives, first birth when the patient is under the age of 25, and breast feeding by the patient. All of these activities inhibit ovulation.

Hereditary ovarian cancer syndromes

Three familial or hereditary ovarian cancer syndromes have been described and together account for about 0.05% (5:10,000) of all cases. They have autosomal dominant inheritance patterns through either the maternal or paternal genes and tend to be diagnosed in younger women. The lifetime risk of ovarian cancer in these women approaches 50%. The syndromes are[1,2]:

1. Site-specific ovarian cancer syndrome
2. Hereditary breast-ovarian cancer syndrome, which is characterized by a predisposition to ovarian and breast cancer
3. Lynch syndrome II, which is characterized by a predisposition to ovarian cancer, endometrial cancer, colon cancer, upper gastrointestinal cancers, and urothelial cancers

Staging

Staging of ovarian cancer is as follows:

Stage I	Limited to one or both ovaries
Stage II	Limited to the pelvis
Stage III	Has spread to the peritoneal cavity
Stage IV	Involves the liver or has spread outside the peritoneal cavity

The 5-year survival rates for stage I are 75% to 80%; for stage II, 60% to 65%; for stage III, 23% to 35%; and for stage IV, less than 10%. Unfortunately, most women are in the more advanced stages at diagnosis.

Screening or case finding

Screening modalities such as regular pelvic examinations, transabdominal or transvaginal sonography, or CA-125 measurement have not been shown to alter the mortality rate of ovarian cancer.[2]

CA-125 is a monoclonal antibody that reacts with an antigen found in serous ovarian adenocarcinomas. The CA-125 level is elevated in 80% of patients with advanced ovarian cancer (mainly the serous variants) but in only 25% to 50% of those with early ovarian cancer. It is not specific for the ovary and may be elevated in some benign conditions such as benign ovarian cysts, endometriosis, menstruation, and pregnancy. It may also be elevated with some breast, lung, and gastrointestinal malignancies.[3]

CA-125 is not a good screening test for the general population. In one large British study of more than 20,000 postmenopausal women, the relative risk of ovarian cancer within 1 year in women with a CA-125 level greater than 30 U/ml was increased 35 fold. The overall sensitivity of the test was 75% at 1 year and 54% at 5 years. However, the positive predictive value was only 3.1%, which means that 96.9% of women who had positive tests did not have development of ovarian cancer but suffered the psychological trauma inherent in false-positive tests. The impact of CA-125 screening on mortality is unknown.[4] Whether this test is useful in women with a strong family history of ovarian cancer is also unknown.

The Canadian Task Force on the Periodic Health Examination advises against using any of these modalities[5] for the general population ("D" recommendations), as do the U.S. Preventive Services Task Force[6] and the American College of Physicians.[7] Patients with family ovarian cancer syndrome need a specialist's care.

Response to chemotherapy is increased if the residual tumor mass is small. Therefore the first stage of treatment is "debulking." The usual chemotherapy regimen involves three to six cycles of cisplatin (Platinol) and cyclophosphamide (Cytoxan) at 3- to 4-week intervals.[8,9] In one recent study paclitaxel (Taxol) plus cisplatin gave a better remission rate than did cyclophosphamide and cisplatin.[10] There are also studies showing that intraperitoneally adminstered cisplatin is more effective than intravenously administered cisplatin.[11]

REFERENCES

1. Carlson K, Skates SJ, Singer DE: Screening for ovarian cancer, *Ann Intern Med* 121:124-132, 1994.
2. NIH Consensus Development Panel on Ovarian Cancer: Ovarian cancer: screening, treatment, and follow-up, *JAMA* 273: 491-497, 1995.
3. Westhoff C, Randall MC: Ovarian cancer screening: potential effect on mortality, *Am J Obstet Gynecol* 165:502-505, 1991.
4. Jacobs IJ, Skates S, Davies AP, et al: Risk of diagnosis of ovarian cancer after raised serum CA 125 concentration: a prospective cohort study, *BMJ* 313:1355-1358, 1996.
5. Canadian Task Force on the Periodic Health Examination: *Clinical preventive health care,* Ottawa, 1994, Canadian Communication Group—Publishing.
6. US Preventive Services Task Force: *Guide to clinical preventive services: an assessment of the effectiveness of 169 interventions,* Baltimore, 1989, Williams & Wilkins, pp 81-85.
7. American College of Physicians: Screening for ovarian cancer; recommendations and rationale, *Ann Intern Med* 121:142-143, 1994.
8. Cannistra S: Cancer of the ovary, *N Engl J Med* 329:1550-1558, 1993.
9. Mann WJ: Diagnosis and management of epithelial cancer of the ovary, *Am Fam Physician* 49:613-618, 1994.
10. McGuire WP, Hoskins WJ, Brady M, et al: Cyclophosphamide and cisplatin compared with paclitaxel and cisplatin in patients with stage III and stage IV ovarian cancer, *N Engl J Med* 334:1-6, 1996.
11. Alberts DS, Liu PY, Hannigan EV, et al: Intraperitoneal cisplatin plus intravenous cyclophosphamide versus intravenous cisplatin plus intravenous cyclophosphamide for stage III ovarian cancer, *N Engl J Med* 335:150-155, 1996.

PELVIC INFLAMMATORY DISEASE

(See also sexually transmitted diseases)

More than 50% of cases of pelvic inflammatory disease (PID) are caused by *Chlamydia trachomatis* or *Neisseria gonorrhoeae.*[1-3] *Mycoplasma hominis* is reported in 5% to 20% of cases, and anaerobes are important pathogens in more severe cases.[3] Mild cases are usually caused by *Chlamydia*, whereas moderately severe cases are caused by *Chlamydia* or gonococci and are often complicated by anaerobic infection. Gonorrhea is more common in patients with an infected sex partner, in street youths, and in sex trade workers. In most parts of North America 5% to 15% of gonococcal isolates are resistant to tetracycline. Both gonococcal and chlamydial infections are more likely to begin during the first half of the menstrual cycle.

The most important clinical criteria for PID according to the Centers for Disease Control and Prevention are lower abdominal tenderness, adnexal tenderness, and cervical motion tenderness.[4] The presence of these three together is sufficient to justify empirical therapy if other diseases have been effectively ruled out.[4] Other important criteria are mucopurulent cervical discharge, increased numbers of leukocytes (10 white blood cells per high-power field) in the cervical discharge,[3] and a temperature greater than 38.3° C (101.8° F).[4] About one third of patients with physical signs of PID do not have laparoscopic evidence of the disease, but many cases would be missed if patients were not treated on the basis of clinical suspicion.

Infertility rates after PID are quoted as being 8% after one episode, 19.5% after two, and 40% after three or more.[5] Other complications are recurrent episodes of PID in 20% to 25% of cases,[6] chronic abdominal pain in 18%,[7] and a two to ten times greater risk of ectopic pregnancies.[8]

Recommendations published in *Medical Letter* for the outpatient treatment of PID are cefoxitin (Mefoxin) 2 g intramuscularly once plus probenecid 1 g po once, or ceftriaxone (Rocephin) 250 mg intramuscularly once, either of which is followed by doxycycline (Vibra-Tabs, Doxycin) 100 mg po bid for 14 days. Alternatives to doxycycline are ofloxacin (Floxin) 400 mg po bid plus metronidazole (Flagyl) 500 mg po bid for 14 days, or clindamycin (Cleocin, Dalacin) 450 mg po qid for 14 days.[1]

REFERENCES

1. Drugs for sexually transmitted diseases, *Med Lett* 37:117-122, 1995.
2. MCormack WM: Pelvic inflammatory disease, *N Engl J Med* 330:115-118, 1994.
3. Megran DW: Treat PID effectively in four simple steps, *Patient Care Can* 6:16-26, 1995.
4. 1993 Sexually transmitted diseases treatment guidelines, *MMWR* 42(RR-14):77, 1993.
5. Westrom L, Joesoef R, Reynolds G, et al: Pelvic inflammatory disease and fertility: a cohort study of 1,844 women with laparoscopically verified disease and 657 control women with normal laparoscopic results, *Sex Transm Dis* 19:185-192, 1992.
6. Soper DE: Diagnosis and laparoscopic grading of acute salpingitis, *Am J Obstet Gynecol* 164(5 Pt 2):1370-1376, 1991.
7. Westrom L: Incidence, prevalence, and trends of acute pelvic inflammatory disease and its consequences in industrialized countries, *Am J Obstet Gynecol* 138(7 Pt 2):880-892, 1980
8. Walker CK, Kahn JG, Washington AE, et al: Pelvic inflammatory disease: meta-analysis of antimicrobial regimen efficacy, *J Infect Dis* 168:969-978, 1993.

PREMENSTRUAL DYSPHORIC DISORDER

The nature or even the existence of the premenstrual syndrome is controversial. This uncertainty is inevitable when more than 150 symptoms of the disorder have been described in the medical literature. Even its nomenclature is in a state of flux. A now obsolete term is "late-luteal-phase dysphoric disorder."[1] In the *Diagnostic and Statistical Manual of Mental Disorders,* edition 4 (DSM-IV), it is called "premenstrual dysphoric disorder."[2]

As might be expected for an entity whose existence is uncertain, the epidemiology of premenstrual syndrome is confusing. Its prevalence rate is reported as anywhere from 2% to 70% of menstruating women. If the syndrome exists, the probable prevalence rate is about 2% to 10%.

Although multiple etiological theories have been proposed, evidence is increasing that this condition is a variant of a mood disorder. In fact, in DSM-IV it is labeled "premenstrual dysphoric disorder" under the broad category "depressive disorders not otherwise specified."[2] The major symptoms are those of classic depression, but they are limited to the premenstrual period. To supply sufficient data as a basis for diagnosis, the patient must prospectively rate her symptoms in a log for at least three cycles because retrospective ratings have proved inaccurate.

For practical purposes, selective serotonin reuptake inhibitor (SSRI) antidepressants, particularly fluoxetine (Prozac) and paroxetine (Paxil), have been the only effective medications.[1,3-6] The usual dose of fluoxetine is 20 to 40 mg/day. Adverse effects with 60 mg/day caused many women to drop out of one study.[5] All the major studies to date have used antidepressants on a daily basis throughout the cycle, but studies on their use only in the late luteal phase are in progress.[5]

A 1995 study of premenstrual syndrome compared placebo, progesterone, and alprazolam (Xanax) given during the luteal phase for three cycles. Dosage was on a flexible schedule. Overall results showed significant improvement in 30% of the placebo group, 29% of the progesterone group, and 37% of the alprazolam group. When the alprazolam group was divided according to doses received, improvement was seen in 50% of those receiving 1.25 mg or less per day compared with only 24% of those receiving higher doses.[7]

Treatments shown to be ineffective include complex diets, large quantities of nutritional supplements, progesterone, synthetic progestins, oral contraceptives, vitamin B, evening primrose oil (gamma-linolenic acid), and bromocriptine.

REFERENCES

1. Robinson G: Determining which patients have premenstrual syndrome, *Can J Diagn* 11:73-81, 1994.
2. American Psychiatric Association: *Diagnostic and statistical manual of mental disorders,* ed 4, Washington, DC, 1994, American Psychiatric Association, pp 715-718.
3. Stone AB, Pearlstein TB, Brown WA: Fluoxetine in the treatment of late luteal phase dysphoric disorder, *J Clin Psychiatry* 52:290-293, 1991.
4. Menkes DB, Taghavi E, Mason PA, et al: Fluoxetine treatment of severe premenstrual syndrome, *BMJ* 305:346-347, 1992.
5. Steiner M, Steinberg S, Stewart D, et al (Canadian Fluoxetine/Premenstrual Dysphoria Collaborative Study Group): Fluoxetine in the treatment of premenstrual dysphoria, *N Engl J Med* 332:1529-1534, 1995.
6. Eriksson E, Hedberg MA, Andersh B, Sundblad C: The serotonin re-uptake inhibitor, paroxetine, is superior to the adrenalin re-uptake inhibitor, maprotiline in the treatment of premenstrual syndrome, *Neuropsychopharmacology* 12:167-176, 1995.
7. Freeman, EW, Rickels K, Sondheimer SJ, Polansky M: A double-blind trial of oral progesterone, alprazolam, and placebo in treatment of severe premenstrual syndrome, *JAMA* 274:51-57, 1995.

VAGINISMUS

Vaginismus is caused by spasm of the levator muscles, which can be detected on pelvic examination (pelvic examination should not be performed if the patient is too frightened to allow it or it is too painful). The essence of treatment is a behavioral one in which the patient is first taught Kegel exercises and then reverse Kegel exercises. The goal of the latter is longer and longer periods of relaxation after the initial contraction. As the patient gains confidence, she may insert one lubricated finger into the vagina to sense the tightening and relaxation of the levators, and with time she may be able to insert two or three fingers. The purpose of finger insertion is not to dilate the vagina manually, which is now an obsolete concept, but to monitor the efficacy of voluntary relaxation of the muscles. Once the patient can accomplish these exercises effectively, she may try coitus in which she is in the superior position.[1]

REFERENCES

1. Lamont JA: Vaginismus: reflex response out of control, *Patient Care Can* 7(2):75-78, 1996.

VAGINITIS AND VULVITIS

(See also drugs and chemicals in pregnancy; inflammatory Papanicolaou smears)

The differential diagnosis of vaginitis should include contact dermatitis of the vulva. This has been reported with Always sanitary napkins.[1]

Candidiasis

Candida is present in the vaginas of one fourth of all women, and at least half of these are asymptomatic. In candidiasis the vaginal pH is usually less than 4.5. Table 29 lists drugs commonly used in the treatment of vaginal yeast infections. Vaginal preparations are available as creams or vaginal tablets. The latter vary in dose; the more potent preparations are generally given for 1 or 3 days and the less potent for a week. Single-dose intravaginal regimens are probably not as effective as longer treatment programs.[2] A single oral dose of 150 mg of fluconazole (Diflucan) is as effective as intravaginal treatments of vulvovaginal candidiasis.[3,4]

When a patient has recurrent vaginal yeast infections, underlying precipitants such as diabetes mellitus, antibiotic use, and HIV infection should be ruled out. In addition, the diagnosis should be reevaluated to make sure some unrelated condition such as vulvar lichen sclerosus et atrophicus has not been misdiagnosed as candidiasis. If the infection is always related to antibiotic therapy, a 3-day course of a vaginal anticandidal preparation or a single oral dose of 150 mg of fluconazole (Diflucan) may be given near or at the end of the antibiotic treatment.[5] Fluconazole may also be particularly useful if relapses are frequent.[6] In this circumstance one dose of 100 or 150 mg per week or per month may be tried.[2] Another option for recurrent infections is to use a vaginal preparation once or twice weekly for prophylaxis. Whether yogurt has any value is doubtful. According to one report the daily oral consumption of 8 ounces of unpasteurized yogurt containing *Lactobacillus acidophilus* decreased the incidence of recurrent vaginal yeast infections.[7] However, placebo-controlled studies have not confirmed the efficacy of this agent.

Table 29 Vaginal Yeast Infections

Generic name	Trade names
Topical Imidazoles	
Clotrimazole	Canesten, Gyne-Lotrimin, Mycelex
Miconazole	Monistat
Terconazole	Terazol
Oral Agents	
Fluconazole	Diflucan

Bacterial Vaginosis

Gardnerella vaginalis is associated with bacterial vaginosis. The cause of this infection is probably polymicrobial, with anaerobes playing a significant role. *G. vaginalis* can be cultured from 50% of women with no symptoms of vaginal disease, so vaginal cultures are not clinically useful.[2] There is no proof that bacterial vaginosis is an STD, and treating the partners is of no value.

Studies have shown that pregnant women with bacterial vaginosis have an increased risk of preterm deliveries[8,9] and that treating the condition in women at high risk of premature delivery with oral erythromycin or metronidazole reduces the risk.[9,10] However, bacterial vaginosis is only one of several risk factors for preterm delivery. Others include a previous history of preterm delivery (a major risk factor), smoking, black race, first pregnancy, and history of previous abortion.[8] Further studies on both high- and low-risk women are needed to determine who if anyone should be screened and treated for bacterial vaginosis in pregnancy.[10] Other reported complications in patients with bacterial vaginosis are an increased incidence of PID after first-trimester abortion, an increased incidence of endometritis after Cesarean section, and an increased rate of vaginal cuff cellulitis after vaginal hysterectomy.[11]

Classic findings in patients with bacterial vaginosis are a fishy odor before or after potassium hydroxide is added to a smear of vaginal secretions, more than 20% clue cells in a wet smear, and a vaginal pH greater than 4.5.[11]

Symptomatic patients should be treated, and in general, asymptomatic patients should not. However, culture studies and treatment of women positive for bacterial vaginosis may be advisable before Cesarean section, first-trimester abortion, or hysterectomy.[11] Three standard treatment modalities for bacterial vaginosis are oral metronidazole, intravaginal metronidazole gel, and intravaginal clindamycin cream. In a comparative study of these three regimens all were equally effective, although patient satisfaction was greatest with the intravaginal products.[12] Specific treatment regimens include metronidazole (Flagyl) tablets 500 mg bid for 7 days or, as an alternative that may be less effective, 2 g as a single dose; 0.75% metronidazole vaginal gel (MetroGel-Vaginal) bid for 5 days; or 2% clindamycin vaginal cream (Cleocin, Dalacin), 1 application qhs for 7 days.[2,11] Clindamycin 300 mg bid po for 7 days is also effective.[11]

Trichomoniasis

Although metronidazole is generally considered to be contraindicated during the first trimester of pregnancy,[2] the evidence for this is tenuous. A metaanalysis of patients exposed to orally administered metronidazole in the first trimester found no increased risk of teratogenicity.[13] The usual treatment of trichomoniasis is 2 g as a single oral dose or 500 mg po bid for 7 days.

REFERENCES

1. Eason EL, Feldman P: Contact dermatitis associated with the use of Always sanitary napkins, *Can Med Assoc J* 154:1173-1176, 1996.
2. Drugs for sexually transmitted diseases, *Med Lett* 37:117-122, 1995.
3. Oral fluconazole for vaginal candidiasis, *Med Lett* 36:81-82, 1994.
4. Sobel JD, Brooker D, Stein GE, et al: Single oral dose fluconazole compared with conventional clotrimazole topical therapy of candidal vaginitis, *Am J Obstet Gynecol* 172:1263-1268, 1995.
5. Steinberg WM: Avoiding recurrent yeast infections, *Patient Care Can* 5:11, 1994.
6. Patel HS, Peters MD 2nd, Smith CL: Is there a role for fluconazole in the treatment of vulvovaginal candidiasis? *Ann Pharmacother* 26:350-353, 1992.
7. Hilton E, Isenberg HD, Alperstein P, et al: Ingestion of yogurt containing *Lactobacillus acidophilus* as prophylaxis for candidal vaginitis, *Ann Intern Med* 116:353-357, 1992.
8. Hillier SL, Nugent RP, Eschenbach DA, et al: Association between bacterial vaginosis and preterm delivery of a low-birth-weight infant, *N Engl J Med* 333:1737-1742, 1995.
9. Hauth JC, Goldenberg RL, Andrews WW, et al: Reduced incidence of preterm delivery with metronidazole and erythromycin in women with bacterial vaginosis, *N Engl J Med* 333:1732-1736, 1995.
10. Hack M, Merkatz IR: Preterm delivery and low birth weight—a dire legacy (editorial), *N Engl J Med* 333:1772-1173, 1995.
11. Society of Obstetricians and Gynaecologists of Canada: Clinical practice guidelines: committee opinion; bacterial vaginosis, *J SOGC* 19(5):528-533, 1997.
12. Ferris DG, Litaker MS, Woodward L, et al: Treatment of bacterial vaginosis—a comparison of oral metronidazole, metronidazole vaginal gel, and clindamycin vaginal cream, *J Fam Pract* 41:443-449, 1995.
13. Burtin P, Taddio A, Ariburnu O, et al: Safety of metronidazole in pregnancy: a meta-analysis, *Am J Obstet Gynecol* 172:525-529, 1995.

HEMATOLOGY

Topics covered in this section

ANEMIA

(See also adverse effects of aspirin; bleeding peptic ulcers; diarrhea and hematochezia in runners; elderly; fecal occult blood screening; hemorrhoids; restless legs syndrome; vitamin B_{12})

Microcytic Anemias

The differential diagnosis of microcytic anemias includes iron deficiency anemia, thalassemia, and the anemia of chronic disease (usually normocytic but microcytic in 20% to 30% of cases). Classic findings of these anemias on laboratory examinations are as follows[1]:

Iron deficiency	Mean corpuscular volume (MCV) usually <80, red blood cell distribution width index (RDW) >15, decreased reticulocytes, decreased ferritin level, elevated iron binding capacity, low serum iron level
Thalassemia	MCV often <70, normal RDW, normal reticulocyte count, target cells in peripheral smear
Anemia of chronic disease	Hemoglobin level usually >90 g/L (9 g/dl), MCV normal or low but >72, ferritin level normal or elevated

Iron deficiency anemias

Sequence of laboratory changes. The usual sequence of changes as iron deficiency develops is the following[1]:

1. Decreased ferritin
2. Decreased MCV
3. Decreased hemoglobin
4. Subjective symptoms (usually when the hemoglobin level reaches 8 g/dl [80 g/L])

Some patients with mild iron deficiency have normal red blood cell indices.[2] The most useful test for diagnosing iron deficiency is the serum ferritin level.[3] In one study of elderly patients, ferritin levels less than 18 μg/L (18 ng/ml) were almost pathognomonic of iron deficiency, while levels above 100 μg/L (100 ng/ml) virtually ruled it out.[4]

Ferritin is an acute-phase reactant that tends to rise in cases of inflammatory or neoplastic disease and is therefore usually elevated in the anemias associated with chronic diseases. Patients with iron deficiency anemias in addition to neoplastic or other chronic disease may have a normal or elevated ferritin level. In such situations a bone marrow examination may be necessary to assess iron stores.

Sources of gastrointestinal bleeding in iron deficiency anemia. Gastrointestinal lesions are a common cause of chronic iron deficiency anemia, although 38% of adults with this condition have no demonstrable gastrointestinal lesions. According to one review, if patients with chronic iron deficiency anemia have specific gastrointestinal symptoms, the physician should first investigate the area suggested by the symptoms, and if a lesion is found, further investigation is not warranted. If no localizing symptoms are present and the patient is old, the most useful initial investigation is a colonoscopy; if a colon lesion is found, upper gastrointestinal endoscopy is not needed.[5] This perspective is not shared by other workers, who have found that the chance of detecting the cause by upper gastrointestinal investigation is three times as great as by lower gastrointestinal assessment.[6,7] However, a case can be made for investigating both the upper and lower intestinal tracts regardless of what is found during the initial procedure. A review of this approach performed for iron deficiency anemia in 89 patients over the age of 60 found that close to half of the 13 with colon cancer also had reasonable upper gastrointestinal causes for their anemia.[8]

Symptoms. Does iron deficiency anemia cause symptoms? The literature on this subject is sparse, and the only community-based study I could find, done by the British Medical Research Council in Wales in the 1960s, was on 20- to 64-year-old women with hemoglobin levels between 8 and 12 g/dl (80 to 120 g/L) as a result of iron deficiency. Symptoms including fatigue, dizziness, and breathlessness did not correlate with levels of hemoglobin, and patients randomly assigned to receive iron therapy experienced no greater subjective improvement than those given placebo.[9] However, hemoglobin levels less than 7.5 g/dl (75 g/L) appear to be related to symptoms including fatigue and shortness of breath, at least in patients undergoing dialysis therapy; erythropoietin significantly relieved symptoms in this group of patients.[10] The message for family physicians is that complaints of fatigue in mildly anemic but otherwise well patients may not be related to the anemia and may not resolve with iron therapy.

Iron therapy. Numerous formulations of oral iron preparations are available for the treatment of iron deficiency anemia. The three major ones are ferrous sulfate, ferrous fumarate, and ferrous gluconate. The amount of elemental iron varies among these products. In general elemental iron makes up 20% to 30% of ferrous sulfate, 30% of ferrous fumarate, and 11% of ferrous gluconate. Doses should be calculated on the basis of elemental iron. For the treatment of iron deficiency anemia, adults usually require elemental iron 100 to 200 mg/day in divided doses, and children 3 mg/kg/day in divided doses.

Upper gastrointestinal tract discomfort, constipation, and sometimes diarrhea are the most frequent adverse effects of iron therapy,[11] and their severity depends on the dose of elemental iron.[12] Methods of minimizing these effects are to take the medication with meals, to increase the dose gradually, and to keep the total daily dose as low as possible.[12] Ferrous gluconate has been said to be tolerated better than ferrous sulfate; this may simply be a dose-related phenomenon. A standard dose of ferrous sulfate is 300 mg tid, which gives a daily dose of elemental iron of approximately 200 mg, whereas 300 mg of ferrous gluconate tid gives approximately 100 mg of elemental iron per day. In general, treatment for iron deficiency anemia should be continued for 4 to 6 months or until the serum ferritin level reaches 50 μg/L (50 ng/ml).[13]

Treatment with iron should cause reticulocytosis to begin within 3 to 5 days. If no such response is seen, the patient is not being compliant or the diagnosis is wrong.[1] Treatment with ferrous sulfate should raise the hemoglobin level by 20 g/L (0.2 g/dl) per day if there is no continued blood loss.[13]

Macrocytic Anemias

The following are some of the more important causes of macrocytic anemia:

1. Vitamin B_{12} deficiency (pernicious anemia)
2. Folate deficiency (often nutritional in elderly; celiac disease in younger patients)
3. Liver disease (alcoholism)
4. Hypothyroidism
5. Myelodysplasia (refractory anemia, sideroblastic anemia)
6. Acute bleeding or hemolysis with reticulocytosis (reticulocytes are larger than mature red blood cells)

Myelodysplasia is a common cause of macrocytic anemia in the elderly and usually has little clinical import; in a few cases the condition progresses to leukemia, aplastic anemia, neutropenia, or thrombocytopenia.

Megaloblastic anemias often have oval macrocytosis and an MCV greater than 115 fL (μm^3). In chronic liver disease the macrocytosis is generally between 100 and 110 fL and oval macrocytes are not seen in the peripheral smear.[1]

REFERENCES

1. Yeo EL: Anemia: a practical approach, *Can J Diagn* 13:79-92, 1996.
2. Macdonald D: How to recognize real deficiencies of iron, folate, vitamin B_{12}, *Patient Care Can* 7:6, 1996.
3. Guyatt GH, Oxman AD, Ali M, et al: Laboratory diagnosis of iron-deficiency anemia: an overview, *J Gen Intern Med* 7:145-153, 1992.
4. Guyatt GH, Patterson C, Ali M, et al: Diagnosis of iron-deficiency anemia in the elderly, *Am J Med* 88:205-209, 1990.
5. Rockey DC, Cello JP: Evaluation of the gastrointestinal tract in patients with iron-deficiency anemia, *N Engl J Med* 329:1691-1696, 1993.
6. Calvey HD, Castleden CM: Gastrointestinal investigations for anaemia in the elderly: a prospective study, *Age Aging* 16:399-404, 1987.

7. Ward MC, Gundroo D, Bailey RJ: Effect of investigation on the management of elderly patients with iron deficiency anemia, *Age Aging* 19:204-206, 1990.
8. Till SH, Grundman MJ: Prevalence of concomitant disease in patients with iron deficiency anaemia, *BMJ* 314:206-208, 1997.
9. Elwood P, Water WE, Greene WJ, et al: Symptoms and circulating haemoglobin level, *J Chronic Dis* 21:615-628, 1969.
10. Canadian Erythropoietin Study Group: Association between recombinant human erythropoietin and quallity of life and excercise capacity of patients receiving hemodialysis, *BMJ* 300:573-578, 1990.
11. Swerdlow PS: A tradition of testing ironclad practices (editorial), *JAMA* 267:560-561, 1992.
12. Wingard RL, Parker RA, Ismail N, et al: Efficacy of oral iron therapy in patients receiving recombinant human erythropoietin, *Am J Kidney Dis* 25:433-439, 1995.
13. Swain RA, Kaplan B, Montgomery E: Iron deficiency anemia: when is parenteral therapy warranted? *Postgrad Med* 100:181-182, 185, 188-193, 1996.

ANTICOAGULANTS

(See also atrial fibrillation; myocardial infarction; thrombophlebitis; prosthetic valves; cerebrovascular accidents; transient ischemic attacks)

A portable prothrombin time monitor that uses fingerprick capillary blood has been marketed in the United States (Coumatrack, DuPont Pharmaceutical Co., Wilmington, Delaware). A study of 20 patients who used this device for about 4 years and modified their own medication doses found that these patients maintained better therapeutic ranges of prothrombin time (PT) than did control subjects whose PT levels were monitored in the traditional way.[1]

Both diet and drugs can influence warfarin (Coumadin) levels.[2,3] Vitamin K, which is found predominantly in green leafy vegetables and certain legumes, antagonizes the action of warfarin. Thus if persons taking warfarin suddenly increase their intake of vegetables such as avocados, broccoli, Brussels sprouts, or lettuce, their international normalized ratio (INR) levels may drop. Conversely, if they normally eat a lot of these vegetables and suddenly decrease the intake of these products, their INR levels may rise.[2]

Many drugs potentiate or antagonize the effects of warfarin. Some of the more common agents that tend to increase the INR are erythromycin, metronidazole (Flagyl), isoniazid, some nonsteroidal antiinflammatory drugs, cimetidine (Tagamet), and omeprazole (Prilosec, Losec). Drugs that tend to lower the INR include barbiturates, carbamazepine (Tegretol), chlordiazepoxide (Librium), cholestyramine (Questran), and sucralfate (Sulcrate).[3]

Desirable levels of INR for patients taking warfarin are shown in Table 30. Approximate INR-PT ratios are listed in Table 31.

If a patient is to receive anticoagulatants as an outpatient, one common method is to start with warfarin 10 mg/day for 2 to 4 days controlled by frequent INR or PT readings. Effective anticoagulation is achieved almost as quickly and with less

Table 30 Desirable Levels of INR for Anticoagulation with Warfarin

Desirable INR level	Clinical condition
0.8-1.2	Normal
2.1-3*	All other conditions including mechanical heart valves[4] (some authors recommend that for mechanical heart valves the levels be 2.5 to 3.5[5])

INR, International normalized ratio.
*As indicated, the therapeutic levels of warfarin for most conditions, including atrial fibrillation, are those that maintain an INR of 2 to 3. This is roughly equivalent to a prothrombin time ratio of 1.3 to 1.5.

Table 31 Approximate INR–Prothrombin Time Equivalencies

INR	Prothrombin time ratio
2	1.3
3	1.5
4	2.0

INR, International normalized ratio.

risk if 5 mg of warfarin is used from the beginning of treatment.[6] Traditionally, initial INR readings have been obtained daily; this is illogical because the full effect of a change in a warfarin dose does not manifest itself for 36 to 72 hours.[7] A better system is to begin measuring the INR on day 2 and continue with readings every 48 hours until control is achieved. Thereafter the intervals between INR readings are increased.[8]

If a patient is found to have an elevated INR and is not bleeding, administration of parenteral vitamin K is unnecessary. Temporarily withholding warfarin and then lowering the dose is safe.[9]

REFERENCES

1. Ansell JE, Patel N, Ostrovsky D, et al: Long-term patient self-management of oral anticoagulation, *Arch Intern Med* 155:2185-2189, 1995.
2. Macdonald D: Advice on diet, anticoagulation, *Patient Care Can* 7:18, 1996.
3. Wells PS, Holbrook AM, Crowther NR, et al: Interactions of warfarin with drugs and food, *Ann Intern Med* 121:676-683, 1994.
4. Saour JN, Sieck JO, Mamo LA, et al: Trial of different intensities of anticoagulation in patients with prosthetic heart valves, *N Engl J Med* 322:428-432, 1990.
5. Hirsh J, Dalen JE, Deykin D, et al: Oral anticoagulants: mechanism of action, clinical effectiveness and optimal therapeutic range, *Chest* 102(suppl):312S-326S, 1992.
6. Lamb GC: Loading dose of warfarin, *JAMA* 277:1196, 1997.
7. Brigden ML: Oral anticoagulant therapy, newer indications and an improved method of monitoring, *Postgrad Med* 91:285-296, 1992.
8. Hanna MM, Meuser J: Time to change: rationalizing the daily PT, daily Coumadin order, *Can Fam Physician* 42:513, 1996.
9. Glover JJ: Conservative treatment of overanticoagulated patients, *Chest* 108:987-990, 1995.

BLEEDING DISORDERS

Bleeding disorders are suspected on the basis of personal and family history and confirmed by laboratory tests. Standard investigations are a complete blood count and smear, PT, partial thromboplastin time (PTT), thrombin time or fibrinogen level, and bleeding time.[1]

Hemophilia

Two types of hemophilia are recognized. The classic form, or hemophilia type A, is caused by factor VIII deficiency, and the type B form, or Christmas disease, is caused by factor IX deficiency. Between 80% and 85% of cases are type A. Laboratory tests show a prolonged PTT and a normal PT and bleeding time. Both variants of the disease are sex-linked recessive. For optimal treatment of bleeding episodes, therapy should be initiated at the immediate onset of each incident. This is best done with home therapy in which the parents are trained to give replacement therapy preparations. The effective organization of such a program usually requires a specialized team.[2]

Von Willebrand's disease

Von Willebrand's disease is the most common inherited coagulopathy with an incidence of about 1%. It is caused by an abnormality or reduction of von Willebrand's factor, which has the dual function of stabilizing factor VIII levels and promoting normal platelet functioning. The disease has an autosomal dominant inheritance, and most cases are mild. Bruising, nosebleeds, profuse bleeding from cuts, and hemorrhage after dental extractions are common, but hemarthroses are rare. When hemarthroses do occur, the bleeding begins immediately, whereas with coagulation defects such as hemophilia it is often delayed 12 to 24 hours. Classically the bleeding time is prolonged, and levels of factor VIII and von Willebrand factor are low. Repeated testing may be required to detect these abnormalities.[1,2]

REFERENCES

1. Hampton KK, Preston FE: ABC of clinical haematology: bleeding disorders, thrombosis and anticoagulation, *BMJ* 314:1026-1029, 1997.
2. Association of Hemophilia Clinic Directors of Canada: Hemophilia and von Willebrand's disease. 1. Diagnosis, comprehensive care and assessment, *Can Med Assoc J* 153:19-25, 1995.

LEUKEMIAS

Childhood Leukemias

Acute lymphoblastic leukemia (ALL) is five times as common as acute myeloid leukemia (AML) in children.[1] ALL accounts for 85% of childhood leukemias, and the peak age of incidence is 3 to 4 years.[2] Although claims have been made that long-term exposure to magnetic fields from high-tension power lines is a risk factor, a large case-control study failed to find such a correlation.[3] The cure rate for ALL is about 70%, whereas that for AML is 30% to 40%. The risk of second cancers in cured children is about seven times that in control children who have not had leukemia. Cranial irradiation has particularly serious sequelae; the incidence of brain tumors is markedly increased, and many children are short and obese and have neuropsychiatric disorders. Chemotherapy alone has relatively little adverse effect on growth and development.[1]

Chronic Lymphocytic Leukemia

The median age of persons with chronic lymphocytic leukemia (CLL) is 65 years, and only 10% to 15% of patients are younger than 50. The prognosis of CLL is variable. The median survival is 9 years. Patients with early stable disease do not require treatment. When the disease is more advanced, chlorambucil is usually the drug of first choice.[4]

Chronic Myeloid Leukemia

Chronic myeloid leukemia usually affects adults between the ages of 40 and 60 years. After an initial stable phase lasting a number of years, the disease progresses gradually or suddenly to an acute blastic phase. The average survival time after diagnosis is 5 to 6 years, but the range is considerable. The chronic phase is usually treated with interferon, although bone marrow transplant may be considered for a few patients. About 30% of patients in the advanced phase revert to the chronic phase after treatment with hydroxyurea (Hydrea) or busulphan (Myleran).[5]

REFERENCES

1. Pui C-H: Childhood leukemias, *N Engl J Med* 332:1618-1630, 1995.
2. Liesner RJ, Goldstone AH: The acute leukaemias, *BMJ* 314: 733-736, 1997.
3. Linet MS, Hatch EE, Kleinerman RA, et al: Residential exposure to magnetic fields and acute lymphoblastic leukemia in children, *N Engl J Med* 337:1-7, 1997.
4. Rozman C, Montserrat E: Chronic lymphocytic leukemia, *N Engl J Med* 333:1052-1057, 1995.
5. Goldman J: Chronic myeloid leukaemia, *BMJ* 314:657-660, 1997.

LYMPHOMAS

The Ann Arbor staging system for lymphomas is as follows[1]:

Stage I	Single lymphoid or extranodal site
Stage II	Two lymphoid or extranodal sites on the same side of the diaphragm
Stage III	Lymphoid areas (including spleen) on both sides of the diaphragm
Stage IV	Diffuse involvement of extranodal organs (e.g., bone marrow, liver)

Symptoms of lymphomas are categorized as A if the patient has no systemic symptoms or B if the patient has weight loss, fever, or drenching night sweats.[1]

Hodgkin's Disease

Localized Hodgkin's disease is generally treated with radiation therapy, and more widespread disease with chemotherapy. The overall cure rate is 70% to 80%.[1]

Second tumors are common among children treated for Hodgkin's disease.[1-3] In one study the cumulative risk was 7% by 15 years.[1] The incidence of leukemia reached a plateau by 14 years, but such a leveling off was not seen with solid tumors. Breast cancer was the most common solid tumor, with a relative risk 75 times that of the normal population. The risk was related to radiation and was greatest in girls treated between the ages of 10 and 16 (when breast tissue was proliferating). Other solid tumors were thyroid cancers, basal cell carcinomas of the skin, brain tumors, bone tumors, and colorectal cancers.[1-3]

Non-Hodgkin's Lymphoma

Low-grade non-Hodgkin's lymphoma is a disease of the elderly. Ninety percent of patients are over the age of 50. Most of the follicular lymphomas fall into the non-Hodgkin's lymphoma group. These neoplasms have a similar epidemiology and natural course to chronic lymphocytic leukemia. The tumors are often widespread but indolent with slow progression over many years. The median survival is 5 to 8 years, and cure is rarely possible. Patients without symptoms do not necessarily require treatment. As the disease progresses, chemotherapy may be offered, often in the form of chlorambucil (Leukeran) with or without steroids.[1]

Intermediate-grade non-Hodgkin's lymphoma affects all age groups. The most common form is a diffuse large cell lymphoma that is a B cell neoplasm. These tumors are rapidly progressive, are often associated with type B symptoms, and require therapy. The cure rate is about 40%.[1]

High-grade non-Hodgkin's lymphomas make up only 5% of the non-Hodgkin's lymphomas. The high-grade form is primarily a disease of children and young adults.[1] The cure rate for non-Hodgkin's lymphoma in children is about 70%.[4]

REFERENCES

1. Mead GM: ABC of clinical haematology: malignant lymphomas and chronic lymphocytic leukaemia, *BMJ* 314:1103-1106, 1997.
2. Bhatia S, Robison LL, Oberlin O, et al: Breast cancer and other second neoplasms after childhood Hodgkin's disease, *N Engl J Med* 334:745-751, 1996.
3. Donaldson SS, Hancock SL: Second cancers after Hodgkin's disease in childhood (editorial), *N Engl J Med* 334:792-793, 1996.
4. Sandlund JT, Downing JR, Crist WM: Non-Hodgkin's lymphoma in childhood, *N Engl J Med* 334:1238-1248, 1996.

MULTIPLE MYELOMA

(See also bisphosphonates for bone pain)

In multiple myeloma the neoplastic plasma cells may grow diffusely in the bone marrow or, less commonly, form neoplastic tumors within the bone. They generally produce monoclonal peaks of IgG or IgA. The tumor induces osteoclastic activity, which results in diffuse osteoporosis, lytic lesions, and fractures. Bone pain is the initial complaint of about 60% of patients, and lassitude is another important symptom. The latter is thought to be due to anemia, hypercalcemia, or dehydration. Dehydration is a frequent complication of the disease and is due to proximal tubular dysfunction caused by damage from light chain excretion. Bacterial infections are common.[1,2]

Frequent laboratory abnormalities include normocytic anemia, elevated creatinine and calcium levels, and the presence of monoclonal bands (paraproteins) as determined by electrophoretic evaluations of blood or urine. Both blood and urine should be assessed for paraproteins, since monoclonal immunoglobulins are detectable in the blood of only 80% of patients.[1] Bone scans are often negative in multiple myeloma. This is because the lesions are predominantly lytic and new bone formation is necessary for a bone scan to be positive.[3]

A major differential diagnosis of patients with serum M-protein peaks and no symptoms, signs, or other laboratory abnormalities suggesting multiple myeloma is benign monoclonal gammopathy or monoclonal gammopathy of undetermined significance (MGUS).[1,2] Monoclonal gammopathy of undetermined significance is characterized by an M-protein level less than 3 g/dl (30 g/L) that stays stable over time, less than 10% plasma cells in the bone marrow, no or very little M-protein in the urine (Bence Jones proteinuria), and absence of other clinical or laboratory findings typical of multiple myeloma. A 20- to 35-year follow-up of 241 patients with MGUS at the Mayo Clinic found that serious hematological disorders developed in one fourth of the patients (multiple myeloma in most cases, but also Waldenström's macroglobulinemia and other lymphoproliferative disorders) after a median follow-up of 22 years. The actuarial rate of the development of hematological malignancies was 17% after 10 years and 33% after 20 years. Patients with MGUS require no treatment but should have follow-up examinations at regular intervals.[4]

Patients experience considerable anxiety when told they have something wrong with their plasma cells that is not really serious but could become cancer after many years. The physician should not look for M-proteins without a good reason to suspect that the patient has multiple myeloma.

The standard treatment of myeloma depends on the symptoms and laboratory findings. Patients who are asymptomatic and who do not have significant anemia, renal failure, or severe bone lesions on x-ray examination are classified as having "smoldering" disease that may be followed without treatment. Other patients are treated with a high fluid intake of 3 L/day plus a chemotherapy regimen. The traditional regimen is melphalan (Alkeran) plus prednisone. Other protocols include combinations of multiple chemotherapeutic agents.[1,2]

Berenson and associates[5] in a study of patients with multiple myeloma who had at least one lytic bone lesion reported that 90 mg of pamidronate (Aredia) given as an IV infusion over 4 hours every 4 weeks for nine cycles decreased pain significantly compared with control subjects. Few adverse effects were reported.

REFERENCES

1. MacLennan IC, Drayson M, Dunn J: Multiple myeloma, *BMJ* 308:1033-1036, 1994.
2. Bataille R, Harousseau J-L: Multiple myeloma, *N Engl J Med* 336:1657-1664, 1997.
3. Jacobson AF: Musculoskeletal pain as an indicator of occult malignancy: yield of bone scintigraphy, *Arch Intern Med* 157:105-109, 1997.
4. Kyle RA: Monoclonal gammopathy of undetermined significance, *Blood Rev* 8:135-141, 1994.
5. Berenson JR, Lichtenstein A, Porter L, et al (Myeloma Aredia Study Group): Efficacy of pamidronate in reducing skeletal events in patients with advanced multiple myeloma, *N Engl J Med* 334:529-530, 1996.

SEDIMENTATION RATE

(See also laboratory investigations for connective tissue diseases; polymyalgia rheumatica)

Various reference values have been proposed for the upper limits of normal for sedimentation rates (Westergren method). Higher normal ranges are usually between 20 and 30 mm/hr. The sedimentation rate rises with age and is higher in women than men. It is also increased by anemia, pregnancy, obesity, and renal failure. Most cases of elevated sedimentation rates are not associated with significant disease, and these elevations may persist for prolonged periods.[1]

The sedimentation rate is not an appropriate screening test for asymptomatic individuals and is rarely of value in identifying serious disease in patients with nonspecific symptoms. Diseases in which measuring the sedimentation rate is useful in establishing the diagnosis are polymyalgia rheumatica (although close to one fourth of such patients may have normal values[2]) and temporal arteritis. It may also be helpful in following the course of these diseases but is not as reliable for this as is the clinical evaluation. It may be useful for following the course of rheumatoid arthritis and plays a role in determining the prognosis of Hodgkin's disease.[1]

REFERENCES

1. Zlonis M: The mystique of the erythrocyte sedimentation rate: a reappraisal of one of the oldest laboratory tests still in use, *Clin Lab Med* 13:787-800, 1993.
2. Helfgott SM, Kieval RI: Polymyalgia rheumatica in patients with a normal erythrocyte sedimentation rate, *Arthritis Rheum* 39:304-307, 1996.

THROMBOCYTOPENIA

A low platelet count as reported by an automated counter may be an artifact caused by platelet clumping. This is easily determined by ordering a smear. If present, the platelet clumps will be seen.[1]

Immune thrombocytopenic purpura (ITP), which is also called idiopathic thrombocytopenic purpura, may occur as an acute (acute ITP) or chronic (chronic ITP) disorder. The chronic form is more common in adults and is often detected incidentally when a low platelet count is reported in a complete blood count.[1,2] Splenomegaly is rare.[2] About three fourths of adult cases are in women, and most are in persons under 40.[2] The prognosis for adult cases is excellent.[3]

A harmless, self-limited form of thrombocytopenia is incidental thrombocytopenia of pregnancy. It occurs in the third trimester and does not cause maternal or fetal bleeding.[1]

Other causes of thrombocytopenia include drugs, some viral infections, hypersplenism, thrombotic thrombocytopenic purpura, autoimmune diseases such as lupus, lymphoproliferative disorders, and myelodysplasia.[2]

Bleeding after trauma or surgery may occur with platelet counts less than 50×10^9/L (50,000/mm^3), and serious spontaneous bleeding develops at levels less than 20×10^9 (20,000/mm^3).[1] Massive gastrointestinal bleeding and intracerebral bleeding are most often seen with levels less than 5×10^9/L (5000/mm^3).[4]

Treatment of chronic ITP is necessary only if the platelet count decreases to dangerous levels, which are somewhere around 20 to 30×10^9/L (20,000 to 30,000/mm^3). Prednisone at a dose of 1 mg/kg is the first line of therapy. Some patients require a splenectomy.[2] Nonbleeding patients rarely require platelet transfusions if the counts are above 5×10^9/L (5000/mm^3).[4]

A patient with thrombocytopenia must never be given aspirin.[4]

REFERENCES

1. Goldstein KH, Abramson N: Efficient diagnosis of thrombocytopenia, *Am Fam Physician* 53:915-920, 1996.
2. George JN, el-Harake MA, Raskob GE: Chronic idiopathic thrombocytopenic purpura, *N Engl J Med* 331:1207-1211, 1994.
3. Kirchner JT: Acute and chronic immune thrombocytopenic purpura: disorders that differ in more than duration, *Postgrad Med* 92:112-118, 125-126, 1992.
4. Beutler E: Platelet transfusion: the 20,000/microL trigger, *Blood* 81:1411-1413, 1993.

TRANSFUSIONS

A 1996 paper calculated that in the United States the risk of acquiring viral infections from transfusions was 1:493,000 for HIV, 1:103,000 for hepatitis C, and 1:63,000 for hepatitis B. The authors stated that the rates should decrease as newer screening tests shorten the window periods of these diseases.[1] This has indeed happened, and as of 1997 a revised estimate for HIV-1 is 1:641,000.[2] In looking at risk figures such as this, the practitioner must be aware of the variation in risk between urban and rural areas. In one Canadian study the risk of HIV transmission from a single unit of blood in a large urban area (Montreal) was calculated to be about 1:400,000, whereas for Canada as a whole it was assessed as about 1:1,000,000.[3]

Since erythropoietin was synthesized by recombinant DNA technology, it has become commercially available for subcutaneous or IV use in the form of epoetin alfa (Epogen, Procrit, Eprex). It has numerous uses, including short courses for patients before elective surgery either alone or in combination with autologous blood transfusions.[4]

REFERENCES

1. Schreiber GB, Busch MP, Kleinman SH, Korelitz JJ (Retrovirus Epidemiology Donor Study): The risk of transfusion-transmitted viral infections, *N Engl J Med* 334:1685-1690, 1996.
2. Guidelines for red blood cell and plasma transfusion for adults and children: report of the Expert Working Group, *Can Med Assoc J* 156(suppl 11):S1-S24, 1997.
3. Remis RS, Delage G, Palmer RW: Risk of HIV infection from blood transfusion in Montreal, *Can Med Assoc J* 157:375-382, 1997.
4. Goodnough LT, Monk TG, Andriole GL: Erythropoietin therapy, *N Engl J Med* 336:933-938, 1997.

VITAMIN B_{12}

(See also macrocytic anemia)

Serum vitamin B_{12} is frequently measured in patients with dementia on the grounds that a deficiency is a remediable cause of that disorder. An evaluation of nondemented persons 75 to 85 years of age revealed that low vitamin B_{12} levels were common in this age group but that persons with these findings were no more likely to become demented than were those with normal levels.[1]

REFERENCES

1. Crystal HA, Ortof E, Frishman WH, et al: Serum vitamin B-12 levels and incidence of dementia in a healthy elderly population—a report from the Bronx longitudinal aging study, *J Am Geriatr Soc* 42:933-936, 1994.

IMMUNIZATIONS

(See also *Haemophilus* B; hepatitis A; hepatitis B; infectious diseases; meningococcal disease; pediatrics; tropical medicine)

Topics covered in this section

Storage and Shipping of Vaccines
Immunization Schedules for Children
Haemophilus b
Hepatitis B
Influenza
Measles-Mumps-Rubella Vaccine
Pertussis Vaccine
Pneumococcal Vaccine
Polio Vaccines
Rubella
Tetanus Immunization
Typhoid Fever
Rabies
Varicella Vaccine

STORAGE AND SHIPPING OF VACCINES

Many vaccines can be inactivated if they are exposed to high temperatures or if they are frozen. The jargon for the former phenomenon is "breaking the cold chain." Vaccine inactivation through breaking the cold chain probably occurs frequently in physicians' offices and may also occur during shipping, especially to remote regions. Apparently the Sabin oral polio vaccine can be frozen and thawed without affecting its potency. Some of the specific recommendations for maintaining the cold chain are as follows[1]:

1. Most vaccines should be stored between 2° and 8° C.
2. Refrigerators containing vaccines should have temperature monitors.
3. Refrigerators containing vaccines should not be used for other purposes.
4. The temperature in the refrigerator should be monitored and recorded twice a day.
5. Only vaccines should be kept in the refrigerator; food should be in another refrigerator so that temperature variations from frequent opening and closing of the door are avoided.
6. Vaccines should not be kept in the door of the refrigerator.
7. There should be space between vaccine vials to allow air circulation.
8. Vaccines should be removed from the refrigerator only to draw up a dose and should be returned to the refrigerator immediately.

REFERENCES

1. Laboratory Centre For Disease Control: National guidelines for vaccine storage and transportation, *Can Med Assoc J* 154:3534-3554, 1996.

IMMUNIZATION SCHEDULES FOR CHILDREN

(See also *Haemophilus* b; hepatitis A; hepatitis B; measles-mumps-rubella vaccine; pertussis; polio vaccines; tetanus immunization; typhoid fever; rabies; varicella)

The recommended immunization schedules for children in Canada and the United States differ in only minor details, many of which involve the exact timing of booster doses.[1,2] In 1994 three organizations in the United States came out with common recommendations for childhood immunizations.[2] These organizations are the Advisory Committee on Immunization Practices, the American Academy of Family Physicians, and the American Academy of Pediatrics. Updates are made regularly. Some of the U.S. recommendations and the way they differ from Canadian recommendations are as follows[2]:

1. Hepatitis B immunizations. For infants born to hepatitis B surface antigen (HBsAg)-negative mothers, three vaccinations are recommended, the first at birth if possible, the second between 1 and 4 months (at least 1 month after the first dose), and the third at least 2 months after the second but not before 6 months of age.

In Canada hepatitis B immunization is usually given to children of HBsAg-negative mothers in elementary school because the risk of acquiring the infection becomes significant only in adolescence and because of concern that immunizations given in infancy may not be fully effective by the time the child passes through puberty.

2. Diphtheria-tetanus-pertussis (DTP) or diphtheria–tetanus–acellular pertussis (DtaP). The fourth dose may be given anytime between 15 and 18 months. In Canada it is given at 18 months. In the United States and Canada, DTaP is preferred to DTP. It is available under the trade names Acel-Imune Infantrix or Tripedia. If a series was started with DTP, it may be completed with DTaP.
3. Booster tetanus-diphtheria toxoid (Td). The booster Td dose may be given anytime between 11 and 16 years. In Canada it is given between 14 and 16 years.
4. *Haemophilus influenzae* type b (Hib). The three Hib vaccines licensed for infant vaccinations in the United States are considered interchangeable. If immunization is started with one brand, a different one may be used for booster doses.
5. Measles-mumps-rubella (MMR). An initial MMR dose may be given anytime between 12 and 15 months, and a second dose is recommended between 4 and 6 years. In Canada the initial dose is given at 12 months and (as of 1996) a second dose is recommended at 18 months or 4 to 6 years plus a catch-up reimmunization program with either MMR or single-antigen measles vaccine for all primary and secondary school students.
6. Polio. U.S. recommendations include any one of three protocols involving inactivated polio vaccine (IPV) for all doses, oral polio vaccine (OPV) for all doses, or IPV for the initial two doses and OPV for subsequent doses.
7. Varicella. Varicella immunization is recommended as a routine vaccination of children between the ages of 12 and 18 months, preferably at the time of the MMR injection. If a child has not been immunized at this age and does not have a reliable history of chickenpox, he or she should be immunized between 11 and 12 years of age, although the vaccine can be given anytime after the age of 12 months. Varicella vaccination is not recommended as a routine immunization in Canada.

Adolescents who have not had or completed a primary series of vaccinations may need catch-up immunizations. This is ideally done at the 11- or 12-year-old checkup when Td is given.[2]

REFERENCES

1. *Canadian immunization guide,* ed 4, Ottawa, 1993, Minister of Supply and Services Canada.
2. Centers for Disease Control and Prevention: Recommended childhood immunization schedule—United States, 1988, *JAMA* 279:495-496, 1998.

HAEMOPHILUS b

(See also immunization schedules for children)

Until the introduction of immunization programs, *Haemophilus influenzae* type b (Hib) was the most common cause of bacterial meningitis in infants and young children. The case-fatality rate for meningitis was about 5%. Severe neurological sequelae occurred in 10% to 15% of survivors and deafness in 20%. Other diseases caused by Hib are acute epiglottitis, pneumonia, bacteremia, cellulitis, and septic arthritis.[1]

A variety of Hib conjugated vaccines are available in the United States and Canada, including Hib TITER, Pedvax-HIB, ProHIBiT, and Act HIB. Hib TITER is available in combination with DTP under the trade name TETRAMUNE, Act HIB is available in Canada in combination with DPT and polio vaccines as Penta,[2] and PedvaxHIB is available in combination with the hepatitis B vaccine Recombivax HB as COMVAX.[3] ProHIBiT, which is available in the United States, is used as a single injection without boosters in children 15 months or older.

The recommended schedules for the different vaccine brands vary somewhat. After 18 months of age nonimmunized children require only one dose of Hib vaccine for adequate protection.[1]

Rifampin prophylaxis is not required for contacts of Hib infection who are over the age of 5 years or for those under 5 if all contacts under 5 have been adequately immunized for their age. If one or more contacts under the age of 5 have not been adequately immunized for age or are immunocompromised, rifampin prophylaxis should be given to everyone in the family or day care group.

The usual regimen for prophylaxis against Hib infections is a 4-day course of 600 mg q12h for adults, 20 mg/kg/day in 2 divided doses for children over the age of 1 month, and 10 mg/kg/day in 2 divided doses for children under the age of 1 month.

REFERENCES

1. *Canadian immunization guide,* ed 4, Ottawa, 1993, Minister of Supply and Services Canada.
2. Supplementary statement on newly licensed *Haemophilus influenzae* type B (HIB) conjugated vaccines in combination with other vaccines recommended for infants. From Canada Communicable Disease Report 20:157-160, 1994, *Can Med Assoc J* 152:527-529, 1995.
3. Centers for Disease Control and Prevention: FDA approval for infants of a *Haemophilus influenzae* type b conjugate and hepatitis B (recombinant) combined vaccine, *JAMA* 277:620-621, 1997.

HEPATITIS B

(See also immunization schedules for children)

Primary Immunization

Two recombinant DNA hepatitis B vaccines are available in Canada and the United States (Recombivax HB and Engerix-B), and a combined hepatitis B–*Haemophilus* b vaccine

(Comvax) is available in the United States. Comvax is a combination of the Hib conjugated vaccine Pedvax HIB and the Hib recombinant vaccine Recombivax HB (see immunization schedules for children).[1]

The two hepatitis B (HB) vaccines Recombivax HB and Engerix-B can be used interchangeably. Boosters should be given 1 and 6 months after the primary dose. If the schedule is interrupted, it can be taken up again where it was left off. The third dose is always given 3 to 5 months after the second dose. The dosage should be checked for each product and varies with age. Injections are given intramuscularly into the deltoid of adults and into the anterolateral thigh of children. Gluteal injections should be avoided because in this location the vaccine may be inadvertently deposited in the fat, resulting in lower effectiveness.[2] Comvax should be given at 2, 4, and 12 to 15 months and should not be given before 6 weeks.[1] Evaluation of antibody and antigen status before immunization against HB is not necessary.

Response rates to HB immunization vary with age. For those under 2 years it is 95%, for those 2 to 19 it is 99%, and for those over the age of 60 it is 50% to 75%.[2] Protection against both clinical disease and the carrier state has been documented to persist for 10 years, but whether such immunity will persist for longer periods is unknown. Response rates are lower in immunocompromised persons. Booster doses for these patients are not recommended, even if measured titers are low.[2]

In Canada routine immunization of children against HB is generally recommended during the elementary school years. In the United States immunization is usually given in early childhood (see immunization schedules for children).[2]

Postexposure Prophylaxis for Hepatitis B

All pregnant women should be screened for hepatitis B surface antigen (HBsAg). If a pregnant woman is HBsAg negative but her partner is a hepatitis B carrier, the pregnant woman should be immunized. The risks to the baby from immunization are far outweighed by the risks of acquiring hepatitis B if the mother is not immunized. Infants born to HBsAg-positive mothers should receive 0.5 ml hepatitis B immunoglobulin (HBIG) at birth plus a course of active immunization. If the mother is identified as a carrier after the infant is 7 days old, only active immunization is given.[2]

Sexual contacts of a person with acute hepatitis B should receive HBIG and active immunization. Household contacts need not be immunized except for infants under 1 year of age when the index case is the caretaker. HBIG in doses of 0.06 ml/kg and active immunization can be given at the same time but at different sites. HBIG (HyperHep, H-BIG) is indicated if given within 14 days of exposure. Administering it within 48 hours is most desirable. The efficacy decreases with time, and no reliable data have shown efficacy after 7 days.[2] Sexual and household contacts of chronic carriers should be immunized.[2]

If a health care worker is subject to a percutaneous or mucosal exposure to blood or other body fluids, the risk level for hepatitis B and the HBsAg status of the patient involved should be determined, as well as the anti–hepatitis B surface antigen (anti-HBs) level of the exposed health care worker. It is safe to wait up to 48 hours for the results of anti-HBs levels before deciding on a course of action. If the patient is HBsAg negative, the health care worker needs no immediate treatment but should receive a full vaccination course to avoid future risks. If the patient's HBsAg status cannot be determined but he or she is known to be at low risk, treating the exposed health care worker is not usually necessary.[3] If the patient is at high risk or is known to be HBsAg positive and the anti-HBs level of the health care worker is unknown or is less than 10 IU/L, the health care worker should receive one dose of HBIG immediately and start a full three-dose vaccination course. Complete protocols covering a variety of permutations should be consulted as necessary.[2]

REFERENCES

1. Centers for Disease Control and Prevention: FDA approval for infants of a *Haemophilus influenzae* type b conjugate and hepatitis B (recombinant) combined vaccine, *JAMA* 277:620-621, 1997.
2. Centers for Disease Control and Prevention: Report of the Hepatitis B Working Group, *Can Med Assoc J* 151:1294-1297, 1994.
3. Friedman G, Sherker AH: The ABCs of hepatitis, *Can J Diagn* 13:85-97, 1996.

INFLUENZA

(See also serotonin syndrome)

Vaccines

Eighty percent of influenza epidemics are cause by influenza type A. Whole virus and split virus vaccines are available. The split virus has fewer side effects and should be used for children 13 years of age or younger. The dosage of whole and split viruses is 0.5 ml intramuscularly except for children between the ages of 6 to 35 months, when it is 0.25 ml. The efficacy of the vaccine is reported to be between 65% and 85% in healthy young adults but much lower among nursing home residents (19% to 26%). Some of the strains of influenza in the community change from year to year, and for this reason the vaccines are reformulated annually.[1] The strains for 1997-1998 are A/Johannesburg/82/96, A/Nanchang/933/95, and B/Harbin/07/94.[2] Vaccination during pregnancy is safe and is often indicated because complications of influenza increase in frequency during the last two trimesters of pregnancy.[2]

The recommendations of the Canadian Task Force on the Periodic Health Examination[3] and the U.S. Preventive Services Task Force for immunization with influenza vaccine are as follows[4]:

1. High-risk groups (persons who are over 65 years, are institutionalized, have chronic debilitating diseases, or are immunocompromised) ("B" recommendation)

2. Health care providers in general in Canada and health care providers of high-risk patients in the United States ("B" recommendation)
3. General population under 65 years in Canada ("C" recommendation); no recommendations for this age group in the United States

Chronic diseases for which influenza vaccination is recommended include chronic cardiopulmonary disorders, diabetes, hemoglobinopathies, renal failure, and immunosuppression.[4]

A group from Minneapolis randomly assigned healthy working adults between the ages of 18 and 64 to receive either influenza vaccine or placebo. At the end of the influenza season those who received the vaccine had significantly fewer upper respiratory tract infections, days off work, and visits to physicians' offices for upper respiratory tract infections.[5]

A randomized placebo-controlled study of healthy working adults found that arm soreness was the only adverse effect occurring more frequently in the cohort receiving the flu vaccine. About one third of both the placebo and flu vaccine cohorts reported fever, myalgias, fatigue, malaise, or headache.[6]

Amantadine and Rimantadine

Prophylaxis with amantadine (Symmetrel) or rimantadine (Flumadine) is 70% to 90% effective against influenza A when started before exposure.[7] It is recommended for all patients in nursing homes during outbreaks of influenza in the institution whether or not they have been vaccinated. For prophylaxis the drug is given for the duration of the outbreak or until 2 weeks after active immunization.[8] Both drugs may also be used to treat influenza A infections if given with 24 to 48 hours of the onset of the disease. For adults the usual dosage of either drug for prophylaxis or treatment is 200 mg/day as a single dose or 100 mg bid.[7]

The Canadian Task Force on the Periodic Health Examination gives an "A" recommendation for treating unimmunized high-risk patients exposed to an index case of influenza disease with amantadine.[3] The U.S. Preventive Services Task Force gives a "B" recommendation for this intervention using either amantadine or rimantadine.[4]

REFERENCES

1. Fiebach N, Beckett W: Prevention of respiratory infections in adults: influenza and pneumococcal vaccines, *Arch Intern Med* 154:2545-2577, 1994.
2. Influenza vaccine, 1997-1998, *Med Lett* 39:85-86, 1997.
3. Canadian Task Force on the Periodic Health Examination: *Canadian guide to clinical preventive health care,* Ottawa, 1994, Canada Communication Group—Publishing, pp 743-751.
4. US Preventive Services Task Force: *Guide to clinical preventive services,* ed 2, Baltimore, 1996, Williams & Wilkins, pp 791-814.
5. Nichol KL, Lind A, Margolis KL, et al: The effectiveness of vaccination against influenza in healthy, working adults, *N Engl J Med* 333:889-893, 1995.
6. Nichol KL, Margolis KL, Lind A, et al: Side effects associated with influenza vaccination in healthy working adults: a randomized, placebo-controlled trial, *Arch Intern Med* 156:1546-1550, 1996.
7. Drugs for non-HIV viral infections, *Med Lett* 39:69-76, 1997.
8. Canada communicable disease report: statement on influenza vaccination for the 1995-96 season, *Can Med Assoc J* 153:591-597, 1995.

MEASLES-MUMPS-RUBELLA VACCINE

(See also immunization schedules for children)

Giving MMR to children who have proven egg allergy appears to be safe, but this should be done in a setting where they can be observed for 90 minutes and treated appropriately if necessary.[1] In 1996 a combined attenuated measles-rubella vaccine free of egg protein (MoRu-Viraten) became available in Canada.

To eliminate measles from the population, more than a single early childhood vaccination is necessary. According to one study, maximum antibody levels are obtained if the initial immunizations are not given before 1 year of age and if booster doses are given before entry to elementary school (ages 4 to 6) rather than before entry to middle school (ages 11 to 12).[2]

REFERENCES

1. James JM, Burks W, Roverson PK, Sampson HA: Safe administration of the measles vaccine to children allergic to eggs, *N Engl J Med* 332:1262-1266, 1995.
2. Poland GA, Jacobson RM, Thampy AM, et al: Measles reimmunization in children seronegative after initial immunization, *JAMA* 277:1156-1158, 1997.

PERTUSSIS VACCINE

(See also pertussis)

Immunization of infants against pertussis produces immunity in 80% to 90% of recipients. However, the acquired immunity wanes in time. Loss of protection begins within 3 to 5 years, and no antibodies are detectable after 10 to 12 years. New acellular pertussis vaccines have been developed that are at least as effective as whole-cell vaccines and have fewer side effects.[1]

REFERENCES

1. Edwards KM, Decker MD: Acellular pertussis vaccines for infants (editorial), *N Engl J Med* 334:391-392, 1996.

PNEUMOCOCCAL VACCINE

Traditional indications for pneumococcal vaccination include everyone over the age of 65 and patients who have had a splenectomy, have sickle cell disease, or have a chronic disease such as HIV infection, diabetes, cirrhosis, multiple myeloma, lymphoma, or chronic cardiac, pulmonary, or renal disease.

The efficacy of pneumococcal vaccine has been questioned by some authors because of a lack of adequate controlled trials in high-risk populations.[2] Most workers, while acknowledging this fact, attribute the failure of positive results to inadequate power and interpret the current evidence as supporting immunization of high-risk groups.[3-5]

Specific recommendations vary tremendously. At one extreme is the view that almost no one should receive the vaccine,[2] while at the other are proposals to expand its use to the general population.[3] The specific recommendations of the Canadian Task Force on the Periodic Health Examination are as follows[5]:

1. To be immunized ("A" recommendations)
   a. Patients who have had a splenectomy or patients with sickle cell disease
   b. Immunocompetent elderly patients living in institutions
   c. Adults living or working in crowded conditions.
2. Uncertain whether immunization is of value ("C" recommendation)
   a. Persons over the age of 55 living independently
3. Not to be immunized ("D" and "E" recommendations)
   a. The general population of adults and children ("E" recommendation)
   b. Immunocompromised individuals ("D" recommendation); this assessment is based on evidence that immunocompromised individuals do not respond to the vaccine

The recommendations of the U.S. Preventive Services Task Force are[6]:

1. To be immunized ("B" recommendations)
   a. All immunocompetent individuals aged 65 or over
   b. All high-risk groups (institutionalized individuals 50 years of age or over, patients with chronic pulmonary or cardiac disease, diabetes mellitus, or anatomical asplenia [excluding sickle cell disease])
2. Uncertain whether immunization is of value ("C" recommendation)
   a. Immunocompromised individuals (e.g., HIV, sickle cell disease, malignancy, renal failure, alcoholism, cirrhosis)

The 1997 guidelines of the U.S. Public Health Service recommend 23 valent pneumococcal vaccination of all HIV-positive patients.[7]

Adults at very high risk should be revaccinated every 6 years,[4,8] even though *Drug Facts and Comparisons* and the *Canadian Compendium of Pharmaceuticals and Specialties* (CPS) advise against doing so.

REFERENCES

1. Recommendations of the Immunization Practices Advisory Committee: pneumococcal polysaccharide vaccine, *MMWR* 38: 64-76, 1989.
2. Hirschmann JV, Lipsky BA: The pneumococcal vaccine after 15 years of use, *Arch Intern Med* 154:373-377, 1994.
3. Fedson DS, Shapiro ED, LaForce FM, et al: Pneumococcal vaccine after 15 years of use: another view, *Arch Intern Med* 154: 2531-2535, 1994.
4. Fiebach N, Beckett W: Prevention of respiratory infections in adults: influenza and pneumococcal vaccines, *Arch Intern Med* 154:2545-2577, 1994.
5. Canadian Task Force on the Periodic Health Examination: *Canadian guide to clinical preventive health care,* Ottawa, 1994, Canada Communication Group—Publishing, pp 385-395.
6. US Preventive Services Task Force: *Guide to clinical preventive services,* ed 2, Baltimore, 1996, Williams & Wilkins, pp 791-814.
7. USPHS/IDSA Prevention of Opportunistic Infections Working Group: 1997 USPHS/IDSA guidelines for the prevention of opportunistic infections in persons infected with human immunodeficiency virus, *MMWR* 46(RR-12):1-46, 1997.
8. *Canadian immunization guide,* ed 4, Ottawa, 1993, Minister of Supply and Services Canada.

POLIO VACCINES

(See also immunization schedules for children; postpolio syndrome)

One of the fears concerning poliomyelitis (polio) immunization is that the live virus vaccine may itself cause paralytic polio. This complication has been particularly common in Romania in the latter part of the twentieth century. The reason appears to be intramuscular injections of other drugs, usually antibiotics, within 30 days of receiving oral live polio vaccine.[1,2] This phenomenon was noted in the pre–polio vaccine era when it was known that polio developing in a child after tonsillectomy and adenoidectomy was likely to be bulbar, whereas polio striking a child who had had intramuscular injections was likely to cause paralysis of the limb in which the injection was given.[2]

Polio vaccines have been extraordinarily effective in eradicating the disease. No cases of wild polio infection have been reported in the Americas since October 1991, and the disease was declared eradicated from this area by the World Health Organization.[3]

The incidence of polio has dropped dramatically in the rest of the world, and since 1996 the Pacific countries have been free of the disease.[4] Africa remains the continent with the highest incidence.[4]

Since wild polio has been eliminated in North and South America, the only paralytic polio in these regions is the extremely rare case of paralytic polio secondary to the live Sabin polio vaccines (about 1 case per 2.6 million vaccinations). To avoid this complication many health authorities are recommending that henceforth (as of 1996) all polio immunization be done with the enhanced Salk vaccine, which gives high antibody titers against all three strains of wild polio vaccine. In Canada it is available not only as a single agent, but also in the combination DPT-polio-Hib under the trade name Penta.

REFERENCES

1. Strebel PM, Ion-Nedelcu N, Baughman AL, et al: Intramuscular injections within 30 days of immunization with oral poliovirus vaccine—a risk factor for vaccine-associated paralytic poliomyelitis, *N Engl J Med* 332:500-506, 1995.
2. Wright PF, Karzon DT: Minimizing the risks associated with the prevention of poliomyelitis (editorial), *N Engl J Med* 332:528-529, 1995.

3. Expanded programme on immunization: certification of poliomyelitis eradication—the Americas, 1994, *Wkly Epidemiol Rec* 69:293-295, 1994.
4. Foege WH: Polio eradication—how near? (editorial), *JAMA* 275:1682-1683, 1996.

RUBELLA

Acute arthralgias occur in about one fourth of women receiving rubella vaccination.[1] Reports have suggested an increased incidence of chronic arthritis after such vaccination, but recent studies have not verified this risk.[1,2]

REFERENCES

1. Ray P, Black S, Shinefield H, et al: Risk of chronic arthropathy among women after rubella vaccination, *JAMA* 278:551-556, 1997.
2. Tingle AJ, Mitchell LA, Grace M, et al: Randomised double-blind placebo-controlled study on adverse effects of rubella immunisation in seronegative women, *Lancet* 349:1277-1281, 1997.

TETANUS IMMUNIZATION

(See also immunization schedules for children)

Tetanus immunization of children is widespread. Booster doses for adults are not so well distributed. Only about one fourth of persons in the United States over the age of 70 were found to have protective antibodies against tetanus.[1]

REFERENCES

1. Gergen PJ, McQuillan GM, Kiely M, et al: A population-based serologic survey of immunity to tetanus in the United States, *N Engl J Med* 332:761-766, 1995.

TYPHOID FEVER

(See also immunization schedules for children)

Immunization for typhoid fever is often indicated for travelers. The traditional typhoid vaccines (Typhoid Vaccine H-P or AKD) is given as two subcutaneous doses 1 month apart with boosters every 3 years as needed. Two new vaccines, Typhim VI and Vivotif Berna, have recently become available. Both have a low incidence of side effects; their efficacy is about 70%.[1] Typhim VI is an inactivate vaccine given as a single intramuscular injection. Booster doses are recommended every 2 years in the United States and every 3 years in Canada. Vivotif Berna is a live oral attenuated vaccine. The usual dose is a total of four capsules given as one capsule every second day (days 1, 3, 5, 7). The vaccine is known to be efficacious for 7 years. This form of vaccine should not be given to pregnant women or immunocompromised patients. The timing of booster doses has not been established, but a working recommendation is every 5 years.

REFERENCES

1. Keystone JS: Typhoid vaccination—update, *Can J Infect Dis* 6: 231, 1995.

RABIES

(See also immunization schedules for children)

Some of the animals known to carry rabies are dogs, cats, cattle, foxes, skunks, raccoons, and bats. Infection from cattle is extremely rare. Animals that do not carry rabies in Canada and the United States are hamsters, guinea pigs, gerbils, rats, mice, squirrels, chipmunks, other rodents, rabbits, and hares.[1] Raccoons accounted for about half of reported wildlife animal rabies in the United States in 1995, but so far cases of human rabies have been reported to result from contact with these animals. At present raccoon rabies in the United States is found primarily in the East.[2]

Rabies can be acquired only if a person has direct contact with saliva through a bite or through mucous membrane contact; the virus cannot be transmitted by petting a rabid animal or through contact with its blood, urine, or feces.[3]

Between 1980 and 1995, 25 documented cases of rabies were acquired from bats in the United States; in only six instances was there a clear history of being bitten.[4] Even casual contact with bat variants of rabies may lead to infection, and therefore postexposure immunization should be considered for all bat contacts.[4] Vampire bats are a serious public health problem in the deep Amazonian jungles of Peru. About one in five bats is infected with the rabies virus, and they have caused numerous deaths in children. Vampire bats do not swoop down on their victims but rather use their wings to make a waddling approach along the floor. They pierce the skin with their fangs and lap up the blood that flows from the wounds. Vampire bats avoid all light, so even a candle by the bedside is a reasonably effective protective device.[5]

Postexposure vaccine in nonimmunized individuals consists of five 1-ml intramuscular doses of human diploid cell vaccine (HDCV) given on days 0, 3, 7, 14, and 28. In addition, rabies immune globulin (RIG) should be given at a dose of 20 IU/kg. Half the dose is infiltrated around the wound, and the other half is given intramuscularly in the gluteal or thigh region. Postexposure immunization of previously immunized persons is identical if the antibody titer is unknown. If the titer is known to be adequate, only two doses of HDCV on days 0 and 3 need be given.[1]

Preexposure vaccination is given to high-risk persons as a series of three shots on days 0, 7, and 14. Titers should be checked every 2 years and boosters given as necessary.[1]

REFERENCES

1. *Canadian immunization guide,* ed 4, Ottawa, 1993, Minister of Supply and Services Canada.
2. Centers for Disease Control and Prevention: Update: raccoon rabies epizootic—United States, 1996, *JAMA* 277:282-283, 1997.
3. Rabies prevention—United States, 1991: recommendations of the Immunization Practices Advisory Committee (ACIP), *MMWR* 40(Rr-3):1-19, 1991.

4. Centers for Disease Control and Prevention: Human rabies—Washington, 1995, *JAMA* 274:1187, 1995.
5. Scrutton A: Killer bats no joke in jungle, *Toronto Globe and Mail,* Feb 5, 1996, p A7.

VARICELLA VACCINE

(See also immunization schedules for children; varicella; varicella in children)

A live varicella vaccine (Varivax) became available in the United States in 1995; it must be stored in a freezer until reconstituted. Recommended dosage is 0.5 ml subcutaneously for children 12 months to 12 years of age. Children over 13 and adults should also receive 0.5 ml subcutaneously but with a booster dose of 0.5 ml at 4 to 8 weeks. The *Medical Letter* recommends that all healthy children over the age of 1 year receive the vaccine. If this is implemented, unvaccinated children will be more likely to be exposed when they are adults and when the disease is more serious. How long immunity from the vaccine will last is unknown.[1] The American Academy of Family Physicians[2] and the American Academy of Pediatrics[3] recommend routine use of the vaccine between the ages of 12 and 18 months, preferably at the same visit that MMR is given. Children between the ages of 18 months and 13 years who have not previously been infected or vaccinated may receive a single dose of the vaccine at any time. Children over the age of 13 and adults require two immunizations at 4- to 8-week intervals.[3]

An adult who gives a history of chickenpox is almost certainly seropositive. Most adults who give no history of chickenpox or who have an uncertain history of the disease are also seropositive. If vaccination is being considered for persons in this category, a serological test to determine whether they have had the disease is probably cost effective, since the test is usually less expensive than the two doses of vaccine.[4]

REFERENCES

1. Varicella vaccine, *Med Lett* 37:55-56, 1995.
2. AAFP updates childhood immunization schedule, *Am Fam Physician* 51:2031, 1995.
3. American Academy of Pediatrics Committee on Infectious Diseases: Recommendations for the use of live attenuated varicella vaccine, *Pediatrics* 95:791-796, 1995.
4. Ventura A: Varicella vaccination guidelines for adolescents and adults, *Am Fam Physician* 55:1220-1224, 1997.

IMMUNOLOGY

Topics covered in this section

ALLERGIC RHINITIS

(See also topical ophthalmic medications)

Environmental Control

Some ways of decreasing exposure to airborne pollens are to avoid cutting the grass, going camping, or going on picnics, to wear wraparound sunglasses, and to close the car and bedroom windows.[1]

Pharmacotherapy

The two major drug classes used for treating allergic rhinitis are oral antihistamines and topical nasal corticosteroids.[1-3] Maximum efficacy for both is seen if they are started before contact with the offending allergen and are given continuously throughout the period of exposure; they are less effective as "rescue" medications.[4] Both antihistamines and corticosteroids are effective in controlling nasal itching and sneezing. Antihistamines are reasonably effective for rhinorrhea but are not effective for nasal obstruction. Nasal steroids (Table 32) are very effective for rhinorrhea and moderately effective for nasal obstruction; their maximum efficacy is seen only after 1 to 2 weeks of treatment.[1] In general, topical steroids are slightly more effective than antihistamines,[1,2] but many patients require a combination of drugs from both groups to control symptoms.[2,3] Intranasal sodium cromoglycate (Rynacrom) controls nasal itching, sneezing, or rhinorrhea in some patients but is not as potent as the antihistamines or nasal steroids.[1] This drug is also available as ophthalmic drops (Crolom, Opticrom). Ipratropium bromide (Atrovent Nasal) is effective for rhinorrhea.[1]

Table 32 Topical Nasal Steroids

Drug	Usual adult dose
Beclomethasone dipropionate (Beconase, Vancenase)	Two sprays each nostril bid
Budesonide (Rhinocort)	Two doses each nostril once daily
Flunisolide (Rhinalar, Nasarel, Nasalide)	Two sprays each nostril bid
Fluticasone propionate (Flonase)	Two sprays each nostril once daily
Triamcinolone acetonide (Nasacort)	Two sprays each nostril once daily

tients.[7] Clinically significant renal disease occurs in 40% to 75% of cases.[7,8]

Patients with lupus are at increased risk for the antiphospholipid-antibody syndrome, which is characterized by arterial and venous thrombosis, thrombocytopenia, and recurrent fetal loss.[7,8]

Takayasu's Arteritis

Takayasu's arteritis involves inflammation and stenosis of large and intermediate-sized arteries, especially in the region of the aortic arch. Most affected are women in their teens or early twenties.

Temporal Arteritis

Temporal arteritis is primarily a disease of elderly whites. Headache, jaw claudication, weight loss, malaise, and fever are common symptoms. In about 15% of patients the initial manifestation is fever of unknown origin. Visual symptoms, which can include partial or complete visual loss, diplopia, and ptosis, are less common but are important harbingers of complete visual loss. Between one fourth and one half of the patients have symptoms of polymyalgia rheumatica. An association has been described between temporal arteritis and the later development of thoracic aneurysms.[9]

The diagnosis of temporal arteritis is confirmed by temporal artery biopsy. At times other cranial arteries may be chosen as the biopsy site. If the biopsy cannot be performed before steroid therapy begins, it may still be done within the next 2 weeks with reasonable expectation of showing positive results if the patient has the disease.[9]

Treatment of temporal arteritis is prednisone, usually starting with a dose of 40 to 60 mg/day. In most cases the daily dose may be decreased by about 10 mg after 2 weeks and by another 10 mg 2 weeks later. Thereafter it may be lowered by a maximum of 10% every 1 to 2 weeks, depending on symptoms and the sedimentation rate or C-reactive protein levels. As the dose of prednisone decreases, the frequency and magnitude of further decrements diminish. Many patients can be weaned from prednisone within 2 years.[9]

Wegener's Granulomatosis

Wegener's granulomatosis is a granulomatous vasculitis that involves the upper and lower respiratory tract and sometimes causes glomerulonephritis. The typical clinical presentation is persistent inflammation of the nasal passages or sinuses in conjunction with fever, malaise, and migratory arthritis. The presence of autoantibodies against certain cytoplasmic proteins in neutrophils (c-ANCA or ANCA) offers strong support for the diagnosis, since they are found in 80% to 85% of cases. Other diseases in which patients may be positive for c-ANCA include the Churg-Strauss syndrome, Henoch-Schönlein purpura, and Kawasaki syndrome. Therapy for Wegener's granulomatosis is generally steroids and cyclophosphamide, which produce good remissions. Bladder cancer is a complication of cyclophosphamide therapy.[10] In some patients who are in remission, trimethoprim-sulfamethoxazole (Septra, Bactrim) given daily decreases the relapse rate.[11]

REFERENCES

1. Moore PM, Pope J: Investigating connective tissue disease. I. An overview, *Can J CME,* June, 6:39-49, 1994.
2. Slater CA, Davis RB, Shmerling RH: Antinuclear antibody testing: a study of clinical utility, *Arch Intern Med* 156:1421-1425, 1996.
3. Taubert KA: Epidemiology of Kawasaki disease in the United States and worldwide, *Prog Pediatr Cardiol* 6:181-185, 1997.
4. Shackelford PG, Strauss AW: Kawasaki syndrome (editorial), *N Engl J Med* 324:1664-1666, 1991.
5. Mason WH, Burns JC: Clinical presentation of Kawasaki disease, *Prog Pediatr Cardiol* 6:193-201, 1997.
6. Sundel RP, Newburger JW: Management of acute Kawasaki disease, *Prog Pediatr Cardiol* 6:203-209, 1997.
7. Mills JA: Systemic lupus erythematosus, *N Engl J Med* 330:1871-1879, 1994.
8. Cockwell P, Savage CO, Owen JJ, et al: Systemic lupus erythematosus complicated by lupus nephritis and antiphospholipid antibody syndrome, *BMJ* 314:292-295, 1997.
9. Hunder GG: Giant cell arteritis and polymyalgia rheumatica, *Med Clin North Am* 81:195-219, 1997.
10. Sneller MC: Wegener's granulomatosis, *JAMA* 273:1288-1291, 1995.
11. Stegeman CA, Tervaert JW, de Jong PE, et al (Dutch Co-Trimoxazole Wegener Study Group): Trimethoprim-sulfamethoxazole (co-trimoxazole) for the prevention of relapses of Wegener's granulomatosis, *N Engl J Med* 335:16-20, 1996.

HIV AND AIDS

(See also poverty; sexually transmitted diseases)

The first case of acquired immunodeficiency syndrome (AIDS) was reported in 1981, and the virus was isolated in 1984. The pandemic of AIDS is caused by strains of human immunodeficency virus type 1 (HIV-1) that are called group M viruses. However, a few of the cases in West Africa are caused by group O viruses, and one such case in a recent immigrant from Africa was reported in the United States in 1996.[1] The clinical importance of this is that the current enzyme linked immunosborbent assay (ELISA) for HIV-1 does not always detect group O HIV-1 viruses.[1]

The survival time of patients with AIDS correlates directly with the experience of their physicians in managing this disease. In one study the median survival of patients looked after by inexperienced physicians was 14 months compared with 26 months for those cared for by experienced physicians.[2] Part of the problem appears to be that inexperienced physicians are unfamiliar with ancillary support services.[3] Help for health professionals inexperienced in the care of HIV-positive patients may be obtained in the United States by calling the National HIV Telephone Consultation Service "Warmline" at (800) 933-3413[4] and in Canada by calling the Canadian HIV and AIDS Mentorship Program (CHAMP) at (800) 773-5575.[3]

Another factor that determines the prognosis of patients with AIDS is the nature of the initial AIDS-defining illness. Survival is longer for those with esophageal candidiasis or

Kaposi's sarcoma and shorter for those with *Pneumocystis carinii* pneumonia or other AIDS-associated illness such as cytomegalovirus disease. In one series the median survival was 20 months.[5]

The frequency of specific opportunistic infections varies with geographical location. *P. carinii* pneumonia is common in the developed world, whereas tuberculosis is a far more frequent event in developing nations. Furthermore, because patients in the industrialized world are surviving longer, infections associated with more advanced degrees of immunosuppression such as cytomegalovirus retinitis and *Mycobacterium avium* complex infection are becoming more common.[6]

REFERENCES

1. Centers for Disease Control and Prevention: Identification of HIV-1 group O infection—1996, *JAMA* 276:521-522, 1996.
2. Kitahata MM, Koepsell TD, Deyo RA, et al: Physicians' experience with the acquired immunodeficiency syndrome as a factor in patients' survival, *N Engl J Med* 334:701-706, 1996.
3. Klein A: Beyond biases and outdated perceptions: HIV prevention and mentoring (editorial), *Can Fam Physician* 43:133-134, 1997.
4. Montauk SL, Gebhardt B: Opportunistic infections and psychosocial stress in HIV, *Am Fam Physician* 56:87-96, 1997.
5. Mocroft A, Youle M, Morcinek J, et al (Royal Free/Chelsea and Westminster Hospitals Collaborative Group): Survival after diagnosis of AIDS: a prospective observational study of 2625 patients, *BMJ* 314:409-413, 1997.
6. Beiser C: Recent advances: HIV infection—2, *BMJ* 314:579-583, 1997.

Transmission and Epidemiology of HIV Infection

(See also progression of HIV infection; transfusions)

In 1995 one third of reported AIDS cases in the United States were directly or indirectly (through heterosexual contact or pregnancy) associated with IV use of illicit drugs.[1] Worldwide, 75% to 85% of HIV infections are sexually transmitted.[2]

Acute Retroviral Syndrome

In 30% to 60% of persons with HIV an infectious mononucleosis–like syndrome called acute retroviral syndrome or seroconversion syndrome develops. It is characterized by fever, myalgia, lymphadenopathy, and a maculopapular rash. Some patients also have oral ulcers and oral candidiasis. During this phase of the infection patients usually have leukopenia, reduced CD4 counts, and high viral plasma loads. As the acute infection subsides, the plasma viral load decreases and the CD4 counts rebound, but not to the preinfection level. Progression to AIDS is more rapid among patients who have a prolonged acute retroviral syndrome.[3]

Occupational Exposure

The risk of HIV infection from a needlestick injury is estimated to be 0.36%.[4] The risk is greater if the exposure is from an object visibly contaminated with blood of the HIV-positive patient or from a needle that was in a vein or artery and if the injury is a deep one. The risk is also higher if the patient is in a terminal phase of AIDS and thus has a higher titer of HIV in the blood. Postexposure use of zidovudine (ZDV) in doses of approximately 1000 mg/day for 3 to 4 weeks appears to decrease the risk by about 80%.[5]

A U.S. Public Health Service interagency working group on the management of occupational exposure has recommended the following[6]:

1. When possible, an expert on retroviral diseases should be consulted.
2. Postexposure prophylaxis should be offered to persons exposed to body fluids or tissues known or suspected to be infectious. Blood is the most infectious, but other fluids associated with risk are semen, vaginal secretions, cerebrospinal fluid, and body cavity and joint fluids. Urine and saliva are not listed in this category.
3. Postexposure prophylaxis should be started as soon as possible after exposure, preferably within 1 to 2 hours, and is probably not effective if started after 24 to 36 hours. However, in a case of high-risk exposure, treatment may be worth attempting if started within 2 weeks.
4. All prophylactic regimens include zidovudine (Retrovir) because this drug has been shown to be beneficial in such cases.
5. In the highest risk exposures, be they percutaneous needlesticks, mucosal exposure, or skin exposure, recommended treatment is 4 weeks of combination therapy with two nucleoside analogue antiretroviral drugs, zidovudine (Retrovir) and lamivudine (3TC, Epivir), as well as the protease inhibitor indinavir (IDV, Crixivan) or, if it is not available, saquinavir (Invirase).
6. Factors leading to the characterization of highest risk include deep injury, visible blood on the injuring device, injury from an intravascular needle, exposure from a patient thought to have a high HIV titer, prolonged or massive exposure of the skin to the infecting agent, and exposure of portions of the skin whose integrity has been compromised.
7. For intermediate-risk exposures 4 weeks of combination therapy with the two nucleoside analogue antiretroviral drugs, zidovudine (Retrovir) and lamivudine (3TC, Epivir), is recommended.
8. No postexposure prophylaxis is recommended for exposure to other body fluids such as urine.
9. Regimens for postexposure prophylaxis should continue for 4 weeks. The recommended dosages are:

Zidovudine, ZDV (Retrovir)	200 mg tid
Lamivudine, 3TC (Epivir)	150 mg bid
Indinavir, IDV (Crixivan)	800 mg tid
Saquinavir (Invirase)	600 mg tid

Sexual Transmission

A variety of factors affect the risk of acquiring HIV through sexual contacts. Infectivity is greatest in the few weeks after HIV is acquired (before HIV serological tests become positive) and again in the late stages of the disease. In both these situations, viral blood titers are high. Chances of acquiring HIV are greater in persons with genital ulcers or sexually transmitted diseases such as gonorrhea, *Chlamydia* infection, and trichomoniasis. Intercourse during menstruation increases the risk of infection for both men and women. Circumcised men are less likely to acquire HIV or transmit it to their partners than are uncircumcised men. Condoms offer good protection, but whether nonoxynol-9 affects transmission of HIV is unknown.[2] Male-to-female transmission occurs at about twice the rate of female-to-male transmission,[7] but because many more males than females in the North American population are HIV infected, the overall risk that a North American female will be infected through heterosexual intercourse has been estimated to be 12 times greater than the risk that a male will be infected in this manner.[8] A few persons appear to have a genetic resistance to infection.[2]

The risk of acquiring HIV from a single act of unprotected vaginal intercourse has been estimated as less than 1%.[9] Among 124 couples in which only one partner was HIV positive, no HIV transmission was recorded after 15,000 episodes of intercourse using condoms. In a similar situation in which condoms were used only intermittently, there was about a 5% conversion rate after 1 year with an estimated cumulative conversion rate of 13% at 2 years.[10]

There are case reports of HIV transmission through oral sex. The risk is low, but the actual risk is unknown.[10]

Should postexposure treatment be given to individuals exposed to HIV through an isolated sexual or shared needle exposure? No data are available on which to base an answer; Katz and Gerberding[10] argue that treatment should be provided if continued exposure is unlikely and that such treatment can be started within 24 hours. Treatment is the same as for occupational exposure.

Blood Transfusions

A 1996 U.S. paper calculated the risk of acquiring HIV from transfusions as 1:493,000.[11]

Household Contacts

HIV transmission through household contacts is rare. As of May 1994, eight such cases in the United States had been reported to the CDC. These were probably the result of contact with blood or body fluids.[12]

Pregnancy

The rate of transmission of the HIV virus from a mother to her offspring is estimated to be 15% to 30% in the industrialized world and 25% to 40% in the developing world.[13] The additional risk of breast-feeding a baby is about 14%.[13] If the fetus is not born until 4 hours or more from the time the membranes rupture, the risk of HIV transmission to the fetus is increased.[14] In one study Cesarean section (with membranes intact in 80% of cases) was associated with a decreased rate of transmission of the disease.[15] Treatment of HIV-positive women with zidovudine during pregnancy and of their neonates with the same drug for 6 weeks has reduced transmission of the virus to the fetus by two thirds.[16] The beneficial effects of zidovudine are seen in women with both high and low viral loads and high and low CD4 counts.[17]

REFERENCES

1. Centers for Disease Control and Prevention: AIDS associated with injecting-drug use—United States, 1995, *JAMA* 275: 1628-1629, 1996.
2. Royce RA, Sena A, Cates W Jr, et al: Sexual transmission of HIV, *N Engl J Med* 336:1072-1078, 1997.
3. Cohn FA: Recent advances: HIV infection—1, *BMJ* 314:487-491, 1997.
4. Tokars JI, Marcus R, Culver DH, et al: Surveillance of HIV infection and zidovudine use among health care workers after occupational exposure to HIV-infected blood, *Ann Intern Med* 118:913-919, 1993.
5. Centers for Disease Control and Prevention: Case-control study of HIV seroconversion in health-care workers after percutaneous exposure to HIV-infected blood—France, United Kingdom, and United States, January 1988–August 1994, *JAMA* 275:274-275, 1996.
6. Centers for Disease Control and Prevention: Update: Provisional Public Health Service recommendations for chemoprophylaxis after occupational exposure to HIV, *JAMA* 276:90-92, 1996.
7. Nicolosi A, Leite ML, Musicco M, et al: The efficiency of male-to-female and female-to-male sexual transmission of the human immunodeficiency virus: a study of 730 stable couples, *Epidemiology* 5:570-575, 1994.
8. Padian NS, Shiboski S, Jewell N: The effect of the number of exposures on the risk of heterosexual HIV transmission, *J Infect Dis* 161:883-887, 1990.
9. Katz MH, Gerberding JL: Postexposure treatment of people exposed to the human immunodeficiency virus through sexual contact or injection-drug use, *N Engl J Med* 336:1097-1100, 1997.
10. De Vincenzi I (European Study Group on Heterosexual Transmission of HIV): A longitudinal study of human immunodeficiency virus transmission by heterosexual partners, *N Engl J Med* 331:341-346, 1994.
11. Schreiber GB, Busch MP, Kleinman SH, et al (Retrovirus Epidemiology Donor Study): The risk of transfusion-transmitted viral infections, *N Engl J Med* 334:1685-1690, 1996.
12. Human immunodeficiency virus transmission in household settings—United States, *MMWR* 43:347, 353-356, 1994.
13. Oxtoby MJ: Vertically acquired HIV infection in the United States. In Pizzo PA, Wilfert CM, eds: *Pediatric AIDS: the challenge of HIV infection in infants, children and adolescents,* ed 2, Baltimore, 1994, Williams & Wilkins, pp 3-20.
14. Landesman SH, Kalish LA, Burns DN, et al: Obstetrical factors and the transmission of human immunodeficiency virus type 1 from mother to child, *N Engl J Med* 334:1617-1623, 1996.
15. European Collaborative Study: Caesarean section and risk of vertical transmission of HIV-1 infection, *Lancet* 343:1464-1467, 1994.

16. Connor EM, Sperling RS, Gelber R, et al: Reduction of maternal-infant transmission of human immunodeficiency virus type 1 with zidovudine treatment, *N Engl J Med* 331:1173-1180, 1994.
17. Sperling RS, Shapiro DE, Coombs RW, et al: Maternal viral load, zidovudine treatment, and the risk of transmission of human immunodeficiency virus type 1 from mother to infant, *N Engl J Med* 335:1621-1629, 1996.

HIV Testing

After infection there is a serological window during which AIDS antibodies are not detectable. Ninety-five percent of infected persons become seropositive within 3 months, and 99% within 6 months.[1] The screening test is ELISA. If it is positive, the serum is tested twice more with ELISA and, if positive, is further tested with Western blot, immunoblot, radioimmunoprecipitation, or immunofluorescence. Most results are positive or negative, but a few are indeterminate; in the latter situation the patient should be retested no sooner than 6 weeks after the initial blood was obtained.[1] Antibodies can be detected in saliva, and a commercially available system for doing this is OraSure. It has good sensitivity and specificity. Urine tests are not as sensitive or specific.[2]

REFERENCES

1. Expert Working Group on HIV Testing, Canadian Medical Association: *Counselling guidelines for HIV testing,* Ottawa, 1995, Canadian Medical Association.
2. Diagnostic tests for HIV, *Med Lett* 39:81-83, 1997.

Initial Laboratory Investigations for Patients with HIV

Initial laboratory investigations of a patient who is found to be HIV positive should include the following:

1. CBC and differential, smear, platelets (drugs that may be used can affect the hemogram)
2. Absolute CD4 lymphocyte count
3. Plasma viral load
4. Vitamin B_{12} and folate (AZT may cause macrocytosis)
5. Blood urea nitrogen, creatinine, liver function, electrolytes
6. Hepatitis B and C screening
7. *Toxoplasma* titer
8. Chest x-ray examination (as a screening for tuberculosis)
9. Tuberculin skin test (repeated annually)
10. Papanicolaou smear
11. Swabs and serological tests for sexually transmitted diseases

Progression of HIV Infection

(See also antiretroviral strategies; transmission and epidemiology of HIV infection)

The average time from HIV infection to death is 10 years. However, about 5% of infected individuals have a more prolonged course and maintain their CD4 counts in the normal range.[1] The rate of progression seems to be the same for men and women.[2] However, a Swedish study of HIV-positive homosexual men determined that progression was significantly more rapid in those who had a glandular fever (infectious mononucleosis) type of illness at the time of conversion than in those who had no symptoms or only minor symptoms. The authors estimated that a glandular fever–type syndrome occurs in about half of men who become HIV positive.[3]

A surrogate measure of HIV progression is the CD4 lymphocyte count. On average this decreases by 50 to 100 cells per year. Opportunistic infections usually develop in persons with CD4 counts less than 200/mm^3.[4]

Another prognostic factor appears to be the plasma viral load measured 1 to 3 years after HIV conversion (early chronic HIV-1 infection). In a study of HIV-positive persons with hemophilia, progression to AIDS at 10 years correlated with the viral load measured between 12 and 36 months.[5] Patients with fewer than 1000 RNA copies per milliliter of serum had no progression after 10 years.[5] If plasma viral load is used as a criterion for antiretroviral therapy, the usual threshold for starting treatment is 5000 to 10,000 HIV RNA copies per milliliter.[4]

REFERENCES

1. Baltimore D: Lessons from people with nonprogressive HIV infection (editorial), *N Engl J Med* 332:259-260, 1995.
2. Lepri AC, Pezzotti P, Dorrucci M, et al: HIV disease progression in 854 women and men infected through injecting drug use and heterosexual sex and followed for up to nine years from seroconversion, *BMJ* 309:1537-1542, 1994.
3. Lindback S, Brostrom C, Karlsson A, et al: Does symptomatic primary HIV-1 infection accelerate progression to CDC stage IV disease, CD4 count below 200 × 10 (6) /1, AIDS, and death from AIDS? *BMJ* 309:1535-1537, 1994.
4. Goldschmidt RH, Moy A: Antiretroviral drug treatment for HIV/AIDS, *Am Fam Physician* 54:574-580, 1996.
5. O'Brien TR, Blattner WA, Waters D, et al: Serum HIV-1 levels and time to development of AIDS in the Multicenter Hemophilia Cohort Study, *JAMA* 276:105-110, 1996.

Immunizations for HIV-Positive Patients

(See also prophylaxis of opportunistic infections)

With the possible exception of measeles-mumps-rubella vaccine, patients with AIDS should not receive live vaccines such as oral polio, oral typhoid, or yellow fever. Asymptomatic HIV-positive patients with normal lymphocyte counts may receive such vaccines if they are clinically indicated.[1] Regular immunizations for HIV-positive patients should include the following:

1. Inactivated polio vaccine (IPV, Salk) every 10 years
2. Diphtheria-tetanus vaccine (d_2T_5) every 10 years
3. Influenza vaccine annually
4. Pneumococcal vaccine
5. Hepatitis B vaccine for patients at risk
6. Measles-mumps-rubella (MMR) vaccine (if seronegative for these agents)
7. *Haemophilus* b vaccine (optional)

For travel, patients may receive, as indicated:

1. Inactivated polio vaccine
2. Inactivated typhoid vaccine
3. Gamma globulin
4. Japanese encephalitis vaccine
5. MMR vaccine

REFERENCES

1. Canadian Communicable Disease Report: statement on travellers and HIV/AIDS, *Can Med Assoc J* 152:379-380, 1995.

Antiretroviral Strategies

The three main classes of antiretroviral drugs are nucleoside analogue reverse transcriptase inhibitors (NRTIs), protease inhibitors (PIs), and nonnucleoside reverse transcriptase inhibitors (NNRTIs) (Table 34).

Until recently the monitoring of disease progression in HIV-positive patients and the determination of when to start therapy were based largely on CD4 counts. The 1996 guidelines of the USA panel of the International AIDS Society recommended that all symptomatic patients be treated and that treatment be started for most asymptomatic patients when the CD4 counts were less than 0.50×10^9/L (500/µl) and for virtually all patients when the CD4 counts were less than 0.35×10^9/L (350/µl).[1] In the 1997 update of the guidelines these criteria were still recommended for use when the new laboratory tool that measures HIV RNA in the plasma and thus determines viral load is not available. Since current evidence suggests the existence of a linear relationship between the level of HIV RNA (viral load) and prognosis, with no lower limit, the 1997 recommendations are that all asymptomatic patients with HIV RNA concentrations greater than 5000 to 10,000 copies per milliliter be treated regardless of CD4 count but that serious consideration be given to treating patients who have any measurable level of HIV RNA. If patients are at low risk of progression (relatively high CD4 counts and relatively low HIV RNA level) and are reluctant to begin multiple-drug therapy immediately, treatment may be deferred with monitoring every 3 to 6 months. Symptomatic patients are always treated.[2]

Whether HIV can be eradicated so that the patient is "cured" is unknown. However, in preliminary studies of a very small number of patients aggressively treated with combination therapies within a short time of HIV conversion, viral load has become undetectable.[3]

Because of the risk of developing viral resistance, HIV-positive patients almost always receive combination therapy rather than monotherapy.[1,2,4] The recommendations of the International AIDS Society—USA panel are to use a regimen that is likely to lower and maintain the HIV RNA levels below detectable levels, which is in the range of 400 to 500 copies per milliliter. The first choice is two nucleoside analogue reverse transcriptase inhibitors (NRTIs) plus one protease inhibitor (PI). An alternative is two NRTIs plus one nonnucleoside reverse transcriptase inhibitor (NNRTI). In some cases 3 to 6 months may be needed to achieve full viral suppression.[2] So far, treatment regimens with two PIs or with one NRTI, one PI, and one NNRTI are experimental.[2,3]

Table 34 Antiretroviral Drugs

Drug	Usual dose
Nucleoside Analogue Reverse Transcriptase Inhibitors	
Zidovudine (ZDV), azidothymidine (AZT) (Retrovir)	500-600 mg/day in divided doses
Zalcitabine, dideoxycytidine (ddC) (Hivid)	0.375-0.750 mg tid
Didanosine, dideoxyinosine (ddI) (Videx)	200 mg bid (varies with weight)
Stavudine (Zerit)	40 mg bid
Lamivudine, 3TC (Epivir)	150 mg bid
Protease Inhibitors	
Saquinavir (Invirase)	600 mg tid with food
Ritonavir (Norvir)	600 mg bid with food
Indinavir (IDV) (Crixivan)	800 mg tid on empty stomach
Nelfinavir mesylate (Viracept)	750 mg tid with food
Nonnucleoside Reverse Transcriptase Inhibitors	
Nevirapine (Viramune)	200 mg bid

As of 1997 five nucleoside analogue antiretroviral agents were used in North America; stavudine (Zerit) and lamivudine (Epivir) are recent additions to the armamentarium (Table 34).[5] Nucleoside analogues act against the virus early in its life cycle within the host cell, whereas protease inhibitors work at a later stage (see later discussion).[3]

Four protease inhibitors (saquinavir [Invirase], ritonavir [Norvir], indinavir [Crixivan], and nelfinavir [Viracept]) are approved and available in North America.[5] The least potent at current doses is saquinavir (Invirase) because it has poor bioavailability,[5] and that with the most adverse effects is ritonavir (Norvir).[3,4] Protease inhibitors act on the intracellular virion toward the end of its normal cycle within the host cell. After invading the cell the viral RNA undergoes reverse transcription to produce DNA, a process that may be inhibited by nucleoside analogues. The viral genome is then incorporated into the host cell DNA and undergoes a series of changes whereby large inactive viral polyproteins are produced. For the virus to become active, escape from the cell, and invade other cells, these polyproteins must be broken down into smaller units by HIV-1 protease. Protease inhibitors arrest this step in the viral life cycle.[3,5]

REFERENCES

1. Carpenter CC, Fischl MA, Hammer SM, et al: Antiretroviral therapy for HIV infection in 1996: recommendations of an international panel, *JAMA* 276:146-154, 1996.
2. Carpenter CC, Fischl MA, Hammer SM, et al: Antiretroviral therapy for HIV infection in 1997: updated recommendations of the International AIDS Society–USA Panel, *JAMA* 277:1962-1969, 1997.

3. Deeks SG, Smith M, Holodniy P, et al: HIV-1 protease inhibitors: a review for clinicians, *JAMA* 277:145-153, 1997.
4. New drugs for HIV infection, *Med Lett* 38:35-38, 1996.
5. McDonald CK, Kuritzkes DR: Human immunodeficiency virus type 1 protease inhibitors, *Arch Intern Med* 157:951-959, 1997.

Prophylaxis of Opportunistic Infections

(See also immunizations for HIV-positive patients)

In 1995 the U.S. Public Health Service issued guidelines for the prophylaxis of opportunistic infections in HIV patients,[1] and these were revised in 1997.[2] The recommendations are evidence based and classified in A to E levels such as those found in publications of the U.S. Preventive Services Task Force and Canadian Task Force on the Periodic Health Examination. "A" represents strong evidence for implementing, "C" insufficient evidence to support a recommendation, and "E" good evidence for lack of efficacy or overwhelming adverse effects of an intervention.[1,2] The 1997 recommendations give "A" ratings for chemoprophylaxis against *Pneumocystis carinii* pneumonia (PCP), toxoplasmic encephalitis, tuberculosis, and disseminated *Mycobacterium avium* complex (MAC) disease among HIV-positive patients meeting specified criteria. An "A" rating is also given to vaccinating all adult and adolescent patients who are HIV positive with pneumococcal vaccine. "B" recommendations (moderate evidence of efficacy) are given to hepatitis B and influenza immunizations of HIV-positive patients.[2]

Pneumocystis carinii *pneumonia*

No way of preventing exposure to *P. carinii* is known. Evidence is insufficient ("C" rating) to support a recommendation that a patient with HIV not share a room with someone who has PCP.[2]

PCP prophylaxis is recommended for all HIV-positive patients with a CD4 count less than 0.2 × 10⁹/L (200/μl), signs of immunosuppression such as thrush or hairy leukoplakia, or an unexplained fever (higher than 37.7° C or 100° F) of at least 2 weeks' duration. The drug of choice is trimethoprim-sulfamethoxazole (Bactrim, Septra) one double-strength (DS) tablet daily or, if it is poorly tolerated, 1 regular strength tablet daily. In some cases one DS tablet may be given three times a week. These regimens give cross-protection against toxoplasmosis and other bacterial infections. Alternatives are dapsone (Avlosulfon) 50 mg bid or 100 mg/day plus pyrimethamine (Daraprim) 50 mg po once weekly plus leucovorin (Wellcovorin) 25 mg po once weekly or aerosolized pentamidine 300 mg monthly via Respirgard II.[2] A 1996 metaanalysis concluded that sulfamethoxazole-trimethoprim was the optimal regimen and that efficacy could be maintained and adverse effects diminished with one double-strength tablet three times a week.[3]

Toxoplasmosis

Patients who are HIV positive, especially those who do not have antibodies to *Toxoplasma*, should be advised to wash their hands after handling raw meat and to avoid eating rare (pink) or raw meat, especially lamb, pork, or venison. After gardening or other contact with soil, hands should be thoroughly washed. Cats can transmit the organisms. Strays should be avoided, and pet cats should be kept indoors, never be fed raw or rare meat, and have their kitty litter changed daily, preferably by someone who is HIV negative.[6]

AIDS-related *Toxoplasma* encephalitis is usually caused by reactivation of the disease. Approximately 20% of the general North American population is serologically positive for toxoplasma, and *Toxoplasma* encephalitis develops in 38% of AIDS patients who are seropositive for the organism.[4] Patients who are seropositive for *Toxoplasma* and have a CD4 count below 0.10 × 10⁹ (100/μl) should receive prophylactic trimethoprim-sulfamethoxazole or dapsone-pyrimethamine-leucovorin in the regimens recommended for PCP prophylaxis (see earlier discussion).[2]

Tuberculosis

All patients who are HIV positive, have a purified protein derivative test showing an induration greater than 5 mm, and do not have active tuberculosis are at high risk for active disease.[5] They should receive antituberculosis prophylaxis for 12 months in the form of isoniazid (INH) 300 mg/day plus pyridoxine 50 mg/day, or INH 900 mg twice a week plus pyridoxine 50 mg twice a week (see discussion of tuberculosis).[1]

Mycobacterium avium-intracellulare

Mycobacterium avium is omnipresent in soil and water, and there are no known means of preventing exposure.[2] About half of North American patients with AIDS acquire *M. avium* infection.[6] Prophylaxis should be given to all HIV patients when the CD4 count drops below 0.05 × 10⁹ (50/ml). The drugs of choice are clarithromycin (Biaxin) 500 mg bid or azithromycin (Zithromax) 1200 mg once weekly.[2]

Esophageal candidiasis

Fluconazole (Diflucan) 200 mg/day is an effective agent for the prevention of esophageal candidiasis in patients with advanced HIV disease.[7] However, prophylaxis is not recommended save in exceptional cirumstances because the acute disease can be easily treated, whereas continued prophylaxis may lead to drug interactions and resistant organisms.[2] If prophylaxis is given, it should be with fluconazole 100 to 200 mg/day po in selected patients with a CD4 count less than 0.50 × 10⁹/L (50/μl).[2]

Cytomegalovirus

Nearly half of North American patients with AIDS are likely to acquire cytomegalovirus (CMV) infection.[8] The most common sequela of CMV infection in patients with AIDS is retinitis with subsequent blindness, but the virus may also cause encephalitis, polyradiculitis, and gastroenteritis.[8] One study found that the incidence of these infections decreased when oral prophylaxis with ganciclovir (Cytovene) in doses of 1000 mg tid was given to patients with advanced AIDS (CD4 count less than or equal to $0.05 \times 10^9/L$ [50/μl]), or less than or equal to $0.10 \times 10^9/L$ [100/μl] if the patient had a history of AIDS-defining opportunistic infection).[8] However, a subsequent unpublished study showed no clear benefit.[6] At present the effectiveness of oral prophylaxis with ganciclovir has not been established.[2,6]

REFERENCES

1. USPHS/IDSA Prevention of Opportunistic Infections Working Group: 1997 USPHS/IDSA guidelines for the prevention of opportunistic infections in persons infected with human immunodeficiency virus: disease-specific recommendations, *Clin Infect Dis* 2(suppl):S32-S43, 1995.
2. USPHS/IDSA Prevention of Opportunistic Infections Working Group: USPHS/IDSA guidelines for the prevention of opportunistic infections in persons infected with human immunodeficiency virus, *MMWR* 46(RR-12):1-46, 1997.
3. Ioannidis JP, Cappelleri JC, Skolnik PR, et al: A meta-analysis of the relative efficacy and toxicity of *Pneumocystis carinii* prophylactic regimens, *Arch Intern Med* 156:177-188, 1996.
4. Montauk SL, Gebhardt B: Opportunistic infections and psychosocial stress in HIV, *Am Fam Physician* 56:87-96, 1997.
5. Girardi E, Antonucci G, Ippolito G, et al: Association of tuberculosis risk with the degree of tuberculin reaction in HIV-infected patients, *Arch Intern Med* 157:797-800, 1997.
6. Beiser C: Recent advances: HIV infection-2, *BMJ* 314:579-583, 1997.
7. Powderly WG, Finkelstein DM, Feinberg J, et al: A randomized trial comparing fluconazole with clotrimazole troches for the prevention of fungal infections in patients with advanced human immunodeficiency virus infection, *N Engl J Med* 332:704-705, 1995.
8. Spector SA, McKinley GF, Lalezari JP, et al: Oral ganciclovir for the prevention of cytomegalovirus disease in persons with AIDS, *N Engl J Med* 334:1491-1497, 1996.

Treatment of Specific AIDS-Related Disorders

The treatment of specific AIDS-related disorders is a vast topic, and only a few entities are covered here.

Aphthous ulcers

Aphthous ulcers in patients with AIDS can become progressively larger and deeper, causing severe pain and difficulty eating. A randomized prospective trial found that thalidomide 200 mg/day po ameliorated or healed these lesions. This effect is thought to be mediated through the drug's immune-modulating capacity.[1]

Diarrhea

Diarrhea in patients with AIDS has many causes. Aside from the usual organisms to which everyone is subject, these include *M. avium,* cytomegalovirus, *Clostridium difficile, Cryptosporidium, Isospora belli* (requiring acid-fast staining of stool for diagnosis), and *Microsporidia* (requiring a modified trichrome stain of stool for diagnosis). In clinical practice, if the diarrhea is mild or moderate without blood, investigations may be limited to a routine stool culture and symptomatic treatment may be instituted. Further investigations can be deferred unless the patient's condition deteriorates. Symptomatic treatment consists of short-term bowel rest with clear fluids, bulking agents such as psyllium, and drugs such as diphenoxylate (Lomotil), loperamide (Imodium), or codeine alone or in combination. For patients with uncontrolled profuse diarrhea, octreotide (Sandostatin) in subcutaneous doses of 50 to 100 mg tid may be effective.

Esophageal candidiasis

The initial treatment of eosphageal candidiasis may be instituted on the basis of clinical suspicion. Endoscopy is reserved for patients who do not respond. The most effective medication at present appears to be fluconazole (Diflucan) 100 to 200 mg/day as a single dose for 3 weeks or for 2 weeks after symptoms have resolved; alternatives are itraconazole (Sporanox) 200 mg/day for 2 to 3 weeks and ketoconazole (Nizoral) 200 to 400 mg/day for 2 to 3 weeks.[2]

Weight loss

Megestrol (Megace) in doses of 800 mg/day has been helpful in stimulating the appetite, countering the weight loss of AIDS, and improving the patient's sense of well-being.[3,4]

REFERENCES

1. Jacobson JM, Greenspan JS, Spritzler J, et al: Thalidomide for the treatment of oral aphthous ulcers in patients with human immunodeficiency virus infection, *N Engl J Med* 336:1487-1493, 1997.
2. Drugs for AIDS and associated infections, *Med Lett* 37:87-94, 1995.
3. Oster MH, Enders SR, Samuels SJ, et al: Megestrol acetate in patients with AIDS and cachexia, *Ann Intern Med* 121:400-408, 1994.
4. von Roenn JH, Armstrong D, Kotler DP, et al: Megestrol acetate in patients with AIDS-related cachexia, *Ann Intern Med* 121:393-399, 1994.

INSECT STINGS

(See also urticaria and angioedema)

Types of Stinging Insects

Most stinging insects are members of the Hymenoptera order of the class Insecta. They include yellow jackets, hornets, wasps, honeybees, and bumblebees. The fire ant, *Solenopsis invicta,* is also a member of the Hymenoptera order but does not have wings. Only the females of these species sting. The insects that most commonly cause stings in the United States are yellow jackets. The stingers of the honeybees have multiple barbs and tend to detach and remain in the skin, while the stingers of other insects do not remain in the skin. The venom of Africanized honeybees or "killer bees" is no more toxic and no more likely to induce anaphylaxis than is the venom of other members of the Hymenoptera order. However, the

Africanized honeybee is more aggressive and more likely to sting than its docile cousin. Anaphylaxis may result from stinging insects but rarely from biting insects.[1]

Removal of Bee Stingers

Traditional advice for the immediate management of bee stings is to scrape out the embedded stinger rather than to pluck it out with fingers or forceps. The reason for this is the fear that plucking will compress the stinger and inject more venom into the victim. In fact, this is not so. The longer the stinger remains in the skin, the more venom is liberated. Therefore the stinger should be plucked out as rapidly as possible.[2]

Local Reactions to Insect Stings

Reactions to stings vary. In most cases localized pain, swelling, and erythema develop and then subside in a few hours. More extensive localized reactions are common, may reach a maximum size after 48 hours, and may last for up to a week. Extensive erythema is also common and may be mistaken for cellulitis, which in fact is a rare complication of stings.[1]

Treatment of large local reactions is acetylsalicylic acid 650 mg q4h prn plus an antihistamine. If the reaction is disabling, prednisone 40 mg/day may be given for 2 or 3 days. Persons who have had large local reactions are likely to have similar reactions if stung again; their risk of anaphylaxis with a future sting is 5% per episode. They are not candidates for immunotherapy and therefore are not candidates for venom skin tests. Tetanus prophylaxis is not necessary for insect stings.[1]

Anaphylactic Reactions

Anaphylactic reactions most often occur in persons under 20 and are twice as common in males, probably because they have greater exposure to stings. The most common symptoms are generalized urticaria, flushing, and angioedema. More serious reactions are upper airway edema, bronchospasm, and circulatory collapse. Most deaths occur in adults. In unselected patients who have had an anaphylactic reaction and are subsequently stung (without having had venom immunotherapy), only 50% to 60% have a second anaphylactic reaction. The incidence of second anaphylactic reactions is much lower in children, particularly if the initial manifestation was dermal.[1]

Treatment of an acute anaphylactic reaction is 0.2 to 0.5 ml of 1:1000 epinephrine subcutaneously repeated every 30 minutes prn. If necessary, aerosolized bronchodilators and IV fluids should be added. In most cases acute symptoms subside in 30 minutes. In the rare cases in which they persist, IV steroids should be given followed by prednisone 60 mg/day for 2 days.[1]

Prophylaxis Against Insect Stings

Clothes that cover the body, including gloves when gardening, are helpful. Clothes should be dark colored. Perfumes, cosmetics, and hair sprays should be avoided. Food odors attract yellow jackets.[1]

Epinephrine is available in kit form either as an EpiPen or as an ANA-kit. The EpiPen comes as preloaded syringes of epinephrine. The adult form contains 2 ml of epinephrine 1:1000, and the children's version (EpiPen Jr) contains 2 ml of epinephrine 1:2000. The ANA-Kit contains a preloaded syringe of epinephrine, a tourniquet, alcohol swabs, and two 4-mg chewable chlorpheniramine tablets (Chlor-Trimeton, Chlor-Tripolon). Because epinephrine is relatively unstable, it should be stored in the dark and not used after its expiration date.[3] Antihistamines help with hives and angioedema.

Venom immunotherapy is a long-term proposal, involving regular injections over several years. It is indicated for patients who have had severe symptoms of anaphylaxis and have positive venom skin tests. It is not indicated for children (or probably for adults) who have had only dermal reactions, and it is probably not indicated for individuals with relatively mild symptoms such as urticaria plus some shortness of breath. The Canadian Society of Allergy and Clinical Immunology currently recommends that immunotherapy be given every 4 to 6 weeks for 5 years.[4]

REFERENCES

1. Reisman RE: Insect stings, *N Engl J Med* 331:523-527, 1994.
2. Visscher PD, Vetter RS, Camazine S: Removing bee stings, *Lancet* 348:301-302, 1996.
3. Stability of drugs in solution, *Med Lett* 38:90, 1996.
4. Canadian Society of Allergy and Clinical Immunology: Guidelines for the use of allergen immunotherapy, *Can Med Assoc J* 152:1413-1419, 1995.

INFECTIOUS DISEASES

(See also HIV and AIDS; immunizations; malaria; tropical medicine)

Topics covered in this section

Cat Scratch Disease
Common Cold
Ehrlichiosis
Food Poisoning
Hantavirus
Herpes Simplex
Herpes Zoster
Histoplasmosis
Infectious Mononucleosis
Lyme Disease
Meningitis
Meningococcal Disease
Necrotizing Fasciitis

Parasitology
Pertussis
Polio
Salmonella Infection
Sexually Transmitted Diseases
Streptococcal Infections
Tuberculosis
Varicella

CAT SCRATCH DISEASE

Cat scratch disease usually occurs in children. The disease is transmitted by cat (or more often kitten) scratches, licks, or bites. A localized papule is found 2 to 3 days after the contact, and within a week or two, tender regional adenopathy develops that may persist for weeks or months. In about 6% of cases the site of the inoculum is the conjunctiva and the initial sign is a polypoid lesion of the palpebral conjunctiva, often associated with preauricular adenopathy. This is called Parinaud's oculoglandular syndrome.[1] Rarely patients have central nervous system involvement, often manifested as seizures.[1] The organism responsible for most cases is *Bartonella henselae* (previously called *Rochalimaea henselae*) of the order Rickettsiales, although *Afipia felis* may account for some.[1,2] Serological methods are available in some laboratories to detect *R. henselae,* but the significance of positive results has not been fully elucidated.[2] The disease is self-limited, and antibiotic treatment is usually not required.[1,2] Cats need not be treated because they are merely carriers of the organism.[1]

REFERENCES

1. Smith DL: Cat-scratch disease, *Am Fam Physician* 55:1785-1789, 1997.
2. Adal KA, Cockerell CJ, Petri WA Jr: Cat scratch disease, bacillary angiomatosis, and other infections due to *Rochalimaea, N Engl J Med* 330:1509-1516, 1994.

COMMON COLD

(See also antibiotic resistance; topical nasal anticholinergics; topical nasal vasoconstrictors)

In experimental situations in which various cold-causing viruses were inoculated into the nasal passages of volunteers, the incidence and severity of colds showed a linear relationship to the degree of psychological stress of each individual.[1] This is presumably because stress seems to inhibit a number of immunological functions.[2] A subsequent study found that a related risk factor for colds is social isolation; persons with a wide social network were less likely to have colds after nasal injection of rhinoviruses than more isolated individuals.[3] Other risk factors identified in this investigation were lack of exercise, decreased quality of sleep, and smoking. Moderate alcohol intake was protective.[3]

Treatment of the common cold is generally symptomatic. A study from the Cleveland Clinic found that when given within 24 hours of the onset of symptoms, lozenges containing 13.3 mg of zinc in the form of zinc gluconate taken q2h while awake decreased the time to complete resolution (4.4 days versus 7.6 for control subjects), as well as diminishing the amount of coughing, hoarseness, nasal congestion or drainage, and sore throat. Side effects included nausea and an unpleasant taste in the mouth.[4] Ipratropium bromide (Atrovent Nasal) has been shown to reduce the amount of nasal secretions during upper respiratory tract infections, but not the degree of nasal congestion.[5]

Over-the-counter products for the symptomatic relief of colds often include ephedrine or related alkaloids such as phenylpropanolamine and pseudoephedrine. Serious adverse reactions, including psychoses, seizures, and stroke, may occur, particularly if combinations of these drugs are used.[6]

REFERENCES

1. Cohen S, Tyrell DA, Smith AP: Psychological stress and susceptibility to the common cold, *N Engl J Med* 325:606-612, 1991.
2. Herbert TB, Cohen S: Stress and immunity in humans: a meta-analytic review, *Psychosom Med* 55:364-379, 1993.
3. Cohen S, Doyle WJ, Skoner DP, et al: Social ties and susceptibility to the common cold, *JAMA* 277:1940-1944, 1997.
4. Mossad SB, Macknin ML, Medendorp SV, et al: Zinc gluconate lozenges for treating the common cold—a randomized double-blind, placebo-controlled study, *Ann Intern Med* 125:81-88, 1996.
5. Hayden FG, Diamond L, Wood PB, et al: Effectiveness and safety of intranasal ipratropium bromide in common colds—a randomized, double-blind, placebo-controlled trial, *Ann Intern Med* 125:89-97, 1996.
6. Centers for Disease Control and Prevention: Adverse events associated with ephedrine-containing products—Texas, December 1993–September 1995, *JAMA* 276:1711-1712, 1996.

EHRLICHIOSIS

Ehrlichiosis is a tick-borne, *Rickettsia*-like bacterial disease with cases reported from 30 U.S. states. The disease usually occurs between April and September with the peak incidence from May through July. More than 80% of patients report a tick bite within 3 weeks before the onset of illness. Symptoms are those of a generalized febrile illness and most commonly include fever, chills, malaise, headache, and myalgia. Upper respiratory tract symptoms are rare, and rash is uncommon and often evanescent. Inclusion bodies or morulae may be found in the cytoplasm of monocytes or granulocytes.[1]

REFERENCES

1. Weinstein RS: Human ehrlichiosis, *Am Fam Physician* 54:1971-1976, 1996.

FOOD POISONING

(See also cryptosporidiosis; cyclosporiasis; giardiasis; infectious diarrhea; travelers' diarrhea)

Only a few causes of food poisoning are discussed here. Some of the other causes are dealt with elsewhere in the text.

Infectious Diseases

Ciguatera Fish Poisoning

Ciguatera fish poisoning is the most common illness caused by the ingestion of finned fish. The principal toxin is ciguatoxin-1, which is not inactivated by cooking or freezing. The toxin is produced by single-celled free-swimming dinoflagellates and is concentrated as it goes up the food chain. The distribution of the disease is worldwide but is generally limited to tropical and subtropical regions. It is particularly prevalent in the Caribbean and the South Pacific islands. However, it can also occur in temperate climates from the ingestion of affected imported fish.[1]

Fish most likely to cause ciguatera fish poisoning in North America and the Caribbean are grouper, red snapper, jack, and barracuda. Large fish are far more likely to harbor the toxin than are small ones. Of the fish listed above, barracuda are the worst offenders and should never be eaten.[1]

Major symptoms of ciguatera fish poisoning are gastrointestinal and neurological. A few patients also have cardiovascular symptoms. Gastrointestinal symptoms are usually the first to appear. Within 3 to 6 hours of eating affected fish, patients often have abdominal cramps, watery diarrhea, and vomiting. The gastrointestinal symptoms usually last 1 to 2 days. Typical neurological symptoms are paresthesias of the extremities and peroral region, a reversal of the sensations of hot and cold, and generalized or localized pruritus. These symptoms are aggravated by alcohol and usually persist for 2 to 3 weeks. In some unfortunate persons they last for months. Other possible symptoms are pains in the extremities or teeth, dysuria, and pain in the penis.[1]

Specific treatment for the disorder is an IV infusion of mannitol in a dose of 1 g/kg over 30 to 45 minutes. This should be administered within 24 hours of the onset of symptoms.[1]

Tetrodotoxin Poisoning

Tetrodotoxin poisoning is common in Japan but rare elsewhere. It has been reported in the United States from eating illicitly imported fugu, or puffer fish. The toxin is heat stable. Symptoms come on rapidly and include paresthesias, lightheadedness, and weakness. An ascending paralysis leads to death in about 60% of cases.[2]

Shellfish Food Poisoning

Shellfish can cause food poisoning with the usual bacterial and viral organisms such as *Salmonella, Shigella, Campylobacter, Vibrio,* hepatitis A, and Norwalk-like viruses. Cooking does not always prevent viral infections of this nature.[3] In addition, a number of forms of shellfish intoxication affect the central nervous system. Shellfish-borne toxins are produced by marine dinoflagellates (a significant component of plankton). Toxin levels rise during rapid multiplication of the dinoflagellates ("red tides"). Paralytic shellfish poisoning causes circumoral paresthesias, numbness of the tongue, paresthesias of the fingers and toes, a feeling of floating, and weakness of the limbs. The case-fatality rate (related to respiratory failure) is 8% to 10%. Symptoms of neurotoxic shellfish poisoning include circumoral paresthesias, paresthesias of the fingers, reversal of hot and cold sensation, ataxia, nausea, and vomiting. No deaths have been reported.

Escherichia coli O157:H7

Infection with *E. coli* O157:H7, which is also called hamburger disease and hemorrhagic colitis, is caused by a verotoxin produced by *E. coli* O157:H7. Many cases involve hamburgers prepared at home. Although eating undercooked meat explains some of the cases, others may have resulted from contamination of other foods or utensils by the persons who prepared the hamburgers if they failed to wash their hands with soap and water immediately after handling the raw meat.[4]

Mushroom Poisoning

Most cases of mushroom poisoning are caused by species of *Amanita.* The toxin, which results in hepatitis, is not destroyed by cooking and is tasteless. Symptoms develop after a latent period of 6 to 12 hours and consist of severe diarrhea and vomiting followed by hepatic and renal failure. Treatment is gastric lavage, activated charcoal, and fluid and electrolyte replacement.[5]

REFERENCES

1. Lange WR: Ciguatera fish poisoning, *Am Fam Physician* 50:579-584, 1994.
2. Centers for Disease Control and Prevention: Tetrodotoxin poisoning associated with eating puffer fish transported from Japan —California, 1996, *JAMA* 275:1631, 1996.
3. McDonnell S, Kirkland KB, Hlady G, et al: Failure of cooking to prevent shellfish-associated viral gastroenteritis, *Arch Intern Med* 157:111-116, 1997.
4. Mead PS, Finelli L, Lambert-Fair MA, et al: Risk factors for sporadic infection with *Escherichia coli* O157:H7, *Arch Intern Med* 157:204-208, 1997.
5. Hoey J, Todkill AM: Gather ye rosebuds while ye may—but avoid the mushrooms, *Can Med Assoc J* 157:431, 1997.

HANTAVIRUS

The hantavirus has been known for many years to cause an epidemic hemorrhagic fever with renal failure. The mortality rate associated with this form of the disease is about 10%. Another syndrome caused by the organism is the hantavirus pulmonary syndrome (HPS), which was first described in 1993. Symptoms are fever, myalgia, and acute respiratory difficulties. The death rate is about 60%.[1] Hantavirus infection is found predominantly in the American Southwest, but cases have been reported from 24 U.S. states, Canada, Argentina, and Brazil.[2] The mean age of U.S. patients with HPS is 35 years.[2] The natural habitat for the virus is rodents (in most cases deer mice), and it is found in their urine and saliva. It is spread to humans through direct contact or inhalation.[1] As of 1995 five cases of hantavirus pulmonary syndrome had been reported in Canada; all the cases were in Alberta or British Columbia, and those affected had had contact with mice.[3]

REFERENCES

1. CDC update: hantavirus pulmonary syndrome United States, *JAMA* 270:2287-2288, 1993.
2. Centers for Disease Control and Prevention: Hantavirus pulmonary syndrome—United States, 1995-1996, *JAMA* 275:1395-1397, 1996.
3. From the CCDR: hantavirus pulmonary syndrome in Canada; update, *Can Med Assoc J* 153:1303-1305, 1995.

HERPES SIMPLEX

In one study 239 immunocompetent patients with a history of recurring genital herpes simplex virus infections (more than 12 episodes per year) received continuous acyclovir for 6 or more years.[1] During the year after stopping therapy, 86% had at least one infection. After 6 years of therapy the frequency of infection decreased in 72% of the patients. Whether this was due to the treatment or was a reflection of the natural history of the disease is unknown. No increase in in vitro resistance to acyclovir was found.[1]

In a study from the University of Washington, women with genital herpes simplex were taught to take daily samples from the vulva, cervix, and rectum for viral culture and to record the presence or absence of symptoms for about a 3-month period.[2] About one third of the episodes of viral shedding were subclinical. The mean duration of shedding when patients were asymptomatic was 1.5 days compared with 1.8 days during clinical recurrences. A subsequent study from the same institution found that daily acyclovir (Zovirax) in doses of 400 mg bid suppressed subclinical shedding.[3] However, there are no studies documenting whether taking acyclovir actually decreases transmission rates.[4]

Transmission of herpes simplex is common and in one study of heterosexual couples occurred in close to 10% per year.[5] Transmission from male to female was more frequent than the reverse, and most cases occurred when no clinical lesions were evident.[5] Patients should be advised that asymptomatic transmission occurs. Patients with few clinical recurrences have few episodes of subclinical shedding.[4]

The usual dose of acyclovir (Zovirax) for the prevention of recurrent herpes infections is 400 mg bid. The standard dose for initial infections is 400 mg tid for 7 to 10 days and for recurrent infections is 400 mg tid for 5 days. Acyclovir is not approved for use in pregnant women, but no evidence of teratogenicity has been presented.[6]

Valacyclovir (Valtrex) is rapidly converted to acyclovir in the body, but it has greater bioavailability and requires only two doses per day. In a placebo-controlled study of nearly 1000 patients with recurrent herpes genitalis, valacyclovir in doses of either 500 or 1000 mg bid decreased the duration of the lesions, the pain or discomfort, and the duration of viral shedding.[7] The *Medical Letter* recommends giving 1 g bid for 7 to 10 days for an initial infection and 500 mg bid for recurrent infections and for prophylaxis.[6]

A multicenter Canadian study of famciclovir (Famvir) in patients with recurrent genital herpes found that patient-initiated treatment with the drug in doses of 125, 250, or 500 mg bid resulted in more rapid resolution of lesions and symptom relief than was seen among control subjects receiving placebo. The lower doses were as effective as the higher doses.[8] In another study famciclovir in doses of 250 mg bid was effective in suppressing recurrent herpes infection over a 4-month period.[9] *Medical Letter* recommendations are that initial infections be treated with 250 mg tid for 5 to 10 days and recurrent infections with 125 mg bid for 5 days and that prophylactic dosage be 250 mg bid.[6]

A randomized double-blind placebo-controlled study of primary herpetic gingivostomatitis in young children found an excellent response to ayclovir 15 mg/kg five times daily for 7 days. Oral lesions resolved in a median of 4 days versus 10 days in control subjects, and fever and difficulty drinking and eating also lasted for a shorter period.[10]

Most studies of topical antiviral agents such as valacyclovir (Valtrex) and acyclovir topical (Zovirax topical) have not shown beneficial results.[11] However, a randomized double-blind placebo-controlled trial of patients with herpes labialis found that the topical application of 1% penciclovir (Denavir) commencing at the onset of symptoms and continuing every 2 hours while awake significantly relieved pain and decreased the time to healing and duration of viral shedding.[12]

REFERENCES

1. Fife KH, Crumpacker CS, Mertz GJ, et al: Recurrence and resistance patterns of herpes simplex virus following cessation of greater-than-or-equal-to-6 years of chronic suppression with acyclovir, *J Infect Dis* 169:1338-1341, 1994.
2. Wald A, Zeh J, Selke S, et al: Virologic characteristics of subclinical and symptomatic genital herpes infections, *N Engl J Med* 333:770-775, 1995.
3. Wald A, Zeh J, Barnum G, et al: Suppression of subclinical shedding of herpes simplex virus type 2 with acyclovir, *Ann Intern Med* 124:8-15, 1996.
4. Patel R, Cowan FM, Barton SE: Advising patients with genital herpes: acyclovir reduces asymptomatic viral shedding, but effect on transmission is unclear (editorial), *BMJ* 314:85-86, 1997.
5. Mertz GJ, Bemedetto JK Ashley R, et al: Risk factors for the sexual transmission of genital herpes, *Ann Intern Med* 116:197-202, 1992.
6. Drugs for non-HIV viral infections, *Med Lett* 39:69-76, 1997.
7. Spruance SL, Tyring SK, DeGregorio B, et al (Valacyclovir HSV Study Group): A large-scale, placebo-controlled, dose-ranging trial of peroral valacyclovir for episodic treatment of recurrent herpes genitalis, *Arch Intern Med* 156:1729-1735, 1996.
8. Sacks SL, Aoki FY, Diaz-Mitoma F, et al (Canadian Famciclovir Study Group): Patient-initiated, twice-daily oral famciclovir for early recurrent genital herpes: a randomized, double-blind multicenter trial, *JAMA* 276:44-49, 1996.
9. Mertz GJ, Loveless MO, Levin MJ, et al (Collaborative Famciclovir Genital Herpes Research Group): Oral famciclovir for suppression of recurrent genital herpes simplex virus infection in women: a multicenter, double-blind, placebo-controlled trial, *Arch Intern Med* 157:343-349, 1997.

10. Amir J, Harel L, Smetana Z, et al: Treatment of herpes simplex gingivostomatitis with aciclovir in children: a randomised double blind placebo controlled study, *BMJ* 314:1800-1803, 1997.
11. De Ruiter A, Thin RN: Genital herpes: a guide to pharmacological therapy, *Drugs* 47:297-304, 1994.
12. Spruance SL, Rea TL, Thoming C, et al: Penciclovir cream for the treatment of herpes simplex labialis: a randomized, multicenter, double-blind, placebo-controlled trial, *JAMA* 277:1374-1379, 1997.

HERPES ZOSTER

Epidemiology

The incidence of herpes zoster is low in children and adolescents, about 0.5 to 1.6:1000 for persons under 20, whereas it is 11:1000 in adults over 80.[1] The incidence is high in HIV-positive patients and those with cancer, including childhood leukemia.[1]

The risk of postherpetic neuralgia is negligible before the age of 50, but the incidence over the age of 60 is nearly 50%. Postherpetic neuralgia is defined in various ways, but a good working definition is persistence of pain for more than a month after the onset of the rash. It is rare in children but occurs in approximately 70% of persons over 70. The pain of postherpetic neuralgia may last for months or years.[1]

Clinical Presentation

The prodromal pain of herpes zoster may last for a few days or weeks.[1] The distribution of the lesions is as follows[2]:

Location	Percentage of cases
Thorax	55
Fifth cranial nerve	15
Lumbar roots	14
Neck	12
Sacral roots	3

Crusting occurs in 7 to 10 days, and resolution of the lesions takes 3 to 4 weeks. The area affected is usually hyperesthetic. The type of pain may be burning or lancinating and is sometimes precipitated by trivial stimuli. Paresthesias and hypesthesia commonly extend beyond the boundaries of the initial skin lesions.[1]

Treatment of Acute Illness

Antiviral agents that have been used for the treatment of herpes zoster include acyclovir (Zovirax), famciclovir (Famvir), and valacyclovir (Valtrex). Administration of these drugs within 72 hours of the onset of the rash is associated with a decrease in the herpetic pain of the acute disease. The standard dose of acyclovir for this purpose is 800 mg q4h (five times daily) for 7 to 10 days, that of famciclovir 500 mg tid for 7 days, and that of valacyclovir 1 g tid for 7 days. Famciclovir and valacyclovir are thought to diminish the incidence of postherpetic neuralgia, but this has not been conclusively proved.[1] For example, in one randomized trial, famciclovir was started within 72 hours of the rash at doses of 500 mg or 750 mg tid and given for 7 days. It decreased the time until healing of the lesions and also decreased the median duration of postherpetic neuralgia by about 2 months.[3] Similar results have been reported in a study in which valacyclovir 1 g tid was used for 7 days.[4] Whether acyclovir started within 72 hours can decrease the severity or duration of postherpetic neuralgia is uncertain.[1] A recent metaanalysis concluded that by 6 months the incidence of residual pain was reduced by 46% in treated patients.[5]

The role of steroids in management of herpetic pain during the acute illness is controversial. Some studies have shown no effect. Others have documented significant reduction of pain during the first month of illness but have not shown any reduction in the pain or incidence of postherpetic neuralgia.[1] One study that showed positive results during the first month (but no difference in postherpetic neuralgia) with a combined prednisone-acyclovir regimen used prednisone 60 mg/day for the first 7 days, 30 mg/day for the next 7 days, and 15 mg/day for the third 7 days.[6]

Treatment of Postherpetic Neuralgia

Aside from analgesics, a number of drugs have been recommended for the treatment of established postherpetic neuralgia. Aspirin and acetaminophen generally have little value. Narcotics are often ineffective in neuropathic pain, although some patients do obtain relief with these drugs.[1]

Two topical treatments that have been assessed are lidocaine gel and capsaicin (Zostrix). In a double-blind trial, 5% lidocaine gel was applied to cranial areas without occlusion for 8 hours and to trunk or limb areas under occlusion for 24 hours. This treatment resulted in significant pain relief.[7] Blinded studies using capsaicin are impossible because of the burning experienced during application of the drug. In a study of 143 patients with postherpetic neuralgia treated with either a 0.075% concentration of the drug or a placebo, significant pain relief was reported in the treated cohort.[8] However, an overview of the literature on capsaicin suggests that although the occasional patient receives significant relief, for most it is minor and for many the burning experienced on applying the drug is unacceptable.[1,9]

The tricyclic antidepressants amitriptyline (Elavil) and desipramine (Norpramin, Pertofrane) have been shown to be effective for the burning neuropathic pain of postherpetic neuralgia while the anticonvulsant carbamazepine (Tegretol) is useful for lancinating but not continuous pain. Selective serotonin reuptake inhibitors are not effective.[1] Although the tricyclic agents are generally believed ineffective for lancinating pain, this is probably not true.[10] The doses of tricyclics for pain relief are usually about half those required for depression, and the effect is seen within days rather than weeks.[10] For amitriptyline and desipramine this dose would be about 75 mg/day.

REFERENCES

1. Kost RG, Straus SE: Postherpetic neuralgia—pathogenesis, treatment, and prevention, *N Engl J Med* 335:32-42, 1996.
2. Mamdani FS: Pharmacologic management of herpes zoster and postherpetic neuralgia, *Can Fam Physician* 40:321-332, 1994.

3. Tyring S, Barbarash RA, Nahlik JE, et al (Collaborative Famciclovir Herpes Zoster Study Group): Famciclovir for the treatment of acute herpes zoster: effects on acute disease and postherpetic neuralgia; a randomized, double-blind, placebo-controlled trial, *Ann Intern Med* 123:89-96, 1995.
4. Beutner KR, Friedman DJ, Forszpaniak C, et al: Valaciclovir compared with acyclovir for improved therapy for herpes zoster in immunocompetent adults, *Antimicrob Agents Chemother* 39:1546-1553, 1995.
5. Jackson JL, Gibbons R, Meyer G, et al: The effect of treating herpes zoster with oral acyclovir in preventing postherpetic neuralgia: a meta-analysis, *Arch Intern Med* 157:909-912, 1997.
6. Whitley RJ, Weiss H, Gnann F, et al: Acyclovir with and without prednisone for the treatment of herpes zoster—a randomized, placebo-controlled trial, *Ann Intern Med* 125:376-383, 1996.
7. Rowbotham MC, Davies PS, Fields HL: Topical lidocaine gel relieves postherpetic neuralgia, *Ann Neurol* 37:246-253, 1995.
8. Watson CP, Tyler KL, Bickers DR, et al: A randomized vehicle-controlled trial of topical capsaicin in the treatment of postherpetic neuralgia, *Clin Ther* 15:510-526, 1993.
9. Watson CP: Topical capsaicin as an adjuvant analgesic, *J Pain Symptom Manage* 9:425-433, 1994.
10. McQuay HJ, Moore RA: Antidepressants and chronic pain: effective analgesia in neuropathic pain and other syndromes (editorial), *BMJ* 314:763-764, 1997.

HISTOPLASMOSIS

Histoplasmosis is endemic in the Mississippi and Ohio river valleys, including the states of Kentucky, Illinois, Indiana, Missouri, Ohio, and Tennessee. Infection is acquired from inhaling the spores of the fungus *Histoplasma capsulatum.* Most cases are asymptomatic, many present as a mild flulike syndrome, some have evidence of pulmonary involvement, and in rare cases the disease is disseminated (in the very young, the very old, and the immunocompromised). A recognized source of outbreaks is bird droppings and bat guano.

REFERENCES

1. Centers for Disease Control and Prevention: Histoplasmosis—Kentucky, 1995, *JAMA* 274:1189, 1995.

INFECTIOUS MONONUCLEOSIS

Infectious mononucleosis is primarily a disease of relatively affluent adolescents and young adults. In developing countries and in lower socioeconomic groups within developed countries, viral spread is common among young children so that most are infected by the age of 4; in this young group the disease is mild or asymptomatic. Infectious mononucleosis is rare in persons over the age of 40.[1,2] Patients who have had infectious mononucleosis acquire lifelong immunity. Although they may acquire other mononucleosis-like illnesses in their lives, these are usually caused by other organisms.[2]

The incubation period of infectious mononucleosis is 1 to 2 months. For most patients the disease is self-limited. The major findings are the classic ones of fever, pharyngitis, and generalized lymphadenopathy. Lymphadenopathy and splenomegaly may persist for weeks. Complications are rare but may be serious: encephalitis, myelitis, Guillain-Barré syndrome, Bell's palsy, cerebellar ataxia, uveitis, thrombocytopenia, hemolytic anemia, and pharyngeal obstruction from enlarged tonsils.[1,2]

Laboratory abnormalities include elevated numbers of white blood cells (in the range of 10 to 15 $\times$ 10^9/L [10,000 to 15,000/mm^3]) with a relative lymphocytosis. About 10% to 30% of the lymphocytes are atypical; these are not specific for infectious mononucleosis and may be seen in cytomegalovirus infections and other viral illnesses. The traditional serological investigation is the heterophile or Paul-Bunnell test or its more modern variant, the Monospot latex agglutination test. In about 10% to 20% of adults with infectious mononucleosis and a higher percentage of very young children the Monospot test is falsely negative. Conversely, 5% to 15% of positive results are false positives caused by other infections such as cytomegalovirus or adenovirus infections and toxoplasmosis. The Monospot test remains positive for several months after the onset of infectious mononucleosis but usually reverts to negative within a year. More specific serological tests for infectious mononucleosis are available, but these are performed principally in reference laboratories.[1,2]

Treatment of infectious mononucleosis is generally symptomatic. Strenuous exercises should be avoided for 3 to 4 weeks and contact sports until splenomegaly has resolved; ultrasonography is often necessary to assess splenic size. Prednisone 60 to 80 mg/day for 5 to 7 days followed by tapering so that the drug is discontinued by 14 days is used for upper airway obstruction and severe hemolytic anemia and thrombocytopenia.[1,2]

REFERENCES

1. Bailey RE: Diagnosis and treatment of infectious mononucleosis, *Am Fam Physician* 49:879-888, 1994.
2. Strauss SE, Cohen JI, Tosato G, Meier J: NIH conference: Epstein-Barr virus infections; biology, pathogenesis and management, *Ann Intern Med* 118:45-58, 1993.

LYME DISEASE

Etiology and Epidemiology

Lyme disease was initially recognized in 1975.[1-3] The name comes from the initial cluster of cases in children around Lyme, Connecticut. The etiological agent of the disease is the spirochete *Borrelia burgdorferi.* It is transmitted by the *Ixodes ricinus (scapularis)* group of ticks. In North America these are *I. dammini* and *I. scapularis* along the Eastern Seaboard and in the Midwest and *I. pacificus* along the Pacific coast. The wood tick or American dog tick *Dermacentor variabilis* is not a competent vector for Lyme disease. The larval and nymph forms feed on white-footed mice, and the adult forms on white-tailed deer. It is the larval form that acquires the spirochetes from white-footed mice and the nymph form that infects mammals, including humans. Human infections may occur from May to November, but the majority occur from May to July.

In the United States Lyme disease is found in New England, the Mid-Atlantic region, the Southeast, small endemic areas of Wisconsin and Minnesota, and California and Oregon.[1-3] In 1995, 92% of reported cases were from eight states, which in order of frequency were Connecticut, Rhode Island, New York, New Jersey, Pennsylvania, Maryland, Wisconsin, and Minnesota.[4] The disease is infrequent even in states reporting the highest incidence.[3] The only areas in Canada where Lyme disease is endemic are Long Point, Lake Erie, Ontario and Vancouver Island and the Gulf Islands in British Columbia.[5] The disease is widespread in northern and central Europe and has also been described in Asia.[3]

Early Clinical Manifestations

Overall, erythema migrans occurs in 50% to 80% of patients with Lyme disease[3]; in one prospective study of children 90% had one or more of these lesions.[6] Multiple lesions occur in about half of patients, and nonspecific viral-like symptoms also occur in about half the patients at this stage of the illness. Erythema migrans is an expanding, annular, erythematous lesion at least 5 cm in diameter with central clearing. It is usually not pruritic or tender. It generally occurs 3 to 30 days after the tick bite (only about one third of patients recall this event), although it may develop after an interval of months, and it usually lasts for 3 to 4 weeks. Serological tests for Lyme disease are often negative at this stage of the disease and should not be ordered; the diagnosis of erythema migrans is a clinical one.[7] Lesions occurring within 48 hours of exposure are hypersensitivity reactions, not erythema migrans.[1-3]

The standard treatment of erythema migrans is a 2- to 4-week course of oral antibiotics. Common regimens for adults are doxycycline 100 mg bid, tetracycline 250 to 500 mg qid, or amoxicillin 250-500 mg qid.[3] Common regimens for children are amoxicillin 40 mg/kg/day in divided doses, erythromycin 30 mg/kg/day in divided doses, or penicillin V 25 to 50 mg/kg/day in divided doses.[3]

With rare exceptions appropriate antibiotic treatment of early Lyme disease prevents the development of late clinical manifestations.[3,6]

Late Clinical Manifestations

The late manifestations of Lyme disease include arthritis and central nervous system and cardiovascular symptoms.[1-3]

In 50% of untreated persons with Lyme disease, recurrent brief attacks (weeks to months) of swelling of one or a few large joints develop. The course may also be chronic progressive arthritis preceded by brief attacks. The onset is a few weeks to 2 years after being infected. In areas of the country where awareness of Lyme disease is high, many cases that elsewhere would be called fibromyalgia are misdiagnosed as Lyme disease.[3]

Between 15% and 20% of persons with untreated Lyme disease have central nervous system involvement. This may be lymphocytic meningitis, cranial neuritis, facial palsy, radiculopathy, and rarely encephalomyelitis.

The cardiovascular system is affected in 4% to 8% of patients. This usually involves acute onset of atrioventricular conduction defects that resolve in days or weeks.

Laboratory Investigations

Serology is used to help confirm a diagnosis of Lyme disease. When the clinical picture is typical, the positive predictive value of the serological test is high. It is important to remember that the serological test is not positive until 6 to 8 weeks after a tick bite and that about 3% to 5% of uninfected persons also test positive. Test findings can remain positive long after a patient has been cured. A positive serological test in an asymptomatic person is of no clinical significance.[3]

Prophylaxis After Tick Bites

Prophylactic antibiotic therapy is probably not indicated after tick bites even in endemic areas because of the low transmission rate. In a metaanalysis of three trials of 600 adults and children no cases of Lyme disease developed in patients given prophylactic antibiotics whereas the rate of infection in the placebo groups was 1.4%. None of the patients who became infected had serious sequelae.[8]

REFERENCES

1. Steere AC: Lyme disease, *N Engl J Med* 321:586-596, 1989.
2. Burdge DR, O'Hanlon D: Lyme disease: review from a Canadian perspective, *Can Fam Physician* 38:1426-1432, 1992.
3. Sigal LH: The Lyme disease controversy: social and financial costs of misdiagnosis and mismanagement, *Arch Intern Med* 156:1493-1500, 1996.
4. Centers for Disease Control and Prevention: Lyme disease—United States, 1995, *JAMA* 276:274, 1996.
5. Hamilton J: Zoonotic diseases in Canada: an interdisciplinary challenge, *Can Med Assoc J* 155:413-418, 1996.
6. Gerber MA, Shapiro ED, Burke GS, et al (Pediatric Lyme Disease Study Group): Lyme disease in children in southeastern Connecticut, *N Engl J Med* 335:1270-1274, 1996.
7. Gerber MA, Shapiro ED: Lyme disease in children (response to letters), *N Engl J Med* 336:1107-1108, 1997.
8. Warshafsky S, Nowakowski J, Nadelman RB, et al: Efficacy of antibiotic prophylaxis for prevention of Lyme disease, *J Gen Intern Med* 11:329-333, 1996.

MENINGITIS

(See also meningococcal disease)

Most cases of meningitis occur in children under 2 years of age with a peak incidence between 3 and 8 months. Mortality rates are 5% to 20% depending on age, and significant sequelae are found in about 30% of cases. Meningitis is the leading cause of acquired deafness in children.[1]

The three main etiological agents of bacterial meningitis except in neonates under 1 month of age are *Streptococcus pneumoniae, Neisseria meningitidis,* and *Haemophilus influenzae.* The most common organism causing bacterial meningitis in neonates is group B *Streptococcus (S. agalactiae).* Until recently *H. influenzae* was the predominant organism among children aged 1 month to 4 years, but with mass vaccination this is changing. In this age group, as well as in older children and adults, *N. meningitidis* and *S. pneumoniae* are now the most frequently found bacterial pathogens.[2] Blood cultures are positive in 90% of meningitis cases caused by *H. influenzae* type b and *N. meningitidis* and in 80% of cases caused by *S. pneumoniae.*[1]

Fever, lethargy, and seizures are the main findings in meningitis in the newborn; nuchal rigidity and meningeal signs are found more often in older children.[1]

An IV broad-spectrum cephalosporin such as cefotaxime (Claforan) or ceftriaxone (Rocephin) is used for all immunocompetent patients with bacterial meningitis, but for infants under 1 year of age and adults over 50 years of age IV ampicillin is given as well.[2]

An area of controversy is whether all patients with suspected bacterial meningitis should have cranial computed tomography before lumbar puncture. In the view of some workers this is unnecessary except for patients with papilledema or focal neurological signs. If it is to be done, empirical antibiotic therapy should be started first.[2]

Although the evidence is inconclusive, adjunctive dexamethasone therapy is probably useful in children over the age of 2 months.[2,3]

REFERENCES

1. Pohl CA: Practical approach to bacterial meningitis in childhood, *Am Fam Physician* 47:1595-1603, 1993.
2. Quagliarello VJ, Scheld WM: Treatment of bacterial meningitis, *N Engl J Med* 336:708-716, 1997.
3. McIntyre PB, Berkey CS, King SM, et al: Dexamethasone as adjunctive therapy in bacterial meningitis: a meta-analysis of randomized clinical trials since 1988, *JAMA* 278:925-931, 1997.

MENINGOCOCCAL DISEASE

(See also meningitis)

Meningococcal disease is largely a disorder of small children. The age-specific incidence in Canada per 100,000 during the period 1986-1992 was 18.8 for children under 1 year, 5.8 for those 1 to 4, 1.9 for those 5 to 19, and 0.5 for those over 20. Of the 13 serogroups of *N. meningitidis,* A, B, C, Y, and W-135 are the most common.[1]

Management of Close Contacts

Close contacts of patients with meningococcal disease are defined as follows[1]:

1. Household members
2. Persons who share sleeping arrangements
3. Day care and nursery school contacts
4. Anyone whose nose or mouth has had a direct contact with oral or nasal secretions from the patient with the disease

Chemoprophylaxis is recommended for close contacts because they have a 300 to 400 times greater relative risk of acquiring the infection. Chemoprophylaxis is not recommended for school contacts, transportation and workplace contacts, or casual social contacts.

Chemoprophylaxis is ideally given within 24 hours of the contact and is unlikely to have any value if given after 10 days. It should be used only if the contact occurred during the infectious period, which is from 7 days before the onset of symptoms to 24 hours after the start of treatment. The prophylactic regimen of choice for close contacts of a patient with meningococcal disease is four doses of rifampin given at 12-hour intervals. Each dose is usually 600 mg for adults and 10 mg/kg for children. Each dose for infants younger than 1 month is 5 mg/kg. Rifampin is contraindicated in pregnancy. Alternatives for patients who cannot take rifampin are ceftriaxone (Rocephin) or ciprofloxacin (Cipro).

Vaccines

The standard meningococcal vaccine is quadrivalent and contains serogroups A, C, Y, and W-135. No vaccine against the B strain is available. Vaccination is indicated for adults and children over the age of 2 who are asplenic, populations at increased risk such as military recruits, travelers to areas where incidence of the disease is high, and selected populations during outbreaks of the disease. Meningococcal epidemics are particularly prevalent in sub-Saharan Africa. For children over 6 years of age and for adults, protection from the vaccine lasts about 5 years.[2]

REFERENCES

1. Laboratory Centre for Disease Control: Guidelines for control of meningococcal disease, *Can Med Assoc J* 150:1825-1831, 1994.
2. *Canadian immunization guide,* ed 4, Ottawa, 1993, Minister of Supply and Services, Canada.

NECROTIZING FASCIITIS

(See also streptococcal infections)

Necrotizing fasciitis, or necrotizing myositis, became well known to Canadians in late 1994 when Lucien Bouchard, leader of the Bloc Québecois party and premier of Quebec, fell victim to it and had a leg amputated. The disease has been known since the time of Hippocrates. Otherwise healthy individuals may be affected, and the mechanism of entry of the organism is uncertain.[1] An associated toxic shock syndrome is present in about half the cases.[2] The causative organisms are often beta-hemolytic streptococci alone or with staphylococci, but in other instances mixed aerobic and anaerobic organisms of gut origin are responsible.[3] Case reports suggest that the use of nonsteroidal antiinflammatory drugs may mask the symptoms and delay diagnosis, as well as alter the immune response to the detriment of the patient.[4] Rare cases of secondary infection have been reported in close contacts.[2] Treatment involves antibiotics, surgery, and in a few cases, including that of Monsieur Bouchard, massive doses of IV immune globulins.[5]

Infectious Diseases

REFERENCES

1. Barza MJ: Case Records of the Massachusetts General Hospital. Case 21-1995, *N Engl J Med* 333:113-119, 1995.
2. Bisno AL, Stevens DL: Streptococcal infections of skin and soft tissues, *N Engl J Med* 334:240-245, 1996.
3. Kingston D, Seal DV: Current hypotheses on synergistic microbial gangrene, *Br J Surg* 77:260-264, 1990.
4. Browne BA, Holder EP, Rupnick L: Nonsteroidal anti-inflammatory drugs and necrotizing fasciitis, *Am J Health Syst Pharm* 53:265-269, 1996.
5. Lamothe F, Damico P, Ghosn P, et al: Clinical usefulness of intravenous human immunoglobulins in invasive group A streptococcal infections—case report and review, *Clin Infect Dis* 21: 1469-1470, 1995.

PARASITOLOGY

(See also diarrhea; food poisoning; malaria; travelers' diarrhea; tropical medicine)

Ascaris lumbricoides

The *Medical Letter* recommendations for treatment of *Ascaris lumbricoides,* or round worm infestation, are mebendazole (Vermox) 100 mg bid for 3 days for both children and adults or pyrantel pamoate (Combantrin) 11 mg/kg as a single dose.[1]

Babesiosis

Babesiosis is transmitted by the same tick that transmits Lyme disease, *Ixodes dammini.* The bite is usually by the nymph, which measures only 3 mm in diameter when fully engorged, so most persons are unaware of being bitten. The pathogen is *Babesia microti,* usually found in white-footed mice and voles. The prevalence is high on Nantucket Island; in the 1970s the disease was called "Nantucket fever." Babesiosis is limited to the northeastern United States and a small endemic area in Wisconsin. *B. microti* is an intraerythrocytic parasite. Cases peak in July. The incubation period is 3 to 5 weeks or longer. Symptoms are fever, shaking chills, myalgia, fatigue, and sometimes hemoglobinuria.[2]

Cryptosporidiosis

Cryptosporidiosis, which is caused by the parasitic organism *Cryptosporidium parvum,* is a common cause of diarrhea and vomiting in immunocompetent children and adults. The diarrhea lasts 1 to 20 days, with an average of 10.[3] Oocysts are relatively resistant to water purification programs. Transmission has been reported to occur from animal to person, person to person, food, contaminated surface and ground water,[4] and a wave pool.[5] Laboratory diagnosis of this disease requires specific techniques, such as acid-fast staining, that are not routinely part of investigations for ova and parasites. If cryptosporidiosis is suspected, the laboratory should be specifically asked to check for it.[6]

Cutaneous Larva Migrans

Cutaneous larva migrans results from erratic migration in the skin of the larvae of the dog or cat hookworm. These cause serpiginous inflammatory skin lesions that change shape from day to day. The larvae hatch from ova eliminated with the feces of dogs or cats and lie in the soil or sand waiting to invade the skin of their definitive hosts. Humans are accidental hosts, and in Canada and the northern United States most cases occur in travelers returning from beach holidays in southern climes.

Cutaneous larva migrans is treated with thiabendazole (Mintezol).[1] The usual treatment is 22 mg/kg/dose (10 mg/lb/dose) given as two doses at 12-hour intervals for 1 or 2 days. The tablets should be well chewed before swallowing.

Cyclosporiasis

Cyclosporiasis is a diarrheal disease caused by the parasitic organism *Cyclospora cayetanensis.* It is rare in North America and is usually reported in patients who have traveled to developing countries or in some cases in those who have eaten fruits imported from such countries. Transmission is through contaminated food or water. The incubation period is days to weeks, and the duration of symptoms if untreated is 1 to 7 weeks. Trimethoprim-sulfamethoxazole appears to be efficacious, but the quinolones are not.[7] As with cryptosporidiosis, laboratory diagnosis requires special techniques and skills that are not part of a routine investigation for ova and parasites.

Cysticercosis

Cysticercosis results from ingestion of the eggs of *Taenia solium,* the pork tapeworm, in food or water or through hand to mouth contamination from infested persons. The larval forms migrate preferentially to muscle and brain. The most common clinical presentation is one of central nervous system symptoms (neurocysticercosis), since the muscle cysts are usually asymptomatic. The disease is common in Mexico, South America, Africa, India, Asia, and Eastern Europe.[8] It has been reported in New York among religious Jews who acquired the disease from Central American servants in their employ who were infested with the *T. solium* tapeworm as a result of eating infected pork.[9]

The value of antihelminthic therapy with drugs such as praziquantel (Biltricide) or albendazole (Zentel) plus steroids is controversial. Albendazole is probably the drug of choice. One randomized trial found more short- and long-term sequelae in patients receiving antihelminthic therapy than in control subjects who received only prednisolone.[8] However, other workers interpret the literature as indicating that treatment should be given to patients with numerous viable cysts (in contrast to inactive disease manifested by calcified cysts), solitary cysts and seizures, or meningitis.[10]

Enterobius vermicularis

The *Medical Letter* recommendations for treatment of pinworms are pyrantel pamoate (Combantrin) 11 mg/kg once, repeated after 2 weeks, or mebendazole (Vermox) 100 mg as a single dose for persons over 2 years, repeated after 2 weeks.[1]

Giardiasis

Giardia duodenalis (G. lamblia) has a worldwide distribution and infects wild animals, domestic animals, including cows, and humans. A colloquial synonym is "beaver fever" because beavers (and muskrats) are frequently infected.[11] Water is a common source of human infection. Cysts are not killed by chlorination but are generally eliminated if the water supply is filtered.[12] Treatment is not needed for asymptomatic persons, except perhaps for food handlers, day care workers, and children in day care.[1] *Medical Letter* recommendations for pharmacotherapy are metronidazole (Flagyl) 250 mg tid for 5 days. The pediatric dose is 15 mg/kg/day in three doses for 5 days.[1]

REFERENCES

1. Drugs for parasitic infections, *Med Lett* 37:99-108, 1995.
2. Case Records of the Massachusetts General Hospital: weekly clinicopathological exercises. Case 28-1993. A 63-year-old man with fever, sweats, and shaking chills, *N Engl J Med* 329: 194-199, 1993.
3. Centers for Disease Control and Prevention: Outbreak of cryptosporidiosis at a day camp—Florida, July-August 1995, *JAMA* 275:1790, 1996.
4. Centers for Disease Control and Prevention: Foodborne outbreak of diarrheal illness associated with *Cryptosporidium parvum*—Minnesota, 1995, *JAMA* 276:1214, 1996.
5. McAnulty JM, Fleming DW, Gonzaliz AH: A community-wide outbreak of cryptosporidiosis associated with swimming at a wave pool, *JAMA* 272:1597-1600, 1994.
6. Navin TR: Detecting cryptosporidiosis as a cause of diarrheal illness: implications for clinicians (letter), *JAMA* 277:1355-1356, 1997.
7. Brennan MK, MacPherson DW, Palmer J, et al: Cyclosporiasis: a new cause of diarrhea, *Can Med Assoc J* 155:1293-1296, 1996.
8. Carpio A, Santillán F, León P, et al: Is the course of neurocysticercosis modified by treatment with antihelminthic agents? *Arch Intern Med* 155:1982-1988, 1995.
9. Schantz PM, Moore AC, Munoz JL, et al: Neurocysticercosis in an orthodox Jewish community in New York City, *N Engl J Med* 327:727-728, 1992.
10. Liu LX, Weller PF: Antiparasitic drugs, *N Engl J Med* 334: 1178-1184, 1996.
11. Hamilton J: Zoonotic diseases in Canada: an interdisciplinary challenge, *Can Med Assoc J* 155:413-418, 1996.
12. Juckett G: Intestinal protozoa, *Am Fam Physician* 53:2507-2516, 1996.

PERTUSSIS

(See also cough; immunization schedules for children; pertussis vaccines)

The classic clinical picture of pertussis is a cough lasting 2 weeks or longer that is often paroxysmal and that may end in vomiting or an apneic episode. There may also be an inspiratory "whoop," especially in infants. The usual clinical course of uncomplicated disease is 6 to 10 weeks.[1] According to the World Health Organization definition a paroxysmal cough lasting at least 21 days is required as a basis for the diagnosis. Serological testing has shown that cough lasting longer than 2 weeks in adults is caused by pertussis in 12.4%[2] to 21%[3] of cases. Adults with pertussis have cough that lasts weeks. Whoops are rare, but vomiting or choking after coughing has been reported in about half the cases in one series. In addition, many patients have upper respiratory tract symptoms.[4]

The immunity acquired from vaccination wanes in time, and antibodies are usually not detectable after 10 to 12 years. This is one of the reasons that pertussis outbreaks continue to occur even in well-immunized populations. Another reason is that although immunization protects against the disease within the first few years after its administration, it does not prevent colonization or transmission of *Bordetella pertussis*.[5] Adult pertussis is an important reservoir of infection for children.[6]

Laboratory diagnosis of *B. pertussis* is traditionally based on nasopharyngeal aspirations or a nasopharyngeal swab made with a calcium alginate swab. Cotton swabs are not effective, and oropharyngeal swabs are useless.[1] A negative specimen does not rule out the disease. In one study of adults with serologically proven pertussis, the diagnosis could not be reliably made on the basis of nasopharyngeal cultures or lymphocytosis.[3]

Standard treatment of affected patients and prophylaxis of contacts (see below) is with erythromycin, 40 to 50 mg/kg/day for 10 days. For those unable to tolerate erythromycin, trimethoprim-sulfamethoxazole may be used. Whether antibiotics shorten or ameliorate clinical symptoms is questionable, but they do kill the organisms and so limit the spread of the disease. There is no point giving antibiotics after 21 days of illness because by that time the organisms have cleared spontaneously.[1] A recent study from Japan found that clarithromycin (Biaxin) 10 mg/kg/day in two divided doses for 7 days or azithromycin (Zithromax) 10 mg/kg/day as a single dose for 5 days was as effective as erythromycin in eradicating the organism from infants and children with culture-proven pertussis.[7]

Chemoprophylaxis is generally reserved for nonimmunized contacts and infants under 1 year of age. It should be started within 14 days of initial contact with the primary case. In most cases decisions about chemoprophylaxis and exclusion from school or work (see below) should be made in conjunction with public health authorities.[1]

Patients with pertussis should be kept home until they have had the disease for 3 weeks, have stopped coughing, or have completed 5 days of a 10-day course of antibiotics. Close contacts should be kept away from day care for 14 days. Keeping close contacts away from regular schools is pointless because there are almost certainly many other unrecognized sources of infection in that milieu.[1]

REFERENCES

1. National Advisory Committee on Immunization, Advisory Committee on Epidemiology, Canadian Paediatric Society: Statement on management of persons exposed to pertussis and pertussis outbreak control, *Can Med Assoc J* 152:712-716, 1995.
2. Nennig ME, Shinefield HR, Edwards KM, et al: Prevalence and incidence of adult pertussis in an urban population, *JAMA* 275:1672-1674, 1996.
3. Wright SW, Edwards DM, Decker MD, Zeldin MH: Pertussis infection in adults with persistent cough, *JAMA* 273:1044-1046, 1995.
4. Postels-Multani S, Schmitt HJ, Wirsing von Konig CH, et al: Symptoms and complications of pertussis in adults, *Infection* 23: 139-142, 1995.
5. Edwards KM, Decker MD: Acellular pertussis vaccines for infants (editorial), *N Engl J Med* 334:391-392, 1996.
6. Aoyama T, Takeuchi Y, Goto A, et al: Pertussis in adults, *Am J Dis Child* 146:163-166, 1992.
7. Aoyama T, Sunakawa K, Iwata S, et al: Efficacy of short-term treatment of pertussis with clarithromycin and azithromycin, *J Pediatr* 129:761-764, 1996.

POLIO

(See also immunization schedules for children; polio vaccines and the risk of paralytic polio)

Postpolio Syndrome

The postpolio syndrome develops in between one fourth[1] and two thirds[2] of patients who have had paralytic poliomyelitis. Its onset occurs between 20 and 40 years after the initial infection,[1] and it is more likely to affect those who had a severe initial infection but made a good recovery.[3,4] The symptoms include fatigue, muscle weakness, joint and muscle pain, psychological distress, cold intolerance, respiratory insufficiency, and difficulty in swallowing.[5]

REFERENCES

1. Ramlow J, Alexander M, LaPorte R, et al: Epidemiology of the post-polio syndrome, *Am J Epidemiol* 136:769-786, 1992.
2. Windebank AJ, Litchy WJ, Daube JR, et al: Late effects of paralytic poliomyelitis in Olmstead County, Minnesota, *Neurology* 41:501-507, 1991.
3. Jubelt B, Drucker J: Post-polio syndrome: an update, *Semin Neurol* 13:283-290, 1993.
4. Halstead LS: Assessment and differential diagnosis for post-polio syndrome, *Orthopedics* 14:1209-1217, 1991.
5. Matheson MJ: Practical tips on postpolio syndrome, *Can Fam Physician* 41:669-672, 1995.

SALMONELLA INFECTION

Salmonellosis has long been known to be associated with pet turtles; it may also be transmitted by other reptiles such as iguanas and snakes. Ninety percent of asymptomatic reptiles carry *Salmonella* species in their stools. Transmission to humans may be by direct contact with the animals or through cleaning their cages or aquaria. Children under 5 years, pregnant women, and immunocompromised persons are at high risk for severe complications of *Salmonella* infections such as septicemia and meningitis.[1]

REFERENCES

1. Centers for Disease Control and Prevention: Reptile-associated salmonellosis—selected states, 1994-95, *JAMA* 273:1898-1899, 1995.

SEXUALLY TRANSMITTED DISEASES

(See also HIV and AIDS; inflammatory Papanicolaou smears; pelvic inflammatory disease; Reiter's syndrome; septic arthritis)

Gonorrhea

Quinolones are contraindicated in prepubertal adolescents, in pregnancy, and during lactation. Erythromycin estolate is contraindicated in pregnancy. Spectinomycin (Trobicin) 2 g intramuscularly as a single dose is recommended only for pregnant patients allergic to beta-lactams. It is not effective against pharyngeal gonococcal infections.[1]

Sexually transmitted diseases are hyperendemic in many parts of the developing world, and penicillin-resistant strains of gonorrhea are found in about 50% of isolates in some studies from Africa and Asia. Condoms are said to have a protective efficacy of 40% to 70%. They should be used with spermicides, which also have an antibacterial effect.[2]

The recommended treatment for gonococcal urethritis, cervicitis, proctitis, or pharyngitis is ceftriaxone (Rocephin) 125 mg intramuscularly as a single dose, ofloxacin (Floxin) 400 mg po as a single dose, ciprofloxacin (Cipro) 500 mg po as a single dose, cefixime (Suprax) 400 mg po as a single dose, or, if the patient is pregnant and allergic to beta-lactams, spectinomycin (Trobicin) 2 g intramuscularly as a single dose. Spectinomycin is not effective against pharyngeal gonococci. In addition, all patients should receive treatment for chlamydial infection as outlined below.[1]

Chlamydia Infection

Chlamydia is the most frequent cause of sexually transmitted diseases in North America. Chlamydial infection outstrips gonorrhea by a ratio of 2:1 to 5:1. Between 60% and 80% of cases in females are asymptomatic, but serious consequences of the disease, particularly PID, infertility, and ectopic pregnancy, are well known.[3-5] The prevalence of asymptomatic male carriers has been reported to be as high as 25%.[5] The following women are at high risk of acquiring a chlamydial infection[3-5]:

1. Sexually active women less than 25 years of age
2. Women who have a new partner or have had two or more partners in the last year
3. Women using nonbarrier contraception
4. Women with symptoms or signs of chlamydial infection

Symptoms and signs of chlamydial infection include intermenstrual bleeding, a friable cervix, mucopurulent cervical discharge, and symptoms or signs suggesting endometritis, pelvic inflammatory disease, postabortion sepsis, or perihepatitis.[3-5]

One of the main goals of screening for *Chlamydia* is to reduce the incidence of pelvic inflammatory disease, and such a benefit has been recently documented.[6] The U.S. Preventive Services Task Force recommends screening all sexually active adolescents and other women at high risk ("B" recommendation) but gives a "D" recommendation to the screening of low-risk adults.[5] For pregnant women it recommends screening only those at high risk, which includes all women under 25.[5] The current recommendations of the Canadian Task Force on the Periodic Health Examination are that all women at high risk and all pregnant women in the first trimester be screened ("B" recommendations) but that screening of the general population should not be undertaken ("D" recommendation).[3,4]

The sensitivity of cell cultures for *Chlamydia* is less than that of polymerase chain reaction techniques. A comparison of the two methods in patients from one sexually transmitted disease clinic found a 50% increase in the detection rates by the polymerase chain reaction technique; the increase was greater in males than females.[7] Chlamydial infection is highly communicable; in one study polymerase chain reaction testing for *Chlamydia* was positive in two thirds of both the male and female partners of infected patients. On this basis the authors recommend routine contact tracing and treatment for all partners of *Chlamydia*-infected persons.[7]

Recommendations for the treatment of chlamydial infections in nonpregnant patients are azithromycin (Zithromax) 1 g as a single dose, doxycycline 100 mg bid × 7 days, tetracycline 500 mg qid × 7 days, or minocycline 100 mg bid. Alternatives are ofloxacin 300 mg po bid × 7 days, erythromycin 500 mg qid × 7 days, or amoxicillin 500 mg po tid × 10 days.[1] In pregnancy both erythromycin and amoxicillin are effective, but patients tolerate amoxicillin much better.[8]

Epididymitis

The usual cause of acute epididymitis in men under the age of 35 is *N. gonorrhoeae* or *C. trachomatis.* Older men may have non–sexually transmitted infections caused by gram-negative rods, and these infections may be treated with ofloxacin or another quinolone for 10 days.[1] *Medical Letter* recommendations for the treatment of sexually transmitted epididymitis are ofloxacin 300 mg po bid × 10 days or, as an alternative, ceftriaxone (Rocephin) 250 mg intramuscularly as a single dose followed by doxycycline 100 mg po bid × 10 days or minocycline 100 mg bid × 10 days or tetracycline 500 mg qid × 10 days.[1]

Syphilis

The recommended treatment regimen for early syphilis, defined as primary, secondary, or latent of less than 1 year's duration, is benzathine penicillin G 2.4 million units intramuscularly as a single dose. (Some experts recommend repeating the dose after 1 week, especially if the patient is HIV positive.) An alternative regimen is doxycycline 100 mg bid × 14 days.[1]

REFERENCES

1. Drugs for sexually transmitted diseases, *Med Lett* 37:117-122, 1995.
2. Canadian communicable disease report: statement on travellers and sexually transmitted diseases, *Can Med Assoc J* 152:1826-1828, 1995.
3. Canadian Task Force on the Periodic Health Examination: *Canadian guide to clinical preventive health care,* Ottawa, 1994, Canada Communication Group—Publishing, pp 732-742.
4. Davies HD, Wang EE (Canadian Task Force on the Periodic Health Examination): Periodic health examination, 1996 update. 2. Screening for chlamydial infections, *Can Med Assoc J* 154:1631-1644, 1996.
5. US Preventive Services Task Force: *Guide to clinical preventive services,* ed 2, Baltimore, 1996, Williams & Wilkins, pp 325-334.
6. Scholes D, Stergachis A, Heidrich FE, et al: Prevention of pelvic inflammatory disease by screening for cervical chlamydial infection, *N Engl J Med* 334:1362-1366, 1996.
7. Quinn TC, Gaydos C, Shepherd M, et al: Epidemiologic and microbiologic correlates of *Chlamydia trachomatis* infection in sexual partnerships, *JAMA* 276:1737-1742, 1996.
8. Turrentine MA, Newton ER: Amoxicillin or erythromycin for the treatment of antenatal chlamydial infection: a meta-analysis, *Obstet Gynecol* 86:1021-1025, 1995.

STREPTOCOCCAL INFECTIONS

(See also antibiotic resistance; necrotizing fasciitis; tonsillectomy)

The incidence of strep throat is relatively low over the age of 35 and under the age of 3. The positive predictive value of clinical criteria for the diagnosis of group A beta-hemolytic streptococcal tonsillitis or pharyngitis varies with the prevalence of disease in the community, but even under the best of circumstances it is not very good. Criteria are less specific for young children. The main criteria are as follows[1,2]:

1. Fever or history of documented fever of over 38° C (101° F)
2. Tonsillar exudate
3. Swollen tender anterior cervical nodes
4. Absence of cough

Observational studies have found that in general practice about half of patients with a sore throat have none or only one of these criteria; the chance that these patients will have a positive culture is less than 10%. In contrast, 10% to 15% of patients have all four criteria, and about 50% of them will have a positive culture. Among those with two or three of the criteria, only about 30% will have positive cultures. McIsaac and associates[2] recommend no cultures or antibiotic treatment for patients with no or one criterion, cultures and delayed treatment as needed for those with two or three of the criteria, and cultures and immediate treatment for those with all four criteria. Perkins[3] suggests no cultures or treatment for patients with all four criteria or for patients with sore throats who are household contacts of someone with a documented streptococcal infection.

Rapid streptococcal screening tests have a sensitivity of about 50% to 90% but a specificity of 90%.[4] The false-negative rate of a single throat culture sent to a capable microbiology laboratory is about 5%. Between 15% and 20% of children and 5% to 10% of adults are carriers of beta-hemolytic streptococci, as are up to 25% of patients adequately treated with penicillin. Carriers do not appear to be a source of transmission and are not at risk for the complications of streptococcal disease. Further cultures are not needed after treatment.[4]

Treatment of strep throat with antibiotics prevents about 75% of the cases of rheumatic fever that would follow this infection. However, the actual numbers prevented by such a strategy are low because, except in epidemics, in which the risk of rheumatic fever is higher, rheumatic fever would be expected to develop in only about 3 to 4 persons per 1000 with untreated group A beta-hemolytic streptococcal pharyngitis. Furthermore, since many patients with streptococcal sore throats do not seek medical attention, only a small percentage of cases of rheumatic fever in the community could be prevented, even if every case of streptococcal pharyngitis seen by a physician were diagnosed and treated. Treating streptococcal disease does not prevent glomerulonephritis.[5]

Several papers published over the past decade have shown that antibiotic treatment of strep throat hastens symptom improvement by about 1 to 2 days compared with control subjects given placebo. This has been confirmed by prospective placebo-controlled double-blind randomized trials in general practice.[6,7] Whether this gain is worth the possible risk of adverse effects from penicillin, the possible failure to develop immunity (there is some evidence that treating infection early rather than delaying treatment by 48 to 72 hours leads to more recurrent strep throats by preventing the initial immune response), the risk of facilitating bacterial resistance to antibiotics in the community, and the reinforcement in patients' minds that antibiotics are necessary to treat sore throats[8] is debatable.[4,5,8]

Antibiotics take about 24 hours to eradicate the organisms. A good working rule is to keep children home from school for 24 hours after beginning antibiotics.[9]

REFERENCES

1. Centor RM, Witherspoon JM, Dalton HP, et al: The diagnosis of strep throat in adults in the emergency room, *Med Decis Making* 1:239-246, 1981.
2. McIsaac WJ, Goel V, Slaughter PM, et al: Reconsidering sore throats. 2. Alternative approach and practical office tool, *Can Fam Physician* 43:495-500, 1997.
3. Perkins A: An approach to diagnosing the acute sore throat, *Am Fam Physician* 55:131-138, 1997.
4. Kiselica D: Group A beta-hemolytic streptococcal pharyngitis: current clinical concepts, *Am Fam Physician* 49:1147-1154, 1994.
5. McIsaac WJ, Goel V, Slaughter P, et al: Reconsidering sore throats. 1. Problems with current clinical practice, *Can Fam Physician* 43:485-493, 1997.
6. De Meyere M, Mervielde Y, Verschraegen G, et al: Effect of penicillin on the clinical course of streptococcal pharyngitis in general practice, *Eur J Clin Pharmacol* 43:581-585, 1992.
7. Dagnelie CF, van der Graaf Y, Melker RA: Do patients with sore throat benefit from penicillin? A randomized double-blind placebo-controlled clinical trial with penicillin V in general practice, *Br J Gen Pract* 46:589-593, 1996.
8. Little P, Williamson I, Warner G, et al: Open randomised trial of prescribing strategies in managing sore throat, *BMJ* 314:722-777, 1997.
9. Snellman LW, Stang HJ, Stang JM, et al: Duration of positive throat cultures for group A streptococci after initiation of antibiotic therapy, *Pediatrics* 91:1166-1170, 1993.

TUBERCULOSIS

History

Tuberculosis has been identified in Egyptian mummies and is known to have been present in pre-Columbian native peoples and in ancient Greece ("phthisis"). Koch[1] identified the tubercle bacillus in 1882.

Tuberculosis was epidemic in Europe in the late 17th, the 18th, and the first half of the 19th centuries (Industrial Revolution), accounting for 25% of the total death rate. A decline in incidence and mortality began around 1850 for unknown reasons. There was a dramatic decline throughout the first half of the 20th century before introduction of antibiotic therapy.[1]

Specific pharmacotherapy for tuberculosis became available with the development of streptomycin and paraaminosalicylate in 1946, isoniazid (INH) in 1952, and rifampin in 1970. Before then, one of the chief therapeutic modalities was climatic therapy. In the early 19th century warm climates were in vogue, whereas in the late 19th century a cold climate was considered more therapeutic. The Saranac sanitarium in New York State was founded in 1884 (Dr. Norman Bethune was treated there), and the first Canadian sanitorium was started in Muskoka in 1896.[1]

Epidemiology

About one fourth of clinical cases of tuberculosis diagnosed in the United States in the period 1986 to 1994 were among immigrants, mostly from Latin America, including Haiti, and Southeast Asia. Among this group, incidence is high in both recent arrivals and long-term residents of the United States. About half the cases occur in persons under 35 years of age.[2]

Method of Transmission

Tuberculosis is not transmitted via fomites. Transmission is airborne, through the ingestion of contaminated milk, or rarely through abrasions ("prosector's wart").[3-5]

Risk Factors for Infection

Close contacts of a tuberculous patient are at increased risk. Close contact is defined as contact with someone who is expectorating bacilli for several minutes in an enclosed space when masks are not being worn. The risk of infection is much higher if the smear from the person with the index case is positive for acid-fast bacilli. In various studies of such cases, 27% to 80% of contacts of patients with positive smears have purified protein derivative (PPD) conversion compared with only about 5% if the smear is negative. Medical risk factors for tuberculosis include AIDS, silicosis, gastrectomy, chronic renal failure, diabetes, corticosteroid use, immunosuppression, and malignancy. The risk of infection after PPD conversion is discussed in the following paragraphs.[3-5]

Purified Protein Derivative

Whether a PPD test is positive and whether a positive reaction requires treatment are determined by a variety of factors, as discussed in the following paragraphs.[3,5-10]

The only standardized form of PPD is 5 TU (tuberculin units). The physician should not use 1 TU or 250 TU because norms for interpreting the results of such tests have not been established. If the initial PPD test is negative, it should be repeated in 1 week to assess the "booster effect." If the patients are truly tuberculin positive but reactivity has waned over the years, they could have an initially negative PPD; a second PPD test a week or more later would then be positive. Repeated PPD testing cannot by itself induce sensitization. If the PPD test is negative, the practitioner should remember that it takes 3 to 12 weeks after exposure to tuberculosis for the test to become positive. If tuberculosis is suspected on clinical grounds but the PPD test is negative (e.g., in AIDS patients), the possibility of anergy should be considered and a Multitest performed. Twenty-five percent of patients with active tuberculosis are anergic to 5 TU tests.

Bacille Calmette-Guérin (BCG) inoculations may result in PPD readings of 10 mm or greater even after 25 years, but this is rare; in most cases the tuberculin reaction wanes after 5 years. In 1990 the American Thoracic Society recommended that for individuals who had received BCG in the past, an induration of 10 mm or greater with PPD testing should be interpreted as evidence of present or past tuberculous infection.

The risk of active infection after PPD conversion in an adult is greatest in the first 2 years; it is 3.3% in the first year and 5% to 15% in a person's lifetime. The risk for an infant less than 6 months is 80%. The risk decreases between the ages 3 or 4 and puberty and increases again in adolescence. The risk peaks again in the elderly. Children are at higher risk for tuberculous meningitis than adults.

The definition of a positive PPD reading depends on risk factors and varies from 5 to 15 mm of induration measured in the greatest diameter (Table 35).

Adults over the age of 35 who are PPD positive but otherwise healthy, who have normal chest x-ray findings, and who are not known to have seroconverted within 2 years do not require INH. Management in adults between 20 and 35 years of age presenting a similar scenario is controversial; some experts recommend treatment and others do not.

Table 35 Purified Protein Derivative Readings and Clinical Circumstances Determining the Need for Chemoprophylaxis with Isoniazid in Patients with No Evidence of Active Tuberculosis

PPD	Clinical circumstances
Negative	Children and adolescents who are close contacts: treat for 3 months and repeat PPD. If negative after 3 months of treatment, discontinue treatment. Some authors advise a similar protocol for adults.[6]
5-9 mm	Close contacts, HIV positive, upper lobe fibrotic lesion: treat for 12 months.
10-14 mm	High-incidence groups: treat those under 35 for 6 months. IV drug users (HIV negative) and high–medical risk groups: treat all ages for 6-12 months.
15 mm +	Low-risk group: treat those under 35 for 6 months.
Converts within 2 years (10 mm)	Treat those under 35 for 6-12 months.
Converts within 2 years (15 mm)	Treat all patients for 6-12 months.

Chemoprophylaxis

The usual method of administering chemoprophylaxis is to give isoniazid at a dose of 300 mg/day for adults and 10 mg/kg to a maximum of 300 mg/day for children. The indications for treatment and the duration of treatment are outlined in Table 35. Hepatitis and peripheral neuropathy are important side effects of isoniazid therapy. Patients over the age of 35 or any patients who have a history of alcoholism, liver disease, or IV drug use should have liver function studies at the initiation of therapy and monthly for the first 2 to 4 months of treatment and should be advised to avoid alcohol and acetaminophen. A doubling of the alanine aminotransferase or aspartate aminotransferase level is a reason for considering discontinuation of therapy. Peripheral neuropathy is often manifested as paresthesias of the hands or feet, and patients should be advised to report these symptoms. Some workers recommend giving prophylactic pyridoxine (vitamin B_6) in doses of 6 to 25 mg/day for all patients taking isoniazid.[10]

Treatment of Active Disease

All patients with active tuberculosis should be initially treated with a three-drug regimen of isoniazid, rifampin (Rifadin, Rimactane, Rofact), and pyrazinamide. In addition, patients at high risk of multidrug-resistant disease should receive ethambutol (Myambutol) or streptomycin. After 8 weeks of treatment with three of four drugs the regimen may be cut to isoniazid and rifampin provided that cultures have not shown resistance to these drugs. These two should be continued for another 16 weeks for a total treatment time of 24 weeks or approximately 6 months. Many workers suggest adding pyridoxine with the hope of decreasing the risk of neuropathy caused by isoniazid. Monthly red/green color discrimination and visual acuity testing is advised for patients taking ethambutol. Regular liver function tests are indicated for the other drugs.[10]

HIV-infected patients with tuberculosis should be treated for more than 9 months because of a high relapse rate after only 6 months of treatment.[11]

REFERENCES

1. Warren CPW: Cold and consumption: Canada and the climatic treatment of tuberculosis, *Ann RCPSC* 26:178-181, 1993.
2. Zuber PL, McKenna MT, Binkin NJ, et al: Long-term risk of tuberculosis among foreign-born persons in the United States, *JAMA* 278:304-307, 1997.
3. LaFlamme P-J, Lavergne M: La tuberculose en 1993. I, *Clinicien* 8:61-74, 1993.
4. LaFlamme P-J, Lavergne M: La tuberculose en 1993. II, *Clinicien* 8:105-118, 1993.
5. Anderson C, Menzies R: Meeting the challenges of tuberculosis, *Can J Diagn* 10:97-109, 1993.
6. Chittock DR, McCormack DG: Interpreting the tuberculin skin test, *Can J Diagn* 10:31-42, 1993.
7. Ball JB JR, Farer LS, Hopewell PC, et al: Treatment of tuberculosis and tuberculosis infection in adults and children, *Am J Respir Crit Care Med* 149:1359-1374, 1994.
8. The use of preventive therapy for tuberculosis infection in the United States: recommendations of the Advisory Committee for the Elimination of Tuberculosis, *MMWR* 39(RR-8):9-12, 1990.
9. Pennie RA: Mantoux tests: performing, interpreting, and acting upon them, *Can Fam Physician* 41:1025-1029, 1995.
10. McColloster P, Neff NE: Outpatient management of tuberculosis, *Am Fam Physician* 53:1579-1594, 1996.
11. Pulido F, Peña K, Rubio R, et al: Relapse of tuberculosis after treatment in human immunodeficiency virus-infected patients, *Arch Intern Med* 157:227-232, 1997.

VARICELLA

(See also varicella in children; varicella vaccine)

Varicella is infectious for 48 hours before the onset of the rash, and infectivity persists until the last vesicles crust over (about 1 week). The infection is transmitted via the respiratory route. The usual incubation period is 10 to 21 days. Secondary attack rates of susceptible individuals within a family are 70% to 90%. The absolute risk of congenital anomalies being caused by varicella infection of the mother in the first 20 weeks of pregnancy is about 2%.[1]

Treatment of varicella in otherwise healthy children with acyclovir (Zovirax) is controversial. If medication is started within 24 hours of the onset of rash, defervescence may occur 1 to 2 days earlier than in untreated persons and fewer skin lesions develop. However, treatment does not decrease the rate of transmission of the infection within the household, decrease complications, or cause less scarring.[2,3] Theoretical objections to treatment are that it might foster the development of viral resistance to the drugs used and that either humoral or cellular immunity might be inhibited by treatment. To date, no evidence has been presented that either of these has occurred.[2-4] One factor that may influence the decision about treatment is the probable severity of the disease. It is greater in adolescents and in secondary household contacts (probably as a result of larger inocula of virus).[3]

Treatment of varicella in otherwise healthy adults with acyclovir (Zovirax) starting within 24 hours of the onset of the rash decreases the time to complete crusting by 1.5 to 2 days, as well as reducing the duration of fever by about the same amount. The usual dosage is 800 mg po 5 times a day for 5 to 7 days.[5,6]

The value of treating uncomplicated chickenpox in immunocompetent individuals is controversial. At present there is no consensus.[3,7,8]

REFERENCES

1. Pastuszak AL, Levy M, Schick B, et al: Outcome after maternal varicella infection in the first 20 weeks of pregnancy, *N Engl J Med* 330:901-905, 1994.
2. Balfour HH Jr, Kelly JM, Suarez CS, et al: Acyclovir treatment of varicella in otherwise healthy children, *J Pediatr* 116:633-639, 1990.
3. Feldman S: Acyclovir therapy for varicella in otherwise healthy children and adolescents, *J Med Virol* 1(suppl):85-89, 1993.
4. Levin MJ, Rotbart HA, Hayward AR: Immune response to varicella-zoster virus 5 years after acyclovir therapy of childhood varicella (letter), *J Infect Dis* 171:1383-1384, 1995.
5. Wallace MR, Bowler WA, Oldfield EC 3d: Treatment of varicella in the immunocompetent adult, *J Med Virol* 1(suppl):90-92, 1993.
6. Choo DC, Chew SK, Tan EH, et al: Oral acyclovir in the treatment of adult varicella, *Ann Acad Med Singapore* 24:316-321, 1995.
7. Balfour HH Jr: Acyclovir for childhood chickenpox: no reason not to treat, *BMJ* 310:109-110,1995.
8. McKendrick MW: Acyclovir for childhood chickenpox: cost is unjustified, *BMJ* 310:108-109, 1995.

LOCOMOTOR SYSTEM

Topics covered in this section

Table 36 Muscle Relaxants

Drug	Usual doses
Chlorzoxazone (Paraflex, Parafon Forte DSC)	250-500 mg tid-qid
Chlorzoxazone + acetaminophen (Parafon Forte)	1-2 tablets tid-qid
Chlorzoxazone + acetaminophen + codeine (Parafon Forte C8)	1-2 tablets tid-qid
Cyclobenzaprine HCl (Flexeril)	10 mg tid po
Methocarbamol (Robaxin)	1-2 g tid-qid
Methocarbamol + acetaminophen (Robaxacet)	1-2 tablets tid-qid
Methocarbamol + acetaminophen +codeine (Robaxacet-8)	1-2 tablets tid-qid
Orphenadrine citrate (Norflex)	100 mg bid
Orphenadrine HCl (Disipal)	50 mg tid

Table 37 Nonsteroidal Antiinflammatory Drugs

Drug	Usual doses
Indolacetic Acids (Acetic Acid Derivatives)	
Indomethacin (Indocid, Indocin)	25-50 mg bid to tid
Ketorolac tromethamine (Toradol)	10 mg q4-6h; 10-30 mg IM
Sulindac (Clinoril)	200 mg bid
Tolmetin sodium (Tolectin)	400 mg tid
Phenylacetates	
Diclofenac sodium (Voltaren)	25-50 mg tid
Diclofenac sodium + misoprostol (Arthrotec)	1 tablet bid or tid
Oxicams	
Piroxicam (Feldene)	10 mg bid or 20 mg/day
Tenoxicam (Mobiflex)	20 mg/day
Propionic Acid Derivatives	
Fenoprofen calcium (Nalfon)	50-100 mg tid-qid
Flurbiprofen (Ansaid, Froben)	50-100 mg tid-qid
Ibuprofen (Motrin, Advil)	400-600 mg tid-qid
Ketoprofen (Orudis, Oruvail Actron)	50 mg tid-qid
Naproxen (Naprosyn)	250-500 mg tid-qid
Naproxen sodium (Anaprox, Aleve, Naprelan)	275-550 mg tid-qid
Oxaprozin (Daypro)	1200 mg once daily
Tiaprofenic acid (Surgam)	100-200 mg tid
Salicylic Acids	
Acetylsalicylic acid, ASA (Aspirin)	325-650 mg qid
Diflunisal (Dolobid)	500 mg bid
Salsalate (Disalcid)	500-750 mg bid
Fenamates	
Mefenamic acid (Ponstan)	250 mg qid
Alkanone Derivatives	
Nabumetone (Relafen)	1000 mg/day as a single dose
Pyranocarboxylic Acid	
Etodolac (Ultradol, Lodine)	200-300 mg bid

MUSCLE RELAXANTS

Whether muscle relaxants are useful in low back pain is controversial. Some of the drugs available in this class are listed in Table 36.

NONSTEROIDAL ANTIINFLAMMATORY DRUGS

(See also dementia; nonsteroidal antiinflammatory drug gastropathy; nonsteroidal antiinflammatory drugs and hypertension; nonsteroidal antiinflammatory drugs in the treatment of renal colic; nonsteroidal antiinflammatory drugs, topical, ophthalmic; prescribing habits and the elderly; primary prevention of colon cancer)

A practical reason for dividing nonsteroidal antiinflammatory drugs (NSAIDs) into their different chemical classes is that if a drug from one class is ineffective, replacing it with one from another class is often better than with another from the same class (Table 37). So far, studies have failed to show any consistent evidence that one NSAID is superior to another.[1] However, preliminary data suggest that two of the newer NSAIDs, etodolac (Ultradol, Lodine) and nabumetone (Relafen), may be less toxic to both the gastrointestinal tract and the kidneys. This is because these drugs have a less inhibitory effect on cyclooxygenase 1 (COX-1), which is protective in the stomach and kidneys, than cyclooxygenase 2 (COX-2), which aggravates inflammation in joints.[2]

Since adverse effects from NSAIDs are common in the elderly; these drugs should be avoided when possible, or dosages should be as low as possible. Although gastrointestinal erosions and ulcers are the most common adverse effects of these drugs, they also increase the risk of acute renal failure, particularly in the elderly.[3]

Patients who require NSAIDs but who have had an allergic reaction to them such as angioedema or asthma may be able to take salsalate (Disalcid).

Pain, not inflammation, is the primary indication for ketorolac (Toradol).

REFERENCES

1. Bellamy N: Treating musculoskeletal disease with NSAIDs: practitioner's guide, *Can Fam Physician* 42:482-492, 1996.
2. Tannenbaum H, Davis P, Russell AS, et al: Canadian NSAID Consensus Participants: an evidence-based approach to prescribing NSAIDs in musculoskeletal disease: a Canadian Consensus, *Can Med Assoc J* 155:77-88, 1996.
3. Gutthann SP, Rodriguez LA, Raiford DS, et al: Nonsteroidal anti-inflammatory drugs and the risk of hospitalization for acute renal failure, *Arch Intern Med* 156:2433-2439, 1996.

ORTHOPEDICS

(See also prosthetic joint infection prophylaxis)

Stress Fractures

Most stress fractures occur in the lower extremities, most commonly at the necks of the second and third metatarsals. The reported incidence varies considerably from one report to an-

Locomotor System

other and is higher in more recent publications, probably because bone scans were used to make the diagnosis. In some reports of military recruits the incidence during basic training was as high as 31%. Women, especially those who are oligomenorrheic, are more likely to have this disorder than men. The incidence is lower in blacks and Hispanics.[1] Stress fractures are rare in children.[2] A change in exercise pattern or training often precedes the onset of symptoms by a few weeks.[1]

The two most common locations of stress fractures in athletes are the tibia and the metatarsals. Any portion of the tibia may be involved, whereas in the case of metatarsals the shaft and neck of the second and third metatarsals are the usual sites. About 5% of stress fractures occur in the femoral neck; diagnosing these and obtaining an orthopedic consultation are important because of the high rate of progression to complete femoral neck fractures. Stress fractures of the shaft of the femur also occur but are relatively rare.[1]

Pain is the complaint of patients with stress fractures. Initially it comes on after physical activity or late during the activity, but as the condition worsens, pain begins earlier. There may be some swelling, but point tenderness is the most common physical finding. X-ray films usually fail to reveal the lesions early in the course of the disease and are often normal even after several weeks or months. The gold standard for making a specific diagnosis is the bone scan, which can be positive within a few days of the onset of symptoms. However, the specificity of this test is relatively low.[1]

In general, the management of stress fractures involves rest, pain control, and exercises to prevent deconditioning. These are followed by gradual reintroduction of the causative exercise activity.[1]

REFERENCES

1. Monteleone GP Jr: Stress fractures in the athlete, *Orthop Clin North Am* 26:423-432, 1995.
2. Griffin LY: Common sports injuries of the foot and ankle seen in children and adolescents, *Orthop Clin North Am* 25:83-93, 1994.

Hip

(See also osteoarthritis; osteoporosis; septic arthritis; stress fractures)

Apophyseal injuries

Apophyseal injuries similar to Osgood-Schlatter disease occur in the region of the hip, anterior superior iliac spine, anterior inferior iliac spine, iliac crest, and ischial tuberosity. Rest, ice, and NSAIDs are usually effective.[1]

Hip fractures

Many but not all of the risk factors for hip fracture parallel those for osteoporosis. Current alcohol use is a risk factor for hip fracture,[2,3] as are long- and short-acting benzodiazepines.[4] High rates of prescription medication use also correlate with hip fractures.[4,5] A prospective multicenter U.S. study of hip fractures in white women found that most had multiple risk factors; weight gain after the age of 25 was protective.[6]

The type of surgery selected for hip fractures depends on a number of variables. Nondisplaced femoral neck fractures in patients over 70 or even displaced fractures in those under 70 may be treated with internal fixation. The rate of nonunion and femoral head necrosis in displaced femoral neck fractures in patients over 70 is high, and these are usually treated with a prosthesis. Intertrochanteric fractures are usually managed by internal fixation.[7]

Mortality rates after hip fractures are reported to be between 14% and 36%. Between 50% and 65% of patients regain their previous ambulatory status, 10% to 15% can ambulate only in the home, and 20% become nonambulatory. Recovery of ambulation is more likely among patients who are male, nondemented, and relatively young.[7] In many cases mortality associated with hip fractures appears to be due to serious underlying conditions that in themselves contribute to the fractures; it is doubtful that measures to prevent fractures (such as hormone replacement therapy) would significantly affect the mortality of this group of patients.[8]

The long-term results of hip prostheses are excellent even after 20 years.[9,10] One of the original problems with hip arthroplasty was aseptic loosening of the femoral component, but with advances in cementing techniques this is now a rare complication. However, loosening of cemented acetabular components remains a significant problem.[10]

Transient synovitis

Transient synovitis of the hip is the most common cause of hip pain in children aged 3 to 10 years. It affects males twice as often as females. The most important differential diagnosis is septic arthritis. Clues to septic arthritis are severe hip pain and spasm, fever, tenderness, and an elevated sedimentation rate. However, the absence of these criteria does not rule out infection. Patients with transient synovitis have usually improved spontaneously within a week to 10 days. Other joints may also be affected by transient synovitis; after the hip, the knee is the most frequently involved joint.[11]

REFERENCES

1. Peck DM: Apophyseal injuries in the young athlete, *Am Fam Physician* 51:1891-1895, 1995.
2. Felson DT, Kiel DP, Anderson JJ, Kannel WB: Alcohol consumption and hip fractures; the Framingham Study, *Am J Epidemiol* 128:1102-1110, 1988.
3. Grisso JA, Kelsey JL, Strom BL, et al: Risk factors for hip fracture in black women, *N Engl J Med* 330:1555-1559, 1994.
4. Gerings RM, Stricker BH, de Boer A, et al: Benzodiazepines and the risk of falling leading to femur fractures: dosage more important than elimination half-life, *Arch Intern Med* 155: 1801-1807, 1995.
5. Davidson W, Molloy DW, Bédard M: Physician characteristics and prescribing for elderly people in New Brunswick: relation to patient outcomes, *Can Med Assoc J* 152:1227-1234, 1995.
6. Cummings SR, Nevitt MC, Browner WS, et al: Risk factors for hip fracture in white women, *N Engl J Med* 332:767-773, 1995.

7. Zuckerman JD: Hip fracture, *N Engl J Med* 334:1519-1525, 1996.
8. Browner WS, Pressman AR, Nevitt MC, Cummings SR (Study of Osteoporotic Fractures Research Group): Mortality following fractures in older women, *Arch Intern Med* 156:1521-1525, 1996.
9. Schulte KR, Callaghan JJ, Kelley SS, Johnston RC: The outcome of Charnley total hip arthroplasty with cement after a minimum twenty-year follow-up: the results of one surgeon, *J Bone Joint Surgery [Am]* 75:961-975, 1993.
10. Mulroy RD, Harris WH: The effect of improved cementing techniques on component loosening in total hip replacement, *J Bone Joint Surg [Br]* 72:757-760, 1990.
11. Hart JJ: Transient synovitis of the hip in children, *Am Fam Physician* 54:1587-1591, 1996.

Knee

(See also ankle trauma; foot trauma; osteoarthritis; Sever's disease)

Apophyseal injuries

Osgood-Schlatter disease of the tibial tuberosity is the best known apophyseal disorder in the knee region. A similar phenomenon about the inferior patella is called the Sindig-Larsen-Johansson syndrome, and about the heel the condition is called Sever's disease.[1]

Knee trauma

Clinical decision rules for ordering knee x-ray studies after trauma (Ottawa knee rules) are any of the following[2]:

1. Age greater than 55
2. Inability to walk four consecutive steps immediately after injury or in the emergency room (two steps on each limb)
3. Inability to flex 90 degrees
4. Tenderness over the head of the fibula
5. Isolated tenderness over the patella (no tenderness of bone elsewhere on knee)

Use of these rules was 100% sensitive for detecting fractures and had the potential for decreasing the number of radiographs by 28%.[2]

REFERENCES

1. Peck DM: Apophyseal injuries in the young athlete, *Am Fam Physician* 51:1891-1895, 1995.
2. Stiell IG, Greenberg GH, Wells GA, et al: Prospective validation of a decision rule for the use of radiography in acute knee injuries, *JAMA* 275:611-615, 1996.

Ankle

(See also foot trauma; knee trauma; stress fractures)

Ankle trauma

Refined clinical decision rules for ordering ankle radiographs apply only if there is pain in the region of either malleolus plus:

1. Inability to bear weight both immediately after the injury and for four steps in the emergency department *or*
2. Bone tenderness at the tip of either malleolus or over the posterior tibia or fibula in the regions 6 cm proximal to the tips of the malleoli

With use of these techniques sensitivity was virtually 100%.[1-3] Approximately 20% fewer radiographs are required, patient costs are lower, and time spent in the emergency room is less.[2]

The initial treatment for an ankle sprain is the standard RICE (relative rest, ice, compression, and elevation) therapy, but in short order this should be followed by an active rehabilitation program. Initially the ankle should be iced before any exercise is tried. One set of recommendations that should be instituted on a progressive basis is as follows[4]:

1. Alphabet drawing. Have the patient draw the alphabet on the floor with the foot.
2. Towel exercises. Have the patient place the foot on a towel that has been laid out on the floor. Keeping the heel on the floor, the patient should move the towel back and forth with inversion and eversion movements of the ankle and foot.
3. Stretching exercises of the gastrocnemius and soleus. Initially this is done by having the patient sit on the floor with the legs extended. A towel is looped around the sole of the forefoot of the affected side, and the two ends are held in the patient's two hands. Gentle pulling on the ends of the towel causes dorsiflexion of the ankle. As the patient improves, he or she can stretch the calves by standing facing a wall and then leaning toward it with the heel kept on the floor.
4. Proprioception or balance exercises. The patient stands on one foot and then extends the other one forward, laterally, backward, and back down. This should be repeated 10 times.

REFERENCES

1. Stiell IG, Greenberg GH, McKnight RD, et al: Decision rules for the use of radiography in acute ankle injuries: refinement and prospective validation, *JAMA* 269:1127-1132, 1993.
2. Stiell IG, Wells K, Laupacis A, Brison R, et al (Multicentre Ankle Rule Study Group): Multicentre trial to introduce the Ottawa ankle rules for use of radiography in acute ankle injuries, *BMJ* 311:594-597, 1995.
3. Stiell I: Ottawa ankle rules, *Can Fam Physician* 42:478-480, 1996.
4. Vopicka AA: Acute ankle sprain: getting patients back on their feet, *Can J Diagn* 11:57-71, 1994.

Foot

(See also ankle trauma; knee trauma; apophyseal injuries in the knee region in adolescents; stress fractures)

Plantar fasciitis

Traditional treatment of plantar fasciitis is rest, heel pads, NSAIDs, occasionally steroid injections, and very rarely surgery.[1,2] Most patients with plantar fasciitis have associated tightness of the Achilles tendon, and the resultant limitation of dorsiflexion on heel strike strains the plantar fascia. In addition, the condition tends to make the patient sleep with the feet in plantar flexion, which causes contractures of the plantar fascia. Therapeutic modalities include stretching of the Achilles tendon (keeping the heel on the floor while leaning forward)[1] and the plantar fascia (with the heel on the floor and toes on wall, putting weight on the foot),[2] full or three-quarter length off-the-shelf orthoses of relatively soft material giving a good arch support, shoes with cushioned heels, and in many cases night splints that maintain the feet and toes in about 5% of dorsiflexion.[1]

Freiberg's disease

Freiberg's disease is an osteochondritis of bone involving the distal portion of one of the metatarsals. It is seen most often in girls between the ages of 12 and 15. Two thirds of the cases involve the second metatarsal, most of the remainder the third, and about 5% the fourth. Patients have pain, swelling, and tenderness, and the x-ray picture is typical. Treatment involves metatarsal pads or orthotics to decrease weight bearing on the area.[3]

Sever's disease

Sever's disease is a traction apophysitis of the posterior calcaneus and is thus similar to Osgood-Schlatter disease of the knee. The disease usually affects girls between the ages of 8 and 10 and boys between 10 and 12. The patients complain of unilateral or bilateral heel pain that comes on after weight bearing and often after starting a new sport. They usually have no pain on arising in the morning, and the pain, when present, is relieved by rest. On examination there may be tenderness both over the posterior insertion of the Achilles tendon to the calcaneus and along the medial and lateral borders of the calcaneus near its posterior border (the line of junction of the posterior epiphysis of the calcaneus and the body of the calcaneus). The maneuver that reveals this pain is called the squeeze test. Initial treatment is ice, rest, and heel lifts. These are followed by heel cord, calf, and hamstring stretching exercises, as well as ankle dorsiflexion strengthening exercises. Sever's disease is not associated with long-term sequelae.[4]

Foot trauma

According to refined clinical decision rules for the efficient use of radiography, foot radiographs are necessary only if the patient has pain in the midfoot plus either inability to bear weight immediately after the injury and for four steps in the emergency department or bone tenderness at the navicular or the base of the fifth metatarsal.[5] One study using these criteria found them to be 100% sensitive for 19 foot fractures.[5]

REFERENCES

1. Ryan J: Use of posterior night splints in the treatment of plantar fasciitis, *Am Fam Physician* 52:891-898, 1995.
2. Singh D, Angel J, Bentley G, et al: Plantar fasciitis, *BMJ* 315: 172-175, 1997.
3. Griffin LY: Common sports injuries of the foot and ankle seen in children and adolescents, *Orthop Clin North Am* 25:83-93, 1994.
4. Madden CC, Mellion MB: Sever's disease and other causes of heel pain in adolescents, *Am Fam Physician* 54:1995-2000, 1996.
5. Stiell IG, Greenberg GH, McKnight RD, et al: Decision rules for the use of radiography in acute ankle injuries: refinement and prospective validation, *JAMA* 269:1127-1132, 1993.

Shoulder

(See also detrimental effects of investigations)

Dislocation

In a Swedish prospective study of 247 anterior dislocations the patients were assigned at random to three forms of initial treatment: immobilization for 3 to 4 weeks by binding the arm to the torso, sling for pain relief that was discontinued when the patient was comfortable, and immobilization for various durations. At 10 years recurrent dislocations requiring surgical treatment occurred in about one fourth of the patients. Another 22% had at least two recurrences in the first 2 to 5 years, but then the condition stabilized with no further recurrences. The rate of recurrent dislocations was unrelated to the initial treatment. In this study 18% of patients under 30 had a dislocation of the opposite shoulder whereas the rate of contralateral dislocation for those between 30 and 40 was only 3%.[1]

Imaging studies of shoulder

Magnetic resonance imaging (MRI) of the dominant shoulder was conducted on 96 persons with no shoulder complaints and with normal findings on examination of the shoulder. Of the 46 subjects over 60 years of age, 28% had complete rotator cuff tears and 26% had partial tears. Those between the ages of 40 and 60 demonstrated fewer abnormalities, with 4% having complete tears and 24% partial tears.[2] This study reconfirms the fundamental clinical principle that abnormal results from investigative procedures may be irrelevant to the patient's clinical condition.

Physiotherapy for soft tissue injuries of the shoulder

A systematic review of the literature failed to find any benefit from ultrasound therapy. Few of the reviewed trials found physiotherapy to be effective, but methodological errors were so common that it remains unknown whether such treatment modalities as exercise, mobilization, heat or cold applications, low-level laser therapy, or electrotherapy are of any value.[3]

REFERENCES

1. Hovelius L, Augustini BG, Fredin H, et al: Primary anterior dislocation of the shoulder in young patients—a ten-year prospective study, *J Bone Joint Surg [Am]* 78A:1677-1684, 1996.
2. Sher JS, Uribe JW, Posada A, et al: Abnormal findings on magnetic resonance images of asymptomatic shoulders, *J Bone Joint Surg* 77A:10-15, 1995.

3. van der Heijden GJ, Van der Windt DA, de Winter AF: Physiotherapy for patients with soft tissue shoulder disorders: a systematic review of randomised clinical trials, *BMJ* 315:25-35, 1997.

Elbow

Apophyseal injuries

A medial epicondylitis in the elbow region similar to Osgood-Schlatter disease of the tibial tuberosity occurs about the medial epicondyle in adolescent pitchers.[1]

Supracondylar fractures

Supracondylar fractures are the most common elbow fractures of children. The mechanism of injury is a fall that causes hyperextension of the elbow, and most cases occur between the ages of 5 and 8. Neurovascular damage is an important complication. Splinting in 20 to 30 degrees of flexion often relieves brachial artery obstruction.[2]

Tennis elbow

In more than 95% of patients tennis elbow has nothing to do with tennis.[3] In most young persons it is caused by sports and in older persons by occupation.[4]

REFERENCES

1. Peck DM: Apophyseal injuries in the young athlete, *Am Fam Physician* 51:1891-1895, 1995.
2. Townsend DJ, Bassett GS: Common elbow fractures in children, *Am Fam Physician* 53:2031-2041, 1996.
3. Chop WM Jr: Tennis elbow, *Postgrad Med* 86:301-304, 307-308, 1989.
4. Gellman H: Tennis elbow (lateral epicondylitis), *Orthop Clin North Am* 23:75-82, 1992.

Hand

Boxer's fracture

Treatment of boxer's fracture varies from one surgeon to another. Unless the angulation of the distal fragment is greater than 45 degrees, reduction is unnecessary. Pain can be relieved with a tensor bandage.[1]

Skier's thumb

Skier's or gamekeeper's thumb is a laxity of the ulnar collateral ligament of the metacarpophalangeal ligament of the thumb. It is an occupational disorder resulting from repetitive strain such as occurs when killing snared small game by forcefully hyperextending their heads using the thumb and forefinger. At present most injuries to this ligament take place as a result as forced abduction during sports injuries, particularly skiing accidents. If the patient has a complete tear of the ligament, surgical repair is indicated because in at least 50% of cases the proximal end is trapped in such a way that healing cannot take place. It is important to distinguish ligamentous tears from avulsion fractures. Before stress is placed on the ligament, x-ray examination should be performed; if a small avulsion fracture is found and the displacement is less than 5 mm, conservative treatment with a short arm or even glove-type spica cast for 4 to 6 weeks will suffice. If the gap is greater than 5 mm or the fragment involves more than 25% of the joint surface, surgical repair is indicated.[2]

If no fracture is seen on the x-ray film, the joint should be stressed for the assessment of a complete ligamentous tear. This maneuver should not be performed if the patient has an avulsion fracture because it may cause displacement of the fragment. The ligament is at maximum tension when the metacarpophalangeal joint is fully flexed, so that is the position that should be used for stressing. If the degree of angulation exceeds 30 degrees, or if it is 15 degrees more than on the unaffected side, surgical consultation is indicated. In many cases local anesthesia is necessary so the physician can adequately stress the joint.[1]

REFERENCES

1. Ford MH: What's best for "boxer's fracture," *Patient Care Can* 7:15, 1996.
2. Richard JR: Gamekeeper's thumb: ulnar collateral ligament injury, *Am Fam Physician* 53:1775-1780, 1996.

Cervical Spine

(See also head restraints)

Whiplash injury

Between 20% and 40% of persons with whiplash injury have persistent debilitating symptoms that may last for years. Although claims have been made that such patients have psychological problems or financial incentives for persistent illness, many workers believe that this is unlikely.[1]

Carette[2] emphasizes the importance of conservative management and the maintenance of function in patients with whiplash injury. Although analgesic or antiinflammatory drugs are useful in the early stages, the wearing of a collar is counterproductive if done for more than a few days. Patients should be encouraged to mobilize the neck in spite of pain and reassured that this will not aggravate the condition. Prolonged physiotherapy may simply reinforce patients' images of themselves as sick. Steroid injections into apophyseal joints have not been shown to be valuable.

Is there a role for MRI in patients with whiplash injury? In a series of 100 patients with whiplash injury, normal neurological findings, and normal plain radiographs, MRI performed within 3 weeks of injury revealed no clinically significant abnormalities.[3]

REFERENCES

1. Radanov BP, Di Stefano G, Schnidrig A, et al: Role of psychosocial stress in recovery from common whiplash, *Lancet* 328:712-715, 1991.
2. Carette S: Whiplash injury and chronic neck pain (editorial), *N Engl Med J* 330:1083-1084, 1994.
3. Ronnen HR, Dekorte PJ, Brink PR, et al: Acute whiplash injury —is there a role for MR imaging: prospective study of 100 patients, *Radiology* 201:93-96, 1996.

Lumbar Spine

Low back pain

(See also ankylosing spondylitis; detrimental effects of investigations; medical economics; muscle relaxants)

Epidemiology. The annual incidence of acute low back pain leading to medical attention or loss of time from work is 2% to 5%. The lifetime prevalence is 80% to 85%. Chronic low back pain is the most common cause of disability in people under the age of 45 and the third most common for those aged 45 to 64. The peak age for low back pain is about 40. In some studies low back pain is second only to respiratory tract complaints as a reason for visiting office-based physicians. The incidence of low back disability has increased markedly in Western societies from the 1950s through the 1970s.[1]

The likelihood in family medicine that patients with low back pain have underlying systemic or visceral disease is low. Figures vary but range from about 0.05% to 0.1% for neoplasms and about half that for infectious disorders.[2,3] An association has been reported between smoking and low back pain, but whether this is causal is uncertain.[4]

Diagnosis. For up to 85% of cases of low back pain, a definite pathophysiological diagnosis (substantive diagnosis) cannot be made. Instead nominative diagnoses such as "lumbar strain," "nonspecific low back pain," or "mechanical disorder of the back" are given.[1]

Inflammatory back pain (ankylosing spondylitis) is a rare but important cause of low back pain in those under 40. Findings suggesting this diagnosis are discussed under "Ankylosing Spondylitis."[1] Malignancy as a cause of low back pain is most likely to occur in persons over 50, and infection as a cause of back pain is most often seen in IV drug abusers.[1]

One of the main diagnostic roles of the family physician faced with a patient who has low back pain is to rule out a visceral cause (e.g., malignancy, infection, aortic aneurysm), to rule out an acute cauda equina syndrome (incontinence of urine or stool, difficulty walking, bilateral lower limb neurological signs, saddle anesthesia, and decreased rectal tone), and to look for objective evidence of nerve root irritation.

Imaging. Lumbosacral spine x-rays have been estimated to be the largest single source of gonadal radiation in the United States. According to one report the amount of gonadal radiation from lumbosacral spine x-rays is equivalent to that received from a daily chest x-ray over 6 years.[5]

The yield of lumbar spine x-rays is low, and many abnormal x-ray findings have no or only questionable clinical significance (e.g., spondylosis, spondylolysis, single disk narrowing, apophyseal joint abnormalities, Schmorl's nodes, and mild to moderate scoliosis).[6]

Patients who have not improved over 2 to 4 weeks from the time of the initial visit should probably have x-ray examination of the lumbosacral spine. The following specific indications for ordering x-rays on the first visit are suggested[7]:

1. Age over 50
2. Fever
3. Findings suggestive of ankylosing spondylitis
4. History of previous malignancy or striking weight loss
5. Significant trauma
6. Moderate neurological deficits (including cauda equina syndrome)
7. Intended litigation or compensation
8. Use of corticosteroids
9. Drug or alcohol abuse

Disk bulging or disk protrusions are extremely common in individuals without back pain. In one MRI study of the lumbar spine in persons aged 20 to 80 (mean 42) with no back pain, 52% of the subjects had a bulge at least one level, 27% had a protrusion, and 1% an extrusion.[8] The implication of this and other similar studies is that abnormalities found by imaging may mislead clinicians into thinking that what is detected is necessarily a cause of the patient's symptoms. The potential for unnecessary surgery is great in such situations.

In most cases computed tomography or MRI should be ordered for patients with back pain only if they have signs and symptoms of radiculopathy that have not responded to conservative therapy over a 6-week period and if they are now being considered as candidates for surgery.[9]

Prognosis and Management. More than 90% of cases of low back pain resolve spontaneously within 3 months, and the vast majority of patients return to work within 6 weeks. According to Waddell,[1] in most cases there is no evidence that any form of treatment is better than time and placebo effect.

Only 1% of patients with acute low back pain require surgery, and these are almost all patients who have proven disk protrusion with nerve root irritation that has not responded to conservative therapy. Of patients with proven disk protrusions causing neurological symptoms, only 5% to 10% require surgery.[1]

Even during the acute phase of low back pain it is questionable whether rest is useful.[1] One study of army recruits showed a benefit,[10] but this has not been replicated in other studies.[11] In a comparison of 2 days versus 7 days of bed rest for acute low back pain without neurological deficits, no advantage was found for the longer period.[12] In a Finnish study of patients with low back pain (without evidence of nerve root compression) patients were randomly assigned to three groups: 2 days of bed rest, back mobilizing exercises, and continuation of normal activities as tolerated. The group that continued normal activities did better than the other two.[13] A Dutch study also found that physiotherapy for acute low back pain did not shorten the time until return to work.[14]

Patients with disk herniation and nerve root compression may benefit from slightly more prolonged bed rest, but the maximum period should be 1 week.[15] Most patients with nerve root compression can stand and walk by the third day, and by day 7 they should be able to walk 20 minutes for every 3 hours spent supine. They should be encouraged in these activities even if the pain is aggravated, and as soon as possible they should move on to low-impact aerobics such as bicycling, swimming, or speed walking.[16] Given time a herniated nucleus pulposus shrinks; this was demonstrated in a prospective MRI study that found substantial shrinkage in 36% of patients at 6 weeks and in 60% of patients at 6 months after presentation.[17]

Physically fit persons have fewer and shorter episodes of low back pain than do the physically unfit.[16,18] Psychosocial factors are important issues in low back pain.[1,19-21] In a prospective study of industrial injury claims for low back pain, the only positive predictors were job dissatisfaction and distress as reported on scale 3 (indicating tendencies to somatize and deny emotional distress) on the Minnesota Multiphasic Personality Inventory.[19]

A randomized double-blind controlled (with sham traction) trial of traction for nonspecific low back pain failed to show any benefit.[22] Patients with root compression who do not respond to conservative therapy may be treated with a number of interventions. Some of the newer ones include laser disk decompression[23] and microlumbar diskectomy, which may be performed as an outpatient procedure.[24]

An observational study from North Carolina found that for patients with low back pain who did not require surgery, the times to functional recovery, return to work, and complete recovery were identical for patients treated by primary care physicians, orthopedic surgeons, and chiropractors. The cost of care was highest for orthopedic surgeons and chiropractors (the latter because of multiple visits) and least for primary care physicians. However, patient satisfaction was greatest when patients were treated by chiropractors.[25]

Prevention. A large-scale controlled trial of an educational program taught by physiotherapists (such as is used in "back schools") failed to demonstrate any long-term benefits.[26]

REFERENCES

1. Waddell G: A new clinical model for the treatment of low-back pain (1987 Volvo Award in Clinical Sciences), *Spine* 12:632-644, 1987.
2. Liang M, Komaroff AL: Roentgenograms in primary care patients with acute low back pain: a cost-effectiveness analysis, *Arch Intern Med* 142:1108-1112, 1982.
3. Deyo RA, Diehl AK: Lumbar spine films in primary care: current use and the effects of selective ordering criteria, *J Gen Intern Med* 1:20-25, 1986.
4. Leboeufyde C, Yashin A: Smoking and low back pain—is the association real? *J Manip Physiol Ther* 18:457-463, 1995.
5. Hall FM: Back pain and the radiologist, *Radiology* 137:861-863, 1980.
6. Nachemson AL: The lumbar spine: an orthopedic challenge, *Spine* 1:59-71, 1976.
7. Deyo RA: Early diagnostic evaluation of low back pain, *J Gen Intern Med* 1:328-338, 1986.
8. Jensen MC, Brant-Zawadzki MN, Obuchowski N, et al: Magnetic resonance imaging of the lumbar spine in people without back pain, *N Engl J Med* 331:69-73, 1994.
9. Deyo RA: Magnetic resonance imaging of the lumbar spine: terrific test or Tar Baby? (editorial), *N Engl J Med* 331:115-116, 1994.
10. Wiesel SW, Cuckler JM, Deluca F, et al: Acute low back pain; an objective analysis of conservative therapy, *Spine* 5:324-330, 1980.
11. Gilbert JR, Taylor DW, Hildebrand A: Clinical trial of common treatments for low back pain in family practice, *BMJ* 291:791-794, 1985.
12. Deyo RA, Diehl AK, Rosenthal M: How many days of bed rest for acute low back pain? *N Engl J Med* 315:1064-1070, 1986.
13. Malmivaara A, Häkkinen U, Aro T, et al: The treatment of acute low back pain—bed rest, exercises, or ordinary activity? *N Engl J Med* 332:351-355, 1995.
14. Faas A, van Eijk JT, Chavannes AW, et al: A randomized trial of exercise therapy in patients with acute low back pain: efficacy on sickness absence, *Spine* 20:941-947, 1995.
15. Deyo RA, Loeser JD, Bigos SJ: Herniated lumbar intervertebral disk, *Ann Intern Med* 112:598-603, 1990.
16. Biering-Soresen P: Physical measurements as risk indicators for low back trouble over a one year period, *Spine* 9:106-119, 1984.
17. Modic MT, Ross JS, Obuchowski NA, et al: Contrast-enhanced MR imaging in acute lumbar radiculopathy: a pilot study of the natural history, *Radiology* 195:323-324, 1995.
18. Cady L, Bischoff D, O'Connel E: Strength and fitness and subsequent back injuries in firefighters, *J Occup Med* 21:269-272, 1979.
19. Bigos SJ, Battie MC, Spengler DM, et al: A longitudinal, prospective study of industrial back injury reporting, *Clin Orthop Rel Res* 279:21-34, 1992.
20. Frymoyer JW: Predicting disability from low back pain, *Clin Orthop Rel Res* 279:101-109, 1992.
21. Nachemson AL: Newest knowledge of low back pain, *Clin Orthop Rel Res* 279:8-20, 1992.
22. Beurskens AJ, de Vet HC, Köke AJ, et al: Efficacy of traction for non-specific low back pain: a randomised clinical trial, *Lancet* 346:1596-1600, 1996.
23. Ohnmeiss DD, Guyer RD, Hochschuler SH: Laser disc decompression: the importance of proper patient selection, *Spine* 19:2054-2058, 1994.
24. Zahrawi F: Microlumbar discectomy: is it safe as an outpatient procedure? *Spine* 19:1070-1074, 1994.
25. Carey TS, Garrett J, Jackman A, et al: The outcomes and costs of care for acute low back pain among patients seen by primary care practitioners, chiropractors, and orthopedic surgeons, *N Engl J Med* 333:913-917, 1995.
26. Daltroy LH, Iversen MD, Larson MG, et al: A controlled trial of an educational program to prevent low back injuries, *N Engl J Med* 337:322-328, 1997.

Scoliosis

Evidence is limited regarding the effectiveness of scoliosis screening and treatment, and the natural history of the disease is uncertain.[1,2] Most patients with scoliosis seen in family medicine have curvatures of less than 10 degrees, and few of these progress.[3] Even more frustrating is that although bracing effectively straightens out many curvatures in the short run, long-term studies have shown that much of the benefit is lost with time.[3] In addition, screening and treatment are associated with significant psychological and physical morbidity.[1] Because of these factors both the Canadian Task Force on the Periodic Health Examination[1] and the U.S. Preventive Services Task Force[2] have given screening of adolescents for scoliosis a "C" recommendation. On the other hand, numerous American organizations recommend the screening of adolescents for scoliosis. These include the American Academy of Pediatrics and the American Academy of Orthopedic Surgeons. In addition, 15 U.S. states require screening by law. As might be expected, the British Orthopaedic Association and the British Scoliosis Society advise against a national policy of screening.[1]

REFERENCES

1. Canadian Task Force on the Periodic Health Examination: *Clinical preventive health care,* Ottawa, 1994, Canadian Communication Group—Publishing, pp 345-354.
2. US Preventive Services Task Force: *Guide to clinical preventive services,* ed 2, Baltimore, 1996, Williams & Wilkins, pp 517-529.
3. Diguiseppi CG, Woolf SH: The family physician's role in adolescent idiopathic scoliosis (editorial), *Am Fam Physician* 53: 2268-2272, 1996.

Reflex Sympathetic Dystrophy

Reflex sympathetic dystrophy is usually precipitated by trauma; the severity of the trauma does not correlate with the incidence of the disease. Women are more commonly affected than men and whites more than other races. Symptoms occur more often in the lower than the upper extremity. The cardinal symptom is pain, and this is accompanied by tenderness of the affected limb. Some patients find light touch as occurs with bed clothing intolerable. In the early stages patients may have edema; later, dystrophic changes are found with smooth shiny skin and mottling and coolness of the extremity. The cornerstone of treatment is pain relief and physiotherapy. Some patients require sympathetic blockade or even a sympathectomy. Drugs that may be useful aside from analgesics or NSAIDs are calcium channel blockers or in some cases parenteral injections of calcitonin.[1]

REFERENCES

1. Drake WT, Anderson K: Reflex sympathetic dystrophy: what are the signs? *Can J Diagn* 12:67-81, 1995.

RHEUMATOLOGY

(See also hemochromatosis; Lyme disease; nonsteroidal antiinflammatory drugs)

Crystal-Induced Arthritis

For patients who cannot take NSAIDs, prednisone 30 to 50 mg/day tapered over 7 to 10 days is effective in cases of crystal-induced arthritis.[1]

Gout

In gout the most frequently affected joints are the first metatarsophalangeal joints, ankles, midfoot joints, and knees. Put another way, gout usually involves the joints of the lower extremities, excluding the hips.[1-3] The wrists are also sometimes involved.[2] An initial attack usually comes on suddenly and involves only one joint.[1-3] Males are affected seven times as often as females.[4]

An acute attack of gout may be precipitated by minor trauma, systemic illnesses, surgery, or anything causing either a rapid rise in the uric acid level (thiazides, other diuretics, low-dose aspirin, and alcohol) or a rapid decrease in uric acid (high-dose aspirin, allopurinol [Zyloprim], probenecid [Benemid], or sudden cessation of alcohol).[4]

The risk of gout increases with increasing levels of serum urate. The risk is 5% per year for persons with a urate level of 9 mg/dl or 535 µmol/L (normal is 2 to 7 mg/dl or 120 to 420 µmol/L). There is no clinical indication for treating asymptomatic hyperuricemia, but it would seem advisable to identify, and if possible modify, known causes of this condition such as myeloproliferative disorders, low-dose salicylates, thiazides, loop diuretics, excessive alcohol consumption, high-purine diets, and obesity.[1] Common foods with high purine content are all meats (including organ meats), gravies, meat extracts, seafood, yeast, yeast extracts, beer, other alcoholic beverages, asparagus, beans, cauliflower, lentils, mushrooms, oatmeal, peas, and spinach.[1]

The drugs of choice for acute gout are NSAIDs. The agent used most frequently is indomethacin (Indocin) in doses of 150 to 300 mg/day (usually 50 mg tid or qid) with gradual reduction of the dose as symptoms resolve.[1-3] Other NSAIDs such as naproxen, ketoprofen, and ibuprofen have also been used starting with maximum doses and tapering as symptoms resolve.[3] Some degree of pain relief usually occurs within 2 to 4 hours if the drug is started reasonably soon after the onset of symptoms. Alternatives to NSAIDs are oral prednisone starting at 30 to 50 mg/day and tapering gradually over 7 to 10 days or, if only one joint is involved, intraarticular injection of steroid. Colchicine can also be used. Best results with colchicine are obtained if the drug is started within 24 hours; it is ineffective if started after 5 days. The initial dose is 1 mg, and this is followed by 0.5 mg every 2 hours until the patient has diarrhea or abdominal cramps or until a total of 8 mg has been administered. Pain relief usually begins 12 to 18 hours later if the drug has been started reasonably soon after the onset of symptoms.[1-3] A few patients with recurrent episodes of gout are able to abort acute attacks if they recognize the initial symptoms and immediately take 1 to 1.2 mg of colchicine.[3]

Prophylaxis is indicated if the patient has recurrent attacks of gout or has tophi. Colchicine in doses of 0.5 to 1 mg/day is often effective in preventing recurrent attacks and should be continued for about a year after the last attack. If a patient with recurrent attacks is hyperuricemic or has tophi, urate-lowering drugs should also be used. The usual drug is allopurinol (Zyloprim). Allopurinol and other drugs that lower serum uric acid may precipitate acute attacks of gout, a risk that may be decreased by starting with low doses (allopurinol 50 to 100 mg/day, increasing weekly up to 300 mg/day in most cases but up to 600[4] or even 800 mg/day[3] in a few), by avoiding use of these drugs until several weeks since the last acute attack, and by giving prophylactic medications such as low-dose colchicine (0.5 to 1 mg/day) before and concurrently with the allopurinol. Lifelong treatment is often needed, and the goal is to maintain the uric acid level below 6 mg/dl (360 µmol/L) unless there are tophi, in which case the target is less than 5 mg/dl (300 µmol/L).[1]

Pyrophosphate arthropathy

Pyrophosphate arthropathy (chondrocalcinosis, calcium pyrophosphate deposition disease [CPPD]) is also called pseudogout if the onset of the illness is acute and mimics gout. It is caused by the intraarticular precipitation of pyrophosphate dihydrate crystals. CPPD is usually a disease of the elderly, and the most commonly affected joint is the knee. Other joints that are commonly inflamed are the wrist, elbow, shoulder, ankle, and metacarpophalangeal joints. Pseudogout may have an acute onset, affecting one or two joints. The onset of the acute disease is not quite as dramatic as that of gout but requires 2 hours to 3 days for the pain to reach maximum intensity.[2,5] As with gout, acute episodes of CPPD may be precipitated by minor trauma, surgery, or systemic illness.[4] A more common presentation of CPPD is that of chronic arthritis involving several joints and thus mimicking osteoarthritis.[2,4]

The acute disease can usually be controlled by NSAIDs. Other therapeutic modalities are IV colchicine (1 to 2 mg as a single dose IV on day 1 and 0.5 mg q6h IV on day 2 and sometimes day 3), oral colchicine (which is not as reliably effective as the IV route), aspiration of the joint without steroid instillation (to remove the crystals), and aspiration of the joint with steroid injection. For recurrent attacks prophylactic colchicine 0.6 mg bid is effective.[5] NSAIDs are usually given for the chronic disease; no way is known to prevent calcium pyrophosphate dihydrate crystals from forming or to remove them from the tissues.[2]

REFERENCES

1. Emmerson BT: The management of gout, *N Engl J Med* 334:445-451, 1996.
2. Beutler A, Schumacher HR Jr: Gout and "pseudogout": when are arthritic symptoms caused by crystal deposition? *Postgrad Med* 95:103-120, 1994.
3. Schumacher HR Jr: Crystal-induced arthritis: an overview, *Am J Med* 100(suppl 2A):46S-52S, 1996.
4. Joseph J, McGrath H: Gout or "pseudogout": how to differentiate crystal-induced arthropathies, *Geriatrics* 50:33-39, 1995.
5. Handy JR: Pyrophosphate arthropathy in the knees of elderly persons, *Arch Intern Med* 156:2426-2432, 1996.

Fibromyalgia

(See also chronic fatigue syndrome; depression; multiple chemical sensitivities)

Fibromyalgia, chronic fatigue syndrome, and multiple chemical sensitivities are three conditions whose very existence is controversial. Believers search ever more intensely for organic causes, while unbelievers attribute the symptoms to psychiatric disorders such as depression or personality disorders. There is considerable overlap in the symptoms and epidemiology of the three conditions[1]; many patients with fibromyalgia also meet the criteria of chronic fatigue syndrome.[2]

The diagnostic criteria for fibromyalgia vary somewhat from article to article.[3,4] The detailed 1990 criteria of the American College of Rheumatology include the following[4]:

1. History of widespread pain involving at least three sites, one of which must be the axial spine. The axial spine is defined as including the cervical, thoracic, or lumbar spine and the anterior chest.
2. Tenderness over 11 of 18 tender points. These points are all bilateral and include the following:
   a. Suboccipital
   b. Midpoint of sternocleidomastoid muscles
   c. Medial portion of supraspinatus muscles above spines of scapulae
   d. Midpoint of upper border of trapezius muscles
   e. Second costochondral junctions
   f. Lateral epicondyles
   g. Upper outer buttocks
   h. Greater trochanters
   i. Medial fat pad of knees proximal to joint line

Fibromyalgia, like chronic fatigue syndrome and multiple chemical sensitivities, is predominantly a disorder of middle-aged women.[1,3,4] Aside from the rheumatological symptoms and signs just listed, a variety of symptoms are found in patients with this diagnosis. In most series well over 50% have sleep disturbances, fatigue, muscle weakness, and cognitive changes such as memory loss.[1] When patients with fibromyalgia have been assessed for psychiatric disorders, at least two thirds have been found to have or have had an affective or anxiety disorder.[5] If the symptoms of fibromyalgia had been scored as symptoms of somatization disorder, 25% of patients would have fulfilled the criteria for that condition.[5]

Tricyclic antidepressants have been recognized as effective over the short term for some patients with fibromyalgia.[3,6] The usual doses given have been between 25 and 75 mg/day.[3,6,7] A 1996 crossover study compared 25 mg of amitriptyline (Elavil) daily, 20 mg of fluoxetine (Prozac) daily, a combination of the two antidepressants, and placebo, each given over a 4- to 6-week period. All of the regimens that included antidepressants caused improvement compared with placebo, but the combination of amitriptyline and fluoxetine worked best.[8]

The reason that more patients have not responded to antidepressants may be that what is really being treated is depression with somatic manifestations; 25 to 75 mg of most tricyclic agents is inadequate for the treatment of depression.

REFERENCES

1. Buchwald D, Garrity D: Comparison of patients with chronic fatigue syndrome, fibromyalgia, and multiple chemical sensitivities, *Arch Intern Med* 154:2049-2053, 1994.

2. Hudson JI: Comorbidity of fibromyalgia with medical and psychiatric disorders, *Am J Med* 92:363-367, 1992.
3. Goldenberg DL: Fibromyalgia syndrome: an emerging but controversial condition, *JAMA* 257:2782-2787, 1987.
4. Wolfe F, Smythe HA, Yunus MB, et al: The American College of Rheumatology 1990 criteria for the classification of fibromyalgia: report of the multicenter criteria committee, *Arthritis Rheum* 33:160-172, 1990.
5. Hudson JI, Goldenberg DL, Pope HG, et al: Comorbidity of fibromyalgia with medical and psychiatric disorders, *Am J Med* 92:363-367, 1992.
6. Carette S, Bell MJ, Reynolds WJ, et al: Comparison of amitriptyline, cyclobenzaprine, and placebo in the treatment of fibromyalgia: a randomized, double-blind clinical trial, *Arthritis Rheum* 37:32-40, 1994.
7. Goodnick PJ, Sandoval R: Psychotropic treatment of chronic fatigue syndrome and related disorders, *J Clin Psychiatry* 54:13-20, 1993.
8. Goldenberg D, Mayskiy M, Mossey C, et al: A randomized, double-blind crossover trial of fluoxetine and amitriptyline in the treatment of fibromyalgia, *Arthritis Rheum* 39:1852-1859, 1996.

Osteoarthritis

(See also nonsteroidal antiinflammatory drugs; prescribing habits and the elderly; nonsteroidal antiinflammatory drug gastropathy)

Epidemiology

Osteoarthritis is a disease of the elderly, and the incidence of the disease in various joints varies with race. Osteoarthritis of the hips is common in whites but rare in Chinese and blacks. On the other hand, osteoarthritis of the knees is more common in black American women than white American women.[1]

Clinical presentation

Joints frequently and rarely involved by osteoarthritis are listed in Table 38.

Table 38 Joint Involvement in Osteoarthritis

Frequently involved	Rarely involved
Upper Extremity	
Distal interphalangeal joints of fingers (Heberden's nodes)	Metacarpophalangeal joints of fingers
Proximal interphalangeal joints of fingers (Bouchard's nodes)	Wrists
First carpometacarpal joints	Elbows
Acromioclavicular joints	Glenohumeral joints
Lower Extremity	
Hips	
Knees	
First metatarsophalangeal joints	Ankles (unless previous trauma)
Spine	
Cervical spine	Thoracic spine
Lumbar spine	

Prognosis

Osteoarthritis is not always a progressive disease, and patients with hip and knee pain may experience remissions. Osteoarthritis of the hands usually does not impair function.[1]

Management

Management of osteoarthritis centers on pain control. Simple measures for those with hip pain include splitting heavy loads or carrying the load on the side of the affected hip. Physical activity is important because the health of cartilage depends on normal loads being applied to joints. There is no good evidence that NSAIDs are better than simple analgesics, and theoretically some NSAIDs may actually damage cartilage (see discussion of NSAIDs below). Surgery is indicated for patients who cannot function adequately after a reasonable trial of conservative management.[1] Some specific therapeutic modalities are discussed below.

Hylin injections. Hylins are derivatives of hyaluronan; both agents form an elastoviscous fluid and have been advocated for the treatment of osteoarthritis of the knees through repeated intraarticular injections. Some workers think that formulations with higher molecular weight may have better therapeutic results, but this is not universally accepted.[2] This form of treatment has been available in Europe for two decades, and reports from there are positive; one author from Paris stated that the response rate was 65% to 80% compared with a response rate of 30% to 35% in control subjects.[3] Other workers have found the treatment to be no better than placebo.[4] Hylin G-F 20 is commercially available in Canada as Synvisc.

Nonsteroidal antiinflammatory drugs. The role of inflammation in the pathophysiology of osteoarthritis is unproved, and any symptomatic relief from NSAIDs is probably due to their analgesic effects rather than their antiinflammatory actions.[5] One study comparing acetaminophen 4000 mg/day and ibuprofen 1200 and 2400 mg/day for the treatment of osteoarthritis of the knees found no difference in the efficacy of the two drugs,[6] and another comparing naproxen and acetaminophen for the same condition concluded that neither drug was very effective.[7] It seems reasonable to emphasize nonpharmacological therapy for patients with osteoarthritis such as exercises, braces, canes, walkers, heat, ultrasound, and ice.[8] In view of these findings many patients could probably be managed as effectively and more safely with simple analgesics rather than NSAIDs.[9]

Weight loss. In the Framingham Study women who lost weight decreased their risk for osteoarthritis of the knees. A weight loss of 5.1 kg over the previous 10 years decreased the relative risk of clinical osteoarthritis of the knee by 50%.[10]

Exercise. A 1992 study found that an 8-week program of fitness walking for patients with osteoarthritis of the knees not only increased their functional status but also decreased the amount of pain experienced and the use of medications.[11]

A 1997 investigation of 439 elderly patients living in the community who had osteoarthritis of the knees reported similar outcomes. Aerobic exercises (walking) and to a lesser extent resistance exercises of major muscle groups decreased pain and increased mobility.[12]

REFERENCES

1. Sack KE: Osteoarthritis: a continuing challenge, *West J Med* 163:579-586, 1995.
2. Aviad AD, Houpt JB: The molecular weight of therapeutic hyaluronan (sodium hyaluronate): how significant is it? *J Rheumatol* 21:276-301, 1994.
3. Peyron JG: Intraarticular hyaluronan injections in the treatment of osteoarthritis: state-of-the-art review, *J Rheumatol* (suppl 39):S10-S15, 1993.
4. Henderson EB, Smith EC, Pegley F, et al: Intra-articular injections of 750 kD hyaluronan in the treatment of osteoarthritis: a randomised single centre double-blind placebo-controlled trial of 91 patients demonstrating lack of efficacy, *Ann Rheum Dis* 53:529-534, 1994.
5. Pinals RS: Pharmacologic treatment of osteoarthritis, *Clin Ther* 14:336-346, 1992.
6. Bradley JD, Brandt KD, Katz BP, et al: Comparison of an anti-inflammatory dose of ibuprofen, an analgesic dose of ibuprofen and acetaminophen in the treatment of patients with osteoarthritis of the knee, *N Engl J Med* 325:87-91, 1991.
7. Williams HJ: Comparison of naproxen and acetaminophen in the treatment of osteoarthritis of the knees, *Arthritis Rheum* 34 (suppl):S84, 1991.
8. Mazanec DJ: Conservative treatment of rheumatic disorders in the elderly, *Geriatrics* 46:41-45, 1991.
9. Dieppe PA, Frankel SJ, Toth B: Is research into the treatment of osteoarthritis with non-steroidal anti-inflammatory drugs misdirected? *Lancet* 341:353-354, 1993.
10. Felson DT, Zhang Y, Anthony JM, et al: Weight loss reduces the risk for symptomatic knee osteoarthritis in women: the Framingham Study, *Ann Intern Med* 116:535-539, 1992.
11. Kovar PA, Allegrante JP, MacKenzie CR, et al: Supervised fitness walking in patients with osteoarthritis of the knee: a randomized, controlled trial, *Ann Intern Med* 116:529-534, 1992.
12. Ettinger WH Jr, Burns R, Messier S, et al: A randomized trial comparing aerobic exercise and resistance exercise with a health education program in older adults with knee osteoarthritis: the Fitness Arthritis and Senior Trial (FAST), *JAMA* 277: 25-31, 1997.

Paget's Disease

Paget's disease is common in Europe and North America and rare in Asia. Although it may be monostotic, usually multiple lesions are present. Sites of predilection are the axial skeleton, long bones, and skull. The vast majority of lesions are asymptomatic. Although the individual lesions of Paget's disease may cause pain, many of the symptoms result from complications of the disease. These include enlargement of the skull, hearing loss, bowing of long bones, pain from secondary osteoarthritis or fractures, osteosarcoma (in less than 1% of cases), and neurological deficits from entrapment of nerves or compression of the spinal cord. The serum alkaline phosphatase level is usually but not always elevated. Bone scans are the investigative procedure of choice.[1]

Treatment is indicated for patients with symptoms or for asymptomatic patients at risk of complications such as hearing loss (lesions at base of skull), spinal cord compression (lesions in vertebrae), and osteoarthritis or fractures (lesions in long bones). The drug of choice in most cases is alendronate (Fosamax) in oral doses of 40 mg/day. Alternatives are etidronate (Didrocal) or calcitonin (Calcimar).[1]

REFERENCES

1. Delmas PD, Meunier PJ: The management of Paget's disease of bone, *N Engl J Med* 336:558-566, 1997.

Polymyalgia Rheumatica

(See also sedimentation rate; temporal arteritis)

The onset of polymyalgia rheumatica can be indolent or sudden. In most cases aching and stiffness of proximal limb muscles, especially the shoulder girdle, are prominent symptoms. Morning stiffness, gelling after activities, malaise, and fatigue are also common. The patient may have pain, especially at night, that makes getting out of bed or in and out of the bathtub difficult. Transient synovitis of joints may occur. Elevated sedimentation rates and a mild normocytic anemia are common findings; slight elevation on liver function tests may also occur.[1] It is important to realize that in one fifth of patients the sedimentation rate will be normal (30 mm/hr or less).[2]

If specimens of temporal artery are obtained for biopsy from patients with polymyalgia rheumatica, many of them will be found to have histological evidence of temporal arteritis. However, this finding is a poor predictor for the development of clinical temporal arteritis. Furthermore, temporal arteritis develops later in a number of patients with negative biopsies. Fortunately, severe sequelae such as vision loss rarely if ever occur as the initial manifestation of temporal arteritis. Therefore temporal artery biopsies should be reserved for patients with suspicious symptoms or signs such as jaw claudication, headaches, visual changes, or tender temporal arteries.[3]

The differential diagnosis of polymyalgia rheumatica includes fibromyalgia, paraneoplastic syndromes, endocarditis, hypothyroid myopathy, polymyositis, systemic lupus erythematosus, monoclonal gammopathies, and rheumatoid arthritis, particularly if it is seronegative. Investigations that may clarify the diagnosis are urinalysis (looking for hematuria), creatine kinase, rheumatoid factor, antinuclear antigen (ANA), thyroid-stimulating hormone, and serum and urine electrophoresis.[1]

An important diagnostic test for polymyalgia rheumatica is a response within 24 to 48 hours to low-dose steroids such as prednisone 10 mg/day. A few other conditions, most commonly seronegative rheumatoid arthritis, respond in the same way.[3]

Locomotor System

The usual treatment of polymyalgia rheumatica is steroids.[1,3] The initial dose, which is titrated to a level that gives complete symptom relief, is usually prednisone 10 to 20 mg/day. This is decreased every 2 to 4 weeks by 2.5 mg until a daily dose of 10 mg is achieved, and thereafter tapering continues by 1-mg decrements every 2 to 4 weeks until a maintenance dose of 5 to 7.5 mg is achieved. Total duration of treatment varies from 2 to 15 years. Between one fourth and one half of patients have a relapse after discontinuation of treatment.[3] Mild symptoms may be successfully managed with NSAIDs.[1]

Patients with polymyalgia rheumatica who have sedimentation rates lower than 40 mm/hr tend to have a milder clinical course. Fever, anemia, and weight loss are less common than in patients with higher sedimentation rates.[4]

REFERENCES

1. Hunder GG: Giant cell arteritis and polymyalgia rheumatica, *Med Clin North Am* 81:195-219, 1997.
2. Helfgott SM, Kieval RI: Polymyalgia rheumatica in patients with a normal erythrocyte sedimentation rate, *Arthritis Rheum* 39:304-307, 1996.
3. Brooks RC, McGee SR: Diagnostic dilemmas in polymyalgia rheumatica, *Arch Intern Med* 157:162-168, 1997.
4. González-Gay MA, Rodriguez-Valverde V, Blanco R, et al: Polymyalgia rheumatica without significantly increased erythrocyte sedimentation rate—a more benign syndrome, *Arch Intern Med* 157:317-320, 1997.

Rheumatoid Arthritis

(See also nonsteroidal antiinflammatory drug gastropathy; steroids and osteoporosis)

Three times more women than men have rheumatoid arthritis. Among the elderly the ratio evens out.[1]

According to the American Rheumatism Association a diagnosis of rheumatoid arthritis can be made if the patient has four or more of the following findings[2]:

1. Morning stiffness for 1 hour or more for at least 6 weeks
2. Soft tissue swelling (arthritis) in three or more locations observed by a physician for at least 6 weeks
3. Swelling of the wrist, metacarpophalangeal joints, or proximal interphalangeal joints for at least 6 weeks
4. Symmetrical joint involvement for at least 6 weeks
5. Rheumatoid nodules
6. Presence of rheumatoid factor
7. X-ray findings consistent with rheumatoid arthritis (erosion or osteopenia of wrist or hand joints)

One of the major issues in the management of rheumatoid arthritis is whether active treatment should be started immediately and if so whether so-called disease-modifying agents such as methotrexate (Rheumatrex) or sulfasalazine (Azulfidine) should be used early in the course of the disease. These issues are discussed in the sections below. However, if early treatment is indeed indicated, the diagnoses must be made early and rheumatological consultations, if appropriate, should be arranged without delay. Until now this has rarely happened.[3]

Nonsteroidal antiinflammatory drugs

NSAIDs have usually been considered the first-line drugs for rheumatoid arthritis. No one drug has been shown to be superior to another. In general a specific NSAID should be tried for 10 to 14 days before a decision is made as to whether it is effective. If one NSAID is ineffective, another should be used. Traditionally this process would be continued until several different NSAIDs had been tried.[4] Some writers suggest using newer NSAIDs such as nabumetone (Relafen) or etodolac (Ultradol, Lodine), which inhibit cyclooxygenase 1 (COX-1) to a lesser extent than cyclooxygenase 2 (COX-2) and thus are less likely to induce a gastropathy (see discussion of nonsteroidal antiinflammatory drugs).[5]

Second-line drugs

Second-line or "disease-modifying" drugs for rheumatoid arthritis include methotrexate (Rheumatrex), sulfasalazine (Azulfidine), hydroxychloroquine (Plaquenil), azathioprine (Imuran), cyclosporine (Sandimmune), gold salts (Myochrysine, Solganal), and penicillamine (Cuprimine, Depen). It is hoped that second-line drugs will alter the basic pathological processes responsible for the inflammation and through this mechanism will prevent deformities and disabilities.[6-10] Whether this is the case is uncertain,[8] although some studies, particularly with methotrexate, are encouraging.[10]

Second-line drugs for rheumatoid arthritis reduce swelling and inflammation in the short run as long as the patient continues the medications. No drug has been definitively shown to have more beneficial effects than another, but at present methotrexate and hydroxychloroquine are considered the drugs of first choice by most North American rheumatologists because they are thought to act more rapidly, reduce the degree of synovitis to a greater degree, and be less toxic than other drugs in this category.[6,7] The most popular drug in Great Britain is sulfasalazine.[9]

There is an increasing tendency to use second-line drugs early in the course of the disease on the grounds that this gives better control of symptoms and perhaps prevents permanent damage to joints; preliminary studies support this approach.[11] An important theoretical reason for starting second-line drugs early (assuming they do in fact modify the disease process) is that permanent damage to joints can develop within months of the onset of the disease.[8] At present the traditional indications for this class of drugs are a failure of NSAIDs or a clinical presentation suggesting a rapidly progressing disease. These indications are challenged by some rheumatologists, who claim that the fact that NSAIDs are effective proves that significant inflammation is present and that therefore second-line drugs are needed immediately.[9] These workers tend to treat patients with newly diagnosed rheumatoid arthritis with second-line drugs from the onset of the disease.[9] Prolonged use of second-line drugs may be necessary to prevent flare-up of disease. In one study patients with rheumatoid arthritis who had been taking second-line drugs for a median of 5 years were randomly assigned to take placebo or continue the second-line drug. At the end of a year the placebo group had twice as many exacerbations, a finding that applied to all the drugs tested except penicillamine.[12]

Several long-term studies of patients taking disease-modifying drugs have shown a high rate of discontinuation of the medications because of toxic side effects or perceived lack of beneficial effect.[13,14] Among all these drugs, methotrexate appears to have the lowest discontinuation rate.[14] In one 5-year study of methotrexate in rheumatoid arthritis, 36% of patients discontinued the medication, 7% because of adverse effects and 7% because of lack of efficacy. However, in the same study, more than two thirds of the patients showed a marked clinical improvement.[13]

When methotrexate is used, it is usually given in small weekly doses in the range of 7.5 to 25 mg. Methotrexate may be given orally or parenterally. The parenteral route is preferred for doses over 20 mg weekly, for patients who cannot tolerate oral medications because of gastrointestinal side effects, and for patients who have not responded to orally administered methotrexate.[13] The most common side effects of methotrexate are gastrointestinal and include anorexia, nausea, diarrhea, and stomatitis. Other adverse reactions are headaches, mood alterations, fatigue, interstitial pneumonitis, leukopenia, and hepatic toxicity. The last is rare with the low doses that are used, but liver function tests should be performed every 2 months. Many of the adverse symptoms of this drug are prevented or alleviated by giving patients a daily supplement of 1 mg of folic acid.[15]

Corticosteroids

Oral steroids are often used as "bridging therapy" when one of the second-line drugs is being started. The duration of such steroid therapy is generally less than 3 months with a maximum dose of prednisone of about 10 mg/day and gradual tapering toward the end of the period.[5]

A 1995 randomized double-blind placebo-controlled study of 128 adults with early-onset rheumatoid arthritis (duration less than 2 years) found that 7.5 mg of prednisolone daily over a 2-year period resulted in less pain and disability in the steroid-treated group and a decreased rate of radiological progression.[16] However, whether this approach will have long-term benefits or whether the risks of steroids will outweigh any possible benefits is unknown. Individual joints are commonly injected with steroids to help control symptoms.[5]

Other drugs

Minocycline (Minocin) in doses of 100 mg bid has been shown in a placebo-controlled double-blind study to reduce pain and swelling in mild to moderately severe rheumatoid arthritis over a 48-week trial period. Whether this is due to its antibacterial or its antiinflammatory effect is not known.[17]

REFERENCES

1. Akil M, Amos RS: Rheumatoid arthritis. I. Clinical features and diagnosis, *BMJ* 310:587-590, 1995.
2. Arnett FC, Edworthy SM, Bloch DA, et al: The American Rheumatism Association 1987 revised criteria for the classification of rheumatoid arthritis, *Arthritis Rheum* 31:315-324, 1988.
3. Chan KA, Felson DT, Yood RA, et al: The lag time between onset of symptoms and diagnosis of rheumatoid arthritis, *Arthritis Rheum* 37:814-820, 1994.
4. Grondin C: L'arthrite rhumatoïde: approche thérapeutique, *Can Fam Physician* 36:487-490, 499, 1990.
5. Morin F, Carette S: A pharmacologic approach to rheumatoid arthritis, *Can J CME* 7:57-65, 1995.
6. Cash JM, Klippel JH: Second-line drug therapy for rheumatoid arthritis, *N Engl J Med* 330:1368-1375, 1994.
7. Drugs for rheumatoid arthritis, *Med Lett* 36:101-106, 1994.
8. Pope RM: Rheumatoid arthritis: pathogenesis and early recognition, *Am J Med* 100(suppl 2A):2A-3S, 7S, 1996.
9. Emery P: Therapeutic approaches for early rheumatoid arthritis. how early? How aggressive? *Br J Rheumatol* 34(suppl 2): 87-90, 1995.
10. Weinblatt ME: Efficacy of methotrexate in rheumatoid arthritis, *Br J Rheumatol* 34(suppl 2):43-48, 1995.
11. van der Heide A, Jacobs JW, Bijlsma JW, et al: The effectiveness of early treatment with second-line antirheumatic drugs—a randomized, controlled trial, *Ann Intern Med* 124:699, 1996.
12. Ten Wolde S, Breedveld FC, Hermans J, et al: Randomised placebo-controlled study of stopping second-line drugs in rheumatoid arthritis, *Lancet* 347:347-352, 1996.
13. Weinblatt ME, Kaplan H, Germain BF, et al: Methotrexate in rheumatoid arthritis: a five-year prospective multicenter study, *Arthritis Rheum* 37:1492-1498, 1994.
14. Pincus T: Long-term outcomes in rheumatoid arthritis, *Br J Rheumatol* 34(suppl 2):59-73, 1995.
15. Weinblatt ME: Methotrexate for chronic diseases in adults, *N Engl J Med* 332:330-331, 1995.
16. Kirwan JR (Arthritis and Rheumatism Council Low-Dose Glucocorticoid Study Group): The effect of glucocorticoids on joint destruction in rheumatoid arthritis, *N Engl J Med* 333: 142-146, 1995.
17. Tilley BC, Alarcón GS, Heyse SP, et al: Minocycline in rheumatoid arthritis: a 48-week, double-blind, placebo-controlled trial, *Ann Intern Med* 122:81-89, 1995.

Septic Arthritis

(See also gonorrhea; transient synovitis of hip)

The most frequent joints affected in nongonococcal septic arthritis are large joints such as the knees and hips. Between 80% and 90% of cases of septic arthritis are monarticular.

Gonococcal arthritis is two to three times more common in women than in men. Migratory tendinitis and arthritis often precede gonococcal monarthritis. One half to three fourths of patients with disseminated gonococcal infections have skin lesions, which usually number less than 30 and are located primarily on the extremities.[1] Ninety percent of patients with disseminated gonococcal infections have arthritis.[1] Disseminated meningococcal disease must be considered in the differential diagnosis because it too can cause skin and joint disease.[2]

REFERENCES

1. Handsfield HH: Disseminated gonococcal infection, *Clin Obstet Gynecol* 18:131-142, 1975.
2. Rompalo AM, Hook WE 3d, Roberts PL, et al: The acute arthritis-dermatitis syndrome: the changing importance of *Neisseria gonorrhoeae* and *Neisseria meningitidis, Arch Intern Med* 147: 281-283, 1987.

Seronegative Spondyloarthropathies

The seronegative spondyloarthropathies are a group of inflammatory arthritides that are rheumatoid factor and ANA negative and that have a much greater frequency in HLA-B27-positive persons than in those who do not carry this histocompatibility antigen. Conditions included in this category are ankylosing spondylitis, psoriatic arthritis, Reiter's syndrome, and arthritis associated with inflammatory bowel disease.[1] Some workers also place Whipple's disease and Behçet's disease into the category of seronegative spondyloarthropathies. Reiter's syndrome and the arthritis of inflammatory bowel disease are often called reactive arthritides.[1]

The clinical characteristics of the seronegative spondyloarthropathies differ, but common findings are a propensity to involve the back and the sacroiliac joints, a tendency to affect only a few peripheral joints, most often in an asymmetrical pattern in the lower extremities, and a tendency for inflammatory reactions to involve the entheses or sites of attachments of ligaments and tendons to bones (enthesopathy). Typical manifestations of enthesopathy are pain and tenderness over the plantar fascia where it inserts on the calcaneus or pain and tenderness over the region where the Achilles tendon inserts onto the calcaneus. Isolated arthritis and tenosynovitis of a single digit of the toes or fingers (dactylitis) occurring as a diffuse sausagelike swelling is particularly characteristic of Reiter's syndrome and psoriatic arthritis.[1]

Extraarticular manifestations are common with the seronegative spondyloarthropathies. Iritis or other inflammatory eye conditions may be seen in all of them, skin lesions in psoriasis and Reiter's syndrome, and urethritis in Reiter's syndrome even when precipitated by a dysenteric syndrome.[1]

Ankylosing spondylitis

Archaic synonyms for ankylosing spondylitis are rheumatoid spondylitis and Marie-Strumpell disease. It used to be thought that males were affected 20 times as often as women. Because of this erroneous belief the diagnosis is often missed. It turns out that women with the disease usually have fewer symptoms, and the true sex ratio is probably about 5:1 in favor of males. Although some persons are disabled by the disease, the majority are not.[1] Inflammatory back pain (ankylosing spondylitis) is a rare but important cause of low back pain in persons under the age of 40. The following findings suggest this diagnosis[2,3]:

1. Insidious onset
2. Onset before age 40
3. Pain for more than 3 months
4. Morning stiffness longer than 30 minutes
5. Pain relief with activity
6. Pain forcing the patient from bed
7. History of psoriasis, Reiter's disease, uveitis, or colitis
8. Chest expansion of less than 2 inches
9. Peripheral joint disease

The first five criteria have a high sensitivity and specificity, but because of the low prevalence of the disorder the positive predictive value is on the order of only 0.04.[3]

The classic physical findings of ankylosing spondylitis are a positive Schober's test, a positive occiput to wall test, and decreased chest expansion (less than 5 to 6 cm).

Schober's test is performed as follows. With the patient standing vertically, the end of a measuring tape is placed over the spinous processes at the level of the posterior superior iliac spines and stretched proximally along the spine. A mark is placed on the skin at the 10-cm level. With the end of the tape kept in place, the patient is asked to flex as fully forward as possible. The distance to the skin mark is measured. Normally it is about 15 cm because of flexion of the lumbar spine. In patients with ankylosing spondylitis it is less because most or all flexion takes place at the hips.

In the occiput to wall test the patient stands with heels against the wall and tries to press the occiput against the wall. Many patients with ankylosing spondylitis cannot do this because of fixed flexion deformity of the spine.

Unfortunately, the defining signs are not usually present in the early stages of the disease. Testing for HLA-B27 is not usually helpful. If the clinical picture is convincing, this study is not necessary (10% of patients with the disease are HLA-B27 negative), and if the diagnosis is unlikely on a clinical basis, the presence of a positive HLA-B27 adds little.[1]

Reiter's syndrome

Reiter's syndrome may be initiated by either urethritis, which is usually chlamydial in origin, or a dysentery-like syndrome caused by a variety of organisms, including *Shigella, Salmonella, Campylobacter,* and *Yersinia.* The postvenereal form of Reiter's syndrome affects about five to nine times as many men as women, whereas the postdysentery form affects the sexes equally. The classic triad is urethritis, conjunctivitis, and arthritis, usually appearing in that order, but only one third of patients have all three entities. Symptoms of urethritis usually develop 2 to 4 weeks after either sexual exposure or a diarrheal illness. Ocular symptoms are reported in about half the cases and are usually the result of a short-lived mild conjunctivitis; some patients have iritis, uveitis, or keratitis. Arthritis develops last. The most frequently affected joints are the knees, ankles, and toes ("sausage" digits). Asymmetrical oligoarthritis is the rule. In half the patients the spine or sacroiliac joints are involved. Enthesopathy, circinate balanitis of the penis, and keratoderma blennorrhagicum of the palms and soles are common. About half of the patients have a prolonged course or recurrences over months or years, but little functional disability. Standard treatment is NSAIDs for symptom relief and antibiotics if active chlamydial infection is still present. Trials of prolonged antibiotic treatment as a treatment for Reiter's syndrome have been conducted, but the results are inconclusive.[1,4]

Psoriatic arthritis

In 85% of patients with psoriatic arthritis, skin lesions develop before the arthritis. In some patients skin stigmata of psoriasis may not be obvious at first glance; patients may have pitting of nails, onycholysis, scalp lesions, or lesions between the buttocks or in the umbilicus. The arthritis is usually asymmetrical and involves only a few joints. Dactylitis of a toe or finger is characteristic of psoriatic arthritis or Reiter's syndrome.[1]

Enteropathic arthropathies

Seronegative arthropathies develop in about 8% of patients with ulcerative colitis and 14% of those with Crohn's disease. Larger joints of the lower extremities are usually involved, and the activity of the arthritis tends to parallel that of the bowel disease.[1]

REFERENCES

1. Osial TA Jr, Cash JM, Eisenbeis CH Jr: Arthritis-associated syndromes, *Primary Care* 20:857-882, 1993.
2. Calin A, Porta J, Fries JF, et al: Clinical history as a screening test for ankylosing spondylitis, *JAMA* 237:2613-2614, 1977.
3. Calin A, Kaye B, Sternberg M, et al: The prevalence and nature of back pain in an industrial complex: a questionnaire and radiographic and HLA analysis, *Spine* 5:201-205, 1980.
4. Kirchner JT: Reiter's syndrome: a possibility in patients with reactive arthritis, *Postgrad Med* 97:111-112, 115-117, 121-122, 1995.

METABOLIC

Topics covered in this section

Adrenal Gland
Diabetes Mellitus
Electrolytes
Hypoglycemia
Lipids
Osteoporosis
Thyroid
Pituitary

ADRENAL GLAND

(See also metastatic breast cancer)

Adrenal Insufficiency

Addison's disease is a rare disease that is more common in females than males and is most frequently diagnosed in young and middle-aged adults. The three cardinal symptoms are weight loss, fatigue, and weakness. Psychiatric and gastrointestinal symptoms are common, and most patients have hyperpigmentation. Hypotension, hyponatremia, and hyperkalemia are frequent findings. The diagnosis may be difficult to make, and some patients undergo extensive workups for such conditions as inflammatory bowel disease. Psychiatric disorders such as anorexia nervosa and bulimia are also part of the differential diagnosis.[1,2] Laboratory abnormalities that may be found in initial screening tests are mild normocytic anemia, mild eosinophilia, hyponatremia, and hyperkalemia.[2] In many cases an 8 AM cortisol determination can confirm or rule out the diagnosis. If the level is 83 nmol/L (3 µg/dl) or less, the diagnosis is confirmed, whereas if the concentration is 525 nmol/L (19 µg/dl) or more, it is ruled out (assuming a normal range to be 165 to 662 nmol/L [6 to 24 µg/dl]).[2]

Treatment of chronic adrenal insufficiency is with glucocorticoids, often oral hydrocortisone or cortisol. The dose varies from one patient to another; most receive cortisone 25 to 37.5 mg/day. Usually two thirds of the daily dose is given in the morning and one third at night, although some patients feel better if the daily dose is given in equal amounts three times a day. In times of stress, such as intercurrent illnesses, injury, or surgery, the maintenance dose is usually doubled. Patients with primary adrenal insufficiency often lose salt and may need to take fludrocortisone (Florinef) 50 to 200 µg as a single daily dose; those with secondary adrenal insufficiency (caused by pituitary disorders) rarely require fludrocortisone.[2,3] The physician should be aware that prednisone, prednisolone, and dexamethasone are not the drugs of choice for Addison's disease because they have little mineralocorticoid activity. In fact, taking these drugs for other reasons may not prevent the development of Addison's disease.[4]

Cushing's Syndrome

The clinical findings in Cushing's syndrome are well known. Rapid weight gain is characteristic. The rounded "moon" facies is due to increased facial fat and the florid complexion to telangiectasias. Whereas a buffalo hump is a common finding with any type of weight gain, filling out of the supraclavicular fat pads is more specific for Cushing's syndrome. Muscle wasting leads to difficulty climbing stairs, getting out of a low chair, or rising from a squatting position.[5]

If Cushing's syndrome is suspected, a 24-hour urine study for free cortisol (plus creatinine to assess the adequacy of collection) should be performed and repeated on 1 or 2 consecutive days.[5] A dexamethasone suppression test is the standard alternative but is not as sensitive for mild cases. The test is performed by giving 1 mg of dexamethasone at 11 PM and measuring the serum cortisol by 9 AM the next day. If the level is less than 135 nmol/L (5 μg/dl), the diagnosis of Cushing's syndrome is ruled out in 99% of cases.

REFERENCES

1. Keljo DJ, Squires RH Jr: Clinical problem-solving: just in time, *N Engl J Med* 334:46-48, 1996.
2. Oelkers W: Adrenal insufficiency, *N Engl J Med* 335:1206-1212, 1996.
3. Werbel SS, Ober KP: Acute adrenal insufficiency, *Endocrinol Metab Clin North Am* 22:303-328, 1993.
4. Cronin CC, Callaghan N, Keaarney PJ, et al: Addison disease in patients treated with glucocorticoid therapy, *Arch Intern Med* 157:456-458, 1997.
5. Orth DN: Cushing's syndrome, *N Engl J Med* 332:791-803, 1995.

DIABETES MELLITUS

(See also endometrial carcinoma)

Until recently the diagnosis of diabetes mellitus was made if two fasting glucose readings were greater than 7.8 mmol/L (140 mg/dl) or if two random glucose readings were greater than 11.1 mmol/L (200 mg/dl).[1] At the 1997 annual meeting of the American Diabetes Association it was recommended that the diagnosis of diabetes be made if the fasting sugar level was 7 mmol/L (126 mg/dl) or over.[2] (To convert SI units [mmol/L] to traditional units [mg/dl], divide by 0.05551. To convert traditional units [mg/dl] to SI units [mmol/L], multiply by 0.05551.)

REFERENCES

1. Expert Committee of the Canadian Diabetes Advisory Board: Clinical practice guidelines for diabetes mellitus in Canada, *Can Med Assoc J* 147:697-712, 1992.
2. Macready N: American Diabetes Association calls for testing all those over 45, *BMJ* 315:11, 1997.

Microvascular Complications of Diabetes Mellitus

Diabetic retinopathy

The development of diabetic retinopathy is related to the length of time the patient has had diabetes. In insulin-dependent diabetes mellitus (IDDM) retinopathy rarely develops before puberty and usually only after the patient has had the disease for 3 to 5 years. After 7 years approximately 50% of patients with IDDM have some degree of retinopathy, and after 20 years more than 90% have the disorder.[1] Pregnancy is a recognized risk factor for the progression of diabetic retinopathy, which is why close ophthalmological follow-up of pregnant diabetic women is advised.[2] Between one fourth and one third of adolescent girls with IDDM also have eating disorders. They tend to omit insulin doses to lose weight, as well as purge and vomit, and their metabolic control is poor (some cases of "brittle diabetes" are probably due to this phenomenon). They are at a much increased risk for retinopathy.[3]

Severe retinopathy with loss of vision may occur in both IDDM and non-insulin-dependent diabetes mellitus (NIDDM) but is more common in IDDM. Patients with NIDDM may have retinopathy at diagnosis, but rarely is it advanced at that time. The incidence of the more severe proliferative retinopathy in NIDDM increases with the duration of the disease. After 20 years 5% of patients treated with diet or hypoglycemic agents have the disorder and 25% of those requiring insulin therapy have it.[4] The incidence of proliferative retinopathy is higher in blacks[5] and Mexican-Americans[6] with NIDDM than in whites. In both IDDM and NIDDM the degree of retinopathy and the risk of progression correlate with the degree of elevation of glycosylated hemoglobin.[7]

Three types of retinal abnormalities are common in diabetes: nonproliferative retinopathy, proliferative retinopathy, and macular edema. Diabetic retinopathy is one of the leading causes of blindness in North American adults. Visual loss is caused by either macular edema or proliferative retinopathy. These two conditions usually develop gradually, and if they are detected and treated by laser photocoagulation, further visual loss can often be arrested.

Nonproliferative retinopathy. The initial and most common manifestation of diabetic retinopathy is microaneurysm formation. Erythrocytes escape from these lesions, leading to dot and blot hemorrhages. Leaking of serous fluid from the capillaries leads to the formation of hard exudates. Microaneurysms, dot and blot hemorrhages, and hard exudates are collectively termed "background retinopathy" or "nonproliferative retinopathy." Nonproliferative retinopathy does not lead to loss of vision unless it occurs near the maculae and causes macular edema.[1]

Proliferative retinopathy. As the diabetic retinal disease progresses, some vessels become occluded, leading to infarcts of the retinae seen as soft or "cotton wool" exudates. In response to ischemia, new vessels develop and proliferate out of the retina into the vitreous. This is proliferative retinopathy. These attenuated fragile vessels tend to bleed, causing vitreous hemorrhages. Vitreous hemorrhages usually resorb in 1 to 3 months, but subsequent fibrous proliferation can lead to retinal detachment and loss of vision.[1] Diabetic patients with proliferative retinopathy have a significantly higher risk of other diabetic complications, including stroke, myocardial infarction, lower limb amputations, and nephropathy. They have an increased mortality rate compared with diabetic patients who do not have proliferative retinopathy.[8]

One concern that some physicians have is whether aspirin is contraindicated in diabetic patients because of a possible increased risk of vitreous hemorrhage. A recent report found no increase in the frequency or severity of vitreous hemorrhages in patients with nonproliferative or early proliferative retinopathy.[9]

Macular edema

Macular edema can occur at any stage of retinopathy and is the most common cause of visual loss in diabetic patients. It rarely develops until 5 to 7 years after the onset of the diabetes. Its detection requires specialized ophthalmological examination (stereoscopic examination), which is not available to most primary care physicians.[10]

Guidelines for ophthalmological care

Recommendations of the American Diabetes Association[11] and the Expert Committee of the Canadian Diabetes Advisory Board[12] are that initial ophthalmological evaluations should be obtained for the following:

1. Patients with IDDM who are at the onset of puberty or older and have had diabetes for 5 or more years
2. Patients over the age of 30 whose diabetes has first been diagnosed
3. Diabetic patients with any other ocular pathological condition
4. Diabetic women in the first trimester of pregnancy
5. Women with IDDM who are planning a pregnancy

Any patient found to have any degree of retinopathy should have annual ophthalmological examinations.

The Canadian Task Force on the Periodic Health Examination gives a "B" recommendation to funduscopy or retinal photography of diabetic patients during the periodic health examination.[13] The U.S. Preventive Services Task Force makes no specific recommendation on this issue.[14]

REFERENCES

1. Nathan DM: Long-term complications of diabetes mellitus, *N Engl J Med* 328:1676-1685, 1993.
2. Klein BE, Moss SE, Klein R: Effect of pregnancy on progression of diabetic retinopathy, *Diabetes Care* 13:34-40, 1990.
3. Rydall AC, Rodin GM, Olmsted MP, et al: Disordered eating behavior and microvascular complications in young women with insulin-dependent diabetes mellitus, *N Engl J Med* 336: 1849-1854, 1997.
4. Klein R, Klein BE, Moss SE: The Wisconsin Epidemiological Study of Diabetic Retinopathy: a review, *Diabetes Metab Rev* 5:559-570, 1989.
5. Careter Center of Emory University: Closing the gap: the problem of diabetes mellitus in the United States, *Diabetes Care* 8: 391-406, 1985.
6. Haffner SM, Fong D, Stern MP, et al: Diabetic retinopathy in Mexican Americans and non-Hispanic whites, *Diabetes* 37: 878-884, 1988.
7. Klein R, Klein BE, Moss SE, et al: Relationship of hyperglycemia to the long-term incidence and progression of diabetic retinopathy, *Arch Intern Med* 154:2169-2178, 1994.
8. Klein R, Klein BE, Moss SE: Epidemiology of proliferative diabetic retinopathy, *Diabetes Care* 15:1875-1891, 1992.
9. Chew EY, Klein ML, Murphy RP, et al: Effects of aspirin on vitreous preretinal hemorrhage in patients with diabetes mellitus—Early Treatment Diabetic Retinopathy Study report no. 20, *Arch Ophthalmol* 113:52-55, 1995.
10. Murphy RP: Management of diabetic retinopathy, *Am Fam Physician* 51:785-796, 1995.
11. American Diabetes Association: Standards of medical care for patients with diabetes mellitus, *Diabetes Care* 20(suppl 1):S5-S13, 1997.
12. Expert Committee of the Canadian Diabetes Advisory Board: Clinical practice guidelines for diabetes mellitus in Canada, *Can Med Assoc J* 147:697-712, 1992.
13. Canadian Task Force on the Periodic Health Examination: *Canadian guide to clinical preventive health care,* Ottawa, 1994, Canada Communication Group—Publishing, pp 932-942.
14. US Preventive Services Task Force: *Guide to clinical preventive services,* ed 2, Baltimore, 1996, Williams & Wilkins.

Diabetic nephropathy

(See also microalbuminuria)

Nephropathy develops in about 35% to 45% of patients with IDDM and less than 20% of those with NIDDM. The first evidence of the process is microalbuminuria, followed by manifest proteinuria. In the case of IDDM the mean duration of the disease from the onset of microalbuminuria to the development of proteinuria is 17 years. In half of diabetic patients with proteinuria, end-stage renal failure develops, and the mean time from the onset of proteinuria to azotemia is 5 years.[1,2]

Microalbuminuria is albuminuria insufficient to be detected by dipstick. It is variously defined as less than 200 or 300 mg/24 hr. Special kits are used to test for it. Diabetic patients with microalbuminuria have a higher incidence of nephropathy, renal failure,[3] retinopathy,[4] and total and cardiovascular mortality[5] than other patients with diabetes. Microalbuminuria also occurs in other renal diseases, such as preeclampsia, immune-related disorders, and multiple myeloma.[6]

Diabetic nephropathy is one of the disorders most commonly necessitating dialysis or renal transplantation. However, the vast majority of patients with end-stage diabetic nephropathy die of cardiovascular disease rather than renal failure. The incidence of diabetic nephropathy in patients with NIDDM is four times as great in blacks and six times as great in Mexican-Americans as in whites.[7] Other risk factors for nephropathy in NIDDM are retinopathy, poor glycemic control, and elevated cholesterol levels.[8]

Good control of hypertension, especially with the use of angiotensin-converting enzyme (ACE) inhibitors, may ameliorate diabetic nephropathy or at least slow its progression. Even in normotensive patients with IDDM, ACE inhibitors have been shown to decrease microalbuminuria, slow the development of frank proteinuria, reduce protein excretion in those with frank proteinuria, and delay the anticipated decline in glomerular filtration rate. A randomized control trial of captopril (Capoten) in patients with IDDM showed a 50% reduction in the risk of the combined endpoints of death, dialysis, and transplantation.[9] A similar study of lisinopril (Prinivil, Zestril) found a decrease in the rate of progression of renal disease in IDDM as measured by the degree of albuminuria.[10] Protection against diabetic nephropathy has also been shown in normotensive patients with NIDDM who were treated with enalapril (Vasotec).[11] At present it seems clear that any diabetic patient with nephropathy should be treated with ACE inhibitors, but whether such treatment should be given before there is evidence of nephropathy remains to be determined.[12] An expert panel of the U.S. National Kidney Foundation says that it should.[13]

Tight control of IDDM has been shown to decrease the incidence of microalbuminuria and proteinuria,[14] but whether this will translate into a decreased incidence of end-stage renal failure is not known.

The Canadian Task Force on the Periodic Health Examination recommends screening for microalbuminuria in patients with IDDM ("A" recommendation),[15] whereas the U.S. Preventive Services Task Force makes no recommendation on the subject.[16]

REFERENCES

1. Nathan DM: Long-term complications of diabetes mellitus, *N Engl J Med* 328:1676-1685, 1993.
2. McCrary RF, Petts TO, Puschett JB: Diabetic nephropathy: natural course, survivorship and therapy, *Am J Nephrol* 1:206-218, 1981.
3. Mogensen CE, Christensen CK: Predicting diabetic nephropathy in insulin-dependent patients, *N Engl J Med* 311:89-93, 1984.
4. Vigstrup J, Mogensen CE: Proliferative diabetic retinopathy: at risk patients identified by early detection of microalbuminuria, *Acta Ophthalmol* 63:530-534, 1985.
5. Dinneen SF, Gerstein HC: The association of microalbuminuria and mortality in non-insulin-dependent diabetes mellitus, *Arch Intern Med* 157:1413-1418, 1997.
6. Konen JC, Shihabi ZK: Microalbuminuria and diabetes mellitus, *Am Fam Physician* 48:1421-1428, 1993.
7. Cowie CC, Port FK, Wolfe RA, et al: Disparities in incidence of diabetic end-stage renal disease according to race and type of diabetes, *N Engl J Med* 321:1074-1079, 1989.
8. Gall M-A, Hougaard P, Borch-Johnsen K, et al: Risk factors for development of incipient and overt diabetic nephropathy in patients with non-insulin dependent diabetes mellitus: prospective, observational study, *BMJ* 314:783-788, 1997.
9. Lewis EJ, Hunsicker LG, Bain RP, et al (Collaborative Study Group): The effect of angiotensin-converting-enzyme inhibition on diabetic nephropathy, *N Engl J Med* 329:1456-1462, 1993.
10. EUCLID study group: Randomised placebo-controlled trial of lisinopril in normotensive patients with insulin-dependent diabetes and normoalbuminuria or microalbuminuria, *Lancet* 349:1787-1792, 1997.
11. Ravid M, Lang R, Rachmani R, et al: Long-term renoprotective effect of angiotensin-converting enzyme inhibition in non-insulin-dependent diabetes mellitus, *Arch Intern Med* 156:286-289, 1996.
12. Remuzzi G, Ruggenenti P: Slowing the progression of diabetic nephropathy (editorial), *N Engl J Med* 329:1496-1497, 1993.
13. Bennett PH, Haffner S, Kasiske BL, et al: Screening and management of microalbuminuria in patients with diabetes mellitus: recommendations to the Scientific Advisory Board of the National Kidney Foundation from an ad hoc committee of the Council on Diabetes Mellitus of the National Kidney Foundation, *Am J Kidney Dis* 25:107-112, 1995.
14. Diabetes Control and Complications Trial Research Group: The effect of intensive treatment of diabetes on the development and progression of long-term complications in insulin-dependent diabetes mellitus, *N Engl J Med* 329:977-986, 1993.
15. Canadian Task Force on the Periodic Health Examination: *Clinical preventive health care,* Ottawa, 1994, Canadian Communication Group—Publishing, pp 436-445.
16. US Preventive Services Task Force: *Guide to clinical preventive services,* ed 2, Baltimore, 1996, Williams & Wilkins.

Diabetic neuropathy

A peripheral symmetrical sensorimotor neuropathy is the most common form of neuropathy in diabetes and is characterized by paresthesias that progress to hypesthesia. A painful lancinating variant of neuropathy occurs but is rare. The pain of diabetic neuropathy has been treated with amitriptyline (Elavil) starting at doses of 25 mg hs and slowly building to 150 to 200 mg/day if necessary. Other tricyclic agents are also effective but perhaps less so than amitriptyline. Carbamazepine (Tegretol) and phenytoin (Dilantin) have been used for lancinating neuropathy,[1,2] but tricyclic drugs are also effective for this form of pain.[3] Capsaicin 0.075% cream (Zostrix H.P.) has been reported to give pain relief.[2]

Focal motor neuropathies occur in diabetes mellitus. These may be cranial or peripheral and usually resolve spontaneously in 2 to 12 months.

Autonomic neuropathies are common. The most frequent manifestation is impotence, which affects more than 50% of men with diabetes. Other features of autonomic neuropathy are diabetic gastroparesis, orthostatic hypotension, and diarrhea.[2] Treatment options for gastroparesis include erythromycin 250 to 500 mg qid or metoclopramide (Maxeran) 10 mg tid ac. In a direct comparison of these two drugs erythromycin was more effective. Domperidone (Motilium) and cisapride (Prepulsid) have also been helpful in some cases. The dose of cisapride is 10 to 20 mg po qid ac. One treatment method for the diarrhea of autonomic neuropathy is one or two doses of tetracycline (200 or 500 mg) at the onset of symptoms. The mechanism of action is unknown. A more traditional treatment is diphenoxylate with atropine (Lomotil). Postural hypotension caused by autonomic neuropathy is difficult to treat; increasing salt intake, wearing elastic tights, and sleeping with the head of the bed elevated might be tried. In some cases fludrocortisone (Florinef) is indicated.[2]

The Diabetes Control and Complications Trial has shown that intensive insulin treatment of patients with IDDM decreases the incidence of neuropathy measured after 5 years (13% versus 5%).[4] A 10-year follow-up of patients with NIDDM showed that 42% had neuropathy (versus 8.3% at baseline) and that the risk of neuropathy correlated with poor glycemic control and low serum insulin levels.[5]

REFERENCES

1. Nathan DM: Long-term complications of diabetes mellitus, *N Engl J Med* 328:1676-1685, 1993.
2. Clark CM Jr, Lee DA: Prevention and treatment of the complications of diabetes mellitus, *N Engl J Med* 332:1210-1217, 1995.
3. McQuay HJ, Moore RA: Antidepressants and chronic pain: effective analgesia in neuropathic pain and other syndromes (editorial), *BMJ* 314:763-764, 1997.
4. Diabetes Control and Complications Trial Research Group: The effect of intensive diabetes therapy on the development and progression of neuropathy, *Ann Intern Med* 122:561-568, 1995.
5. Partanen J, Niskanen L, Lehtinen J, et al: Natural history of peripheral neuropathy in patients with non-insulin dependent diabetes mellitus, *N Engl J Med* 333:89-94, 1995.

Macrovascular Complications of Diabetes Mellitus

Cardiovascular disease is the major cause of the increased morbidity and mortality associated with diabetes. Coronary artery disease and cerebrovascular accidents are increased twofold to threefold in persons with diabetes,[1-3] and coronary heart disease is the leading cause of death in these patients.[4] Peripheral vascular disease is common and often leads to gangrene and amputation. In view of this, the Expert Committee of the Canadian Diabetes Advisory Board recommends instituting intensive treatment of all cardiovascular risk factors, including discontinuation of smoking, careful control of hypertension, and a lipid-lowering program that includes drugs if exercise and diet are unsuccessful.[5] This last measure makes sense, but to my knowledge no conclusive studies have demonstrated that tight lipid control programs have any effect on the morbidity or mortality of diabetes.

REFERENCES

1. Garcia MJ, McNamara PJ, Gordon T, et al: Morbidity and mortality in diabetics in the Framingham population: sixteen year follow-up study, *Diabetes* 23:105-111, 1974.
2. Krolewski AS, Kosinski EJ, Warram JH, et al: Magnitude and determinants of coronary artery disease in juvenile-onset, insulin-dependent diabetes mellitus, *Am J Cardiol* 59:750-755, 1987.
3. Kannel WB, McGee DL: Diabetes and cardiovascular disease: the Framingham Study, *JAMA* 241:2035-2039, 1979.
4. Morrish NJ, Stevens LK, Head J, et al: A prospective study of the mortality among middle-aged diabetic patients (the London cohort of the WHO Multinational Study of Vascular Disease in Diabetics). I. Causes and death rates, *Diabetologia* 33:538-541, 1990.
5. Expert Committee of the Canadian Diabetes Advisory Board: Clinical practice guidelines for diabetes mellitus in Canada, *Can Med Assoc J* 147:697-712, 1992.

Other Complications of Diabetes

Glucose toxicity

Prolonged hyperglycemia can in itself aggravate insulin resistance and impair insulin secretion from the pancreas.[1] Correction of the hyperglycemia by diet, oral agents, or insulin often rapidly improves glucose control.[2] This is why a simple change in diet, such as eliminating refined sugars or stopping the patient from drinking 2 or 3 L of fruit juice a day, can lead to a rapid decline in hyperglycemia without any weight loss. One symptom of marked hyperglycemia is transient decreased visual acuity. This is due to the hyperosmolar effect of high glucose levels on the shape of the crystalline lens. I had one patient who could always tell when his glucose levels were very high because at these times he could not read the channel numbers on his television screen.

REFERENCES

1. Rossetti L, Giacarri A, DeFronzo RA: Glucose toxicity, *Diabetes Care* 13:610-630, 1990.
2. Genuth S: Insulin use in NIDDM, *Diabetes Care* 13:1240-1264, 1990.

Infections

Diabetic patients are at increased risk for a variety of infections, but only the infected diabetic foot is dealt with here. Foot ulcers are common because of neuropathy and ischemia, and they often become infected. The infections may be subclassified into those that are limb threatening and those that are not.

Non-limb-threatening infections are superficial, and the erythema extends less than 2 cm from the edge of the ulcer. Organisms causing non-limb-threatening infections are usually gram-positive cocci, such as streptococci or staphylococci, and may be treated on an outpatient basis if the home situation is adequate and follow-up every 24 to 48 hours can be arranged. Weight bearing must be avoided, and in most cases oral antibiotics such as clindamycin (Cleocin, Dalacin), cephalexin (Keflex), dicloxacillin (Dycill, Dynapen, Pathocil), or cloxacillin (Tegopen, Orbenin) are effective as single agents. Limb-threatening infections are generally polymicrobial, involving gram-positive aerobes, gram-negative aerobes, and anaerobes, and patients with such a condition require hospitalization and IV antibiotics.[1]

With deep ulcers, the presence of an underlying osteomyelitis is often difficult to determine. If bone can be detected in the base of the ulcer by probing with a metal probe, the odds are high that osteomyelitis is present. If the infection is not limb threatening, bone cannot be detected on probing, and initial x-ray findings are negative, the duration of treatment can be that for soft tissue infection (10 to 14 days) with reassessment after it is completed.[1]

REFERENCES

1. Caputo GM, Joshi N, Weitekamp MR: Foot infections in patients with diabetes, *Am Fam Physician* 56:195-202, 1997.

Pregnancy in Women with Insulin-Dependent Diabetes

Patients with IDDM generally are at much higher risk of having children with congenital anomalies and fetal death than nondiabetic women.[1-4] However, when tight control was maintained with monitoring by specialist centers in both the pregestational and gestational periods, these rates were shown to drop to nearly that of nondiabetic control subjects.[4] Unfortunately, such good results have not been achieved in some community settings.[2,3]

REFERENCES

1. Simmons D: Persistently poor pregnancy outcomes in women with insulin dependent diabetes (editorial), *BMJ* 315:263-264, 1997.
2. Casson IF, Clarke CA, Howard CV, et al: Outcomes of pregnancy in insulin dependent diabetic women: results of a five year population cohort study, *BMJ* 315:275-278, 1997.
3. Hawthorne G, Robson S, Ryall EA, et al: Prospective population based survey of outcome of pregnancy in diabetic women: results of the Northern Diabetic Pregnancy Audit, 1994, *BMJ* 315: 279-281, 1997.
4. Diabetes Control and Complications Trial Research Group: Pregnancy outcomes in the diabetes control and complications trial, *Am J Obstet Gynecol* 174:1343-1353, 1996.

Initial and Annual Laboratory Investigations for Diabetic Patients

Initial and annual (and sometimes more frequent) laboratory investigations recommended by the expert committee of the Canadian Diabetes Advisory Board are as follows[1]:

1. Fasting glucose
2. Glycated hemoglobin
3. Fasting plasma lipid levels (total cholesterol, high- and low-density cholesterol, and triglycerides)
3. Serum creatinine
4. Urinalysis including microscopy
5. Microalbuminuria (preferably at the time of diagnosis in patients without proteinuria, and then annually in patients without proteinuria who have had diabetes for more than 5 years)
6. 24-Hour urine protein excretion (in patients with proteinuria)
7. Creatinine clearance (in patients with proteinuria)
8. Electrocardiogram (if indicated)
9. Thyroid-stimulating hormone (for IDDM and, if indicated, for NIDDM)

REFERENCES

1. Expert Committee of the Canadian Diabetes Advisory Board: Clinical practice guidelines for diabetes mellitus in Canada, *Can Med Assoc J* 147:697-712, 1992.

Target Levels for Glucose in the Control of Diabetes Mellitus

Target levels for glucose control as set by various expert committees have become more stringent since the publication of the Diabetes Control and Complications Trial in 1993 (see below). The current position statement of the American Diabetes Association is that the optimal preprandial glucose level is 4.4 to 6.7 mmol/L (80 to 120 mg/dl) and that remedial action should be taken if values are above 7.8 mmol/L (140 mg/dl) or below 4.4 mmol/L (80 mg/dl). Bedtime glucose should be between 5.6 and 7.8 mmol/l (100 to 140 mg/dl), and remedial action is indicated if the levels are below 5.6 mmol/L (100 mg/dl) or above 8.9 mmol/L (160 mg/dl). The ideal hemoglobin A_{1c} level is below 7%.[1] As far as I have been able to determine, there is hope but no good evidence that control of glucose to the recommended levels through the use of oral hypoglycemic agents or insulin will alter long-term morbidity or mortality of patients with NIDDM (see below).

REFERENCES

1. American Diabetes Association: Standards of medical care for patients with diabetes mellitus, *Diabetes Care* 20(suppl 1):S5-S13, 1997.

Intensive Treatment in Preventing Diabetic Complications in Insulin-Dependent Diabetes Mellitus

Diabetologists have almost always favored "tight control" of diabetes on the assumption that this will decrease the complications of the disease. Until recently there was no solid evidence supporting this hypothesis. However, a 1993 seminal study by the Diabetes Control and Complications Trial Research Group (DCCT), published in the *New England Journal of Medicine,* showed that after a mean follow-up of 6.5 years patients with IDDM given intensive therapy had a significant diminution of retinopathy, neuropathy, proteinuria, and microalbuminuria.[1] Specifically, intensive therapy slowed the progression of retinopathy by 54% and reduced the development of proliferative or severe nonproliferative retinopathy by 47%. Clinical neuropathy was reduced by 60%, albuminuria by 54%, and microalbuminuria by 39%. No statistically significant decline occurred in macrovascular disease, but because of the youth of the study population this was not unexpected. However, these dramatic improvements in microvascular complications were achieved at a cost. In the DCCT trial the incidence of severe hypoglycemic reactions increased threefold and patients had significant weight gain. The mean weight gain over 5 years was 4.6 kg (10 lb) greater than in the conventionally treated control subjects. A somewhat similar study from the Karolinska Institute in Stockholm, also published in the *New England Journal of Medicine* in 1993, showed similar results.[2]

REFERENCES

1. Diabetes Control and Complications Trial Research Group: The effect of intensive treatment of diabetes on the development and progression of long-term complications in insulin-dependent diabetes mellitus, *N Engl J Med* 329:977-986, 1993.
2. Reichard P, Nilsson BY, Rosenqvist U: The effect of long-term intensified insulin treatment on the development of microvascular complications of diabetes mellitus, *N Engl J Med* 329:304-309, 1993.

Intensive Treatment in Preventing Diabetic Complications in Non-Insulin-Dependent Diabetes Mellitus

(See also attitudes, physician; pharmacologic treatment of non-insulin-dependent diabetes mellitus)

From the viewpoint of the family physician the practical significance of the DCCT findings is clear enough for patients with IDDM, but whether the findings are relevant to those with NIDDM whose disease cannot be controlled by diet and exercise alone is controversial. Tight control in this group of patients often means insulin therapy, which can aggravate an already existing hyperinsulinemia with all of its attendant risks.[1] As an editorial accompanying the DCCT study points out, the results of that trial do not seem applicable to NIDDM because of the problems of weight gain and hyperinsulinemia.[2] Even the American Diabetic Association, which supports tight control for NIDDM, does so with ambivalence, not only because weight gain (from insulin therapy) may lead to insulin resistance with its adverse effects on blood pressure lipids and coronary artery disease, but also because elderly patients with NIDDM are more vulnerable to the adverse effects of hypoglycemia,[3] one of which is impaired cognitive functioning.[4]

An important question that was not addressed by the DCCT trial is whether intensive insulin treatment decreases the risk of macrovascular disease. Although poor glycemic control has been shown to correlate with an increased risk of coronary artery disease,[5,6] it does not necessarily follow that tight control will improve that risk, and preliminary studies suggest that for the general population with NIDDM it does not.[7,8] A more definitive answer may be forthcoming with the expected publication of the results of the ongoing U.K. Prospective Diabetes Study, which involves approximately 5000 patients with NIDDM who were entered into the trial in 1977.[9]

In a group of patients with NIDDM who had had a myocardial infarction (MI), a prospective randomized trial found that 24 hours of in-hospital insulin infusion followed by ongoing subcutaneous insulin injections four times daily decreased the absolute mortality rate by 11% after 3.6 years. This benefit was particularly marked among low-risk patients with NIDDM who were not taking insulin at the time of their MIs.[10] Withdrawal of other hypoglycemic agents rather than the addition of insulin might account for these results.[11]

In the case of NIDDM it is reasonable to conclude that intensive glucose control will decrease microvascular complications.[12] Unfortunately, most of the morbidity and mortality of NIDDM are caused by macrovascular disease and, except in post-MI patients,[10] this is unlikely to be influenced by tight control. For most patients with NIDDM the safest method of improving control is through weight loss, and physicians should vigorously promote this. Most patients do not lose weight, however, and in this situation the guidelines advise initiation of pharmacotherapy. Physicians will probably do this, but they should not delude themselves that "a little tighter control" will necessarily decrease morbidity or mortality. This is important because "a little tighter control" often diminishes quality of life through increased doses of oral hypoglycemic medications, a switch to insulin, frequent fingerpricks, obsessive attention to the timing of meals, the medical risks outlined previously, and the deleterious psychological effect of being labeled "sick enough to require insulin."

REFERENCES

1. De Fronzo RA, Ferrannini E: Insulin resistance: a multifaceted syndrome responsible for NIDDM, obesity, hypertension, dyslipidemia and atherosclerotic vascular disease, *Diabetes Care* 14:173-194, 1991.
2. Lasker RD: The Diabetes Control and Complications Trial (editorial), *N Engl J Med* 329:1035-1036, 1993.
3. American Diabetes Association: Position statement: implications of the Diabetes Control and Complications Trial, *Diabetes* 42:1555-1558, 1993.
4. Langan JS, Deary IF, Hepburn DA, et al: Cumulative cognitive impairment following recurrent severe hypoglycemia in adult patients with insulin-treated diabetes mellitus, *Diabetologia* 34:337-344, 1991.
5. Andersson DK, Svärdsudd K: Long-term glycemic control relates to mortality in type II diabetes, *Diabetes Care* 18:1534-1543, 1995.
6. Gall M-A, Borch-Johnsen K, Hougaard P, et al: Albuminuria and poor glycemic control predict mortality in NIDDM, *Diabetes* 44:1303-1309, 1995.
7. Zinman B: Diabetes research: are we getting anywhere? (editorial), *Can Med Assoc J* 155:1271-1274, 1996.
8. Meigs JB, Singer DE, Sullivan LM, et al: Metabolic control and prevalent cardiovascular disease in non-insulin-dependent diabetes mellitus (NIDDM)—the NIDDM Patient Outcomes Research Team, *Am J Med* 102:38-47, 1997.
9. United Kingdom Prospective Diabetes Study (UKPDS) 13: Relative efficacy of randomly allocated diet, sulfonylurea, insulin or metformin in patients with newly diagnosed non-insulin-dependent diabetes followed for three years, *BMJ* 310:83-88, 1995.
10. Malmberg K (DIGAMI [Diabetes Mellitus, Insulin Glucose Infusion in Acute Myocardial Infarction] Study Group): Prospective randomised study of intensive insulin treatment on long term survival after acute myocardial infarction in patients with diabetes mellitus, *BMJ* 314:1512-1515, 1997.
11. Nattrass M: Managing diabetes after myocardial infarction: time for a more aggressive approach (editorial), *BMJ* 314:1497, 1997.
12. Ohkubo Y, Kishikawa H, Araki E, et al: Intensive insulin therapy prevents the progression of diabetic microvascular complications in Japanese patients with non-insulin-dependent diabetes mellitus: a randomized prospective 6-year study, *Diabetes Res Clin Pract* 28:103-117, 1995.

Insulin-Dependent Diabetes Mellitus

(See also eating disorders; intensive treatment in preventing diabetic complications in insulin-dependent diabetes mellitus)

Epidemiology

By 20 years of age between 1 in 300 and 1 in 600 individuals has IDDM. IDDM constitutes about 5% of cases of diabetes. The incidence varies with age and is lowest in infants and highest in adolescents. The incidence in increased in those who have a first-degree relative with IDDM (father 6%, mother 2%, sibling 5%, nonidentical twin 5%, identical twin 30% to 50%). In general, the farther from the equator, the higher the incidence of IDDM. The highest incidence in Europe is in Finland, and the lowest incidence in the world is in Japan. The disease most frequently becomes manifest in the spring and autumn. IDDM is more common in children who have not been breast fed or who have been breast fed for only a short period.[1]

REFERENCES

1. Atkinson MA, Maclaren NK: The pathogenesis of insulin-dependent diabetes mellitus, *N Engl J Med* 331:1428-1436, 1994.

Insulin therapy for insulin-dependent diabetes mellitus

(See also glucose monitoring for non-insulin-dependent diabetes mellitus; hypoglycemia; insulin therapy for non-insulin-dependent diabetes mellitus)

Classification of insulins. Trying to keep track of the various types of insulin available in the United States and Canada is a daunting task. Products include short- and long-acting insulins, mixtures of insulins, human insulins, analogues of human insulin, beef insulins, pork insulins, beef-pork insulins, biosynthetic insulins, semisynthetic insulins, insulins in vials, and insulins in pens. The two major manufacturers in North America have different products with different names. Sometimes the names for the same product are different in Canada and the United States.

Commercial insulins are available in Canada or the United States in the following forms, all of which are available as short-, intermediate-, or long-acting formulations:

1. Human insulins (biosynthetic human insulins, semisynthetic human insulins, and analogues of human insulin)
2. Mixtures of beef and pork insulins
3. Pure pork insulins
4. Pure beef insulins

Biosynthetic human insulins are produced by *Escherichia coli* that has been genetically programmed by recombinant DNA techniques to produce human insulin. Semisynthetic human insulin is produced by a chemical modification of highly purified pork insulin. Since the end products are virtually the same, the means of production is not of great clinical significance.

Trade names of human insulins. Trade names of human insulins available in Canada or the United States are Humulin, Novolin, Velosulin, and Humalog. Humalog is the trade name for lispro, which is an analogue of human insulin. It is ultra-short acting (see below).

Trade names of beef and pork insulins. Iletin I in the United States and Iletin in Canada are the trade names of Lilly's beef-pork insulins. Iletin II is Lilly's pure pork insulin in both countries. Pure pork and pure beef insulins are no longer produced by Novo Nordisk, and Lilly is planning to discontinue its production of mixed beef-pork insulin (Iletin, Iletin I) in late 1998.

Choice of human or animal insulins. In many cases physicians are renewing prescriptions for patients who are already taking insulin. In that case the trade name of the insulin the patient is already taking is known and should be used. In other circumstances it is important to specify clearly whether the prescription is for human insulin, mixed beef and pork insulin, or pure pork insulin.

At present most physicians prescribe human insulin, although I am unaware of conclusive evidence that long-term outcomes are better with this product. The Expert Committee of the Canadian Diabetes Advisory Board has recommended that all pregnant women and all patients with newly diagnosed IDDM receive human insulin but that patients whose diabetes is already well controlled with porcine or bovine-porcine insulin do not have to be switched to human insulin.[1]

Patients who are allergic to pork and beef insulins obviously need human insulins. Pork and beef insulins are usually less expensive, which may be an important consideration for some patients. On the other hand, many patients find premixed short- and intermediate-acting insulins convenient to use, and these mixtures are available only as human insulins (see later discussion).

Duration of action of insulins. Both human and animal insulins are subclassified according to their duration of action (Table 39),[2,3] and the figures given vary from one source to another. Table 39 gives a rough approximation of the time of onset, peak effect, and duration of action of various insulin types.

Human insulins have a slightly earlier onset and a slightly shorter duration of action than beef or pork insulins. Thus patients taking human rather than pork or beef intermediate-acting insulins before supper are more likely to be hyperglycemic before breakfast.[2]

Lispro (Humalog), a synthetic analogue of human insulin, was approved by the U.S. Food and Drug Administration (FDA) in 1996. This product can be injected up to 15 minutes before a meal, thus increasing the flexibility of mealtimes for some diabetic patients. The number of hypoglycemic reactions may also be slightly diminished with lispro, but there is no evidence as yet that this agent results in better overall control.[3]

Insulin vials, pens, cartridges, and syringes. All insulins, regardless of the format in which they are supplied and whether they are premixed, contain 100 units/ml.

Mixed pork and beef insulin and pure pork and pure beef insulin are available only in 10-ml multidose vials contain-

Table 39 Classification of Insulins by Time of Action

Type	Time of action in hours		
	Onset	Peak	Duration
Very Short Acting			
Lispro (Humalog)	0.1	0.5-1	3-4
Short Acting			
Regular (Crystalline Zinc Insulin, Toronto)	0.5-2	2-4	3-6
Prompt insulin zinc suspension (Semilente)	1-1.5	5-10	12-16
Intermediate Acting	2-4	4-14	16-24
Isophane insulin (Neutral Protamine Hagedorn [NPH])			
Insulin zinc suspension (Lente)			
Long Acting	6-14	10-30	24-36+
Extended insulin zinc suspension (Ultralente)			
Protamine zinc insulin suspension (PZI)			

ing 100 units/ml of unmixed insulins (e.g., regular, NPH, Ultralente). Human insulins are also available in this format but in addition come as premixed vials containing regular plus NPH insulin in various proportions. In Canada the figures given for mixtures have regular insulin first followed by NPH insulin. Thus 30/70 means 30% regular insulin and 70% NPH. In the United States the order is sometimes reversed so that the above mixture might be written 70/30. The practitioner can avoid confusion by remembering that except for a 50/50 mixture (in which the order does not matter), the smaller figure is always regular insulin and the larger one is NPH. In this text the convention of putting regular insulin first is used. In Canada a full range of mixtures of regular and NPH insulins from 10/90 to 50/50 is available, whereas in the United States only the 30/70 and 50/50 mixtures are marketed.

A variety of cartridges for dial-a-dose insulin pens that contain regular or NPH insulin or mixtures of regular and NPH insulin (30/70 in the United States and in various proportions from 10/90 to 50/50 in Canada) may be purchased. Pens take 1.5-ml cartridges (containing 150 units of insulin) or 3-ml cartridges (containing 300 units of insulin), and the correct dose can be dialed.

Only human regular insulin and human NPH insulin are available in premixed formats, whether as vials, insulin pen cartridges, or disposable dispensing devices. Patients who are receiving beef or pork insulins or Lente or Ultralente insulins (human or animal) and require mixtures of regular and longer acting insulins have to mix their own.

Insulin syringes have a l-ml capacity and are graduated in 0.01-ml portions. Since all commercial insulins are supplied with 100 units/ml, 0.01 ml = 1 unit.

Insulin injection sites. Injection in an extremity that is exercised and massage of the injection site should be avoided because both increase absorption and may lead to hypoglycemia.[4] However, this applies only if the exercise takes place within half an hour of the injection.[5] Sites should be rotated in the same general anatomical area, such as the abdominal wall, rather than using the thigh one day, the arm the next, and so on. Keeping sites in one area improves glycemic control.[4]

Glucose monitoring. Urine dipstick testing for glucose was the original home monitoring method, and it remains an inexpensive, painless, and effective technique.[6] Capillary blood monitoring at home has largely replaced urine testing, but there is no evidence from randomized clinical trials that any form of glucose home monitoring improves glycemic control.[7]

Numerous glucometers are available. Modern ones are compact reflectance meters that are operated in one step and that draw fingertip capillary blood onto the strips by osmosis. They do not require wiping, washing, or timing. Glucose strips that are designed for a particular glucometer must be used. The patient must calibrate each package of glucose strips according to the package instructions before use.

Glucose sticks using a color comparison table are available. They are less expensive but less accurate than reflectance meters. The cost may be decreased even further by cutting each stick in half.[8] Some diabetic patients have decreased blue/yellow color discrimination and therefore may not be able to interpret the colors accurately.[9]

The technique of drawing blood for home glucose monitoring involves the following steps:

1. Wash and dry hands. Do not clean the area of fingerprick with alcohol.
2. Choose the lateral or medial side of the pulp of the fingers as the site for the fingerprick, not the volar surface.
3. Load an autolancet into its carrier, apply the tip of the carrier firmly to the finger, and release the spring.
4. Make sure the drop of blood is adequate to cover the glucose strip.

A common initial routine for home glucose monitoring of IDDM is to test the blood glucose daily before breakfast and before supper. With a twice-daily insulin regimen the goal is to keep the glucose level between 4 and 10 mmol/L (70 to 180 mg/dl) before meals. Patients whose condition is stable may monitor once a day, choosing different times on different days—before each meal, at bedtime, and occasionally in the early hours of the morning. Early morning monitoring is particularly important if the before-supper intermediate-acting insulin dose is increased. If the patient is in an unstable condition, has an intercurrent illness, or changes insulin doses, monitoring should be more frequent.[6]

Glycosylated or glycated hemoglobin is monitored to assess the efficacy of diabetic control over a 2- to 3-month period, whereas fructosamine is used for a 2- to 3-week period. Glycated hemoglobin is measured either as HBA_{1C} or as total glycated hemoglobin. In either case the goal is a level below

0.08 to 0.09 (8% to 9%). Measurements approximately every 3 months are recommended. An elevation of 0.01 (1%) corresponds to about a 1.7 mmol/L (30 mg/dl) rise in the average glucose level.

Urine testing is the least expensive test and glycated hemoglobin the most expensive. However, since the latter is done less frequently and reflects long-term control, it may be more cost effective.[6]

Initial insulin dose

The usual total daily dose of insulin for a patient with IDDM is 0.5 to 1.5 units/kg/day. Therapy should start with 0.3 to 0.5 units/kg/day if the patient is not ketoacidotic and is receiving insulin as an outpatient. The dose is increased according to frequent glucose readings, but the usual maintenance levels are 0.6 to 0.7 unit/kg/day for an adult and 0.9 to 1 unit/kg/day for an adolescent.[2] Usually two thirds of the daily dose is given 30 minutes before breakfast and one third 30 minutes before supper, with the injections given 10 to 12 hours apart. The usual mixture of each dose is 30% crystalline or Toronto insulin and 70% NPH or Lente insulin. As a result of the DCCT trial,[10] tighter control with three or four daily doses may become the norm (see discussion of basal bolus regimen). The ideal goal for glucose control varies from author to author, but an acceptable working guideline is to keep the blood glucose level between 4 and 10 mmol/L before meals.

Adjusting insulin doses

The insulin dose may be increased or decreased at any time by 1 to 2 units (or for higher doses by 10%). The particular insulin to be modified is determined by the blood sugar levels at different times during the day.[2,11,12] Assuming a twice a day insulin regimen with a mixture of regular and NPH insulin at each dose, the theoretical relationship would be as shown in Table 40.

Before insulin doses are adjusted, it is important to ensure that some exogenous factor such as an intercurrent illness, unusual exercise, irregularity of meal and snack schedules, or noncompliance with the insulin doses is not responsible for the inadequate control.

Before-breakfast hyperglycemia

One of the common problems of control in patients with IDDM is hyperglycemia before breakfast.[2,11] This is often seen in patients taking human intermediate-acting insulins, which may not have long enough action to maintain control for the 15 hours from the before-supper dose until breakfast time the next morning. In addition, early morning is a time of relative insulin resistance, probably because of nocturnal surges in growth hormone (the so-called dawn phenomenon).[13] Several alternative management strategies are available for this:

1. The patient could take the same dose of regular insulin before supper but take the intermediate-acting insulin at bedtime. This is probably the option of choice. It usually works well, although it involves a third injection each day. Once the before-breakfast hyperglycemia is controlled, lowering the before-breakfast regular insulin dose may be necessary to prevent hypoglycemia before lunch.
2. The before-supper dose of intermediate-acting insulin could be increased, but the risk would be hypoglycemia in the early hours of the morning. If this course is chosen, the patient must check his or her glucose level a few times early in the morning.
3. Another alternative would be to switch to a regimen of Ultralente and regular insulin, the so-called basal-bolus method. About half the daily requirement is given either as two equal doses of Ultralente at breakfast and supper or as a single dose at bedtime. The remainder is given as rapid-acting or very rapid-acting insulin before the three meals. Usually, more regular insulin is required before breakfast than before lunch, so an acceptable starting regimen would be to give half the total amount of regular insulin before breakfast, one fourth before lunch, and one fourth before supper and then adjust further according to glucose levels. Some patients may not need the dose before lunch if the noon meal is small. Good control is often obtained with this program, but more daily injections are required and premixed insulins are not available for it. An additional advantage of this method is that rigid timing of meals is not critical.
4. A final and inexpensive option is to switch the patient to beef or pork insulin because they tend to be slightly longer acting than human insulins. As in several of the other alternatives, premixed insulins are not available for this program.

Table 40 Relationship Between Glucose Levels and Insulin Dose Adjustments in Patients Taking Mixture of Regular and NPH Insulins

Glucose reading	Responsible insulin
Before lunch	Before breakfast: regular
Before supper	Before breakfast: NPH
Bedtime	Before supper: regular
Before breakfast	Before supper: NPH

"Somogyi" phenomenon

In the past it was thought that prebreakfast hyperglycemia was often due to an excessive counterregulatory response to nocturnal hypoglycemia, the so-called Somogyi phenomenon. The suggested treatment was to decrease the before-supper intermediate-acting insulin. It has now been determined that the usual cause of early morning hyperglycemia is the dawn phenomenon (see above) and that the Somogyi phenomenon is extremely rare. Therefore decreasing the before-supper intermediate-acting insulin is not recommended.[14,15]

Hypoglycemic reactions

Up to 20% of patients with IDDM have severe hypoglycemic episodes. Those whose overall control is near normoglycemia have a three times greater incidence of hypoglycemia than those with less optimal control. Missed meals, exercise without a snack, and erroneous insulin doses are some of the causes. The Somogyi phenomenon is discussed above in the section on before-breakfast hyperglycemia.

First-line treatment of hypoglycemia is sugar by mouth if the patient is conscious or applied to the buccal mucosa if the patient is not. Alternatives are a glucagon injection (1 mg for adults and older children and 0.5 mg for children under 5) or IV glucose.

REFERENCES

1. Expert Committee of the Canadian Diabetes Advisory Board: Clinical practice guidelines for diabetes mellitus in Canada, *Can Med Assoc J* 147:697-712, 1992.
2. Rodgers W: Insulin-dependent (type I) diabetes mellitus, *Can Med Assoc J* 145:1227-1237, 1991.
3. Holleman F, Hoekstra JB: Insulin lispro, *N Engl J Med* 337:176-183, 1997.
4. Bantle JP, Weber MS, Rao SM, et al: Rotation of the anatomic regions used for insulin injections and day-to-day variability of plasma glucose in type I diabetic subjects, *JAMA* 263:1802-1806, 1990.
5. Fahey PF, Stallcamp ET, Kwatra S: The athlete with type I diabetes: managing insulin, diet and exercise, *Am Fam Physician* 53:1611-1617, 1996.
6. Koch B: Glucose monitoring as a guide to diabetes management: critical subject review, *Can Fam Physician* 42:1142-1152, 1996.
7. Gallichan M: Self monitoring of glucose by people with diabetes: evidence based practice, *BMJ* 324:964-966, 1997.
8. Spraul M, Sonnenberg GE, Berger M: Less expensive, reliable blood glucose self-monitoring, *Diabetes Care* 10:357-359, 1987.
9. Bresnick GH, Groo A, Palta M, et al: Urinary glucose testing inaccuracies among diabetic patients: effect of acquired color vision deficiency caused by diabetic retinopathy, *Arch Ophthalmol* 102:1489-1496, 1984.
10. Diabetes Control and Complications Trial Research Group: The effect of intensive treatment of diabetes on the development and progression of long-term complications in insulin-dependent diabetes mellitus, *N Engl J Med* 329:977-986, 1993.
11. Schlossberg AH: Diabetes case and comment: "re-controlling" man, 30, with IDDM, *Patient Care Can,* July-August 1992, 3:20-21.
12. Hirsch I: Intensive insulin therapy. II. Multicomponent insulin regimens, *Am Fam Physician* 45:2141-2147, 1992.
13. Campbell PJ, Bolli GB, Cryer PE, et al: Pathogenesis of the dawn phenomenon in patients with insulin-dependent diabetes mellitus: accelerated glucose production and impaired glucose utilization due to nocturnal surges in growth hormone secretion, *N Engl J Med* 312:1473-1479, 1985.
14. Lerman IG, Wolfsdorf JL: Relationship of nocturnal hypoglycemia to daytime glycemia in IDDM, *Diabetes Care* 11:636-642, 1988.
15. Tordjman KM, Havlin CE, Levandoski LA, et al: Failure of nocturnal hypoglycemia to cause fasting hyperglycemia in patients with insulin-dependent diabetes mellitus, *N Engl J Med* 317:1552-1559, 1987.

Diet and insulin-dependent diabetes mellitus

Daily food intake for patients with IDDM is divided into three regular meals plus two or three snacks at midmorning, midafternoon, and in the evening just before bedtime. The timing and quantity of the meals should be as consistent as possible to avoid large fluctuations in glucose levels.[1] The purpose of the snacks is to prevent hypoglycemia caused by the regular or intermediate-acting insulin the patient is taking. If the patient is taking a mixture of regular and NPH insulin twice a day before breakfast and before supper, the midmorning snack counters the effect of the morning regular insulin, the afternoon snack counters that of the morning NPH, and the evening snack counters that of the before-supper regular insulin. A substantial evening snack may also be a way of obviating early morning hypoglycemia caused by before-supper NPH.

REFERENCES

1. Service FJ, Rizza RA, Hall LD, et al: Prandial insulin requirements in insulin-dependent diabetics: effects of size, time of day, and sequence of meals, *J Clin Endocrinol Metab* 57:931-936, 1983.

Exercise and insulin-dependent diabetes mellitus

An exercise program is important for patients with IDDM because it improves the quality of their lives. However, unlike the case with NIDDM, exercise has not been shown in controlled studies to improve outcome.[1,2]

Whenever possible exercise should be done at regular times. The major risk is hypoglycemia, which may develop during, shortly after, or 6 to 12 hours after exercise. The patient may try to prevent this with a preexercise snack or, when exercising is done on a regular basis, by decreasing the appropriate insulin dose on exercise days. For low- to moderate-intensity exercise of less than an hour's duration, a preexercise snack is usually not required unless the preexercise glucose level is less than 5.6 mmol/L (100 mg/dl). For high-intensity exercises, snacks are advised.[3]

Athletes with IDDM who exercise regularly should, at least initially, monitor their blood sugar before, during, and for several hours after the exercise. If the exercise is performed in the late afternoon or evening, this includes a 2 AM glucose measurement. In general a 30% to 50% reduction in the preprandial insulin dose before exercise is required. In hot weather lower doses may be required than in cold weather. To prevent postexercise nocturnal hypoglycemia, the patient should have only regular insulin before supper and NPH or, even better, Lente, at bedtime.[3]

A danger signal for athletes is a preexercise glucose level greater than 13.9 mmol/L (250 mg/dl). In this situation exercise can aggravate hyperglycemia and even cause ketoacidosis. If the glucose level is between 13.9 mmol/L (250 mg/dl) and 16.7 mmol/L (300 mg/dl) and the urine is free of ketones, participation in the athletic event can proceed. If ketones are present or if the glucose level is above 16.7 mmol/L (300 mg/dl), exercise should be postponed until better control is achieved.[3]

Exercise of the muscle that is the site of an insulin injection increases the rate of absorption and so the risk of hypoglycemia, but only if the exercise takes place within half an hour of the injection.[4] Absorption from the abdomen is greater than from the thigh, so switching from thigh to abdomen may result in hypoglycemia. The practical significance of these findings is that the athlete should rotate insulin injection sites around one anatomical area and not switch from one to another body site. If there is a choice, the abdomen is probably the preferable site.[3]

REFERENCES

1. Zinman B, Zuniga-Guajardo S, Kelly D: Comparison of acute and long-term effects of exercise on glucose control in type I diabetes, *Diabetes Care* 7:515-519, 1984.
2. Expert Committee of the Canadian Diabetes Advisory Board: Clinical practice guidelines for diabetes mellitus in Canada, *Can Med Assoc J* 147:697-712, 1992.
3. Fahey PF, Stallcamp ET, Kwatra S: The athlete with type I diabetes: managing insulin, diet and exercise, *Am Fam Physician* 53:1611-1617, 1996.
4. Kemmer FW: Prevention of hypoglycemia during exercise in type I diabetes, *Diabetes Care* 15:1732-1735, 1992.

Non-Insulin-Dependent Diabetes

Epidemiology

Diabetes affects 4% to 6% of Canadians; about 90% of persons with diabetes have NIDDM and 5% to 10% have IDDM.

The genetic propensity for NIDDM is greater than that for IDDM. A person who has one first-degree relative with the disease has twice the risk, and if the person has two first-degree relatives with the condition, the risk is quadrupled. The concordance rate for identical twins is 60% to 80%.[1] Race is also a risk factor; the disease is twice as common in blacks[1] and two-and-a-half to three times as common in Mexican-Americans as in whites.[2] Diabetes among Native Canadians was virtually unknown before 1947, but it now has a high prevalence rate.[3] This increase is almost certainly due to a marked increase in the incidence of obesity in this population. In the United States the incidence of diabetes in Native Americans is five times that of whites.[2] In the northern Canadian community of Sioux Lookout the prevalence of NIDDM in adolescents under 16 was 2.5:1000. Most patients were asymptomatic obese females with a strong family history of NIDDM.[4]

The major risk factor, which at least in theory can be controlled, is weight gain. In a prospective cohort study of American nurses, a weight gain after the age of 18 of 5 to 7.9 kg increased the risk of diabetes by 1.9 and a weight gain of 8 to 10.9 kg increased the risk by 2.7. A weight loss of more than 5 kg decreased the relative risk by 50%.[5]

Moderate alcohol intake appears to have a protective effect on the development of NIDDM.[6,7] Cigarette smoking increases the risk,[6] and physical exercise decreases it.[7,8]

An estimated 50% of cases of NIDDM in the United States are undiagnosed.[9]

REFERENCES

1. Bennett PH: Epidemiology of diabetes mellitus. In Rifkin H, Porte D Jr, eds: *Ellenberg and Rifkin's diabetes mellitus,* New York, 1990, Elsevier, pp 363-377.
2. Harris MI, Hadden WC, Knowler WC, et al: Prevalence of diabetes and impaired glucose tolerance and plasma glucose levels in the US population, *Diabetes* 36:523-534, 1987.
3. Expert Committee of the Canadian Diabetes Advisory Board: Clinical practice guidelines for diabetes mellitus in Canada, *Can Med Assoc J* 147:697-712, 1992.
4. Harris SB, Perkins BA, Whalen-Brough E: Non-insulin-dependent diabetes mellitus among First Nations children: new entity among First Nations people of northwestern Ontario, *Can Fam Physician* 42:869-876, 1996.
5. Colditz GA, Willett WC, Rotnitzky A, et al: Weight gain as a risk factor for clinical diabetes mellitus in women, *Ann Intern Med* 122:481-486, 1995.
6. Rimm EB, Chan J, Stampfer MJ, et al: Prospective study of cigarette smoking, alcohol use, and the risk of diabetes in men, *BMJ* 210:545-546, 1995.
7. Perry IF, Wannamethee SG, Walker MK, et al: Prospective study of risk factors for development of non-insulin dependent diabetes in middle aged British men, *BMJ* 310:560-564, 1995.
8. Lynch J, Helmrich SP, Lakka TA, et al: Moderately intense physical activities and high levels of cardiorespiratory fitness reduce the risk of non-insulin-dependent diabetes mellitus in middle-aged men, *Arch Intern Med* 156:1307-1314, 1996.
9. Harris MI: Undiagnosed NIDDM: clinical and public health issues, *Diabetes Care* 16:642-652, 1993.

Insulin resistance and the pathogenesis of non-insulin-dependent diabetes mellitus

(See also role of intensive treatment in preventing diabetic complications in non-insulin-dependent diabetes mellitus)

Insulin resistance seems a necessary but not sufficient condition for the development of NIDDM. The theory is that individuals who develop insulin resistance but have good beta cell reserves simply produce more insulin (hyperinsulinemia) to maintain normoglycemia. When the reserves of the beta cells become inadequate, NIDDM supervenes.

Hyperinsulinemia is thought to have a number of adverse effects on human health. It may be responsible for NIDDM, obesity, hypertension, dyslipidemia, and atherosclerotic vascular disease,[1] a group of conditions often lumped together as "syndrome X." This is one reason that many authorities are reluctant to treat NIDDM with insulin.

A clear relationship that is independent of age and obesity

exists between hypertension and NIDDM.[2,3] When a person has both diseases, the hypertension antedates the diabetes eight times more frequently than the reverse sequence.[3] It may be that hyperinsulinemia is responsible for both conditions, or it may be that drugs such as thiazides and beta-blockers used to treat the hypertension aggravate the insulin resistance.[4] However, no empirical evidence has been presented to indicate that classes of antihypertensives that do not adversely affect insulin resistance produce greater benefits than beta-blockers and thiazides in hypertensive patients.[5]

REFERENCES

1. De Fronzo RA, Ferrannini E: Insulin resistance: a multifaceted syndrome responsible for NIDDM, obesity, hypertension, dyslipidemia and atherosclerotic vascular disease, *Diabetes Care* 14:173-194, 1991.
2. Modan M, Halkin H, Almog S, et al: Hyperinsulinaemia: a link between hypertension, obesity and glucose intolerance, *J Clin Invest* 75:809-817, 1985.
3. Teuscher A, Egger M, Herman JB: Diabetes and hypertension: blood pressure in clinical diabetic patients and a control population, *Arch Intern Med* 149:1942-1945, 1989.
4. Lundgren H, Björkman L, Keiding P, et al: Diabetes in patients with hypertension receiving pharmacological treatment, *BMJ* 297:1512, 1988.
5. Yudkin J: Hypertension and non-insulin dependent diabetes (editorial), *BMJ* 303:730-731, 1991.

Screening for non-insulin-dependent diabetes mellitus

(See also screening)

Two expert panels that have reviewed the evidence for screening patients for fasting plasma glucose have come to the same conclusions.[1,2] No evidence supports routine screening of the general population over 50. However, screening may be considered for those with a family history of diabetes, a history of gestational diabetes, or marked obesity, even though early detection has not been shown to affect the ultimate outcome.[1] The Canadian Task Force on the Periodic Health Examination gives screening of the general population for diabetes a "D" recommendation,[1] whereas the U.S. Preventive Services Task Force gives it a "C."[2] However, at its annual meeting in 1997 the American Diabetes Association recommended screening all adults over the age of 45 for diabetes.[3] As far as I know, there is no good evidence that such a move would decrease morbidity or mortality.

REFERENCES

1. Canadian Task Force on the Periodic Health Examination: *Clinical preventive health care,* Ottawa, 1994, Canadian Communication Group—Publishing, pp 602-609.
2. US Preventive Services Task Force: *Guide to clinical preventive services,* ed 2, Baltimore, 1996, Williams & Wilkins, pp 193-208.
3. Macready N: American Diabetes Association calls for testing all those over 45, *BMJ* 315:11, 1997.

Diet and exercise in non-insulin-dependent diabetes mellitus

Diet and exercise are essential components of the treatment of NIDDM because of their value in controlling weight, reducing insulin resistance, and preventing coronary artery disease.[1,2] Except in a few symptomatic patients the initial treatment of patients with NIDDM should be an intensive, individualized diet and exercise program. Only if it is unsuccessful after 3 to 6 months of persistent endeavor should pharmacological treatment be considered.[3,4]

REFERENCES

1. Schneider SH, Amoroso LF, Khachadurian AK, et al: Studies on the mechanism of improved glucose control during regular exercise in type 2 (noninsulin-dependent) diabetes, *Diabetologia* 26:355-360, 1984.
2. Expert Committee of the Canadian Diabetes Advisory Board: Clinical practice guidelines for diabetes mellitus in Canada, *Can Med Assoc J* 147:697-712, 1992.
3. Gerich JE: Oral hypoglycemic agents, *N Engl J Med* 321:1231-1245, 1989.
4. Rodger W: Non-insulin-dependent (type II) diabetes mellitus, *Can Med Assoc J* 145:1571-1581, 1991.

Pharmacological treatment of non-insulin-dependent diabetes mellitus

(See also role of intensive treatment in preventing diabetic complications in non-insulin-dependent diabetes mellitus)

Whether good glucose control in NIDDM decreases either the microvascular or the macrovascular complications of the disease is controversial. The U.K. Prospective Diabetes Study has been set up to answer these questions.[1] Patients in this program have been assigned at random to one of five treatment regimens: diet only, glyburide, chlorpropamide, metformin, or insulin. A preliminary report after 3 years of follow-up showed that 23% of patients assigned to the diet only group maintained fasting sugar levels below 7.8 mmol/L (140 mg/dl) in contrast to 53% of those treated pharmacologically; glycosylated hemoglobin levels were also lower in the pharmacologically treated group. All groups showed weight gain except those on diet only and obese patients who were treated with metformin. Serum insulin levels were raised in all pharmacologically treated groups except for the obese treated with metformin, in whom insulin levels actually dropped. As expected, hypoglycemic reactions were greater in the pharmacologically treated, especially those receiving glyburide or insulin; reactions were more common in those whose pretreatment fasting glucose levels were relatively low. No data were yet available for complication rates, and the authors state that long-term follow-up will be required before rational management conclusions can be drawn.[1]

Oral hypoglycemic agents. The Expert Committee of the Canadian Diabetes Advisory Board for the pharmacological treatment of NIDDM recommends that if 6 weeks of intensive diet and exercise fails to lower the fasting glucose level to below 10 mmol/L (180 mg/dl), treatment with a biguanide or a sulfonylurea should be initiated. If this fails, a second class of oral hypoglycemic agents should be added, and if the fasting sugar level still remains above 10 mmol/L (180 mg/dl), these drugs should be discontinued and insulin started.[2]

One of the main arguments for trying to obtain "good" blood sugar control by such a protocol is that impaired glucose tolerance has been identified as an independent risk factor for coronary artery disease,[3,4] probably because of associated dyslipidemia.[5] However, no evidence has shown that this approach decreases morbidity or mortality, and some have argued that insulin therapy, in particular, may be counterproductive (see discussion of the role of intensive treatment in preventing diabetic complications in non-insulin-dependent diabetes mellitus).

When oral hypoglycemic medications are indicated, the physician has the choice of starting with one of the sulfonylureas, a biguanide, or an alpha-glucosidase inhibitor (Table 41).

The primary action of sulfonylureas is to increase insulin output from the pancreatic beta-cells.[5] These agents may cause hypoglycemic reactions and should not be given to patients who are allergic to sulfonamides. They tend to stimulate the appetite, although the manufacturer of gliclazide (Diamicron) claims that drug does not. The sulfonylureas can be subclassified into first- and second-generation drugs. First-generation sulfonylureas tend to have more drug interactions than second-generation drugs and are now rarely used. Second-generation sulfonylureas include glyburide (DiaBeta, Glynase, Micronase), gliclazide (Diamicron), glimepiride (Amaryl), and glipizide (Glucotrol).

The biguanides, of which the only one currently available in Canada and the United States is metformin (Glucophage), act primarily by decreasing glucose output from the liver but also by increasing the insulin sensitivity of muscle. Metformin leads to weight loss through the preferential diminution of adipose tissue[6]; it decreases triglyceride, total cholesterol, and LDL cholesterol levels,[7] is as effective as the sulfonylureas, and does not induce hypoglycemia.[8] Disadvantages of the drug are that it has to be given two or three times a day and that 5% to 20% of patients have transient gastrointestinal effects, usually diarrhea. Metformin should not be given to persons with impaired liver or renal function because of the risk of lactic acidosis. Specifically, physicians should be wary of prescribing the drug to someone with a creatinine level above 150 mmol/L (1.7 mg/dl).

Acarbose (Prandase, Precose) is an alpha-glucosidase inhibitor that is taken three times daily immediately before meals. It acts by inhibiting the hydrolysis of dietary disaccharides and thus limits the absorption of monosaccharides. It has been used for both IDDM and NIDDM. The main adverse effects are flatulence, distention, cramps, and diarrhea.[9] These tend to diminish with time.[10] Although hypoglycemia is not a complication of acarbose therapy, the drug inhibits the hydrolysis of dietary disaccharides, which means that sucrose or fructose by mouth may not correct hypoglycemic episodes in diabetic patients taking acarbose in addition to insulin or other hypoglycemic agents.[10]

A new class of agents is the thiazolidinediones, one of which, troglitazone (Rezulin), was approved by the FDA in 1997 for addition to the treatment protocol of patients whose NIDDM is inadequately controlled with insulin alone. It acts by increasing insulin sensitivity so that liver and muscle cells increase their consumption of glucose. Although approved only for use with insulin in the United States, it can be administered as monotherapy or with other oral medications. Long-term safety and efficacy have not been fully evaluated.[8]

If adequate control of glucose cannot be obtained with one class of oral hypoglycemic medication, a member of another class can be added.

Table 41 Oral Hypoglycemic Agents

Drugs	Usual doses
Sulfonylureas, Second Generation	
Glyburide (DiaBeta, Glynase, Micronase)	5-10 mg qam or 10 mg bid
Gliclazide (Diamicron)	40-160 mg bid
Glimepiride (Amaryl)	1-8 mg qam
Glipizide (Glucotrol)	5-40 mg qam or 10-20 mg bid
Biguanides	
Metformin (Glucophage)	500 mg tid-qid or 850 mg bid-tid
Alpha-Glucosidase Inhibitors	
Acarbose (Precose, Prandase)	25-100 mg tid
Thaizolidinediones	
Troglitazone (Rezulin)	200-600 mg once daily

REFERENCES

1. United Kingdom Prospective Diabetes Study (UKPDS) 13: Relative efficacy of randomly allocated diet, sulfonylurea, insulin or metformin in patients with newly diagnosed non-insulin-dependent diabetes followed for three years, *BMJ* 310: 83-88, 1995.
2. Expert Committee of the Canadian Diabetes Advisory Board: Clinical practice guidelines for diabetes mellitus in Canada, *Can Med Assoc J* 147:697-712, 1992.
3. Barrett-Connor E, Wingard DL, Criqui MH, et al: Is borderline fasting hyperglycemia a risk factor for cardiovascular death? *J Chron Dis* 37:773-779, 1984.
4. Donahue RP, Abbott RD, Reed DM, et al: Postchallenge glucose concentration and coronary heart disease in men of Japanese ancestry: Honolulu Heart Program, *Diabetes* 36:689-692, 1987.
5. Bressler R, Johnson DG: Pharmacological regulation of blood glucose levels in non-insulin-dependent diabetes mellitus, *Arch Intern Med* 157:836-848, 1997.
6. Stumvoll M, Nurjhan M, Perriello G, et al: Metabolic effects of metformin in non-insulin-dependent diabetes mellitus, *N Engl J Med* 333:550-554, 1995.
7. Bailey CJ, Turner RC: Metformin, *N Engl J Med* 334:574-579, 1996.

8. Troglitazone for non-insulin-dependent diabetes mellitus, *Med Lett* 39:49-51, 1997.
9. Acarbose for diabetes mellitus, *Med Lett* 38:9-10, 1996.
10. Cornish WR: Acarbose: an alpha-glucosidase inhibitor for the management of noninsulin-dependent diabetes mellitus, *Can J Clin Pharmacol* 4:15-23, 1997.

Insulin therapy for non-insulin-dependent diabetes mellitus

(See also attitudes, physician; glucose monitoring for insulin-dependent diabetes mellitus; insulin therapy for insulin-dependent diabetes mellitus; role of intensive treatment in preventing diabetic complications in non-insulin-dependent diabetes mellitus)

Indications. Patients with NIDDM often require temporary insulin therapy if they become pregnant, undergo surgery, or have acute intercurrent illnesses such as myocardial infarction or pneumonia. A widespread hospital practice in such cases is to use sliding insulin scales so that the patient is given regular insulin q6h with the doses calibrated on the basis of regularly measured capillary blood glucose levels. The origin of this practice is unclear, and its net effect is poor control of glycemia; patients are far better off continuing with oral hypoglycemic agents or standard combinations of long- and short-acting insulins.[1,2]

Much more controversial is the question of whether insulin should be prescribed simply because "good" metabolic control is not achieved with other modalities. As stated previously, the Expert Committee of the Canadian Diabetes Advisory Board recommends that insulin therapy be started for any patient with NIDDM if the fasting sugar level does not fall below 10 mmol/L (180 mg/dl) after a full trial of diet, exercise, and oral hypoglycemic agents.[3] The arguments for trying to avoid insulin administration in NIDDM are given in the section "Role of Intensive Treatment in Preventing Diabetic Complications in Non-Insulin-Dependent Diabetes Mellitus."

Method of prescribing insulin. The usual procedure for prescribing insulin therapy for a patient with stable NIDDM is to order a single morning injection of an intermediate- or long-acting insulin in a low dose such as 0.3 unit/kg. Thus the usual initial dose is 15 to 25 units/day. The dose is adjusted according to glucose levels, and many patients require as much as 1 unit/kg/day, particularly if they are obese. If the patient is already taking oral agents, these are stopped on the morning insulin is begun. "Good control" of NIDDM is difficult to achieve and is probably not feasible or necessary for some patients, particularly if they are elderly.[4]

Unnecessary insulin. Even when rather strict criteria are used to define metabolic control, about half of obese diabetic patients who are receiving insulin can stop taking the drug and maintain glycemic control with diet and exercise alone.[1] Reasons for this may be an initial misdiagnosis of IDDM, an inadequate trial of diet, exercise, or oral agents, significant weight loss since starting insulin, or a prescription of insulin that was ordered during a stressful illness and never discontinued.[5] It behooves all family physicians to remember that insulin may not be needed and, where appropriate, to try to discontinue it.

Home glucose monitoring. Glucose monitoring of patients with NIDDM does not seem to improve glycemic control. Although a few patients feel empowered and more in control of their disease when they use this technique, anxiety, helplessness, and guilt are much more common reactions.[6] A comparison of blood and urine glucose monitoring in patients with newly diagnosed NIDDM found no difference between the two in glycosylated hemoglobin levels at 6 and 12 months, although urine testing was six times less expensive.[7]

White coat hyperglycemia. In a British study of patients with NIDDM, glucose levels monitored at home were often lower than those measured in the clinic even when technical errors in home readings were ruled out.[8] The authors labeled this phenomenon "white coat hyperglycemia."

REFERENCES

1. Queale WS, Seidler AJ, Brancati FL: Glycemic control and sliding scale insulin use in medical inpatients with diabetes mellitus, *Arch Intern Med* 157:545-552, 1997.
2. Sawin CT: Action without benefit: the sliding scale of insulin use (editorial), *Arch Intern Med* 157:489, 1997.
3. Expert Committee of the Canadian Diabetes Advisory Board: Clinical practice guidelines for diabetes mellitus in Canada, *Can Med Assoc J* 147:697-712, 1992.
4. Shlossberg AH: Treating non-insulin-dependent diabetes: oral agents or insulin? *Can Fam Physician* 39:119-126, 1993.
5. Genuth S: Insulin use in NIDDM, *Diabetes Care* 13:1240-1264, 1990.
6. Gallichan M: Self monitoring of glucose by people with diabetes: evidence based practice, *BMJ* 324:964-966, 1997.
7. Miles P, Everett J, Murphy J, et al: Comparison of blood or urine testing by patients with newly diagnosed non-insulin dependent diabetes: patient survey after randomised crossover trial, *BMJ* 315:348-349, 1997.
8. Campbell LV, Ashwell SM, Borkman M, et al: White coat hyperglycaemia: disparity between diabetes clinic and home blood glucose concentrations, *BMJ* 305:1194-1196, 1992.

ELECTROLYTES

Potassium

Fist clenching during phlebotomy, with or without the use of a tourniquet, raises the serum potassium level by as much as 1.6 mmol/L (1.6 mEq/L).[1]

REFERENCES

1. Don BR, Sebastian A, Cheitlin M, et al: Pseudohyperkalemia caused by fist clenching during phlebotomy, *N Engl J Med* 322:1290-1292, 1990.

HYPOGLYCEMIA

(See also insulin therapy for insulin-dependent diabetes mellitus)

A number of conditions may cause true hypoglycemia. Insulin reactions in diabetic patients are the most common.

Factitious hypoglycemia from the self-injection of insulin is primarily a disorder of female health care workers. Insulinomas and drugs are other well-recognized causes of hypoglycemia, and Addison's disease, hypopituitarism, and gastric resection may also result in the syndrome.[1,2]

Functional, reactive, or alimentary hypoglycemia is a controversial entity.[1,2] It is characterized by a variety of nonspecific symptoms, such as weakness, palpitations, tremors, sweating, headaches, and hunger, that come on after meals and are relieved by eating.[1] Control has been said to be achievable with a high-protein, low-carbohydrate diet.[1] Primary care physicians should be aware that little scientific evidence supports the existence of functional or alimentary hypoglycemia.[1,2] In studies of patients thought to have this disorder, glucose levels have almost always been normal (greater than 2.8 mmol/L or 50 mg/dl) during the period of symptoms.[1,2] The diagnosis should not be based on a glucose tolerance test, since it is neither sensitive nor specific.[1] The argument that the glucose level may be normal but have dropped rapidly, thereby causing symptoms, does not hold up because this phenomenon is never observed after insulin injections in volunteers.[2] Many patients come to physicians with a diagnosis of hypoglycemia that they have either made themselves or been given by health care workers. A better term for their problem would be idiopathic postprandial syndrome.[2]

REFERENCES

1. Service FJ: Hypoglycemic disorders, *N Engl J Med* 332:1144-1152, 1995.
2. Palardy J, Havrankova J, Lepage R, et al: Blood glucose measurements during symptomatic episodes in patients with suspected postprandial hypoglycemia, *N Engl J Med* 321:1421-1425, 1989.

LIPIDS

Conversion from Systéme International Units to Traditional Units

To convert cholesterol readings from Systéme International (SI) units (mmol/L) to traditional units (mg/dl), divide by 0.0259. To convert cholesterol readings from traditional units (mg/dl) to SI units (mmol/L), multiply by 0.0259.

Epidemiology

(See also adverse effects associated with low cholesterol)

Tremendous variabilities are seen in coronary heart disease (CHD) in different geographical areas, and these are not fully explained by differences in cholesterol levels. For example, men with cholesterol levels in the range of 5.45 mmol/L (210 mg/dl) had CHD mortality rates varying from between 4% and 5% in Japan and Southern Europe to 12% in the United States and 15% in Northern Europe. The reason for this discrepancy is unknown.[1] Within any one culture, CHD risk correlates well with cholesterol levels.[1] Elevated cholesterol levels and low-density lipoprotein cholesterol (LDL-C) levels are also risk factors for women under the age of 65, but not for those over that age.[2] Elevated triglyceride concentrations are a risk factor for MI.[3,4] Whether therapeutic interventions to lower triglycerides are beneficial is unknown.

Hypercholesterolemia is not a good predictor of increased risk of coronary heart disease in the elderly.[5,6] Although one study found that a low high-density lipoprotein cholesterol (HDL-C) level was predictive of an increased morbidity and mortality from CHD in persons over 70,[5] this finding has little practical significance because no studies have shown benefits from lipid-lowering programs in the elderly.[6] Low cholesterol in the elderly has been associated with increased death rates (see discussion of adverse effects associated with low cholesterol).

REFERENCES

1. Verschuren WMM, Jacobs DR, Bloemberg M, et al: Serum total cholesterol and long-term coronary heart disease mortality in different cultures: twenty-five-year follow-up of the seven countries study, *JAMA* 274:131-136, 1995.
2. Walsh JM, Grady D: Treatment of hyperlipidemia in women, *JAMA* 274:1152-1158, 1995.
3. Stampfer MJ, Krauss RM, Ma J, et al: A prospective study of triglyceride level, low-density lipoprotein particle diameter, and risk of myocardial infarction, *JAMA* 276:882-888, 1996.
4. Coresh J, Kwiterovich PO Jr: Small, dense low-density lipoprotein particles and coronary heart disease risk: a clear association with uncertain implications (editorial), *JAMA* 276:914-915, 1996.
5. Corti M-C, Guralnik JM, Salive ME, et al: HDL cholesterol predicts coronary heart disease mortality in older persons, *JAMA* 274:539-544, 1995.
6. Denke MA, Winker MA: Cholesterol and coronary heart disease in older adults: no easy answers (editorial), *JAMA* 274:575-576, 1995.

Variability of Cholesterol Levels

(See also screening; prevention)

A person's cholesterol levels vary substantially from one day to another independent of diet and laboratory testing procedures. In an Ontario study of cholesterol levels any patient whose initial total cholesterol level was greater than 6.2 mmol/L (240 mg/dl) was asked to give a second sample. On the basis of the initial results patients were divided into three risk categories[1]:

Normal risk	<6.2 mmol/L (240 mg/dl)
Moderate risk	6.2-6.9 mmol/L (240-266 mg/dl)
High risk	>6.9 mmol/L (266 mg/dl)

When a second sample was obtained, the two results were averaged and the patient's risk category was reassigned. The results were striking. Fifty percent of patients initially classified as at high risk were reclassified to moderate risk, 10.5% of those initially classified as at moderate risk were reclassified to the normal category, and 4.8% of those initially classified as at moderate risk were moved up to a high-risk category.[1] From the findings of this and other studies, no one should be treated for an elevated cholesterol reading on the basis of one sample. Unfortunately, obtaining a second reading may cause significant psychological morbidity, since the patient will know that the initial cholesterol measurement was "up." Even if subsequent readings are normal, that nagging doubt will not easily be dispelled.

REFERENCES

1. Speechley M, McNair S, Leffley A, Bass M: Identifying patients with hypercholesterolemia: more than one blood sample is needed, *Can Fam Physician* 41:240-245, 1995.

Cholesterol-Lowering Studies in Adults Without Known Coronary Artery Disease

(See also guidelines for cholesterol screening; cholesterol-lowering studies in patients with coronary artery disease; cholesterol screening in children; exercise; medical economics; relative risk reduction)

Table 42 lists seven major cholesterol-lowering studies of persons without known coronary artery disease. Five of these investigations used drugs, and two used diet.

All the studies enrolled primarily middle-aged men without clinical evidence of CAD. A 1993 evaluation that combined the results of these studies (except the 1995 West of Scotland Coronary Prevention Study with pravastatin[6]) found a statistically significant reduction in nonfatal coronary events in the treated groups and a slight but statistically insignificant fall in the number of cardiac deaths. These beneficial results were offset by a significant increase in deaths from noncardiac causes in the treated groups,which resulted in a slight and insignificant excess in the overall death rates. The treated groups had a significant increase in violent deaths and gallbladder disease and an insignificant increase in the number of deaths from cancer.[9] In the WHO clofibrate study, total mortality of the treated group was increased by a relative rate of 47%.[3,4]

The West of Scotland Coronary Prevention Study was the first primary prevention study of cholesterol-lowering drugs to show a decline in the total mortality of the treated group.[6] In addition, this trial showed no evidence of increased mortality in the treated group from suicide, homicide, or accidents,[6] although the power of the study was not sufficient to rule out this phenomenon.[10] In the West of Scotland investigation approximately 3300 middle-aged men without known CAD received pravastatin 40 mg/day for an average of 4.9 years, while an equal number in the control group received a placebo. Prominently presented figures in the abstract of this *New England Journal of Medicine* report were a relative reduction of 31% in definite nonfatal and fatal MIs and a 22% relative reduction in death from all causes in the treated cohort. By careful reading of the text it is possible to calculate that the absolute reduction in definite nonfatal and fatal MIs was 2.4% and that more than 200 men had to be treated for 1 year to prevent one such adverse event. The absolute reduction in total cohort mortality was 0.9%, and this required the treatment of 555 men for 1 year to prevent one death.[6]

Table 42 Seven Cholesterol-Lowering Studies in Patients Without Coronary Artery Disease

Study	Drug
Drug Studies	
Lipid Research Clinics Program Trial (LRC)[1]	Cholestyramine
Helsinki Heart Study (HHS)[2]	Gemfibrozil
World Health Organization (WHO)[3,4]	Clofibrate
Upjohn's Colestipol Study (UCS)[5]	Colestipol
West of Scotland Coronary Prevention Study Group[6]	Pravastatin
Dietary Studies	
Los Angeles Veterans Diet Study (LAVDS)[7]	
Minnesota Coronary Survey (MCS)[8]	

No long-term lipid-lowering studies of young adults have been conducted,[11] and therefore the value of screening young asymptomatic individuals for cholesterol and treating them if it is elevated is unknown. Hulley and associates[12] point out that the mortality rate from cardiovascular disease is so low in persons under 40 that treatment would be unlikely to have beneficial results, whereas the adverse effects of treatment would continue unabated. They argue that delaying treatment until after age 40 would not significantly decrease any possible benefit.

Data on the effects of cholesterol-lowering programs on women are unclear; too few women have been studied to generate enough statistical power to give meaningful results.[13] However, what data are available from primary prevention studies show no evidence that lowering cholesterol affects total mortality.[14]

The West of Scotland Coronary Prevention Study clearly shows that both coronary artery disease deaths and total mortality can be decreased in asymptomatic hypercholesterolemic middle-aged men by prolonged use of high doses of pravastatin. Only a few benefit, but these are important benefits. One problem for clinicians deciding whether to institute more aggressive treatment of their hypercholesterolemic patients with HMG-CoA reductase drugs is that none of these lipid-lowering studies had a control group given a regimen of regular moderate exercise. The benefits of exercise might have equalled or surpassed those of lipid-lowering drugs, although that is merely a hypothesis. Aside from this, evidence for treating young hypercholesterolemic patients (except those with inborn errors of lipid metabolism) or women seems only tenuous. All of the preceding comments apply only to asymptomatic patients; aggressive lipid-lowering strategies seem indicated for patients with proven CAD (see below).

REFERENCES

1. Lipid Research Clinics Coronary Prevention Trial. 1. Reduction in incidence of coronary heart disease, *JAMA* 251:351-374, 1984.

2. Frick MH, Elo O, Haapa K, et al: Helsinki Heart Study: primary prevention trial with gemfibrozil in middle-aged men with dyslipidaemia; safety of treatment, changes in risk factors, and incidence of coronary heart disease, *N Engl J Med* 317: 1237-1245, 1987.
3. Report from the Committee of Principal Investigators: a cooperative trial in the primary prevention of ischaemic heart disease using clofibrate, *Br Heart J* 40:1069-1118, 1978.
4. Heady JA, Morris JN, Oliver MF: WHO clofibrate/cholesterol trial: clarifications, *Lancet* 340:1405-1406, 1992.
5. Dorr AE, Gundersen K, Schneider JC Jr, et al: Colestipol hydrochloride in hypercholesterolemic patients—effect on serum cholesterol and mortality, *J Chron Dis* 31:5-14, 1978.
6. Shepherd J, Cobbe SM, Ford I, et al: Prevention of coronary heart disease with pravastatin in men with hypercholesterolemia, *N Engl J Med* 333:1301-1307, 1995.
7. Dayton S, Pearce ML, Hashimoto S, et al: A controlled clinical trial of a diet high in unsaturated fat in preventing complications of atherosclerosis, *Circulation* 40(suppl II):1-63, 1969.
8. Frantz ID Jr, Dawson EA, Ashman PL, et al: Test of effect of lipid lowering by diet on cardiovascular risk: the Minnesota Coronary Survey, *Atherosclerosis* 9:129-135, 1989.
9. Canadian Task Force on the Periodic Health Examination: The periodic health examination, 1993 update. 2. Lowering the blood total cholesterol level to prevent coronary heart disease, *Can Med Assoc J* 148:521-538, 1993.
10. Oliver MF: Statins prevent coronary heart disease (editorial), *Lancet* 346:1378-1379, 1995.
11. Sox HC Jr: Preventive health services in adults, *N Engl J Med* 330:1589-1595, 1994.
12. Hulley SB, Newman TB, Grady D, et al: Should we be measuring blood cholesterol levels in young adults? *JAMA* 269:1416-1419, 1993.
13. Rich-Edwards JW, Manson JE, Hennekens C, et al: The primary prevention of coronary heart disease in women, *N Engl J Med* 332:1758-1766, 1995.
14. Walsh JM, Grady D: Treatment of hyperlipidemia in women, *JAMA* 274:1152-1158, 1995.

Cholesterol-Lowering Studies in Patients with or at Very High Risk for Coronary Artery Disease

(See also cholesterol-lowering studies in adults without known coronary artery disease; cholesterol screening in children; cholesterol-lowering diets; exercise; prevention; secondary prevention of coronary artery disease; secondary prevention of myocardial infarction; smoking)

Although the evidence supporting the treatment of elevated cholesterol levels in asymptomatic persons is controversial, such treatment clearly benefits patients with known CAD. A Scandinavian randomized trial of patients with a history of angina or MI showed a significant benefit from treatment with the HMG-CoA reductase inhibitor simvastatin.[1] Patients were treated with either simvastatin (Zocor) 20 to 40 mg or a placebo. There was a significant decrease in all-cause mortality (8.2% in the treated group versus 11.5% in the placebo group), which was due almost entirely to a 42% decrease in coronary events. The rates of noncardiovascular deaths were the same in the treatment and placebo groups (no increase in violent deaths occurred in the treated group).[1] A 1995 Dutch study of 885 men with angiographically proven coronary artery disease compared treatment with pravastatin (Pravachol) to a placebo. At the end of 2 years 19% of patients in the placebo group had had vascular events compared with 11% in the treated group and more than twice as many in the placebo group as in the control group required angioplasty.[2]

A 1993 metaanalysis of randomized trials of cholesterol-lowering treatments compared the effects of cholesterol-lowering drugs on high- and low-risk patients. It found that treatment decreased mortality in those at high initial risk of CAD but increased mortality in those at lower initial risk of CAD.[3] High risk was defined as 30:1000 or greater risk of death from CHD within 18 months. Risk was calculated by incorporating into the equation numerous factors such as hypercholesterolemia, hypertension, diabetes, angina, past heart attacks, intermittent claudication, and obesity. Based on these criteria only 0.7% of British men aged 50 to 59 would be classified as at high risk, while for men aged 40 to 49 the number would be 0.1%.[3] If these figures are correct, large numbers of individuals are being inappropriately treated with cholesterol-lowering drugs that may even increase their mortality rate.

In patients with known coronary artery disease, "normal" cholesterol levels may be too high. The Cholesterol and Recurrent Events (CARE) trial showed that cholesterol-lowering drugs were beneficial in post-MI patients with "average" cholesterol and LDL levels. In a 5-year study of more than 4000 patients (mostly men), half were given pravastatin (Pravachol) 40 mg/day and half placebo. At the onset of the study all patients had a cholesterol level less than 240 mg/dl (6.2 mmol/L) with a mean of 209 mg/dl (5.4 mmol/L). At the end of the study the fatal coronary and nonfatal myocardial infarct rates were 10.2% in the pravastatin group and 13.2% in the placebo group for an absolute reduction of risk of 3% (relative risk reduction of 24%). Fewer treated patients required angioplasty or coronary artery bypass surgery, and fewer had strokes.[4]

There are limited data on the benefits of cholesterol-lowering programs in women with proven CAD. On the basis of the information available, this treatment seems to be beneficial.[5]

The key factor in treating elevated lipid levels in patients with proven CAD appears to be lowering the LDL concentration to 2.6 if possible.[6] At present the best drugs for this are considered to be the HMG-CoA reductase inhibitors.[7]

A puzzle of lipid-lowering programs for patients with proven CAD is that in a number of studies the reduction in coronary artery events was much greater than would have been anticipated from the small or negligible regression of coronary artery lesions as determined by angiography.[8-10] Part of the answer may lie in the function of the endothelial cells of the coronary arteries. Normally these cells release endothelium-derived relaxing factor, which causes vasodilation. In the presence of hypercholesterolemia this factor is inhibited so that coronary artery spasm is more likely to occur. One way that elevated cholesterol levels damage endothelium is thought to be through increased oxidative stress (oxygen-derived free radicals).[8-10] If this hypothesis is correct, a major benefit of lowering cholesterol concentrations would be the normalization of endothelial cell function. The hypothesis also supports the benefit of antioxidant therapy.

The efficacy of dietary interventions in patients with CAD is controversial. The effectiveness of diet is suggested by a French study of 302 post-MI patients placed on a Mediterranean diet and 303 post-MI control subjects following a regular diet. At the end of 2 years 59 control patients had died of cardiovascular causes, had another MI, or been found to have unstable angina, stroke, heart failure, or thromboembolism. In the diet cohort only 14 patients experienced similar events. This is a 76% relative reduction rate,[11] a result at least as good as those reported in the 1994 Scandinavian simvastatin study of patients with known CAD.[1] The nature of the Mediterranean diet is discussed below in the section on treatment of elevated cholesterol levels.

REFERENCES

1. Scandinavian Simvastatin Survival Study Group: Randomised trial of cholesterol lowering in 4444 patients with coronary heart disease: the Scandinavian Simvastatin Survival Study (4S), *Lancet* 344:1383-1389, 1994.
2. Jukema JW, Bruschke AVG, Vanboven AJ, et al: Effects of lipid lowering by pravastatin on progression and regression of coronary artery disease in symptomatic men with normal to moderately elevated serum cholesterol levels: the Regression Growth Evaluation Statin Study (REGRESS), *Circulation* 91:2528-2540, 1995.
3. Smith GD, Song F, Sheldon TA: Cholesterol lowering and mortality: the importance of considering initial level of risk, *BMJ* 306:1367-1373, 1993 [Erratum, *BMJ* 306:1648, 1993].
4. Sacks FM, Pfeffer MA, Moye LA, et al: The effect of pravastatin on coronary events after myocardial infarction in patients with average cholesterol levels, *N Engl J Med* 335:1001-1009, 1996.
5. Walsh JM, Grady D: Treatment of hyperlipidemia in women, *JAMA* 274:1152-1158, 1995.
6. National Cholesterol Education Program: The second report of the Expert Panel on Detection, Evaluation, and Treatment of High Blood Cholesterol in Adults (Adult Treatment Panel II), Bethesda, Md, 1993, National Heart, Lung, and Blood Institute, National Institutes of Health, NIH pub no 93-3095.
7. Kantner T: HMG CoA reductase inhibitors for treatment of hyperlipidemia, *Am Fam Physician* 47:1623-1627, 1993.
8. Treasure CB, Klein JL, Weintraub WS, et al: Beneficial effects of cholesterol-lowering therapy on the coronary endothelium in patients with coronary artery disease, *N Engl J Med* 332:481-487, 1995.
9. Anderson TJ, Meredith IT, Yeung AC, et al: The effect of cholesterol-lowering and antioxidant therapy on endothelium-dependent coronary vasomotion, *N Engl J Med* 332:488-493, 1995.
10. Levine GN, Keajney JF Jr, Vita JA: Cholesterol reduction in cardiovascular disease: clinical benefits and possible mechanisms, *N Engl J Med* 332:512-521, 1995.
11. De Lorgeril M, Salen P, Martin J-L, et al: Effect of a Mediterranean type diet on the rate of cardiovascular complications in patients with coronary artery disease—insights into the cardioprotective effect of certain nutriments, *J Am Coll Cardiol* 28:1103-1108, 1996.

Cholesterol-Lowering Studies in Children Without Known Coronary Artery Disease

(See also obesity in childhood)

In 1992 an expert panel on blood cholesterol levels in children and adolescents convened by the National Heart, Lung, and Blood Institute recommended that all Americans over the age of 2 years reduce their dietary fat intake.[1] This same organization sponsored the Dietary Intervention Study in Children (DISC) with the goal of assessing the efficacy and safety of lowering LDL-C levels in pubescent children. The results of the study were reported in 1995.[2]

Dietary Intervention Study in Children

The children enrolled in the DISC study were between the ages of approximately 8 and 11.[2] They were initially assessed by capillary blood cholesterol measurement, and if it was above the 75th percentile, a fasting venous sample for LDL-C was obtained. If the LDL-C level was between the 70th and 99th age- and sex-specific percentiles, a second fasting venous sample was obtained. If the average of the LDL-C levels from the two venous samples was between the 70th and 99th percentiles, the children were randomly assigned to ordinary care or dietary intervention. The parents of children in both groups were told that their children's cholesterol levels were high, and in both groups body mass index was calculated and the hip, waist, and skinfold thickness at various sites were measured. In the dietary intervention group 28% of energy was obtained from fat of which 9% was polyunsaturated. Over the 3-year study period children and families of the intervention group attended approximately 27 group and individual meetings and received monthly phone calls between meetings. Capillary blood cholesterol measurements were obtained periodically during individual meetings, and at the termination of the study venous samples were obtained for the measurement of a variety of parameters. The report does not mention the children's physical activities.[2]

The primary outcome of the DISC study was a decrease in LDL-C in both the intervention group and the ordinary care group. The reduction was 0.09 mmol/L (3.3 mg/dl) greater in the intervention group, which is a statistically significant difference. The intervention group showed no evidence of decreased growth or decreased ferritin levels, and in fact there was no difference in any of the anthropomorphic measurements, including sexual maturation, between the groups. Psychological measurements showed a lower adjusted mean depression score for the intervention children at 3 years.[2]

Psychological harm of screening

Does screening children and finding them hypercholesterolemic cause psychological harm? Some studies have found no evidence of this.[2-4] On the other hand, a 1997 report from Montreal found a much higher rate of behavioral disturbances in children 12 months after they received the diagnosis of hyperlipidemia.[5]

Guidelines for cholesterol screening

The Expert Panel on Blood Cholesterol Levels in Children and Adolescents of the National Heart, Lung, and Blood Institute's National Cholesterol Education Program, the American Academy of Family Physicians, the American Academy of Pediatrics, and the American Medical Association do not recommend universal screening of cholesterol levels in children. However, if the child is over 2 and has a parent with a cholesterol level greater than 240 mg/dl (6.25 mmol/L) or if the parents or grandparents have a history of premature (under age 55) cardiovascular disease, screening is recommended.[6] Both the U.S. Preventive Services Task Force[7] and the Canadian Task Force on the Periodic Health Examination[8] give a "C" recommendation to general cholesterol screening of children and adolescents. The U.S. Preventive Services Task Force qualifies this by stating that a family history of very high cholesterol levels, premature coronary heart disease in a first-degree relative (before age 50 in males and before age 60 in females), or other major risk factors for coronary heart disease may be reasons for measuring cholesterol levels in adolescents or young adults.[7]

Enthusiasm for cholesterol-lowering programs among some segments of the North American medical community seems boundless and at times out of touch with reality. The clinical significance of the DISC trial[2] is hard to comprehend. Healthy children were labeled as having high cholesterol, and a vast amount of time and energy was devoted to altering the diets of the intervention group. One fact is obvious: even if one believed it desirable to measure cholesterol levels in children and institute a dietary program for those with high levels, this clinical trial has no applicability to ordinary clinical practice. What family physician or pediatrician could possibly offer 27 group and individual meetings plus interval phone calls over a 3-year period as part of his or her regular practice? No evidence supports a general cholesterol screening program in children; individual case finding for high-risk adolescents may be justified in some instances.

REFERENCES

1. Expert Panel on Blood Cholesterol Levels in Children and Adolescents: National Cholesterol Education Program report, *Pediatrics* 89(suppl):525-584, 1992.
2. Dietary Intervention Study in Children (DISC): Efficacy and safety of lowering dietary intake of fat and cholesterol in children with elevated low-density lipoprotein cholesterol, *JAMA* 273:1429-1435, 1995.
3. Hanna KJ, Ewart CK, Kwiterovich PO: Child problem solving competence, behavioural adjustment and adherence to lipid-lowering diet, *Patient Educ Couns* 16:119-131, 1990.
4. Rosenthal SL, Knauer-Black S, Stahl MP, et al: The psychological functioning of children with hypercholesterolemia and their families: a preliminary investigation, *Clin Pediatr* 32:135-141, 1993.
5. Rosenberg E, Lamping DL, Joseph L, et al: Cholesterol screening of children at high risk: behavioural and psychological effects, *Can Med Assoc J* 156:489-496, 1997.
6. US Public Health Service: Cholesterol screening in children, *Am Fam Physician* 51:1923-1927, 1995.
7. US Preventive Services Task Force: *Guide to clinical preventive services,* ed 2, Baltimore, 1996, Williams & Wilkins, pp 15-38.
8. Canadian Task Force on the Periodic Health Examination: *Canadian guide to clinical preventive health care,* Ottawa, 1994, Canada Communication Group—Publishing, pp 650-669.

Cholesterol-Lowering Studies and Stroke

An overview of randomized cholesterol-lowering studies involving more than 36,000 persons failed to detect a reduced incidence of strokes.[1] However, an overview of 16 randomized trials of HMG-CoA reductase inhibitors (which are among the most potent cholesterol-lowering agents) by the same authors found a 29% relative reduction in stroke rates.[2]

REFERENCES

1. Hebert PR, Gaziano M, Hennekens CH: An overview of trials of cholesterol lowering and risk of stroke, *Arch Intern Med* 155:50-55, 1995.
2. Hebert PR, Gaziano M, Chan KS, et al: Cholesterol lowering with statin drugs, risk of stroke, and total mortality, *JAMA* 278: 313-321, 1997.

Adverse Effects Associated with Low Cholesterol Levels

(See also abuse; aggression; guns; homicide; suicide; violence against abortion clinics and personnel)

A number of malignancies such as those of the lung, pancreas, rectum, bladder, liver, and kidney, as well as some nonmalignant diseases such as chronic lung disease and strokes, are associated with low cholesterol levels.[1-3] Total mortality in middle-aged and elderly patients is increased among those with the lowest cholesterol levels.[3-5] The accepted explanation for these findings is that the disease processes themselves cause the cholesterol levels to drop. More controversial is the question of whether low cholesterol levels may be causally related to violence in the form of accidents, suicide, homicide, or assaults and whether cholesterol-lowering drugs may be carcinogenic.

Low cholesterol and aggression

A 1990 metaanalysis of controlled trials of cholesterol-lowering diets and medications by Muldoon and associates[6] showed that the incidence of cardiovascular deaths in the treated groups decreased, but not the overall mortality. In the treated groups significantly higher death rates from suicide, accidents, and violence were observed, a finding that was consistent across all studies. Other prospective population studies and cross-sectional studies have shown a correlation between low cholesterol levels and violence, particularly suicide.[7-9] Men arrested more than twice for violent crimes against others were reported to have lower cholesterol levels than control subjects,[10] and experimental studies in monkeys have shown increased contact aggression in those fed a cholesterol-lowering diet.[11] However, not all workers agree that low cholesterol is associated with significant morbidity. Law and associates[12] reviewed 10 large cohort studies and 28 randomized trials as well as other published data and concluded that the only clear-cut adverse effect associated with low cholesterol was hemorrhagic stroke. The Scandinavian simvastatin study, which enrolled men with known CAD, adds an important dimension to this debate because not only did mortality decrease in the treated group (see above), but those taking simvastatin did not have increased mortality from violence.[13] The West of Scotland Coronary Prevention Study using pravastatin in hypercholesterolemic men without known coronary artery disease also demonstrated a decrease in total mortality in the treated cohort with no increase in violent deaths.[14] A large population study in the Netherlands found no increase in noncardiac deaths among persons with low cholesterol levels,[15] and an overview of 16 randomized trials of cholesterol-lowering interventions using statin drugs also failed to find an increased incidence of noncardiovascular deaths.[16] Thus the preponderance of the evidence suggests that lowering cholesterol does not increase the risk of violence.

Carcinogenic potential of cholesterol-lowering drugs

A well-established but rarely discussed aspect of cholesterol-lowering agents is that many of them, including the fibrates such as gemfibrozil and clofibrate and the HMG-CoA reductase inhibitors such as lovastatin and pravastatin, are carcinogenic in rodents. This issue was put in the spotlight by a 1996 article in *JAMA* by Newman and Hulley.[17] They pointed out that almost all human carcinogens are also carcinogenic in rodents but that the specificity of this phenomenon is unknown. Since the latent period between exposure to a carcinogen and the development of cancer may be two decades or more, it will be a long time before it is known whether currently used statins and fibrates are carcinogenic for humans. Newman and Hulley suggest that in the interval niacin or cholestyramine may be safer to use if lipid-lowering drugs are required. A 1997 overview of 16 cholesterol-lowering trials using statins failed to show any increased incidence of cancer, but as the authors state, the mean follow-up time was only 3.3 years and the confidence intervals were wide.[16] The concept that cholesterol-lowering drugs may be carcinogenic has been vehemently challenged in an editorial by Dalen and Dalton,[18] who note that many cholesterol-lowering studies have not shown an increase in cancer deaths in follow-up periods of 4 to 9 years, that even if an increased rate were proved to exist, it would be small, and that animal experiments showing carcinogenicity of lipid-lowering drugs should not be taken too seriously because the doses were many times those used for humans.

Whether statins are carcinogenic in humans is not known. Even if they prove to be, their benefits will probably far outweigh this risk for patients with known CAD. Such may not be the case for asymptomatic persons whose only risk factor for CAD is an elevated cholesterol level. The physician should consider this before writing a prescription for a symptomless patient.

REFERENCES

1. Wannamethee G, Shaper AG, Whincup PH, et al: Low serum total cholesterol concentrations and mortality in middle aged British men, *BMJ* 311:409-413, 1995.
2. Davey Smith G, Shipley MJ, Marmot MG, et al: Plasma cholesterol concentration and mortality: the Whitehall study, *JAMA* 267:70-76, 1992.
3. Manolio TA, Ettinger WH, Tracy RP, et al: Epidemiology of low cholesterol levels in older adults, *Circulation* 87:728-737, 1993.
4. Staessen J, Amery A, Birkenhager W, et al: Is a high serum cholesterol level associated with longer survival in elderly hypertensives? *J Hypertension* 8:755-761, 1990.
5. Forette B, Tortrat D, Wolmark Y: Cholesterol as a risk factor for mortality in elderly women, *Lancet* 1:868-870, 1989.
6. Muldoon MF, Manuck SB, Mathhews KA: Lowering cholesterol concentrations and mortality: a quantitative review of primary prevention trials, *BMJ* 301:309-314, 1990.
7. Linberg G, Råstam L, Gullberg B, et al: Low cholesterol concentration and short term mortality from injuries in men and women, *BMJ* 305:277-279, 1992.
8. Golier JA, Marzuk PM, Leon AC, et al: Low serum cholesterol level and attempted suicide, *Am J Psychiatry* 152:419-423, 1995.
9. Zureik M, Courbon D, Ducimetière P: Serum cholesterol concentration and death from suicide in men: Paris prospective study I, *BMJ* 313:649-651, 1996.
10. Golomb B, Mednick S, Stattin H: *Low cholesterol and violent crime (abstract),* Robert Wood Johnson Clinical Scholars Program, 1996 National Meeting, Key Largo, Fla, November 1996.
11. Kaplan JR, Manuck SB, Shively C: The effects of fat and cholesterol on social behavior in monkeys, *Psychosom Med* 53:634-642, 1991.
12. Law MR, Thompson SG, Wald NJ: Assessing possible hazards of reducing serum cholesterol, *BMJ* 308:373-379, 1994.
13. Scandinavian Simvastatin Survival Study Group: Randomised trial of cholesterol lowering in 4444 patients with coronary heart disease: the Scandinavian Simvastatin Survival Study (4S), *Lancet* 344:1383-1389, 1994.
14. Shepherd J, Cobbe SM, Ford I, et al: Prevention of coronary heart disease with pravastatin in men with hypercholesterolemia, *N Engl J Med* 333:1301-1307, 1995.
15. Verschuren WM, Kromhout D: Total cholesterol concentration and mortality at a relatively young age—do men and women differ? *BMJ* 311:779-783, 1995.

16. Hebert PR, Gaziano M, Chan KS, et al: Cholesterol lowering with statin drugs, risk of stroke, and total mortality, *JAMA* 278: 313-321, 1997.
17. Newman TB, Hulley SB: Carcinogenicity of lipid-lowering drugs, *JAMA* 275:55-60, 1996.
18. Dalen JE, Dalton WS: Does lowering cholesterol cause cancer? (editorial), *JAMA* 275:67-69, 1996.

Guidelines for Cholesterol Screening

Many U.S. medical organizations recommend cholesterol screening for the general population of adults, whereas the recommendations of the Canadian Task Force on the Periodic Health Examination,[1] the U.S. Preventive Services Task Force,[2] and the American College of Physicians[3] are more restrictive. Examples of these guidelines are given in Table 43.

Haq and associates[7] from Sheffield, England, have developed tables that calculate the risk of cardiovascular disease in asymptomatic patients based on sex, age, smoking, hypertension, left ventricular hypertrophy, and diabetes.[7] According to their calculations, which are based primarily on the Framingham data,[8] even extremely high cholesterol levels in the absence of other risk factors pose relatively little threat to health (excluding cases of hereditary lipid abnormalities). Not only does this approach stringently limit the number of patients who would be screened or treated, but it also permits the selection of some patients with multiple risk factors who would merit lipid-lowering treatment even if their cholesterol levels were normal.[7]

The American College of Physicians published its updated recommendations for cholesterol screening in March 1996. The very thorough review of the literature accompanying its recommendations included the West of Scotland Coronary Prevention Study Group report. The College gave conditional approval to screening but stated clearly that there is no proof that lowering cholesterol prolongs life.[9]

Elevated cholesterol level is unquestionably a risk factor for vascular disease. However, it is just one of many. Who should be screened and, if the cholesterol level is elevated, be treated with pharmacotherapy is a matter of controversy. As a family physician who wants to be sure that I am not doing more harm than good (see "Prevention"), I find the Sheffield risk and treatment tables appealing. Even if they are too restrictive for the taste of many of us, they emphasize that significant risk of coronary artery disease is related to multiple risk factors, not just to elevated cholesterol.

Table 43 Variablity of Guidelines for Cholesterol Screening

Organization	Recommendation
American Academy of Family Physicians	Every 5 years starting at age 19[4]
American College of Obstetricians and Gynecologists	All women over 20 and selected high-risk adolescents[5]
American College of Physicians	Appropriate but not mandatory for men aged 35-65 and women aged 45-65; insufficient evidence for or against those 65-75; not recommended for those over 75[3]
National Cholesterol Education Program	At least once every 5 years after age 20[6]
U.S. Preventive Services Task Force	Men aged 35-65 and women aged 45-65 ("B" recommendation); interval of screening uncertain—probably 5 years[2]; insufficient evidence for or against screening those over 65 ("C" recommendation)[2]
Canadian Task Force on the Periodic Health Examination	Case finding in men 30-59 ("C" recommendation)[1]
Sheffield Risk and Treatment Tables	Screening limited to patients with multiple risk factors—sex, age, smoking, hypertension, left ventricular hypertrophy, and diabetes[7]

REFERENCES

1. Canadian Task Force on the Periodic Health Examination: *Canadian guide to clinical preventive health care,* Ottawa, 1994, Canada Communication Group—Publishing, pp 650-669.
2. US Preventive Services Task Force: *Guide to clinical preventive services,* ed 2, Baltimore, 1996, Williams & Wilkins, pp 15-38.
3. American College of Physicians: Clinical guideline. I. Guidelines for using serum cholesterol, high-density lipoprotein cholesterol, and triglyceride levels as screening tests for preventing coronary heart disease in adults, *Ann Intern Med* 124:515-517, 1996.
4. American Academy of Family Physicians: *Age charts for periodic health examination,* Kansas City, Mo, 1994, American Academy of Family Physicians, Reprint No 510.
5. American College of Obstetricians and Gynecologists: *The obstetrician-gynecologist in primary preventive health care: a report of the ACOG Task Force on Primary and Preventive Health Care,* Washington, DC, 1993, American College of Obstetricians and Gynecologists.
6. Expert Panel on Detection, Evaluation, and Treatment of High Blood Cholesterol in Adults: Summary of the second report of the National Cholesterol Education Program (NCEP) Expert Panel on the Detection, Evaluation, and Treatment of High Blood Cholesterol in Adults (Adult Treatment Panel II), *JAMA* 269:3015-3023, 1993.
7. Haq IU, Jackson PR, Yeo WW, et al: Sheffield risk and treatment table for cholesterol lowering for primary prevention of coronary heart disease, *Lancet* 346:1467-1471, 1995.
8. Anderson KM, Odell PM, Wilson PW, et al: Cardiovascular disease risk profiles, *Am Heart J* 121:293-298, 1991.
9. Garber AM, Browner WS, Hulley SB (American College of Physicians): Clinical guideline. II. Cholesterol screening in asymptomatic adults, revisited, *Ann Intern Med* 124:518-531, 1996.

Treatment of Elevated Cholesterol Levels

(See also adverse effects associated with lowering cholesterol levels; antioxidants; cholesterol-lowering studies in patients with coronary artery disease)

Target goals for cholesterol

In treating hypercholesterolemia, what are the target levels? The recommendations of the National Cholesterol Educational Program are as follows[1]:

No CAD and fewer than two risk factors	LDL <4.1 mmol/L (160 mg/dl)
No CAD and two risk factors	LDL <3.4 mmolL (130 mg/dl)
Established CAD	LDL <2.6 mmol/L (100 mg/dl)

Risk factors include age (men ≥45 and women ≥55 or postmenopausal), hypertension, diabetes, smoking, and CHD in a first-degree relative under 55 if male and under 65 if female.

Diet

The usual protocol for lowering blood cholesterol is to begin with a 3- to 6-month trial of diet and to add drugs only if dietary changes are unsuccessful. As far as I know, until the publication of the effects of a Mediterranean diet on patients with known CAD (see discussion of cholesterol-lowering studies in patients with coronary artery disease),[2-4] no studies showed a total cohort decrease in mortality from diet alone. However, numerous studies have shown that diet can reduce cholesterol levels, usually by about 5% to 15%.[5] In almost all of these a small percentage of patients failed to respond or even demonstrated a paradoxical increase in cholesterol levels.[5]

The Mediterranean diet that was so effective in decreasing cardiovascular events and deaths in post-MI patients did not change the serum concentration of total, low-density, or high-density cholesterol.[3,4] The diet was high in linolenic and oleic acid, relatively low in saturated fatty acids and linoleic acid, and high in some antioxidant vitamins.[2-4] The reason for its efficacy is unknown, but constituents such as omega-3 fatty acids, oleic acid, and antioxidant vitamins may be cardioprotective (see discussion of antioxidants).[1,2]

A Mediterranean diet has a high content of oil, particularly olive oil or canola (rapeseed) oil, complex carbohydrates such as bread, and pasta, fruits, vegetables, fish, and poultry. It has a low content of beef and pork and other meats, and the amount of cheese and wine consumed is moderate. More specifically, patients on this diet were instructed to eat the following[3]:

1. More bread
2. More vegetables
3. More fish
4. Less beef, lamb, and pork (to be replaced with poultry)
5. Fruit daily
6. No butter or cream (in the study a special margarine based on canola oil was provided)
7. Olive oil or canola oil (rapeseed without erucic acid) to be used exclusively for preparing foods and salad dressings

In experimental animals, substituting soy protein for animal protein lowers cholesterol. A metaanalysis of 38 controlled clinical trials in humans found that a soy protein intake averaging 47 g/day led to a mean cholesterol reduction of 0.6 mmol/L (23.2 mg/dl). Soy milk and tofu are the most common sources of soy protein.[6]

A margarine enriched with the plant sterol sitostanol decreases the absorption of cholesterol from the gut and has been shown to lower total cholesterol and LDL-C in a 1-year randomized controlled trial of 153 mildly hypercholesterolemic subjects.[7]

Pharmacotherapy

As discussed previously, many of the indications for treating lipid disorders are controversial in part because of possible or proven adverse effects. The bulk of evidence strongly supports the use of cholesterol-lowering drugs in patients with known coronary artery disease, and they are likely to be used more and more frequently for asymptomatic individuals with multiple risk factors for coronary artery disease. For better or worse, they will probably also be used with increasing frequency in asymptomatic patients whose only risk factor is hypercholesterolemia. The National Cholesterol Educational Program estimated that if its recommendations were followed, 7% of U.S. adults would be taking cholesterol-lowering drugs and 30% would be following nonpharmacological regimens to lower cholesterol.[1]

The lipid levels of patients who have had an MI often drop significantly, so lipid-lowering treatment programs should be based on figures obtained 8 weeks after the event.[8] In addition to aiming for LDL-C levels less than 2.6 mmol/L (100 mg/dl) for patients with proven CAD, the goal should be to raise the HDL-C to above 1 mmol/L (40 mg/dl).[1]

A wide variety of lipid-lowering drugs are available (Table 44), and the choice depends on numerous variables. All the lipid-lowering drugs lower LDL-C, and niacin (nicotinic acid), and the fibrates such as gemfibrozil are particularly effective in lowering triglycerides. Whether lowering triglycerides significantly reduces the morbidity or mortality of coronary artery disease is unknown. The HMG-CoA reductase inhibitors are potent and can be taken once daily, but they are more expensive than some of the other drugs. They are the drugs used most frequently at present.[9] Nicotinic acid is inexpensive, available over the counter, and often effective. It not only lowers total cholesterol, LDL-C, and triglycerides, but also is more effective in raising HDL than any other drug.[10] However, for many patients its side effects are unacceptable for long-term treatment. In one study 43% of patients discontinued the drug for this reason.[11] Efficacy is related to dose, but even doses as low as 1.5 g/day may be effective in raising HDL.[12] Flushing caused by nicotinic acid can be diminished by pretreatment with aspirin or ibuprofen (Advil, Motrin).[10] Adaptation to side effects may be improved by initiating treatment with small doses and increasing them gradually.

Table 44 Lipid-Lowering Drugs

Drug	Usual doses
Bile Acid Sequestrants	
Cholestyramine (Questran)	4 g 1-6 times per day
Fibrates	
Bezafibrate (Bezalip)	200 mg tid
Clofibrate (Atromid-S)	Not recommended
Fenofibrate (Lipidil)	100 mg tid with meals
Gemfibrozil (Lopid)	600 mg bid
HMG-CoA Reductase Inhibitors	
Atorvastatin (Lipitor)	20-80 mg/day, with evening meal
Fluvastatin (Lescol)	20-40 mg/day in evening
Lovastatin (Mevacor)	20-80 mg/day with evening meal
Pravastatin (Pravachol)	10-40 mg/day in evening
Simvastatin (Zocor)	20-40 mg/day in evening
Niacin Derivatives	
Niacin, nicotinic acid	1-6 g/day in 2-4 divided doses
Other Lipid-Lowering Drugs	
Probucol (Lorelco)	500 mg bid
Psyllium (Metamucil)	5-15 g/day (1-3 rounded teaspoons)

Use of the fibrate clofibrate (Atromid-S) seems inadvisable, since the WHO clofibrate study found a 47% increase in total mortality among those treated with the drug.[13,14] Probucol (Lorelco) is a weak cholesterol-lowering agent and is no longer available in the United States in part because it lowers HDL as well as LDL.[15] It is, however, a potent antioxidant that significantly decreases the rate of restenosis in patients undergoing angioplasty.[16]

All of the HMG-CoA reductase inhibitors are potentiated by niacin. Short-term studies show no adverse effects of this combination, but long-term safety is unknown. Severe myositis was reported when lovastatin was used with gemfibrozil. Mild elevations of liver transaminase levels and elevations of creatine kinase to two to three times normal are common in patients taking HMG-CoA reductase inhibitors and are usually transient. Therapy need not be discontinued for this degree of elevation, but liver enzyme levels must be monitored. If given in conjunction with a resin such as cholestyramine, the drug should be administered 1 hour before or 4 hours after the resin.

Evidence indicates that soluble fiber such as psyllium (Metamucil) in doses of 5 to 15 g/day (1 to 3 rounded teaspoons) may reduce cholesterol by a small amount.[17-19] The drug appears to be most effective if given with rather than between meals.[20]

REFERENCES

1. National Cholesterol Education Program: *The second report of the Expert Panel on Detection, Evaluation, and Treatment of High Blood Cholesterol in Adults. (Adult Treatment Panel II.)* Bethesda, Md, 1993, National Heart, Lung, and Blood Institute, National Institutes of Health, NIH Pub No 93-3095.
2. de Lorgeril M, Salen P, Martin J-L, et al: Effect of a Mediterranean type of diet on the rate of cardiovascular complications in patients with coronary artery disease: insights into the cardioprotective effect of certain nutriments, *J Am Coll Cardiol* 28:1103-1108, 1996.
3. Renaud S, de Lorgeril M, Delaye J, et al: Cretan Mediterranean diet for prevention of coronary heart disease, *Am J Clin Nutr* 61(suppl):1360S-1367S, 1995.
4. de Lorgeril, Renaud S, Mamelle N, et al: Mediterranean alpha-linolenic acid-rich diet in secondary prevention of coronary heart disease, *Lancet* 343:1454-1459, 1994.
5. Denke MA: Cholesterol-lowering diets: a review of the evidence, *Arch Intern Med* 155:17-26, 1995.
6. Anderson JW, Johnstone BM, Cook-Newell ME: Meta-analysis of the effects of soy protein intake on serum lipids, *N Engl J Med* 333:276-282, 1995.
7. Miettinen TA, Puska P, Gylling H, et al. Reduction of serum cholesterol with sitostanol-ester margarine in a mildly hypercholesterolemic population, *N Engl J Med* 333:1308-1312, 1995.
8. Dafoe W, Huston P: Current trends in cardiac rehabilitation, *Can Med Assoc J* 156:527-532, 1997.
9. Genest J Jr, Leiter LA: When and how to use lipid-lowering drugs, *Patient Care Can,* February 1995, 6:18-26.
10. Choice of lipid-lowering drugs, *Med Lett* 38:67-70, 1996.
11. Gibbons LW, Gonzalez V, Gordon N, et al: The prevalence of side effects with regular and sustained-release nicotinic acid, *Am J Med* 99:378-385, 1995.
12. Martin-Jadraque R, Tato F, Mostaza JM, et al: Effectiveness of low-dose crystalline nicotinic-acid in men with low high-density lipoprotein cholesterol levels, *Arch Intern Med* 156:1081-1088, 1996.
13. Report from the Committee of Principal Investigators: a cooperative trial in the primary prevention of ischaemic heart disease using clofibrate, *Br Heart J* 40:1069-1118, 1978.
14. Heady JA, Morris JN, Oliver MF: WHO clofibrate/cholesterol trial: clarifications, *Lancet* 340:1405-1406, 1992.
15. Libby P, Ganz P: Restenosis revisited—new targets, new therapies (editorial), *N Engl J Med* 337:418-419, 1997.
16. Tardif J-C, Coté G, Lespérance J, et al (Multivitamins and Probucol Study Group): Probucol and multivitamins in the prevention of restenosis after coronary angioplasty, *N Engl J Med* 337:365-372, 1997.
17. Glore SR, Van Treeck D, Knehans AW, et al: Soluble fiber and serum lipids: a literature review, *J Am Dietetic Assoc* 94:425-436, 1994.
18. Wolever TM, Jenkins DJ, Mueller S, et al: Psyllium reduces blood lipids in men and women with hyperlipidemia, *Am J Med Sci* 307:269-273, 1994.
19. Davidson MH, Dugan LD, Burns JH, et al: A psyllium-enriched cereal for the treatment of hypercholesterolemia in children—a controlled, double-blind, crossover study, *Am J Clin Nutr* 63:96-102, 1996.
20. Wolever TM, Jenkins DJ, Mueller S, et al: Method of administration influences the serum cholesterol-lowering effect of psyllium, *Am J Clin Nutr* 59:1055-1059, 1994.

OSTEOPOROSIS

(See also celiac disease; female athletes; hip fractures; hormone replacement therapy; tamoxifen)

Epidemiology

(See also hip fractures)

An estimated 25% of white women over the age of 60 will have an osteoporotic fracture. The common sites for osteoporotic fractures are the distal radius, hip, ribs, and vertebral bodies. Vertebral fractures in women 50 to 60 years of age are 10 times as common as they are in men of similar age, and hip fractures occur twice as often in women as in men. Patients with osteoporotic hip fractures are usually over 75, and the median age for such fractures in postmenopausal women is 80.[1,2] Mortality from hip fractures is between 10% and 25% in the first year, many patients lose mobility, and up to 25% require nursing care.[3]

Peak bone mass is reached at about age 25 and is about 20% less in women than in men. After age 35, bone mass declines by about 0.5% to 1% per year in both men and women. Between ages 50 and 80 a woman's bone density decreases 30%. In the first 10 years after menopause the decline is about 3% to 5% per year. Men lose about two thirds as much bone mass as women; their rate of bone loss increases after age 65.[4]

REFERENCES

1. Lees B, Molleson T, Asnett T: Differences in proximal femur bone density over two centuries, *Lancet* 341:673-675, 1993.
2. Kahn AA: A current approach to osteoporosis, *Can J Diagn*, July 1994, pp 29-42.
3. Kelly PJ, Eisman JA, Sambrook PN: Interaction of genetic and environmental influences on peak bone density, *Osteoporosis Int* 1:56-60, 1990.
4. Scientific Advisory Board, Osteoporosis Society of Canada: Clinical practice guidelines for the diagnosis and management of osteoporosis, *Can Med Assoc J* 155:1113-1133, 1996.

Risk Factors for Osteoporosis

Recognized risk factors for osteoporosis are listed in Table 45. There is a poor correlation between these risk factors and the bone density of individual patients. Some of these risk factors are discussed in more depth below.

Table 45 Risk Factors for Osteoporosis

Race	**Medical Conditions**
White	Surgically induced early menopause
Asian	Hypogonadism
Genetics	Cushing's disease
Female sex	Thyrotoxicosis
Thin habitus	Hyperparathyroidism
Early menopause	Anorexia nervosa
Family history of osteoporosis	Multiple myeloma
Life-Style	Intestinal malabsorption
Sedentary life-style	Gastrectomy
Smoking	Rheumatoid arthritis
Excessive use of alcohol	**Medications**
Excessive exercise causing amenorrhea	Long-term steroid use
Inadequate nutrition causing low weight	Anticonvulsant medications
	Long-term heparin therapy
	Long-term lithium use
	Chemotherapy
	? Thyroid replacement

Body weight

Thin women are at significantly greater risk of hip fracture than are heavy women.[1-4]

Smoking

Smoking is associated with an increased fracture rate in postmenopausal women,[5] probably mediated by decreased bone density.[6] Smoking leads to earlier menopause,[7,8] and some studies have found smoking to be associated with lower serum estrogen levels in postmenopausal women receiving estrogen hormone replacement therapy, probably through increased hepatic metabolism of estrogens.[9] It has been suggested that transdermal estrogen will bypass the hepatic first-pass effect and maintain adequate levels of estrogen in postmenopausal smokers receiving replacement therapy by that modality, but this has not been proved.[10] Not all studies confirm a decreased level of serum estrogens in smokers.[11]

Corticosteroids

Patients receiving long-term steroid therapy lose bone density.[12]

Thyroid replacement therapy

The previously held belief that excessive thyroid replacement therapy could lead to osteoporosis and fractures has not been substantiated by subsequent studies.[13,14]

REFERENCES

1. Kelsey JL, Hoffman S: Risk factors for hip fracture, *N Engl J Med* 316:404-406, 1987.
2. Farmer ME, Harris T, Madans JH, et al: Anthropometric indicators and hip fracture: the NHANES I epidemiologic follow-up study, *J Am Geriatr Soc* 37:9-16, 1989.
3. Pruzansky ME, Tuarano M, Luckey M, et al: Low body weight as a risk factor for hip fracture in both black and white women, *J Orthop Res* 7:192-197, 1989.
4. Grisso JA, Kelsey JL, Strom BL, et al: Risk factors for hip fracture in black women, *N Engl J Med* 330:1555-1559, 1994.
5. Rodysill KJ: Postmenopausal osteoporosis—intervention and prophylaxis: a review, *J Chron Dis* 40:743-760, 1987.
6. Jensen J, Christiansen C, Rødbro P: Cigarette smoking, serum estrogens, and bone loss during hormone-replacement therapy early after menopause, *N Engl J Med* 313:973-975, 1985.
7. Lindquist O, Bengtsson C: Menopausal age in relation to smoking, *Acta Med Scand* 205:73-77, 1979.

8. Andersen FS, Transbol I, Christiansen C: Is cigarette smoking a promotor of the menopause? *Acta Med Scand* 212:137-139, 1982.
9. Michnovicz JJ, Hershcopf RJ, Naganuma H, et al: Increased 2-hydroxylation of estradiol as a possible mechanism for the anti-estrogenic effect of cigarette smoking, *N Engl J Med* 315: 1305-1309, 1986.
10. Jensen J, Christiansen C: Effects of smoking on serum lipoproteins and bone mineral content during postmenopausal hormone replacement therapy, *Am J Obstet Gynecol* 159:820-825, 1988.
11. Cauley JA, Seeley DG, Ensrud K, et al (Study of Osteoporotic Fractures Research Group): Estrogen replacement therapy and fractures in older women, *Ann Intern Med* 122:9-16, 1995.
12. Adachi JD, Bensen W, Brown J, et al: Intermittent etidronate therapy to prevent corticosteroid-induced osteoporosis, *N Engl J Med* 337:382-387, 1997.
13. Solomon BL, Wartofsky L, Burman KD: Prevalence of fractures in postmenopausal women with thyroid disease, *Thyroid* 3:17-23, 1993.
14. Franklyn JA, Betteridge J, Daykin J, et al: Long-term thyroxine treatment and bone mineral density, *Lancet* 340:9-13, 1992.

Bone Density

The following are some of the techniques for measuring bone density:

1. Dual photon absorptiometry (DPA)
2. Dual energy x-ray absorptiometry (DXA, DEXA); by use of a dual beam the absorption caused by soft tissues can be calculated and more accurate bone densities assessed; this is currently the standard technique
3. Quantitative computerized tomography (QCT); this is accurate but causes more radiation and costs more than DXA

Should perimenopausal women be screened for osteoporosis by bone density? The following factors should be borne in mind. No correlation has been established between bone density at the time of the menopause and hip fractures in old age. Many women prescribed hormone replacement therapy probably would not take it or would discontinue it prematurely. Knowledge of bone density at the time of the menopause has not been shown to be a significant factor in determining whether to prescribe hormone replacement therapy.[1] Although assessment of bone density can determine risk categories for future fractures as effectively as can blood pressure measurement for strokes and cholesterol levels for cardiovascular disease, it is not an effective tool for determining which women will have fractures.[2] The arguments against using bone density measurements as a screening tool are that a great overlap exists between the bone densities of those who have fractures and those who do not, compliance with such a screening program is unknown, and the effectiveness of preventive interventions for fractures is not well established.[2] The U.S. Preventive Services Task Force gives a "C" recommendation to bone density screening of all postmenopausal women,[3] while the Canadian Task Force on the Periodic Health Examination gives it a "D" recommendation.[4]

In selected cases bone density measurement may be useful. It may aid the patient and physician in deciding whether to initiate hormone replacement therapy (either postmenopausally or for prolonged amenorrhea in younger women as occurs with anorexia nervosa), or it may be used to monitor treatment programs for established osteoporosis. In the latter instance follow-up bone density measurement should not be performed at intervals of less than a year.[5]

Radiation exposure from DXA is low, about 300 times less than that received from a standard chest x-ray[5] and for that matter considerably less than that experienced on a round-trip transcontinental airplane flight.[6]

REFERENCES

1. Heidrich F: Limitations of bone densitometry, *Am Fam Physician* 48:250-258, 1993.
2. Marshall D, Johnell O, Wedel H: Meta-analysis of how well measures of bone mineral density predict occurrence of osteoporotic fractures, *BMJ* 312:1254-1259, 1996.
3. US Preventive Services Task Force: *Guide to clinical preventive services,* ed 2, Baltimore, 1996, Williams & Wilkins, pp 509-516.
4. Canadian Task Force on the Periodic Health Examination: *Canadian guide to clinical preventive health care,* Ottawa, 1994, Canada Communication Group—Publishing, pp 620-631.
5. Sturtridge W, Lentle B, Hanley DA: The use of bone density measurement in the diagnosis and management of osteoporosis, *Can Med Assoc J* 155:924-929, 1996.
6. Wahner HW, Fogelman I: *The evaluation of osteoporosis,* London, 1994, Martin Dunitz, p 60.

Prevention of Osteoporosis with Calcium and Vitamin D Supplements

(See also exercise for the prevention of osteoporosis; hormone replacement therapy; hormone replacement for the prevention of osteoporosis)

Studies of calcium and vitamin D supplementation

Whether calcium supplementation inhibits the development of osteoporosis is controversial, but the bulk of the evidence suggests that it does. This is particularly evident in women who are at least 5 years postmenopausal, probably because in the immediate postmenopausal years estrogen deficiency–induced bone loss overshadows other etiological factors.[1]

Reid and associates[2] from Auckland, New Zealand, studied 122 healthy women who were at least 2 years postmenopausal and whose mean dietary calcium intake was 750 mg/day. They were treated with calcium supplements of 1000 mg/day. At the end of 2 years the rate of appendicular and axial bone loss was significantly lower in the calcium-treated group. After another 2 years the overall benefit persisted in the 86 women who agreed to continue the study.[3] Similar results have been reported by Dawson-Hughes and co-workers[4] and Aloia and associates.[5] The latter group used 1700 mg of calcium carbonate as the supplemental dose.

Prince and associates[6] from western Australia divided a group of postmenopausal women into three cohorts. One cohort was treated with exercise alone, one with exercise plus calcium supplementation (calcium lactate–gluconate 1 g/day), and one with exercise plus estrogens and progestins. Bone density decreased significantly in the exercise only group, decreased very slightly in the exercise plus calcium group, and increased in the exercise plus hormone replacement group.

Chapuy and associates[7] from Lyon, France, treated elderly women (mean age 84) with 800 IU of vitamin D_3 plus 1.2 g of elemental calcium in the form of tricalcium phosphate over an 18-month period. They did not assess vertebral fractures, but the total number of nonvertebral fractures was reduced by 32% compared with control subjects and the number of hip fractures was reduced by 43%. In addition, bone density measurements of the proximal femur showed an increase of 2% in the calcium–vitamin D_3 treated group and a decrease of 4.6% in the placebo control group. One Dutch study found that 400 IU of vitamin D given to elderly women increased the bone density of the femoral neck (a surrogate outcome for hip fracture),[8] but another from the same center found no decrease in the incidence of hip or peripheral bone fractures in elderly persons taking 400 IU of vitamin D daily over a 3½-year period.[9] In an American 3-year placebo-controlled study of men and women over the age of 65 living in the community, those taking 700 IU of vitamin D_3 plus 500 mg of calcium daily had less bone loss in the femoral neck, spine, and total body than control subjects; there were also fewer nonvertebral fractures in the treated group.[10]

How should family physicians use these data in their practices? There seem to be no significant adverse effects to moderate exercise, calcium, and low-dose vitamin D supplementation. A reasonable program would be to recommend that all postmenopausal women as well as all men over the age of 65 exercise and take daily supplements of 1000 to 1500 of calcium and 400 to 800 IU of vitamin D. Whether a woman should also receive hormone replacement therapy is discussed below and in the section on hormone replacement therapy.

Recommended daily allowances of calcium

The recommended daily allowances of calcium have recently been increased by the National Institutes of Health in the United States. These recommendations are as follows[11]:

Children 1-10 years	800-1200 mg/day
Adolescents and young adults 11-24	1200-1500 mg/day
Pregnant and lactating women	1200-1500 mg/day
Adult men ages 25-65	1000 mg/day
Adult women ages 25-50	1000 mg/day
Postmenopausal women 51-65 on estrogens	1000 mg/day
Postmenopausal women 51-65 not taking estrogens	1500 mg/day
Everyone over the age of 65	1500 mg/day

Dietary sources of calcium

The basic North American diet without dairy products provides a daily intake of 300 to 400 mg of calcium. One 8-ounce (250-ml) glass of 1% or 2% milk contains 300 mg of calcium. Other good sources of calcium, supplying about 300 mg per serving, are firm cheeses (45 g or 1½ ounces), canned salmon (125 ml or ½ cup), and canned sardines (seven medium sized) if the bones are eaten. In addition, 125 ml or ½ cup of tofu has about 150 mg, 250 ml or 1 cup of cooked soy beans about 200 mg, and 125 ml or ½ cup of dry-roasted almonds about 200 mg.[12]

Calcium supplements

A large number of calcium products are available without prescription. Most of them are in the form of calcium carbonate and are displayed in pharmacies along with the vitamins. Calcium carbonate may cause constipation. In prescribing a dose the physician should specify "elemental calcium." Absorption of calcium supplements is most effective if no more than 500 mg is taken at one time and if the tablets are taken with meals.[13] Calcium supplements are available in liquid forms, as tablets to be dissolved in water, as chewable tablets, or as tablets or capsules to be swallowed. Some of the tablets are large, so many patients prefer chewable forms. A few of the chewable calcium carbonate tablets are Tums 500, Os-Cal 500, and Caltrate 600.

Vitamin D supplementation

Most multivitamin compounds contain 400 IU of vitamin D.

REFERENCES

1. Heaney RP: Thinking straight about calcium, *N Engl J Med* 328:503-505, 1993.
2. Reid IR, Ames RW, Evans MC, et al: Effect of calcium supplementation on bone loss in postmenopausal women, *N Engl J Med* 328:460-464, 1993.
3. Reid IR, Ames RW, Evans MC, et al: Long-term effects of calcium supplementation on bone loss and fractures in postmenopausal women: a randomized controlled trial, *Am J Med* 98:331-335, 1995.
4. Dawson-Hughes B, Dallal GE, Krall EA, et al: Controlled trial of the effect of calcium supplementation on bone density in postmenopausal women, *N Engl J Med* 323:878-883, 1990.
5. Aloia JF, Vaswani A, Yeh JK, et al: Calcium supplementation with and without hormone replacement therapy to prevent postmenopausal bone loss, *Ann Intern Med* 120:97-103, 1994.
6. Prince RL, Smith M, Kick IM, et al: Prevention of postmenopausal osteoporosis: a comparative study of exercise, calcium supplementation, and hormone-replacement therapy, *N Engl J Med* 325:1189-1195, 1991.
7. Chapuy MC, Arlot ME, Duboeuf F, et al: Vitamin D_3 and calcium to prevent hip fractures in the elderly women, *N Engl J Med* 327:1637-1642, 1992.
8. Ooms ME, Roos JC, Bezemer PD, et al: Prevention of bone loss by vitamin D supplementation in elderly women—a randomized double-blind trial, *J Clin Endocrinol Metab* 80:1052-1058, 1995.
9. Lips P, Graafmans WC, Ooms ME, et al: Vitamin D supplementation and fracture incidence in elderly persons, *Ann Intern Med* 124:400-406, 1996.

10. Dawson-Hughes B, Harris SS, Krall EA, et al: Effect of calcium and vitamin D supplementation on bone density in men and women 65 years of age or older, *N Engl J Med* 337:670-676, 1997.
11. NIH releases consensus statement on optimal calcium intake, *Am Fam Physician* 50:1385-1387, 1994.
12. Miller A: 10 practical answers in dietary counselling, *Patient Care Can* 6:22-49, 1995.
13. Calcium supplements, *Med Lett* 38:108-109, 1996.

Exercise for the Prevention of Osteoporosis

(See also exercise; hormone replacement therapy; hormone replacement for the prevention of osteoporosis)

Femoral neck bone densities of the skeletons of premenopausal and postmenopausal women buried in the crypt of Christ Church, Spitalfields, London, between 1729 and 1852 were significantly greater than those of present-day women. The probable explanation was a greater degree of physical activity in these 18th and 19th century women.[1] A number of longitudinal and cross-sectional studies of living 20th century women confirm that exercise correlates with greater bone density[2-5] and a decrease in hip fractures.[6-8] Weight-bearing exercise (brisk walking or the equivalent) is an essential part of any osteoporosis preventive program and is particularly important for women, according to one British survey, because they are much less physically active and less fit than men at all ages[9] (which may not be saying a great deal, because men are not especially fit either).

High-intensity strength training exercises have had a striking effect on bone density in postmenopausal women who were not taking hormone replacement therapy. In a study by Nelson and associates[10] the experimental group spent 45 minutes twice a week doing exercises that involved hip extension, knee extension, lateral pull-down, back extension, and abdominal flexion. In addition to increasing bone density, this program increased muscle mass, overall strength, overall physical activity levels, and dynamic balance. Bone density decreased in the control group.

Premenopausal women aged 35 to 45 participating in regular high-impact exercises (jumping and step exercises) over an 18-month period were found to have increased their femoral neck bone densities.[11]

REFERENCES

1. Lees B, Molleson T, Asnett T: Differences in proximal femur bone density over two centuries, *Lancet* 341:673-675, 1993.
2. Kelly PJ, Eisman JA, Sambrook PN: Interaction of genetic and environmental influences on peak bone density, *Osteoporosis Int* 1:56-60, 1990.
3. Pocock NA, Eisman JA, Yeates MG, et al: Physical fitness is a major determinant of femoral neck and lumbar spine bone mineral density, *J Clin Invest* 78:618-621, 1986.
4. Simkin A, Ayalon J, Leichter I: Increased trabecular bone density due to bone-loading exercises in postmenopausal osteoporotic women, *Can Fam Physician* 40:59-63, 1987.
5. Dalsky GP, Stocke KS, Ehsani AA, et al: Weight-bearing exercise training and lumbar bone mineral content in postmenopausal women, *Ann Intern Med* 108:824-828, 1988.
6. Perez CR, Galan Galan F, Dilsen G: Risk factors for hip fracture in Spanish and Turkish women, *Bone* 14(suppl 1):S69-S72, 1993.
7. Jaglal SB, Kreiger N, Darlington G: Past and recent physical activity and risk of hip fracture, *Am J Epidemiol* 138:107-118, 1993.
8. Paganini-Hill A, Chao A, Ross RK, Henderson BE: Exercise and other factors in the prevention of hip fracture: the Leisure World study, *Epidemiology* 2:16-25, 1991.
9. Activity and Health Research: *Allied Dunbar national fitness survey: a report on activity patterns and fitness levels; main findings,* London, 1992, Sports Council and Health Education Authority.
10. Nelson ME, Fiatarone MA, Morganti CM, et al: Effects of high-intensity strength training on multiple risk factors for osteoporotic fractures: a randomized controlled trial, *JAMA* 272:1909-1914, 1994.
11. Heinonen A, Kannus P, Seivanen H, et al: Randomised controlled trial of effect of high-impact exercise on selected risk factors for osteoporotic fractures, *Lancet* 348:1343-1347, 1996.

Hormone Replacement for Prevention of Osteoporosis

(See also calcium and vitamin D for the prevention of osteoporosis; exercise for the prevention of osteoporosis; hip fractures; hormone replacement therapy; surrogate outcomes)

Estrogen replacement therapy started within a few years of menopause not only decreases the rate of bone loss as measured by bone density but, as shown in the 3-year Postmenopausal Estrogen/Progestin Interventions (PEPI) trial[1] and the 2-year Continuous Hormones as Replacement Therapy (CHART) study,[2] may lead to an increase in bone density. Both the PEPI and CHART trials used combinations of oral estrogens and oral progestins; the positive effect on bone density was observed with both intermittent and continuous use of the progestins.[1,2] In a 1-year study, transdermal estrogen was also found effective in decreasing the rate of bone density loss and the number of asymptomatic vertebral fractures in postmenopausal women.[3]

Although short-term studies have clearly shown that postmenopausal hormone replacement therapy improves bone density (a surrogate outcome for fractures), a critical question for physicians and patients is whether this therapy reduces the fracture rate and if so how long the hormones must be given to achieve this goal. Fractures can be reduced by hormone replacement therapy, but the duration required is controversial. It is often stated that fractures will be prevented if therapy is begun within 3 to 5 years of menopause and is continued for 6 to 9 years.[4] This view is challenged by several studies indicating that estrogen taken for even 7 or more years, starting at menopause, may not have much effect on bone density by the time a woman reaches age 75 when her risk of hip fracture becomes much greater.[5-7]

The probable need to continue estrogen therapy indefinitely if it is to be the main modality of preventing osteoporosis is supported by reports showing that current estrogen therapy is associated with a much lower incidence of hip fractures than is past therapy.[6,7] The view that hormonal replacement therapy for fracture protection must be started shortly after menopause and continued indefinitely is supported by a 1995 report from the Study of Osteoporotic Fractures Research Group. The important findings of this prospective cohort study were that hip and wrist fractures were significantly reduced in women who had started taking estrogen replacement therapy within 5 years of menopause and who did not discontinue it. Estrogen combined with a progestin was just as effective as unopposed estrogen, and current smokers were also protected. On the other hand, no significant protection was found among current users who had started hormonal replacement therapy more than 5 years after menopause or among women who had started hormone replacement therapy shortly after menopause, continued it for many years, but were no longer current users.[7]

The failure of estrogens to protect against osteoporosis if started well after menopause has been challenged by a cross-sectional study of women aged 60 to 98 using the surrogate outcomes of bone densities of the distal radius, midshaft radius, hip, and lumbar spine. Although maximum bone densities were observed in women who started taking estrogens at the time of menopause and never discontinued them, almost equal densities were obtained in women who initiated hormone replacement therapy after age 60 and who continued to take the medication indefinitely. In this study, as in others, little protection was noted in women who started taking estrogens at menopause but who discontinued them even after 10 years of use.[8]

An important reason for trying to prevent osteoporosis is the assumption that this in turn will prevent hip fractures with their attendant morbidity and mortality. Although this may be the case for many persons, one study of hip fractures found that serious underlying medical conditions were often a major factor leading to the falls that caused the fractures. In these cases the mortality associated with the fractures was due largely to the underlying medical conditions and would probably not have been altered by preventive interventions such as hormone replacement therapy.[9]

Even if prolonged estrogen replacement therapy is desirable, it may be difficult to achieve. In one British study 39% of the women for whom hormone replacement therapy was recommended because of low bone density either stopped the therapy prematurely or never started it.[10]

One of the most important issues regarding hormone replacement therapy for preventing osteoporosis is the risk/benefit ratio. As noted in the discussion of hormone replacement therapy, about one third of postmenopausal women will die of cardiovascular disease and only about 3% as a result of complications from hip fractures; from the point of view of mortality, the prevention of cardiovascular disease takes precedence. This does not appear to create a conflict, since hormone replacement therapy decreases the risks of both disorders. However, after 10 years of hormone use the risk of breast cancer mortality rises sufficiently to vitiate much of the benefit achieved through a decrease in CAD (see discussion of hormone replacement therapy).[11] Therefore lifetime prescriptions for hormones may do more harm than good.[11,12]

If hormone replacement therapy is prescribed for protection against osteoporosis, the usual recommended dose is 0.625 mg of conjugated estrogens (Premarin) daily or the equivalent (1.25 mg of estropipate [Ogen], 1 mg of estradiol [Estrace], and 0.02 mg of ethinyl estradiol [Estinyl]).[8] However, lower doses may be effective. In the Rancho Bernardo Study, women who began hormone therapy after age 60 took an average of 0.48 mg of conjugated estrogens daily,[8] and Ettinger and associates[13] reported prevention of bone loss with conjugated estrogens 0.3 mg/day in conjunction with calcium 1500 mg/day.[13]

REFERENCES

1. Writing Group for the PEPI Trial: Effects of hormone therapy on bone mineral density: results from the Postmenopausal Estrogen/Progestin Interventions (PEPI) Trial, *JAMA* 276:1389-1396, 1996.
2. Speroff L, Rowan J, Symons J, et al (CHART Study Group): The comparative effect on bone density, endometrium, and lipids of continuous hormones as replacement therapy (CHART Study), *JAMA* 276:1397-1403, 1996.
3. Lufkin EG, Wahner HW, O'Fallon WM, et al: Treatment of postmenopausal osteoporosis with transdermal estrogen, *Ann Intern Med* 117:1-9, 1992.
4. Josse RG: Effects of ovarian hormone therapy on skeletal and extraskeletal tissues in women, *Can Med Assoc J* 155:929-934, 1996.
5. Felson DT, Zhang Y, Hannan MT: The effect of postmenopausal estrogen therapy on bone density in elderly women, *N Engl J Med* 329:1141-1146, 1993.
6. Ettinger B, Grady D: The waning effect of postmenopausal estrogen therapy on osteoporosis, *N Engl J Med* 329:1192-1193, 1993.
7. Cauley JA, Seeley DG, Ensrud K, et al (Study of Osteoporotic Fractures Research Group): Estrogen replacement therapy and fractures in older women, *Ann Intern Med* 122:9-16, 1995.
8. Schneider DL, Barrett-Connor EL, et al: Timing of postmenopausal estrogen for optimal bone mineral density: the Rancho Bernardo Study, *JAMA* 277:543-547, 1997.
9. Browner WS, Pressman AR, Nevitt MC, et al (Study of Osteoporotic Fractures Research Group): Mortality following fractures in older women, *Arch Intern Med* 156:1521-1525, 1996.
10. Ryan PJ, Harrison R, Blake GM, et al: Compliance with hormone replacement therapy (HRT) after screening for post menopausal osteoporosis, *Br J Obstet Gynaecol* 99:325-328, 1992.
11. Grodstein F, Stampfer MJ, Colditz A, et al: Postmenopausal hormone therapy and mortality, *N Engl J Med* 336:1769-1775, 1997.
12. Brinton LA, Schairer C: Postmenopausal hormone-replacement therapy—time for a reappraisal? (editorial), *N Engl J Med* 336:1821-1822, 1997.

13. Ettinger B, Genant HK, Cann CE: Postmenopausal bone loss is prevented by treatment with low-dosage estrogen with calcium, *Ann Intern Med* 106:40-45, 1987.

Prevention of Corticosteroid-Induced Osteoporosis

According to one study, treatment with calcium carbonate 1000 mg/day plus 500 IU of vitamin D_3 to patients receiving long-term corticosteroids prevented bone loss.[1] A similar study showed equivocal benefits.[2] The 1996 American College of Rheumatology Task Force on Osteoporosis Guidelines recommended that all patients likely to be taking corticosteroids on a long-term basis in doses of 7.5 mg or more of prednisone daily should be given preventive therapy. Bone density measurements are indicated for most patients. Everyone should take calcium and vitamin D supplements, maintain a program of weight-bearing exercises, and especially if bone density is low, receive hormone replacement therapy. Thiazide diuretics increase the absorption of calcium from the gastrointestinal tract and decrease its urinary excretion. Therefore the addition of hydrochlorothiazide in doses of 25 mg or less may be helpful, especially in patients excreting more than 300 mg of calcium in their urine over a 24-hour period. The guidelines also suggested that if postmenopausal women were unable to take replacement hormones, consideration should be given to a bisphosphonate such as etidronate (Didronel), alendronate (Fosamax), or calcitonin (Calcimar).[3] A subsequent multicenter randomized placebo-controlled trial studied the effects of cyclical etidronate and calcium on patients beginning a regimen of prednisone 7.5 mg/day or greater for at least 3 months. Study patients received a 2-week course of etidronate 400 mg/day followed by calcium carbonate (elemental calcium 500 mg/day) for 56 days, and this cycle was repeated three times. At the end of a year patients taking etidronate and calcium had an increase in bone density (control subjects had a loss) and suffered far fewer vertebral fractures.[4]

REFERENCES

1. Buckley LM, Leib ES, Cartularo KS, et al: Calcium and vitamin D-3 supplementation prevents bone loss in the spine secondary to low-dose corticosteroids in patients with rheumatoid arthritis—a randomized, double-blind, placebo-controlled trial, *Ann Intern Med* 125:961-968, 1996.
2. Adachi JD, Bensen WG, Bianchi F, et al: Vitamin D and calcium in the prevention of corticosteroid induced osteoporosis—a 3 year follow-up, *J Rheumatol* 23:995-1000, 1996.
3. Hochberg MC, Prashker MJ, Rogers EN, et al: Recommendations for the prevention and treatment of glucocorticoid-induced osteoporosis: American College of Rheumatology Task Force on Osteoporosis guidelines, *Arthritis Rheum* 39:1791-1801, 1996.
4. Adachi JD, Bensen W, Brown J, et al: Intermittent etidronate therapy to prevent corticosteroid-induced osteoporosis, *N Engl J Med* 337:382-387, 1997.

Treatment of Established Osteoporosis

(See also amenorrhea; metastatic breast cancer; multiple myeloma)

Hormone replacement therapy

Estrogen treatment of postmenopausal women with established osteoporosis has been reported to increase bone density[1] and to decrease the incidence of vertebral fractures.[2] The role of estrogen therapy for amenorrheic young women is discussed under "Amenorrhea."

Calcium

The recommended daily requirement for calcium in normally menstruating women is 700 mg/day. Postmenopausal women require 1200 to 1500 mg/day and osteoporotic women 1500 to 2000 mg/day. Calcium supplements are listed above in the discussion of calcium and vitamin D for the prevention of osteoporosis.

Vitamin D

The usual daily requirement of vitamin D for the population at large is 400 IU. Those with osteoporosis should probably receive 800 IU/day. Almost all multivitamins contain 400 IU of vitamin D.

Calcitonin

Calcitonin may give rapid pain relief from compression fractures.[3,4] An intranasal formulation seems to be even more effective than the parenteral route for analgesic effect. The usual dose of the parenteral formulation (Calcimar) is 100 IU subcutaneously or intramuscularly three or four times a week, and that of the nasal spray (Miacalcin) is one spray of 200 IU in one nostril daily (alternate nostrils each day).

Bisphosphonates

Bisphosphonates bind to bone and inhibit osteoclast activity, thus decreasing bone removal. They are indicated for treatment of established osteoporosis but not as yet for prevention of the disorder.[5] In two 3-year trials of postmenopausal osteoporotic women treated with alendronate (Fosamax), bone density increased and the incidence of clinical and radiological vertebral fractures decreased.[6,7] IV infusion of the bisphosphonate pamidronate (Aredia) has proved beneficial for patients with breast cancer metastatic to bone (see "Metastatic Breast Cancer") and those with multiple myeloma (see "Multiple Myeloma").

Etidronate (Didronel) is taken daily (400 mg once daily or 200 mg bid) for a 2-week period four times a year. On all other days of the year the patient should take calcium supplementation.

The usual dose of alendronate (Fosamax) is 10 mg/day taken with water on an empty stomach 30 minutes before breakfast. Calcium supplements should also be taken daily. Esophageal ulceration is a rare complication of swallowing alendronate pills. Taking the pill with a large glass of water and remaining vertical for half an hour afterward may help prevent this problem.[8]

REFERENCES

1. Lindsay R, Tohme JF: Estrogen treatment of patients with established postmenopausal osteoporosis, *Obstet Gynecol* 76:290-295, 1990.
2. Lufkin EG, Wahner HW, O'Fallon WM, et al: Treatment of postmenopausal osteoporosis with transdermal estrogen, *Ann Intern Med* 117:1-9, 1992.
3. Siminoski K, Josse RG: Calcitonin in the treatment of osteoporosis, *Can Med Assoc J* 155:962-965, 1996.
4. Recker RR: Clinical review 41: current therapy for osteoporosis, *J Clin Endocrinol Metab* 76:14-16, 1993.
5. Hodsman A, Adachi J, Olszynski W: Use of bisphosphonates in the treatment of osteoporosis, *Can Med Assoc J* 155:945-948, 1996.
6. Liberman UA, Weiss SR, Broll J, et al: Effect of oral alendronate on bone mineral density and the incidence of fractures in postmenopausal osteoprosis, *N Engl J Med* 333:1437-1443, 1995.
7. Black DM, Cummings SR, Karpf DB, et al: Randomised trial of effect of alendronate on risk of fracture in women with existing vertebral fractures, *Lancet* 348:1535-1541, 1996.
8. de Groen PC, Lubbe DF, Hirsch LJ, et al: Esophagitis associated with the use of alendronate, *N Engl J Med* 335:1016-1021, 1996.

THYROID

Thyroid Tests

In outpatient practice a sensitive thyroid-stimulating hormone (sTSH) measurement is sufficient to screen for a hyperthyroid or hypothyroid state. Free thyroxine (FT_4) determinations are required only if the sTSH result is abnormal.[1]

REFERENCES

1. Bauer DC, Brown AN: Sensitive thyrotropin and free thyroxine testing in outpatients: are both necessary? *Arch Intern Med* 156: 2333-2337, 1996.

Euthyroid Sick Syndrome

The euthyroid sick syndrome occurs in three forms. In all of them triiodothyronine (T_3) or thyroxine (T_4) concentrations are abnormal but the TSH level is normal or near normal. The normal TSH is the clue to the diagnosis.

Low T_3 Syndrome

Normally T_4 is converted in almost equal amounts to T_3 and reverse (inactive) T_3. In severe catabolic states or with carbohydrate restriction, the enzyme catalyzing T_3 formation is inhibited, resulting in increased production of the metabolically inactive reverse T_3. This causes a state of functional hypothyroidism that helps to prevent nitrogen loss during stress. Hypothyroidism is rapidly reversible once the stress (illness, surgery) is removed. In the low T_3 syndrome, the T_4 level is normal and the T_3 level is low. The diagnosis is made by measuring TSH concentraion, which is normal or near normal (except in the rare cases of pituitary or hypothalamic failure as the cause of low T_3).

Low T_3, Low T_4 Syndrome

The low T_3, low T_4 syndrome is seen in severely ill patients and indicates a poor prognosis. Both T_3 and T_4 levels are low, but the TSH level is normal.

High T_4 Syndrome

In the high T_4 syndrome the T_4 level is elevated because of excessive iodine intake, as occurs with gallbladder studies and occasionally from drugs such as amiodarone. The high iodine inhibits the conversion of T_4 to T_3, leading to a buildup of T_4. TSH concentrations are normal or near normal.

Hyperthyroidism

Smokers have an increased incidence of Graves' disease and particularly Graves' ophthalmopathy.[1] Lithium therapy, which is known to be a risk factor for hypothyroidism, may also be associated with an increased risk of hyperthyroidism.[1]

Subclinical hyperthyroidism

Subclinical hyperthyroidism is defined as a low sTSH level in a clinically well person with normal serum thyroid hormone concentrations. Persons over 60 years of age with this condition are at three times greater relative risk for atrial fibrillation over the next decade than those without subclinical hyperthyroidism.[2] However, it does not follow that such individuals should be treated with antithyroid drugs, since the risks of treatment might outweigh the risks of atrial fibrillation.[3]

Overview of the treatment of thyrotoxicosis

Therapy for hyperthyroidism is targeted at either immediate control of symptoms (adjunct treatment), usually with beta-blockers, or modification of the disease through the use of drugs or radioactive iodine.

Beta-blockers and calcium channel blockers. A number of beta-blockers can be used to control the symptoms of tachycardia and palpitations. Examples are propranolol (Inderal) 20 to 40 mg qid, nadolol (Corgard) 80 to 240 mg/day as a single dose, atenolol (Tenormin) 50 to 100 mg/day as a single dose, and metoprolol (Lopresor) 50 to 100 mg bid. Treatment usually starts with low doses that are increased as necessary. Symptomatic beta-blocker treatment should be continued for 4 to 6 weeks, overlapping with the definitive treatment. For patients who cannot take beta-blockers, the calcium channel blocker diltiazem (Cardizem) 30 to 120 mg tid is often effective.[4]

Radioactive iodine. Use of radioactive iodine as the initial definitive treatment for hyperthyroidism is becoming more common in North America, but it is not used nearly as often in Europe or Japan. ^{131}I is particularly indicated in patients with risk factors for relapse such as those with severe symptoms or a large goiter.[4]

Antithyroid drug therapy. The two major antithyroid drugs in use are propylthiouracil (Propyl-Thyracil) and methimazole (Tapazole). Methimazole is the active metabolite of a third antithyroid drug, carbimazole.

The goals of antithyroid drug treatment in Graves' disease are the control of symptoms and the attainment of long-term remission.[4,5] Factors weakly associated with good remissions are small size of goiter and recent onset of hyperthyroidism.[1] More important is the duration of treatment.[6] Long-term remissions have been reported to be much greater after 2 years of treatment than after 6 months of treatment.[7]

In North America antithyroid drugs remain the treatment of first choice in patients under 40 with a first episode of Graves' disease. Older patients, as well as younger ones with a relapse of Graves' disease after treatment with an antithyroid drug, are usually treated definitively with radioactive iodine. Even when use of radioactive iodine is selected, patients may initially be given antithyroid drugs for a short period to control symptoms.[5]

The general policy in North America is to treat patients with antithyroid drugs for 1 to 2 years, since attempts at longer treatment are associated with prolonged monitoring and poor compliance. Relapses are most likely to occur in the 6 months after discontinuing therapy but may take place after many years.[5]

The choice of antithyroid drug seems to be arbitrary. In North America propylthiouracil (Propyl-Thyracil) is used more often than methimazole (Tapazole) for unclear reasons. According to Franklyn,[5] methimazole has several advantages and should be the drug of choice. It requires only once a day dosing and in moderate doses is associated with a lesser risk of agranulocytosis.

The major side effect of both propylthiouracil and methimazole is agranulocytosis. It is an idiosyncratic reaction that is slightly more common in patients over the age of 40. Since it comes on rapidly, routine blood counts are not helpful; instead patients should be warned to report fever or sore throat immediately.[5] A baseline CBC before the initiation of therapy may be helpful.[4]

Propylthiouracil is usually started with doses of 75 to 100 mg tid. After 4 to 6 weeks the dose should be decreased by about one third if the TSH has risen to a normal or above normal level or if the T_4 or T_3 level has returned to normal. After another 4 to 6 weeks the dose may have to be reduced again. The usual maintenance dose is about 50 mg tid. The patient should then be examined clinically and have TSH and T_4 determinations every 2 months for 6 months, then every 3 months for 6 months, then twice a year for 1 year, and then annually. Treatment is generally continued for 1 to 2 years.[4,5]

Treatment with methimazole is usually begun with 10 to 20 mg once a day. After 4 to 6 weeks the dose should be decreased by about one third if the T_4 or T_3 has returned to normal or if the TSH has risen to a normal or above normal level. Since the TSH level may take weeks or even months to return to normal, doses are usually adjusted according to the T_4 and T_3 levels. After another 4 to 6 weeks the dose may have to be reduced once again. The usual maintenance dose is about 5 to 10 mg of methimazole a day. The patient should then have clinical follow-up and TSH and T_4 determinations every 2 months for 6 months, then every 3 months for 6 months, then twice a year for 1 year, and then annually. Treatment is generally continued for 1 to 2 years.[4,5]

REFERENCES

1. Prummel MF, Wiersinga WM: Smoking and risk of Graves' disease, *JAMA* 269:479-482, 1993.
2. Sawin CT, Geller A, Wolf PA, et al: Low serum thyrotropin concentrations as a risk factor for atrial fibrillation in older persons, *N Engl J Med* 331:1249-1252, 1994.
3. Utiger RD: Subclinical hyperthyroidism—just a low serum thyrotropin concentration, or something more? (editorial), *N Engl J Med* 331:302-303, 1994.
4. Singer PA, Cooper DS, Levy EG, et al: Treatment guidelines for patients with hyperthyroidism and hypothyroidism, *JAMA* 273:808-812, 1995.
5. Franklyn JA: The management of hyperthyroidism, *N Engl J Med* 330:1731-1738, 1994.
6. Allannic H, Fauchet R, Orgiazzi J, et al: Antithyroid drugs and Graves' disease: a prospective randomized evaluation of the efficacy of treatment duration, *J Clin Endocrinol Metab* 70:675-679, 1990.
7. Tamai H, Nakagawa T, Fukino O, et al: Thionamide therapy in Graves' disease: relation of relapse rate to duration of therapy, *Ann Intern Med* 92:448-490, 1980.

Hypothyroidism

(See also celiac disease; smoking; thyroiditis; biliary cirrhosis)

Epidemiology

Lithium therapy is an important risk factor for hypothyroidism; 5% of patients receiving lithium have overt hypothyroidism, and 25% have subclinical hypothyroidism.[1] Smoking probably aggravates both the clinical and the biochemical effects of overt hypothyroidism.[2]

Clinical features

An often unrecognized clinical feature of hypothyroidism is myopathy. This may manifest itself as muscle pain or weakness, and levels of muscle enzymes such as creatine kinase may be elevated. Hypercholesterolemia is another clue to the disorder. In a retrospective analysis of hypercholesterolemic patients referred to a lipid disorders clinic, 4.2% were hypothyroid; correction of the hypothyroidism lowered the lipid levels only if the TSH concentration was at least 10 mU/L (10 μU/mL). Put another way, subclinical hypothyroidism is probably not a risk factor for atherosclerosis.[3]

Guidelines for screening

The Canadian Task Force on the Periodic Health Examination recognizes the high prevalence of hypothyroidism among perimenopausal and postmenopausal women but gives screening for this disorder with thyroid function tests a "C" recommendation,[4] and the U.S. Preventive Services Task Force gives screening of asymptomatic adults and children a "D" recommendation.[5] For high-risk groups, including the elderly, the U.S. Preventive Services Task Force gives screening a "C" recommendation.[5]

Treatment

For patients over the age of 50 the usual starting dose of thyroxine (Synthroid, Eltroxin) is 50 µg/day, which is increased after an interval of 3 to 4 weeks to 100 to 150 µg/day. In younger patients (under 30 to 40 years of age[6] or under 50[7]) or those in whom hypothyroidism develops rapidly (postthyroidectomy or post–radioactive iodine treatment), the initial dose may be 100 µg/day.[6,7]

Whether thyroid replacement therapy results in an increased incidence of osteoporosis is controversial. Several studies have failed to show a relationship.[8,9] However, a metaanalysis found that TSH suppressive therapy was associated with increased osteoporosis in postmenopausal women whereas replacement therapy was not.[10] A multicenter prospective study of hip fractures in the United States found that a past history of hyperthyroidism was a risk factor but that thyroid replacement therapy itself was not.[11] The practical point for family physicians is that when hormone replacement therapy is prescribed for hypothyroidism, the TSH level should be kept in the normal rather than the subnormal range.

REFERENCES

1. Prummel MF, Wiersinga WM: Smoking and risk of Graves' disease, *JAMA* 269:479-482, 1993.
2. Müller B, Zulewski H, Huber P, et al: Impaired action of thyroid hormone associated with smoking in women with hypothyroidism, *N Engl J Med* 333:964-969, 1995.
3. Diekman T, Lansberg PJ, Kastelein JJP, et al: Prevalence and correction of hypothyroidism in a large cohort of patients referred for dyslipidemia, *Arch Intern Med* 155:1490-1495, 1995.
4. Canadian Task Force on the Periodic Health Examination: *Canadian guide to clinical preventive health care,* Ottawa, 1994, Canada Communication Group—Publishing, pp 612-618.
5. US Preventive Services Task Force: *Guide to clinical preventive services,* ed 2, Baltimore, 1996, Williams & Wilkins, pp 209-218.
6. Toft AD: Thyroxine therapy, *N Engl J Med* 331:174-180, 1994.
7. Singer PA, Cooper DS, Levy EG, et al: Treatment guidelines for patients with hyperthyroidism and hypothyroidism, *JAMA* 273:808-812, 1995.
8. Solomon BL, Wartofsky L, Burman KD: Prevalence of fractures in postmenopausal women with thyroid disease, *Thyroid* 3:17-23, 1993.
9. Franklyn JA, Betteridge J, Daykin J, et al: Long-term thyroxine treatment and bone mineral density, *Lancet* 340:9-13, 1992.
10. Uzzan B, Campos J, Cucherat M, et al: Effects on bone mass of long term treatment with thyroid hormones: a meta-analysis, *J Clin Endocrinol Metab* 81:4278-4289, 1996.
11. Cummings SR, Nevitt MC, Browner WS, et al: Risk factors for hip fracture in white women, *N Engl J Med* 332:767-773, 1995.

Subclinical hypothyroidism

(See also smoking; thyroiditis)

Subclinical hypothyroidism is two to three times as common as overt hypothyroidism. It occurs frequently in the elderly and is found in 25% of patients receiving lithium therapy,[1] and in some susceptible subjects it may be precipitated by smoking.[2] The most common cause is chronic autoimmune thyroiditis, which is found in 3% of adults and 10% of postmenopausal women.[1]

Whether treatment of subclinical hypothyroidism is indicated is controversial.[3-5] One argument for treatment is that mild reversible target organ damage has been reported with this condition, including impaired left ventricular function, reduced hearing, and increased capillary permeability to protein. Many patients with this disorder are reported to feel better when receiving treatment.[3-5] Although cholesterol levels may be slightly elevated in subclinical hypothyroidism, this does not seem to constitute a significant risk factor for atherosclerosis.[3-6] Another reason for treatment is to prevent progression to overt disease.[3-5] Various risk factors have been described for this, of which two important ones are an elevation of the TSH level to more than twice the upper limit of normal and the combination of elevated TSH and thyroid antibody concentrations. In the latter instance the annual progression rate is 5%.[3] Suggested criteria for treatment include the following[4,5]:

1. The TSH level is unequivocally elevated (greater than twice the upper limit of normal).
2. Goiter is present in the absence of radioactive iodine treatment.
3. There are high levels of microsomal antibodies.
4. An elevated prolactin level is present.
5. A patient at risk for CAD has an elevated cholesterol level.
6. Subtle symptoms of hypothyroidism are present.

REFERENCES

1. Prummel MF, Wiersinga WM: Smoking and risk of Graves' disease, *JAMA* 269:479-482, 1993.
2. Müller B, Zulewski H, Huber P, et al: Impaired action of thyroid hormone associated with smoking in women with hypothyroidism, *N Engl J Med* 333:964-969, 1995.
3. Weetman AP: Hypothyroidism: screening and subclinical disease, *BMJ* 314:1175-1178, 1997.
4. Laryea EA: Subclinical hypothyroidism: to treat or not to treat, *Can Fam Physician* 39:1997-2003, 1993.
5. Toft AD: Thyroxine therapy, *N Engl J Med* 331:174-180, 1994.
6. Diekman T, Lansberg PJ, Kastelein JJP, et al: Prevalence and correction of hypothyroidism in a large cohort of patients referred for dyslipidemia, *Arch Intern Med* 155:1490-1495, 1995.

Thyroid Nodules

(See also effect of screening on apparent prevalence rates)

About 50% of autopsy subjects are found to have thyroid nodules.[1] In most series of living patients only 5% to 8% have clinically palpable nodules and less than 10% of these are cancerous.[2] However, in one California study in which a special effort was made to look for thyroid nodules by palpation in asymptomatic patients, 9% were found to have solitary nodules and 12% had multiple nodules for a total of 21%. When assessed by ultrasound, 67% of these patients were found to have nodules; none was malignant.[3] A Mayo Clinic evaluation comparing palpation and ultrasonography found that nodules less than 1 cm in diameter were rarely palpable and that about 50% of glands thought to have a solitary nodule on palpation were actually multinodular on ultrasonography.[4]

If a low-functioning ("cold") nodule is found in a woman living in an iodine-deficient area, the chance that it is malignant is about 1.5%.[5] A solitary nodule in a 75-year-old man has an almost 60% chance of being malignant.[6] Thyroid nodules are four times as common in females as in males, and their incidence increases in direct proportion to age.[7] The vast majority of thyroid cancers are relatively nonaggressive; about 70% are papillary and 15% follicular.[8] A rare form of thyroid cancer is medullary thyroid cancer, which may be part of the dominantly inherited multiple endocrine neoplasia syndrome. Aside from medullary thyroid cancer, patients with this syndrome may have parathyroid gland hyperplasia and pheochromocytomas. A family history of thyroid disease should be sought in any patient with a thyroid nodule.

Hyperfunctioning ("hot") nodules are almost never malignant, and therefore a thyroid scan is often one of the initial investigations ordered.[2] In most cases, however, fine needle aspiration using a no. 25 needle is the investigative procedure of choice. Correct cytological diagnoses using this technique have been reported in 80% to 90% of undifferentiated carcinomas, medullary carcinomas, and papillary carcinomas and in 40% to 70% of cases of follicular carcinoma.[9] The aspiration is done with a 10- or 25-ml syringe and a 22- to 27-gauge needle. Three to six passes with the needle are generally made to ensure adequate sampling.[2]

About 15% to 25% of aspirated nodules are found to be cysts. Most cysts are benign, but 15% have been reported to be necrotic papillary carcinomas.[7] The chances that a cyst is malignant are increased if it is greater than 4 cm in diameter, is bloody on aspiration, or recurs after repeated aspirations.[8]

Treatment of benign thyroid nodules is controversial. Traditional treatment is levothyroxine with the goal of suppressing TSH to remove any stimulus for the nodule to grow.[2] One study from the Mayo Clinic showed no benefit of such treatment,[10] whereas a report from Italy documents a clear benefit.[11]

If a thyroid nodule is smaller than 1 cm, the chances of its being malignant are very low. In this situation a reasonable management plan is simply follow-up observation.[10]

REFERENCES

1. Mortensen JD, Woolner LB, Bennett WA: Gross and microscopic findings in clinically normal thyroid glands, *J Clin Endocrinol Metab* 15:1270-1280, 1955.
2. Ridgway EC: Clinical review 30: clinician's evaluation of a solitary thyroid nodule, *J Clin Endocrinol Metab* 74:231-235, 1992.
3. Ezzat S, Sarti DA, Cain DR, Braunstein GD: Thyroid incidentalomas: prevalence by palpation and ultrasonography, *Arch Intern Med* 154:1838-1840, 1994.
4. Tan GH, Gharib H, Reading CC: Solitary thyroid nodule: comparison between palpation and ultrasonography, *Arch Intern Med* 155:2418-2423, 1995.
5. Belfiore A, La Rosa GL, La Porta GA, et al: Cancer risk in patients with cold thyroid nodules: relevance of iodine intake, sex, age and multinodularity, *Am J Med* 93:363-369, 1992.
6. Mazzaferri EL: Thyroid cancer in thyroid nodules: finding a needle in the haystack (editorial), *Am J Med* 93:359-362, 1992.
7. Mazzaferri EL: Current concepts: management of a solitary thyroid nodule, *N Engl J Med* 328:553-559, 1993.
8. Boutin J-M: Les nodules thyroïdiens tirés au clair, *Clinicien* 9:93-104, 1994.
9. Miller JM, Kini SR, Hamburger JI: The diagnosis of malignant follicular neoplasms of the thyroid by needle biopsy, *Cancer* 55:2812-2817, 1985.
10. Gharib H, James EM, Charboneau JW, et al: Suppressive therapy with levothyroxine for solitary thyroid nodules, *N Engl J Med* 317:70-75, 1987.
11. La Rosa GL, Lupo L, Giuffrida D, et al: Levothyroxine and potassium iodide are both effective in treating benign solitary solid cold nodules of the thyroid, *Ann Intern Med* 122:1-8, 1995.

Thyroiditis

(See also hypothyroidism; subclinical hypothyroidism)

Classification

Thyroiditis can be classified as follows[1,2]:

1. Acute thyroiditis (bacterial, fungal, or parasitic)
2. Subacute thyroiditis (subacute granulomatous thyroiditis [de Quervain's or painful thyroiditis], painless thyroiditis, postpartum thyroiditis)
3. Chronic lymphocytic thyroiditis (Hashimoto's disease)
4. Riedel's thyroiditis (invasive fibrous thyroiditis or chronic sclerosing thyroiditis)

Acute thyroiditis and Riedel's thyroiditis are very rare. Symptoms of acute infectious thyroiditis are anterior neck pain, swelling, fever, dysphagia, and dysphonia. Riedel's thyroiditis is found in middle-aged or elderly women and consists of a fibrous replacement of the gland that turns the gland into a stony hard mass.

Subacute granulomatous thyroiditis

Subacute granulomatous thyroiditis was described by de Quervain in 1904. It is thought to be secondary to a viral infection. It affects women four times as often as men, most patients are middle aged, and cases are most likely to occur in the summer and fall.[1,2]

The usual symptoms are either those of thyrotoxicosis (about 50% of patients), resulting from the excessive release of thyroid hormone by the damaged gland, or anterior neck pain. In fact, granulomatous thyroiditis is the most common cause of anterior neck pain in the region of the thyroid gland. Patients may have low-grade fever and general malaise. The thyroid gland tends to be firm and tender.[1,2]

The symptoms of pain or thyrotoxicosis often develop rapidly, and this is a distinguishing point from Graves' disease. If the differential between these two conditions is not obvious clinically, it can be resolved by measuring ^{131}I uptake. This is significantly increased in Graves' disease but very low (less than 5%) in granulomatous thyroiditis.[1,2]

The initial phase of inflammation and pain usually lasts 3 to 6 weeks. About one third of patients subsequently enter a hypothyroid stage that persists for several weeks before the euthyroid state is restored. Approximately 5% of patients become permanently hypothyroid.[1,2]

A number of patients have elevated antithyroid antibody levels, which suggests the development of an autoimmune process during the disease.[1,2]

Treatment of granulomatous thyroiditis is symptomatic. Nonsteroidal antiinflammatory drugs are usually effective in relieving the neck pain, but sometimes prednisone 20 to 40 mg/day in divided doses and tapered over 2 to 4 weeks is required. Thyrotoxic symptoms can be controlled by beta-blockers (see discussion of hyperthyroidism), and the subsequent hypothyroid state may need temporary thyroid replacement therapy.[1,2] Antithyroid drugs such as propylthiouracil or methimazole have no role in treating any of the forms of subacute thyroiditis (granulomatous, painless, or postpartum), since the pathogenesis is leakage of preformed hormone, not its excessive production.[1,2]

Painless thyroiditis

Painless thyroiditis may be sporadic or postpartum. Both forms are believed to be autoimmune disorders, since thyroid antibodies are present in 50% of patients with painless thyroiditis and 80% of those with postpartum thyroiditis.[1,2]

The sporadic form of painless thyroiditis is concentrated in the Great Lakes region of North America and accounts for about one third of cases of thyrotoxicosis in this area. Outside of the Great Lakes region it constitutes only about 5% of thyrotoxicosis cases.[1,2]

Like granulomatous thyroiditis, painless thyroiditis affects women four times as often as men and most patients are 40 to 50 years of age. Symptoms are those of thyrotoxicosis and tend to come on abruptly. Patients do not have neck pain. The thyroid gland is slightly enlarged but nontender.[1,2]

Also like granulomatous thyroiditis, painless thyroiditis usually begins with a thyrotoxic phase, passes through a hypothyroid phase, and ends with a recovery phase. In a few patients only the hypothyroid phase is seen. About 6% of patients become permanently hypothyroid, but this may take years to develop. Thus annual TSH testing is indicated for all patients with painless thyroiditis.[1,2]

Painless thyroiditis can be differentiated from Graves' disease by radioactive iodine uptake (RAIU). It is high in Graves' disease and usually less than 3% in painless thyroiditis.[1,2]

Treatment of painless thyroiditis is directed at the symptoms. Some patients require no treatment, whereas others benefit from beta-blockers in the thyrotoxic phase and a temporary course of levothyroxine if symptomatic hypothyroidism ensues.[1,2]

Postpartum thyroiditis

As indicated previously, postpartum thyroiditis is a variant of painless thyroiditis. It occurs in 4% to 5% of women and is usually self-limited. The disorder begins with symptoms of hyperthyroidism, which are classically followed by a period of hypothyroidism and finally a return to the euthyroid state. The entire sine wave cycle may last 6 to 9 months. The syndrome is likely to recur with subsequent pregnancies,[1,2] and about 25% of those who have recovered from the disorder are found to be overtly hypothyroid 4 years later.[3,4]

RAIU scanning shows no or little uptake in patients with postpartum thyroiditis but marked uptake in those with Graves' disease. The test should not be performed if the mother is nursing.[1,2]

Treatment of postpartum thyroiditis is symptomatic. Beta-blockers may be needed in the hyperthyroid stage and short-term levothyroxine in the hypothyroid stage.[1,2]

Chronic lymphocytic thyroiditis

Chronic lymphocytic thyroiditis was described by the Japanese physician Hashimoto in 1912. It is the most common cause of hypothyroidism. Up to 95% of patients are women,[1] and most are over the age of 45 when the diagnosis is made.[5] A small to medium-sized goiter is usually found. Antithyroid antibodies (antimicrosomal or antithyroglobulin) are present in 90% of patients, and the titers of these, particularly the antimicrosomal antibodies, are usually high. The usual replacement dose of levothyroxine (Synthroid, Eltroxin) is 75 to 150 µg/day. Initial doses are low (12.5, 25, and 50 µg), especially in the elderly or those with coronary artery disease. Increments, based on TSH levels, are made every 4 to 6 weeks (see discussion of hypothyroidism above).[1] If a patient with chronic lymphocytic thyroiditis becomes pregnant, she will probably require a dose increase of 25% to 50%.[5]

In one study 11% of patients with Hashimoto's thyroiditis had a spontaneous remission. Levothyroxine was withdrawn after 1 year of treatment, and thyroid function remained normal for up to a year.[6]

REFERENCES

1. Sakiyama R: Thyroiditis: a clinical review, *Am Fam Physician* 48:615-621, 1993.
2. Morrison A: Guidelines for the diagnosis of common thyroid disorders, *Can J CME,* May 1992, pp 79-85.

3. Othman S, Phillips DI, Parkes AB, et al: A long-term follow-up of postpartum thyroiditis, *Clin Endocrinol* 32:559-564, 1990.
4. Tachi J, Amino N, Tamaki H: Long-term follow-up and HLA association in patients with postpartum hypothyroidism, *J Clin Endocrinol Metab* 66:480-484, 1988.
5. Dyan CM, Daniels GH: Chronic autoimmune thyroiditis, *N Engl J Med* 335:99-107, 1996.
6. Comtois R, Faucher L, Lafleche L: Outcome of hypothyroidism caused by Hashimoto's thyroiditis, *Arch Intern Med* 155:1404-1408, 1995.

PITUITARY

Hypopituitarism

Pituitary adenomas, which may be secreting or nonsecreting, are the most common cause of hypopituitarism. Postpartum hemorrhage with hypovolemia may lead to hypopituitarism (Sheehan's syndrome) either immediately or after a delay of several years.[1]

Clinical manifestations

The clinical manifestations of hypopituitarism are often subtle and variable. The variability depends on large part on which target endocrine glands are deficient and whether the deficiency is mild or severe.[1]

Symptoms of corticotropin deficiency include weakness, headache, orthostatic hypotension, fatigue, anorexia, nausea, vomiting, abdominal pain, and weight loss. In long-standing cases patients may have thinning or loss of axillary and pubic hair. On examination the patient often appears pale because of decreased pigmentation, and this contrasts with the hyperpigmentation of Addison's disease. Deficiency of gonadotropins results in decreased libido and erectile function in men and menstrual irregularities or amenorrhea in women. In addition, women may have decreased libido and even hot flashes. Deficiency of TSH results in the symptoms of hypothyroidism. Adults with growth hormone deficiency have nonspecific symptoms such as decreased energy and decreased exercise tolerance.

If the cause of the hypopituitarism is a prolactin-secreting adenoma, the patient may have galactorrhea.[1]

Laboratory investigations

If hypopituitarism is suspected, a family physician may order some initial blood tests as discussed below. Imaging of the pituitary gland and sella is the next level of investigation and is probably best done in conjunction with a consultant.[1]

The most important point about basal serum hormone measurements is that they may be entirely normal even in patients with symptomatic hypopituitarism. They are helpful only if they are abnormal. This is particularly so with hormones secreted in pulsed fashion, such as luteinizing hormone, follicle-stimulating hormone, and growth hormone. Initial blood tests should include complete and differential blood cell counts, electrolytes, prolactin, morning serum cortisol, T_4 and TSH, and follicle-stimulating and luteinizing hormones. Some patients have normocytic normochromic anemia and eosinophilia because of corticotropin deficiencies. Hyponatremia may also be found, but not hyperkalemia as occurs in Addison's disease because the adrenocortical production of aldosterone is not dependent on corticotropin.[1]

REFERENCES

1. Vance ML: Hypopituitarism, *N Engl J Med* 330:1651-1662, 1994.

Pituitary Incidentalomas

(See also effect of screening on apparent prevalence rates)

A pituitary incidentaloma is a lesion of the pituitary gland that is neurologically and endocrinologically inapparent and is discovered incidentally during magnetic resonance imaging or computed tomography. Almost all of them are adenomas, and if they are under 10 mm in diameter, they appear to follow a benign course for at least 6 years.[1] This is not surprising, since it has long been known that up to one fourth of autopsy subjects have small incidental pituitary adenomas.[2]

REFERENCES

1. Donovan LE, Corenblum B: The natural history of the pituitary incidentaloma, *Arch Intern Med* 155:181-183, 1995.
2. McComb DJ, Ryan N, Horvath E, et al: Subclinical adenomas of the human pituitary: new light on old problems, *Arch Pathol Lab Med* 107:488-491, 1983.

MISCELLANEOUS

Topics covered in this section

Pharmaceuticals
Physician-Patient Communications
Prescribing Habits
Risk Analysis
Skepticism
Sleep
Sports Medicine
Surgery
Toxicology
Tropical Medicine
Uncertainty

ALTERNATIVE MEDICINE

(See also antioxidants; nutrition; physician-patient communications; vegetarians; vitamins; vitamin E)

Many terms are encompassed by the term "alternative medicine." An overall encompassing term is "complementary health care services"; synonyms are "unorthodox," "holistic," "unconventional," "questionable," and "new medicine." If such services are offered by qualified physicians, the term "complementary medicine" is used rather than the more encompassing term "complementary health care services," which refers to care administered by physicians or nonphysicians.[1,2]

Some of the specific programs covered under the rubrics "alternative medicine" or "complementary health care services" are classic Chinese medicine (including acupuncture), Indian Ayurveda medicine, chiropractic, massage, homeopathy, mind-body medicine (e.g., biofeedback, visual imagery, meditation, hypnosis, yoga, t'ai chi), pharmacological or biological therapies (e.g., chelation therapy for vascular disease), herbal medicine, naturopathy, reflexology, faith healing, and nutritional therapy.[1,2]

Whether physicians like it or not, alternative medicine plays a major role in the health care systems of the Western world. At least one third of Americans use some form of alternative therapy, and most of them do not tell their physicians they are doing so.[3] From the patient's viewpoint, seeing an alternative medical practitioner does not necessarily preclude conventional medical treatment; many receive both concurrently.[1,2,4] Alternative medicine seems to have a special appeal for cancer patients. An estimated one half of cancer patients seek some form of alternative medicine, and of these half give up standard medical treatment.[4]

Some of the products marketed as "natural" or "herbal" food supplements in the United States have been documented to have serious adverse effects because they contain toxic ingredients. For example, the alkaloid ephedrine, which is found in a number of remedies, has been reported to cause paranoid psychosis, hypertension, coronary spasm, convulsions, coma, and death; such adverse effects are not necessarily dose related.[6] Hepatotoxicity has been reported with germander,[7] jin bu huan,[8] and chaparral (creosote bush, grease-wood).[9]

Appeal of Alternative Medicine

Various reasons have been given to explain why patients seek alternative therapies. Sometimes it is because they have chronic diseases, such as cancer or AIDS, and think that they have exhausted the potential of traditional medicine. Another important reason is that many patients feel they will be given more time, be listened to with more respect, and be treated more as a whole person by alternative practitioners than would be the case with traditional practitioners.[2,10]

Attitudes of Physicians to Alternative Medicine

Many physicians refer patients to alternative practitioners, particularly chiropractors and acupuncturists.[11,12] In a survey of general practitioners in Quebec, 59% referred patients to physicians practicing alternative medicine and 68% to nonmedical practitioners.[11] In a similar study of physicians in Alberta and Ontario, 54% referred patients to alternative practitioners.[12] A survey of 12 studies on the attitudes of physicians toward complementary medicine (in the United Kingdom, Germany, Sweden, The Netherlands, Israel, and New Zealand) found that most considered such practices moderately effective. The studies did not address the issue of whether physicians believed this was because of placebo effect.[13]

Marketing Strategies

A technique some alternative medicine and health food proponents use to promote their products is to impress the consumer with obfuscating scientific jargon. This approach is most successful when one of the many items advocated has some preliminary or proven credibility in the scientific community. A current example is vitamin E and its antioxidant effects.

Another marketing technique is the distribution of videotapes in which "experts" laud the scientific breakthrough of antioxidants, chromium, chelated minerals, and so on. In one such tape I viewed, the expert was introduced as "Director of Surgical Research" in a U.S. medical institution; no statement was made that he had ever done any work in the field he was promoting.

Specific Dietary Supplements

A wide variety of agents, including almost all vitamins and many minerals, are sold in health food stores as dietary supplements. Only selected agents are discussed below. Two examples are described here.

Dehydroepiandrosterone (DHEA) has become an extremely popular "dietary supplement" sold by health food stores. It is reputed to do many things, including improve libido; increase muscle mass; strengthen the immune system; prevent non-insulin-dependent diabetes mellitus, cancer, and heart disease; slow down the process of memory loss; and help in the treatment of Parkinson's disease and Alzheimer's disease. None of these benefits has been demonstrated in large randomized placebo-controlled trials, and the long-term safety of the product is unknown.[14]

The eosinophilia-myalgia syndrome is characterized by myalgia, fatigue, arthralgia, peripheral edema, rash, and eosinophilia. A number of cases developed in 1989 and appeared to be associated with the ingestion of large quantities of contaminated L-tryptophan originating from one manufacturer. This substance, called "peak E," seems to trigger eosinophils and other inflammatory cells and so initiated the disease process.[15] In many cases symptoms persist for months or years.[16-18] With time, however, symptoms abate.[19,20] One study found that within 18 to 24 months most symptoms and physical findings had resolved except for cognitive changes; the only helpful treatment in the acute phase was prednisone.[19]

Chiropractic

A British randomized trial of the management of back pain by chiropractic clinics or hospital outpatient departments found that at 3 years patients treated by chiropractors had more pain relief but that more patients seen by chiropractors were still receiving back pain treatments.[21] A North Carolina observational study found that at 6 months patients with low back pain treated by primary care physicians, orthopedic surgeons, or chiropractors had equally good results. The cost was least for primary care physicians, but satisfaction was greatest for chiropractors and orthopedic surgeons. Chiropractic treatment was expensive because of multiple visits.[22]

Homeopathy

Some individual trials and metaanalyses report that in at least some instances homeopathy is effective.[23-26] On the other hand, many studies fail to show any benefit.[26]

Homeopathy was founded by Samuel Hahnemann in Germany in the late 18th century. Its popularity has waxed and waned over the centuries. At present it is on the upswing in North America but even more so in Europe where many conventional physicians also use homeopathic treatment.[26]

Two of the principles of homeopathic therapy are[26]:

1. An effective drug will produce in normal individuals symptoms similar to those experienced by the patient (law of similars).
2. Before use a drug should be diluted in water and shaken many times (succussion) so the concentration is minuscule. In some cases no molecules of the original drug remain, but to homeopathists this does not matter because in some undefined way the message of the drug is passed on in the water, the so-called memory of water.

In view of the unscientific basis for such therapeutic regimens, many physicians attribute the reported successes of homeopathy, as well as its popularity, to a powerful placebo effect. This is probably brought about in part by the taking of a long and sympathetic history, a procedure that many patients find contrasts sharply with their experience in conventional medical settings.[26]

Herbal Products

Herbal products are widely used, and in Canada and many other countries these products are poorly regulated. Their degree of benefit and of adverse effects is largely unknown because of lack of studies.[27] However, it is clear that serious and sometimes fatal adverse effects do occur.[27,28] Furthermore, even if benefits are proven, standardization of the products is unlikely under current regulatory systems because of biological differences in soil and growth conditions, as well as diverse methods of collection, extraction, and storage.[27]

REFERENCES

1. La Valley JW: Integrating complementary medicine and health care services into practice (editorial), *Can Med Assoc J* 153:45-49, 1995.
2. Gordon JS: Alternative medicine and the family physician, *Am Fam Physician* 54:2205-2212, 1996.
3. Eisenberg DM, Kessler RC, Foster C, et al: Unconventional medicine in the United States: prevalence, costs, and patterns of use, *N Engl J Med* 328:246-252, 1993.
4. Murray RG, Rubel AJ: Physicians and healers: unwilling partners in health care, *N Engl J Med* 326:61-64, 1992.
5. Bourgeault IL: Physicians' attitudes toward patients' use of alternative cancer therapies, *Can Med Assoc J* 155:1679-1685, 1996.
6. Centers for Disease Control and Prevention: Adverse events associated with ephedrine-containing products—Texas, December 1993–September 1995, *JAMA* 276:1711-1712, 1996.
7. Larry D, Vial T, Pauwels A, et al: Hepatitis after germander *(Teucrium chamaedrys)* administration: another instance of herbal medicine hepatotoxicity, *Ann Intern Med* 117:129-132, 1992.
8. Woolf GM, Petrovic LM, Rojter SE, et al: Acute hepatitis associated with the Chinese herbal product jin bu huan, *Ann Intern Med* 121:729-735, 1994.
9. Sheikh NM, Philen RM, Love LA: Chaparral-associated hepatotoxicity, *Arch Intern Med* 157:913-919, 1997.
10. Chung MK: Why alternative medicine? (editorial), *Am Fam Physician* 54:2184-2187, 1996.
11. Goldszmidt M, Leveitt C, Duarte-Franco E, et al: Complementary health care services: a survey of general practitioners' views, *Can Med Assoc J* 153:29-35, 1995.
12. Verhoef MJ, Sutherland LR: Alternative medicine and general practitioners: opinions and behaviour, *Can Fam Physician* 41:1005-1011, 1995.
13. Ernst E, Rexch K-L, White AR: Complementary medicine: what physicians think of it; a meta-analysis, *Arch Intern Med* 155:2405-2408, 1995.
14. Skolnick AA: Scientific verdict still out on DHEA, *JAMA* 276:1365-1367, 1996.
15. Varga J, Uitto J, Jimenez SA: The cause and pathogenesis of the eosinophilia-myalgia syndrome, *Ann Intern Med* 116:140-147, 1992.
16. Kaufman LD: Chronicity of the eosinophilia-myalgia syndrome: a reassessment after three years, *Arthritis Rheum* 37:84-87, 1994.
17. Sack KE, Criswell LA: Eosinophilia-myalgia syndrome: the aftermath, *South Med J* 85:878-882, 1992.

18. Hedberg K, Urbach D, Slutsker L, et al: Eosinophilia-myalgia syndrome: natural history in a population-based cohort, *Arch Intern Med* 152:1889-1892, 1992.
19. Hertzman PA, Clauw DJ, Kaufman LD, et al: The eosinophilia-myalgia syndrome: status of 205 patients and results of treatment 2 years after onset, *Ann Intern Med* 122:851-855, 1995.
20. Sullivan EA, Kamb ML, Jones JL, et al: The natural history of eosinophilia-myalgia syndrome in a tryptophan-exposed cohort in South Carolina, *Arch Intern Med* 156:973-979, 1996.
21. Meade TW, Dyer S, Browne W, et al: Randomised comparison of chiropractic and hospital outpatient management for low back pain: results from extended follow up, *BMJ* 311:349-351, 1995.
22. Carey TS, Garrett J, Jackman A, et al: The outcomes and costs of care for acute low back pain among patients seen by primary care practitioners, chiropractors, and orthopedic surgeons, *N Engl J Med* 333:913-917, 1995.
23. Reilly D, Taylor MA, Beattie NG, et al: Is evidence for homeopathy reproducible? *Lancet* 344:1601-1606, 1994.
24. Kleijnen J, Knipschild P, ter Riet G: Clinical trials of homeopathy, *BMJ* 302:316-323, 1991.
25. Beaulieu M-D: Homéopathie: des résultats reproductibles? *Omnipraticien* 3:1, 8, 10-11, 1995.
26. Ernst E, Kaptchuk TJ: Homeopathy revisited (editorial), *Arch Intern Med* 156:2162-2164, 1996.
27. Kozyrskyj A: Herbal products in Canada: how safe are they? *Can Fam Physician* 43:697-702, 1997.
28. Huxtable RJ: The myth of beneficent nature: the risks of herbal preparations, *Ann Intern Med* 117:165-167, 1992.

ASPIRIN

(See also anemia; asthma; asthma in children; atrial fibrillation; coronary artery disease; myocardial infarction; unstable angina; thrombophlebitis; cerebrovascular accidents; niacin derivatives; transient ischemic attacks; migraines; colon cancer; gout; peptic ulcer; nonsteroidal antiinflammatory drugs)

Aspirin has multiple reputed and proven benefits. It is also well known to have adverse effects on the gastrointestinal tract and to precipitate asthma in susceptible persons. Only a few of these topics are discussed here; others can be found elsewhere in the text.

Prevention of Neoplasms

Evidence suggests that regular aspirin use decreases the risk of several types of cancer. The most striking is colon cancer (see discussion of colon cancer). Other cancer sites where regular aspirin use is said to reduce risk are the esophagus, stomach, rectum, lung, and breast.[1,2] The absolute reduction rates are low, and whether potential benefits outweigh risks has not been established.

Pathophysiology of Antithrombotic Effect

Aspirin irreversibly acetylates and inactivates the enzyme cyclooxygenase. Cyclooxygenase is necessary for the formation of thromboxane A_2, which in turn causes platelet aggregation. This effect is produced within 1 hour by the oral ingestion of 100 mg of aspirin. However, aspirin also irreversibly inhibits endothelial cell prostacyclin, a potent inhibitor of platelet aggregation. Some workers have hypothesized that lower doses of acetylsalicylic acid given at longer intervals may be the most effective prophylactic program against thromboembolic phenomena because they will cause less inhibition of endothelial prostacyclin.[3]

Gastrointestinal Bleeding

One of the major adverse effects of aspirin is an increased incidence of gastrointestinal bleeding. An increased incidence of clinically significant bleeding episodes has been documented even with daily doses as low as 75[4] or 100 mg.[5] The 100-mg study emanating from Australia enrolled 400 men and women with an age range of 70 to 90 years.[5] Over a 1-year period the total percentage of overt bleeding episodes was 3% in treated patients versus none in the control group. In addition, the hemoglobin concentration of the treated group dropped by a mean of 0.33 g/dl (33 g/L), which was statistically significant, but more important, 17.4% of the aspirin-treated group had a reduction of 1 g/dl (100 g/L) or more compared with 9.3% of the control subjects. The mean corpuscular volume increased in the treated group compared with the placebo group, perhaps because of an increase in reticulocytes. Gastrointestinal symptoms were reported by 18% of those taking aspirin and by 12.5% of those given placebo.[5] Similar results have been reported in a Canadian study.[6]

In a British case-controlled study the odds ratio for bleeding peptic ulcer disease in patients taking regular doses of aspirin was 2.3 for 75 mg/day, 3.2 for 150 mg/day, and 3.9 for 300 mg/day. For enteric-coated aspirin it was only 1.1.[7]

Aspirin Sensitivity

Aspirin sensitivity with bronchospasm that is not allergic or IgE mediated occurs in about 20% of persons with asthma.[8]

REFERENCES

1. Thun MJ, Namboodiri MM, Calle EE, et al: Aspirin use and risk of fatal cancer, *Cancer Res* 53:60-74, 1993.
2. Schreinemachers DM, Everson RB: Aspirin use and lung, colon, and breast cancer incidence in a prospective study, *Epidemiology* 5:138-146, 1994.
3. Patrono C: Aspirin as an antiplatelet drug, *N Engl J Med* 330: 1287-1294, 1994.
4. SALT Collaborative Group: Swedish aspirin low-dose trial (SALT) of 75 mg aspirin as secondary prophylaxis after cerebrovascular ischaemic events, *Lancet* 338:1345-1349, 1991.
5. Silagy CA, McNeil JJ, Donnan GA, et al: Adverse effects of low-dose aspirin in a healthy elderly population, *Clin Pharmacol Ther* 54:84-89, 1993.
6. Leibovici A, Lavi N, Wainstok S, et al: Low-dose acetylsalicylic acid use and hemoglobin levels: effects in a primary care population, *Can Fam Physician* 41:64-68, 1995.
7. Weil J, Colinjones D, Langman M, et al: Prophylactic aspirin and risk of peptic ulcer bleeding, *BMJ* 310:827-830, 1995.

8. Manning ME, Stevenson DD: Aspirin sensitivity: a distressing reaction that is now often treatable, *Postgrad Med* 90:227-233, 1991.

ATTITUDES, PHYSICIAN

(See also consensus conferences; detrimental effects of investigations; gestational diabetes mellitus; guidelines for screening or case finding; informed consent; insulin therapy for non-insulin-dependent diabetes mellitus; intensive treatment in preventing diabetic complications in non-insulin-dependent diabetes mellitus; investigations; labeling; risk analysis; practice patterns; prevention; risk assessment in pregnancy; screening; skepticism; uncertainty)

Physicians in their attitudes toward case finding and screening procedures have been categorized by Stephenson as maximalists ("If in doubt, screen") or minimalists ("If in doubt, don't screen").[1] A third category, ritualists ("I was taught it, so I do it") has been added by Jeyapragasan and Morris.[2]

According to Stephenson, the Maximum School is based on three concepts:

1. One must prevent the worst possible eventuality.
2. Interventions are beneficial and do not have serious side effects.
3. The anxiety provoked in physicians by uncertainty can be relieved by accepting protocols or courses of action that by implication guarantee successful outcomes.

The Minimum School is based on three different tenets. These are:

1. Patient care must be based on evidence.
2. "Above all, do no harm," or in more technical terms, avoid malfeasance. In other words, consider the detrimental effects of any intervention.
3. Management should be individualized, and this takes precedence over following protocols.

A similar division was made by Sackett and Holland[3] in 1975; they divided physicians into "advocates" and "methodologists"[3] or, as they later referred to them, "evangelists" and "snails." As Davidoff[4] put it in the context of the cholesterol screening debate, evangelists believe it would be wrong to withhold a preventive program that might be beneficial and that has undemonstrated harm, whereas snails believe it would be wrong to impose an intervention that has undemonstrated benefits and has the potential for harm. There is no right answer here; it is a difference in values that is an inevitable result of scientific uncertainty.[4]

"Practice style" is a term that often reflects physicians' attitudes. An example is the tendency of obstetricians to perform Cesarean deliveries on women with gestational diabetes even when no evidence of macrosomia is present.[5] In some cases it seems that "practice style" is a euphemism for "ritualistic behavior."

Different specialists may hold different attitudes toward the same clinical problem. For example, in a survey of a variety of specialties, cardiologists were found to be the most likely to proceed with cardiopulmonary resuscitation for terminal illnesses and oncologists the least likely to do so.[6]

The training of young physicians in hospitals where errors of omission are considered much more serious than those of commission may foster the attitude that many investigations are better than few and that investigations do no harm.[7]

REFERENCES

1. Stephenson MJ: Gestational diabetes mellitus (editorial), *Can Fam Physician* 39:745-748, 1993.
2. Jeyapragasan M, Morris B: Are you a maximalist, a minimalist, or a ritualist? (letter), *Can Fam Physician* 39:1878, 1881, 1993.
3. Sackett DL, Holland WW: Controversy in the detection of disease, *Lancet* 2:357-359, 1975.
4. Davidoff F: Evangelists and snails redux; the case of cholesterol screening, *Ann Intern Med* 124:513-514, 1996.
5. Naylor CD, Sermer M, Chen E, Sykora K (Toronto Trihospital Gestational Diabetes Investigators): Cesarean delivery in relation to birth weight and gestational glucose tolerance: pathophysiology or practice style? *JAMA* 275:1165-1170, 1996.
6. Hanson LC, Danis M, Garrett JM, Mutran E: Physicians' willingness to use life-sustaining treatment, *Arch Intern Med* 156: 785-789, 1996.
7. Woolf SH, Kamerow DB: Testing for uncommon conditions: the heroic search for positive test results, *Arch Intern Med* 150: 2451-2458, 1990.

AVIATION MEDICINE

(See also cardiopulmonary resuscitation; middle ear effusion; pneumothorax)

Aerotitis Media

A study of 250 volunteers with a history of recurrent ear discomfort when flying were selected at random to receive 120 mg of oral pseudoephedrine (Sudafed) or placebo 30 minutes before departure. Ear discomfort was reported by 32% of those taking pseudoephedrine but 62% of those given placebo.[1]

Spread of Infections on Aircraft

One of the concerns about air travel is the possiblity of increased risk of infection in the cabin environment. An evaluation of the concentration of organisms in the cabin air of domestic and international flights found the levels to be much lower than those in community locations such as buses, shopping centers, or airline terminals.[2]

The number of air exchanges per hour in an aircraft cabin varies with cruise conditions and ranges from 5 to 42. This compares favorably with the 6 air exchanges per hour recommended for hospital isolation rooms housing patients with active tuberculosis.[3] In first-generation jet passenger aircraft all air exchanges used outside compressed air that was heated by the engines to 250° C, compressed, and cooled. In aircraft built since the mid-1980s half of cabin air is fresh and half recirculated, but it is passed through high-efficiency particulate filters.[4]

Many organisms that infect the respiratory tract are spread by large droplets that fall rapidly to the floor. Examples are streptococci, meningococci, and even hemorrhagic fever viruses such as Ebola.[4] Of more concern regarding air travel are organisms spread by tiny aerosol droplets, which in theory could circulate and recirculate in the cabin air for prolonged periods. Examples are measles, influenza, and tuberculosis.[4]

Studies of actual transmission of infections in the aircraft cabin environment are few. One dramatic example was an outbreak of influenza affecting 59% of the occupants of a Boeing 737. The aircraft was delayed on the runway for 3 hours before takeoff, and the ventilation system was defective.[4]

An event widely reported in the popular press was the transmission of tuberculosis from a flight attendant to fellow crew members; the transmission rate correlated with the number of hours of contact. Whether any passengers were affected is uncertain.[6] In 1994 a 32-year-old Korean woman with advanced pulmonary tuberculosis that led to her death 2 weeks later flew from Chicago to Honolulu on a Boeing 747 100 aircraft. She was seated at the back of the rear cabin for the flight, which lasted 8 hours and 45 minutes.[7] Intensive follow-up of the passengers and crew showed no purified protein derivative (PPD) conversion among individuals sitting in other cabin sections. Among those who had been in the same section, six individuals with no other risk factors for tuberculosis had positive PPD tests and four of these were passengers who had sat within two rows of the index case. This study makes it clear that the transmission of the disease was not through the aircraft's recirculation system.[7] As far as I can see, infectious disease transmission as described above could have occurred in many other locations and there is no reason to consider an aircraft cabin a particularly risky environment.

Food poisoning is another uncommon infectious disease risk in commercial air travel. Most cases are caused by *Salmonella* species, and the chances of being affected are much greater among first-class or Concorde (supersonic) passengers than among tourist-class passengers.[8] Bugs as well as people like first-class food.

Flight Emergencies

Major medical emergencies aboard commercial aircraft are rare, an estimated one occurrence in 753 flights.[9] In 1994 British Airways reported 2078 in-flight emergencies; in 559 instances physician or nursing assistance was requested, and in 18 cases unscheduled landings were required.[10] In one emergency a 39-year-old woman on a Hong Kong–London flight became dyspneic because of tension pneumothorax resulting from a motorcycle accident on the way to the airport. Auscultation and percussion were not possible, and the diagnosis was based on the history, severe dyspnea, and deviation of the trachea. A urinary catheter was used as a chest tube, and a coat hanger served as a trocar to insert it into the pleural cavity. An Evian bottle served as an underwater seal and was connected to the catheter with a length of oxygen tubing. The patient did fine.[10]

Semiautomatic external defibrillators that can identify abnormal cardiac rhythms and apply appropriate shocks are available on some airliners. Senior members of the cabin crew are trained to operate them. Qantas Airlines has been a leader in this field and has received the unexpected benefit that aircraft diversions have decreased since the machines were installed.[11]

Jet Lag

Jet lag is a common result of crossing five or more time zones. Adjustment to a new time zone takes longer after an eastward than after a westward flight. Suggested preventive and management protocols are a good night's sleep before the flight, avoidance of alcohol during the flight, ingestion of plenty of fluids to avoid dehydration, and immediate adjustment to the time cycle of the destination. Exposure to several hours of bright outdoor light on arrival seems to be beneficial.[12]

Whether melatonin is effective in controlling jet lag is controversial.[12-15] Secretion of this pineal gland hormone is controlled by the suprachiasmatic nucleus in the hypothalamus, and this in turn is regulated by light. Light inhibits the secretion of melatonin, and darkness fosters its production. Thus the blood levels of melatonin are high at night and low during the day.[13,15] At present its use for jet lag should be considered experimental.[12]

Occupational Risks of Crew

A study of Finnish Airline cabin attendants found an excess of breast cancer and bone cancer (one chondrosarcoma and one malignant chordoma) among women and no significant increase in cancers among men. One hypothesis for this increase is excessive exposure to ionizing radiation.[16]

REFERENCES

1. Csortan E, Jones J, Haan M, et al: Efficacy of pseudoephedrine for the prevention of barotrauma during air travel, *Ann Emerg Med* 23:1324-1327, 1994.
2. Wick RL Jr, Irvine LA: The microbiological composition of airliner cabin air, *Aviat Space Environ Med* 66:220-224, 1995.
3. Centers for Disease Control: Guidelines for preventing the transmission of tuberculosis in health-care settings with special focus on HIV-related issues, *MMWR* 39:1-29, 1990.
4. Wenzel RP: Airline travel and infection (editorial), *N Engl J Med* 334:981-982, 1996.
5. Moser MR, Bender TR, Margolis HS, et al: An outbreak of influenza aboard a commercial airliner, *Am J Epidemiol* 110:1-6, 1979.
6. Driver CR, Valway SE, Morgan WM, et al: Transmission of *Mycobacterium tuberculosis* associated with air travel, *JAMA* 272:1031-1035, 1994.
7. Kenyon TA, Valway SE, Ihle WW, et al: Transmission of multidrug-resistant *Mycobacterium tuberculosis* during a long airplane flight, *N Engl J Med* 334:933-938, 1996.
8. Tauxe RV, Tormey MP, Mascola L, et al: Salmonellosis outbreak on transatlantic flights: foodborne illness on aircraft: 1947-1984, *Am J Epidemiol* 125:150-157, 1987.

9. Cummings RO, Schubach JA: Frequency and types of medical emergencies among commercial air travelers, *JAMA* 261:1295-1299, 1989.
10. Wallace WA, Wong T, O'Bichere A, et al: Managing in flight emergencies, *BMJ* 311:374-376, 1995.
11. Jeffrey S: Aircraft defibrillators save lives, money, *Med Post*, April 22, 1997.
12. Canada communicable disease report: travel statement on jet lag, *Can Med Assoc J* 155:61-63, 1996.
13. Brown GM: Light, melatonin and the sleep-wake cycle, *J Psychiatry Neurosci* 19:345-353, 1994.
14. Arendt J: Melatonin (editorial), *BMJ* 312:1242-1243, 1996.
15. Epstein FH: Melatonin in humans, *N Engl J Med* 336:186-195, 1997.
16. Pukkala E, Auvinen A, Wahlberg G: Incidence of cancer among Finnish Airline cabin attendants, 1967-92, *BMJ* 311: 649-652, 1995.

BED REST COMPLICATIONS

The following are some of the important complications of bed rest[1,2]:

1. Musculoskeletal
   a. Muscle weakness and atrophy. A muscle at complete rest loses 10% to 15% of its strength each week. Nearly 50% of normal strength is lost in 3 to 5 weeks. Strength is recovered at a rate of only 6% per week. Associated with weakness is decreased endurance, manifested as fatigue and muscle atrophy.
   b. Contractures
   c. Disuse osteoporosis
2. Cardiovascular
   a. Increased heart rate. The heart rate increases by 1 beat per minute every 2 days during bed rest. The maximum heart rate resulting from bed rest alone is about 80 beats per minute.
   b. Decreased cardiac output
   c. Orthostatic hypotension. Orthostatic hypotension develops after 3 weeks of bed rest in most adults and sooner in the elderly.
   d. Thromboembolism
3. Respiratory
   a. Decreased ventilation
   b. Atelectasis and pneumonia
4. Metabolic
   a. Glucose intolerance. Glucose intolerance in patients confined to bed is due to increased insulin resistance.
   b. Decreased metabolic rate
   c. Negative nitrogen balance
   d. Hypercalcemia and renal stones (usually with coma or quadriplegia)
5. Gastrointestinal
   a. Anorexia
   b. Constipation
6. Dermatological
   a. Pressure sores
7. Central nervous system
   a. Decreased balance and coordination. Decreased balance and coordination are due not only to muscle weakness but also to deficits in neural control.
8. Social
   a. Social isolation
   b. Dependency

REFERENCES

1. Dittmer DK, Teasell R: Complications of immobilization and bed rest. I. Musculoskeletal and cardiovascular complications, *Can Fam Physician* 39:1428-1432, 1435-1437, 1993.
2. Teasell R, Kittmer DK: Complications of immobilization and bed rest. II. Other complications, *Can Fam Physician* 39:1440-1442, 1445-1446, 1993.

BITES

Cat and Dog Bites

(See also human bites; snake bites)

Epidemiology

Bites account for about 1% of emergency room visits. The incidence varies from one institution to another. Dog bites are responsible for 80% to 90% of all bites assessed by physicians, cat bites for 5% to 15%, and human bites for 3% to 20%.[1] It has been estimated that in the United States each year 2% of the population is bitten by dogs.[2]

In about 90% of dog bite cases the animal belongs to or is known to the victim. Most dog bites involve the extremities except in children under 4, who most commonly have bites to the head and neck. Rates of infection from dog bites are low, between 2% and 20%.[1] Encouraging owners to spay or neuter their animals is an important method of decreasing the incidence of dog bites. Infants and toddlers should never be left alone with a dog. Children should be trained to avoid approaching an unknown dog, to stand still and not to scream if approached by a dog, to avoid eye contact with a dog, and if knocked down by a dog, to roll up into a ball and stay perfectly still.[3]

Cat bites are much more likely than dog bites to become infected (30% to 50%). One reason is that the bites are often puncture wounds and involve the hands, which are more susceptible to infection than many other body parts.[1]

Management principles

Animal bites are managed with meticulous wound irrigation and if indicated debridement, as well as assessment for risk of tetanus and rabies. Some authors recommend suturing low-risk bites (bites that are small, not involving the hands, not clinically infected, and seen within 24 hours), particularly those on the face.[1] Antibiotic prophylaxis is discussed below.

Microbiology of animal bites

Most infections caused by cat or dog bites are polymicrobial. On average three different organisms, both aerobic and anaerobic, are cultured from infected wounds. Organisms most frequently responsible for infections in animal bites are *Pasteurella multocida, Staphylococcus* species, *Streptococcus* species, *Corynebacterium* species, *Capnocytophaga canimorsus,* and anaerobes.[1]

P. multocida is a small, difficult to culture, gram-negative aerobic coccobacillus. It is found in 50% to 80% of cat bite wound infections and about 25% of dog bite wounds.[1] However, not all strains of *P. multocida* are equally virulent, and those native to dogs seem less likely to cause infections than those from cat bites.[3] *P. multocida* is sensitive to penicillin, amoxicillin, amoxicillin-clavulanate (Clavulin, Augmentin), cefuroxime (Ceftin), tetracycline, and ciprofloxacin. It is generally resistant to erythromycin.[1]

C. canimorsus is a rare source of infection after dog bites. It is important because it may cause overwhelming sepsis and death. The vast majority of affected patients have had predisposing conditions such as Hodgkin's disease, splenectomy, idiopathic thrombocytopenic purpura, alcoholism, chronic lung disease, or chronic steroid use. *C. canimorsus* is an aerobic gram-negative rod. It is sensitive to penicillin, which is the drug of choice. It is also sensitive in vitro to amoxicillin, erythromycin, tetracycline, and a variety of other antibiotics.[1]

Anaerobes infecting animal bites rarely produce beta-lactamase and so are sensitive to penicillin. This is not the case with anaerobes infecting human bites (see below).[1]

Antibiotic prophylaxis

Some workers advocate antibiotic prophylaxis for all significant bites; others recommend prophylaxis only for high-risk bites (hand bites, deep puncture wounds, most cat bites, and bites affecting asplenic or immunocompromised patients). More controversial is whether antibiotics should be given for moderate or severe wounds and wounds seen after a delay of 8 hours.[1,4,5] Although a 1994 metaanalysis of dog bites showed that antibiotic prophylaxis after dog bites reduced the relative risk of infection by 44%, this translated into an absolute risk reduction of only 4%. In other words, 25 patients would have to be treated for one patient to benefit.[4] Thus there is general agreement that "minor" bite wounds do not need antibiotic prophylaxis.[1] According to one author, if prophylactic antibiotics are to be given, they should be started in the office or emergency room and not several hours later when, with luck, the patient may have filled his or her prescription.[4]

Broad coverage for most cases of dog or cat bites may be achieved with amoxicillin-clavulanate (Clavulin, Augmentin) 500 mg tid or cefuroxime (Ceftin) 500 mg bid. Alternatives for dog bites are penicillin V 500 mg qid, amoxicillin 250 to 500 mg tid, or, for those allergic to penicillin, doxycycline 100 mg bid. Alternatives for cat bites are penicillin 500 mg qid with or without dicloxacillin (Dycill, Dynapen, Pathocil) 500 mg qid, or, for those allergic to penicillin, doxycycline 100 mg bid. Erythromycin is not a good choice, especially for cat bites, because *P. multocida* is often resistant to it. When given prophylactically, these drugs should be used for 3 to 5 days.[1]

REFERENCES

1. Griego RD, Rosen T, Orengo IF, et al: Dog, cat, and human bite: a review, *J Am Acad Dermatol* 33:1019-1029, 1995.
2. Voelker R: Dog bites recognized as public health problem, *JAMA* 277:278-280, 1997.
3. Centers for Disease Control and Prevention: Dog-bite-related fatalities—United States, 1995-1996, *JAMA* 278:278-279, 1997.
4. Callaham M: Prophylactic antibiotics in dog bite wounds (editorial), *Ann Emerg Med* 23:577-579, 1994.
5. Cummings P: Antibiotics to prevent infection in patients with dog bite wounds: a meta-analysis of randomized trials, *Ann Emerg Med* 23:535-540, 1994.

Human Bites

(See also cat and dog bites; snake bites)

One study found that the infection rate of simple human bites sustained in an institution for developmentally disabled persons was about 18% compared with a rate of 13% for simple lacerations occurring in the same population.[1] Although this infection rate is not very high, the situation is different with bites to the hand. Hand bites may be categorized as clenched fist injuries sustained by punching someone in the teeth or as simple bites. Any bite to the hand carries a greater risk of infection than bites elsewhere on the body, but this is particularly so with clenched fist injuries.[2] The actual skin laceration in hand bites may be small, but in many cases the teeth have penetrated closed hand spaces, tendons, or joints.[3] In clenched fist injuries the laceration is often only a 3- to 8-mm puncture wound on the dorsum of the hand or over the third metacarpophalangeal joint.[2] In view of the high incidence of infection and the complexity of the hand, most human bites of the hand require assessment and management by a hand surgeon.[2,3]

Microbiology of human bites

Like cat and dog bites, infections from human bites are almost always polymicrobial. An average of five different organisms are cultured.[2] The organisms from human bites are those of the oral flora and include alpha-hemolytic streptococci, beta-hemolytic streptococci, *Staphylococcus aureus, Staphylococcus epidermidis, Eikenella corrodens,* and anaerobes.

E. corrodens is a gram-negative facultative anaerobe that can be cultured from about 25% of human bite wounds. It causes serious indolent infections. The organism is sensitive to penicillin, amoxicillin-clavulanate (Clavulin, Augmentin), tetracycline, trimethoprim-sulfamethoxazole (Septra, Bactrim), and ciprofloxacin. It is usually resistant to erythromycin, dicloxacillin, cloxacillin, nafcillin, and first-generation cephalosporins.

Anaerobes can be cultured from nearly 50% of human bite wound infections. Unlike the anaerobes of dog and cat bite infections, many of human origin produce beta-lactamase and are penicillin resistant.

Antibiotic prophylaxis

Whether all human bites (except the most minimal injuries) require prophylactic antibiotics is controversial. However, if the bite involves the hand, prophylactic antibiotics should certainly be given.[1,4] This approach is supported by a prospective study of uncomplicated human bites of the hand that were treated with mechanical wound care alone or accompanied by prophylactic antibiotics. No infections occurred in those who received antibiotics, whereas the infection rate was 47% in those who did not.[4] Other indications for prophylactic antibiotics are similar to those for cat and dog bites.[1]

Broad coverage for most cases of human bites may be achieved by amoxicillin-clavulanate (Clavulin, Augmentin) 500 mg tid or cefuroxime (Ceftin) 500 mg bid. Alternatives are penicillin 500 mg qid (covers *E. corrodens*) plus dicloxacillin (Dycill, Dynapen, Pathocil) 500 mg qid (covers *S. aureus*) or, for those allergic to penicillin, doxycycline 100 mg bid. Erythromycin is not a good choice because *E. corrodens* tends to be resistant to it. When given prophylactically, these drugs should be used for 3 to 5 days.[1]

REFERENCES

1. Lindsay D, Christopher M, Hollenbach J, et al: Natural course of the human bite wound: incidence of infection and complications in 434 bites and 803 lacerations in the same group of patients, *J Trauma* 27:45-48, 1987.
2. Griego RD, Rosen T, Orengo IF, et al: Dog, cat, and human bite: a review, *J Am Acad Dermatol* 33:1019-1029, 1995.
3. Kelly IP, Cunney RJ, Smyth EG, et al: The management of human bite injuries of the hand, *Injury* 27:481-484, 1996.
4. Zubowicz VN, Gravier M: Management of early human bites of the hand: a prospective randomized study, *Plast Reconstr Surg* 88:111-114, 1991.

Snake Bites

(See also cat and dog bites; human bites)

North America has only two families of poisonous snakes. The pit vipers belong to the family Crotalidae and include rattlesnakes, cottonmouths, and copperheads. The Elapidae family includes the coral snakes, which are found only in the southern United States. In Canada the only poisonous snakes are rattlesnakes. The term "pit viper" comes from the presence of a heat-sensitive pit between the eyes and the nostrils. Other identifying features of pit vipers are their vertically elliptical pupils (cat's eye pupils), which contrast with the round pupils of nonvenomous snakes, and in rattlesnakes the presence of a rattle on the tail.[1]

Up to 30% of proven bites are "dry bites" in which no envenomation occurs. Symptoms and signs of pit viper envenomation are severe pain and burning followed by increasing edema, ecchymosis, and constitutional symptoms.

Field therapy for poisonous snake bites consists of immobilizing the bitten appendage, which should be kept below heart level, and removing the patient to an emergency room as quickly as possible. Constricting bands such as elastic bandages should be applied 5 to 10 cm proximal to the bite and kept sufficiently loose to allow the fifth finger to be slipped between the bands and the skin without causing discomfort. The bands should be periodically loosened and readjusted as edema evolves. The purpose of the bands is to decrease lymph flow without obstructing venous return. Incision and suction of the wound in the field are not recommended.

Hospital treatment consists of supportive care, antibiotics, tetanus booster if necessary, and IV administration of 4 to 20 vials of antivenin. Antivenin is made from immune horse serum, so skin testing is mandatory before administration. Wyeth's Crotalidae antivenin covers copperheads, cottonmouths, and rattlesnakes but not coral snakes.

REFERENCES

1. Forks TP: Evaluation and treatment of poisonous snakebites, *Am Fam Physician* 50:123-130, 1994.

CHRONIC FATIGUE SYNDROME

(See also fibromyalgia; multiple chemical sensitivities)

Chronic fatigue syndrome, fibromyalgia, and multiple chemical sensitivities are three conditions whose existence is controversial, and the symptoms and epidemiology of the three entities overlap. Believers search ever more intensely for organic causes such as occult infections or subtle immunological dysfunctions, while unbelievers attribute the symptoms to a variety of functional somatic symptoms that may or may not fit into well-defined psychiatric disorders such as depression, somatoform disorder, or one of the personality disorders.[1,2] Many skeptics are loath to make a diagnosis of "chronic fatigue syndrome," not only because of the lack of scientific evidence supporting its existence, but also because of fear that such a diagnosis would become a self-fulfilling prophecy. On the other hand, many patients who receive the diagnose feel enabled rather than disabled; being labeled as having chronic fatigue syndrome affirms for them that their illness is genuine.[3] Whether chronic fatigue syndrome is a new disorder or simply a new name for "neurasthenia," which was a frequently diagnosed condition in the latter half of the 19th and early decades of the 20th century, is unknown. Abbey and Garfinkel[2] point out striking similarities in the epidemiology and clinical descriptions of the two conditions, and Ware and Kleinman[4] suggest that in both conditions symptoms serve as a metaphor for unacceptable social stresses.

Chronic fatigue syndrome has a variety of definitions. One current example is unexplained (recognized organic and psychiatric disorders having been ruled out) new-onset persistent or recurring fatigue that lasts 6 months or more and substantially reduces the functional level plus four of the following symptoms, which must not have predated the onset of the illness[5]:

1. Self-reported decrease in short-term memory or concentration
2. Sore throat
3. Tender cervical or axillary lymph nodes
4. Muscle pains
5. Multiple arthralgias without swelling or redness
6. Headaches
7. Unrefreshing sleep
8. Postexertional malaise lasting over 24 hours

The chronic fatigue syndrome is most commonly diagnosed in middle-aged women.[1,6,7] One fairly frequent characteristic of the syndrome is its sudden onset coincident with a flulike illness. For believers this is proof positive that the disorder is organic.[6] However, other workers consider psychiatric disorders to be responsible for the symptoms in many patients. In one 1989 study patients who met the extant CDC criteria for chronic fatigue syndrome and who were referred from all over the United States for an acyclovir trial at the National Institutes of Health were assessed psychiatrically; 75% were found to have psychiatric disorders. Over half of the 75% were depressed, and the next most frequent disorders recorded were dysthymia and simple phobias.[7] Another study found that 27% of 565 patients with chronic fatigue syndrome met the clinical criteria for somatoform disorder.[8]

The natural history of chronic fatigue syndrome has not been fully defined. An 18-month follow-up of 298 self-referred patients meeting the criteria of chronic fatigue syndrome found that 3% reported complete recovery and 17% had improvement.[9]

As would be expected, optimal treatment for a condition of unknown etiology is uncertain. A 1996 study from the Netherlands found no benefit from an 8-week treatment regimen of fluoxetine (Prozac) 20 mg.[10] On the other hand, a series of 13[11] or 16[12] weekly or biweekly sessions of cognitive therapy was associated with a satisfactory outcome in about three fourths of treated patients compared with about one fourth of the control subjects who received either relaxation therapy[11] or general medical care from their general practitioners.[12] A randomized controlled trial of graded aerobic exercises versus flexibility exercises and relaxation therapy found a marked improvement with aerobic exercises.[13]

REFERENCES

1. Buchwald D, Garrity D: Comparison of patients with chronic fatigue syndrome, fibromyalgia, and multiple chemical sensitivities, *Arch Intern Med* 154:2049-2053, 1994.
2. Abbey S, Garfinkel P: Neurasthenia and chronic fatigue syndrome: the role of culture in the making of a diagnosis, *Am J Psychiatry* 148:1638-1646, 1991.
3. Woodward RV, Broom DH, Legge DG: Diagnosis in chronic disease: disabling or enabling; the case of chronic fatigue syndrome, *J R Soc Med* 88:325-329, 1995.
4. Ware NC, Kleinman A: Culture and somatic experience: the social course of illness in neurasthenia and chronic fatigue syndrome, *Psychosom Med* 20:35-53, 1992.
5. Fukuda K, Straus SE, Hickie I, et al (International Chronic Fatigue Syndrome Study Group): The chronic fatigue syndrome: a comprehensive approach to its definition and study, *Ann Intern Med* 121:953-959, 1994.
6. Komaroff AL, Buchwald D: Symptoms and signs of chronic fatigue syndrome, *Rev Infect Dis* 13(suppl 1):S8-S11, 1991.
7. Kruese MJ, Dale J, Straus SE: Psychiatric diagnosis in patients who have chronic fatigue syndrome, *J Clin Psychiatry* 50:53-56, 1989.
8. Hickie I, Lloyd A, Hadzi-Pavlovic D, et al: Can the chronic fatigue syndrome be defined by distinct clinical features, *Psychol Med* 25:923-925, 1995.
9. Vercoulen JH, Swanink CM, Fennis JF, et al: Prognosis in chronic fatigue syndrome—a prospective study on the natural course, *J Neurol Neurosurg Psychiatry* 60:489-494, 1996.
10. Vercoulen JH, Swanink CM, Zitman FG, et al: Randomised, double-blind, placebo-controlled study of fluoxetine in chronic fatigue syndrome, *Lancet* 347:858-861, 1996.
11. Deale A, Chalder T, Marks I, et al: Cognitive behavior therapy for chronic fatigue syndrome: a randomized controlled trial, *Am J Psychiatry* 154:408-414, 1997.
12. Sharpe M, Hawton K, Simkin S, et al: Cognitive behaviour therapy for the chronic fatigue syndrome: a randomized controlled trial, *BMJ* 312:22-26, 1996.
13. Fulcher KY, White PD: Randomised controlled trial of graded exercise in patients with the chronic fatigue syndrome, *BMJ* 314:1647-1652, 1997.

CLINICAL PRACTICE GUIDELINES

(See also attitudes, physician; consensus conferences; screening; patient preferences and informed consent; periodic health examination)

Principles

The guiding principles behind the Canadian Clinical Practice Guidelines have been published by the Canadian Medical Association.[1] The 14 guidelines are grouped under three headings: philosophy and ethics, methods and implementation, and evaluation. A few of the important principles enunciated here are that guidelines :

1. Should result in improved health care
2. Must not be so rigid that they inhibit the judgment of individual physicians
3. Should be evidence based and cite the appropriate references
4. Should be reviewed by both experts and users and field tested before implementation

Controversy Over Validity of Guidelines

The merits of clinical practice guidelines are controversial. The raison d'être of such guidelines is to improve the quality of patient care, but some authors fear that health care administrators are using them as cost containment measures. If that happens, clinical practice guidelines may lead to unethical practices.[2] Equally or more important is the question of whether guidelines actually improve patient outcomes. Little research has been done in this area, and what has been published has offered little evidence that they have made a difference in the primary care setting.[3] This may be partly because physicians prefer to use more traditional sources of medical information,[4] but it may also be because physicians are often unaware of the existence of practice guidelines. For example, the U.S. Agency for Health Care Policy and Research (AHCPR) produced and disseminated guidelines on the prevention, diagnosis, and treatment of pressure ulcers in 1992 and 1994, but a survey of family physicians in 1995 found that more than two thirds of the respondents were unaware of them.[5]

There are many reasons for being skeptical about certain guidelines.[6-8] Guidelines are developed by committees of experts, and herein lies the first bias. Who are the experts and how are they chosen? Do they represent a narrow specialty or a broad spectrum of health care workers? Are the recommendations applicable to primary care practice? Who funded the conference, and did this influence the selection or opinions of the participants? Was there political lobbying? Are the final recommendations based on "authoritative opinion" or evidence? Since many organizations produce guidelines, the result is a plethora of often contradictory recommendations. If family physicians favor evidence-based recommendations, they would be wise to put more weight on those from the Canadian Task Force on the Periodic Health Examination or the U.S. Preventive Services Task Force than on those sponsored by specialty societies (e.g., American Urological Association or Society of Obstetricians and Gynecologists of Canada) or disease-specific organizations (e.g., the American Cancer Society).[9,10]

Consensus Conferences

If a consensus conference is held, it usually means that the subjects being dealt with are controversial and therefore that the participants are unlikely to settle the issues no matter how good their intentions. Furthermore, when reading the recommendations of consensus conferences, the physician should realize that unanimity is often not reached. When opinions differ, recommendations are sometimes those of a majority vote,[11] a laudable democratic procedure but one that does not instill confidence about their scientific validity. Finally, it is salutary to remember that expert bodies have on a number of occasions reversed their initial recommendations and that on at least one occasion this seemed to be related to political pressure. In January 1997 a majority report of a National Institute of Health–convened consensus conference stated that evidence was insufficient to recommend universal mammographic screening of women aged 40 to 49. This caused a political furor, and a few months later the National Cancer Institute decreed that women in this age bracket should have screening every 1 to 2 years.[12]

A number of other aspects of consensus conferences may influence the recommendations produced.[6] The most important is probably the membership composition. Often members are chosen for their expertise in a certain area. Their views are already well known, and it is unlikely that they will change during the conference. Does the membership include a balance of disciplines? Have known dissenters or skeptics been invited? Do they have a real voice, or are they token representatives?

The attitudes of the members of a consensus conference are also important.[9,10] Enthusiasts for investigative or therapeutic interventions often take a "maximalist" approach (see discussion of physician attitudes). Maximalists believe that in the face of uncertainty, doing something is always better than doing nothing.[13] This attitude will obviously influence their recommendations.

Aside from the membership composition, knowing the source of financial support for the consensus conference may be important. Does the fact that five pharmaceutical companies, all of which market hormonal products, supported the Canadian Menopause Consensus Conference make a difference, or does it not?[11] In some cases a so-called consensus conference is nothing but a front for drug promotional activities of the sponsoring pharmaceutical industry.[14]

Consensus conferences often produce interesting and useful reports. However, wise physicians read the conclusions both carefully and skeptically. They should not feel obligated to follow the recommendations of a consensus conference if they do not think these are in the best interests of their patients.[6,15,16]

REFERENCES

1. National Partnership for Quality in Health: *Guidelines for Canadian clinical practice guidelines,* Ottawa, 1994, Canadian Medical Association.
2. Berger JT, Rosner F: The ethics of practice guidelines, *Arch Intern Med* 156:2051-2056, 1996.
3. Worrall G, Chaulk P, Freake D: The effects of clinical practice guidelines on patient outcomes in primary care: a systematic review, *Can Med Assoc J* 156:1705-1712, 1997.
4. Hayward RS, Guyatt GH, Moore K-A, et al: Canadian physicians' attitudes about and preferences regarding clinical practice guidelines, *Can Med Assoc J* 156:1715-1723, 1997.
5. Kimura S, Pacala JT: Pressure ulcers in adults: family physicians' knowledge, attitudes, practice preferences and awareness of AHCPR Guidelines, *J Fam Pract* 44:361-368, 1997.
6. Woolf SH: Practice guidelines: what the family physician should know, *Am Fam Physician* 51:1455-1463, 1995.
7. Weingarten S: Practice guidelines and prediction rules should be subject to careful clinical testing (editorial), *JAMA* 277: 1977-1978, 1997.
8. Lewis S: Paradox, process and perception: the role of organizations in clinical practice guidelines development, *Can Med Assoc J* 153:1073-1077, 1995.
9. Czaja R, McFall SL, Warnecke RB, et al: Preferences of community physicians for cancer screening guidelines, *Ann Intern Med* 120:602-608, 1994.
10. Hayward RSA, Steinberg EP, Ford DE, et al: Preventive care guidelines: 1991, *Ann Intern Med* 114:L758-L783, 1991.
11. Canadian Menopause Consensus Conference, *J SOGC* 16:4-40, 1994.

12. Marwick C: Final mammography recommendation? *JAMA* 277:1181, 1997.
13. Stephenson MJ: Gestational diabetes mellitus (editorial), *Can Fam Physician* 39:745-748, 1993.
14. Sheldon TA, Davey Smith G: Consensus conferences as drug promotion, *Lancet* 341:100-102, 1993.
15. Rennie D: Consensus statements, *N Engl J Med* 304:665-666, 1981.
16. The acid test: making clinical sense of the consensus conference on *Helicobacter pylori* (editorial), *JAMA* 272:70-71, 1994.

CONSULTATIONS

(See also practice patterns)

A common form of consultation between primary care physicians and specialists is the "curbside" or "corridor" consultation. These are often done through telephone calls. An analysis by two infectious disease specialists in private practice in the United States found that each had about 25 physician-initiated consultations per month and the average duration was 5 minutes.[1]

Some of the reputed advantages of curbside consultations for the primary care physician are saving of time, verification of correctness of data obtained from manuals or texts, a "free" consultation for the patient, and no fear that the consultant will "steal" the patient. Two advantages for the consultant are a sense of satisfaction in helping colleagues and improving care and the intellectual stimulation of being asked difficult but pertinent questions. For full-time salaried consultants a third advantage is in time management, since curbside consultations take far less time than formal ones.[2]

A disadvantage of curbside consultations is that they are not remunerated for consultants on a fee for service payment system. Even more important, complex problems are difficult to deal with through informal consultations and erroneous advice may be given. A good curbside consultation deals with brief and simple issues, a bad one with complex issues.[1,2] In the study by the infectious disease specialists quoted above, half of the curbside consultations were considered inappropriate because of complexity.[1]

REFERENCES

1. Manian FA, McKinsey DS: A prospective study of 2,092 "curbside" questions asked of two infectious disease consultants in private practice in the Midwest, *Clin Infect Dis* 22:303-307, 1996.
2. Manian FA, Janssen DA: Curbside consultations: a closer look at a common practice, *JAMA* 275:145-147, 1996.

FEVER

(See also febrile seizures; fever in children)

Normal Temperature Values

In young adults rectal temperatures exceeded oral readings by 0.4° C (0.7° F) and these in turn exceeded tympanic readings by 0.4° C (0.7° F). Smoking and mastication have been found to increase oral readings, and this effect persists for longer than 20 minutes. Drinking ice water causes a short-term diminution in temperature readings.[1]

What is a normal temperature, and what is the normal range? Mackowiak and associates[2] studied this in a group of healthy young adult men and women between the ages of 18 and 40. The mean oral temperature was 36.8° C (98.2° F), and 37.7° C (99.9° F) was the upper limit of normal. A diurnal variation with an amplitude of variability of about 0.5° C (0.9° F) was normal with the nadir at 6 AM and the zenith at 4 to 6 PM.[2]

Taking Temperatures

Whether axillary temperatures are accurate is controversial. Shann and Mackenzie[3] from Australia studied temperatures taken by various routes in 120 children of different ages. They concluded that axillary temperatures were accurate. In children over 1 month of age the rectal temperature was very close to 1° C higher than the axillary temperature. During the first 5 weeks of life rectal temperature exceeded axillary temperature by 0.2° C for every week of life. Forehead temperatures were not as accurate as axillary temperatures.[3] However, most other studies have found the axillary route to have a low sensitivity but a high specificity.[4,5] In other words, if the axillary temperature is elevated, the child is febrile, but if it is not, fever cannot be ruled out.

In the past few years noncontact tympanic or external auditory canal thermometers that detect infrared radiation from the tympanic membrane have come into widespread use. How accurate are they? In an emergency room study of children under 4 years the readings of noncontact tympanic thermometers in both the rectal-equivalent mode and the actual-ear mode were compared with rectal temperatures obtained with recently calibrated glass mercury thermometers. With fever defined as at least 38° C (100.4° F) per rectum the noncontact tympanic thermometer in the rectal-equivalent mode had a sensitivity of 75% and a specificity of 96%. In the actual-ear mode the sensitivity dropped to just over 50% while the specificity was 100%.[6] These data show that fever in one fourth or more of young children could be missed if only the noncontact tympanic thermometer was used, but if the instrument indicated "fever," it would rarely be wrong.

Without measuring their temperatures, can parents accurately determine whether young children are febrile? This was assessed in the emergency room study described in the previous paragraph. Parental sensitivity was 82% and parental specificity 77%. The sensitivity of parents' assessment of fever in their children is a bit better than that of the noncontact tympanic thermometer but is considerably less specific; parental opinions should be taken seriously.[6]

Benefits of Fever

Is fever beneficial? Should it be treated? Elevation of body temperature by a few degrees may improve the efficiency of macrophages in killing bacteria, and it impairs the replication of many organisms.[7,8] In addition, during fever there is a transfer from metabolism based on burning glucose, which is an excellent substrate for bacterial growth, to one based on proteolysis and lipolysis. During fever the liver produces acute-phase reactants, some of which bind divalent cations that are necessary for the proliferation of many microorganisms. Temperatures above 40° C (104° F) can damage the central nervous system and other body systems and should certainly be treated. Whether lower degrees of fever should be treated is unknown. A theoretical case exists for not doing so, but there are no critical studies in humans demonstrating that low-grade fever improves the outcome in human infectious diseases.[8]

Treating the Temperature

See discussion of fever in children.

Fever of Unknown Origin

In 10% to 30% of patients who are examined for fever of unknown origin, a diagnosis is never made. The long-term outcome of such patients is good. Nonsteroidal antiinflammatory drugs (NSAIDs) can be used for symptomatic relief if necessary, and the 5-year mortality rate in one study was only 3.2%.[9]

REFERENCES

1. Rabinowitz RP, Cookson ST, Wasserman SS, et al: Effects of anatomic site, oral stimulation, and body position on estimates of body temperature, *Arch Intern Med* 156:777-780, 1996.
2. Mackowiak PA, Wasserman SS, Levine MM: A critical appraisal of 98.6 degrees F, the upper limit of the normal body temperature, and other legacies of Carl Reinhold August Wunderlich, *JAMA* 268:1578-1580, 1992.
3. Shann F, Mackenzie A: Comparison of rectal, axillary and forehead temperatures, *Arch Pediatr Adolesc Med* 150:74-78, 1996.
4. Keeley D: Taking infants' temperatures (editorial), *BMJ* 304: 931-932, 1992.
5. Zengeya ST, Blumenthal I: Modern electronic and chemical thermometers used in the axilla are inaccurate, *Eur J Pediatr* 155:1005-1008, 1996.
6. Hooker EA, Smith SW, Miles T, et al: Subjective assessment of fever by parents—comparison with measurement by noncontact tympanic thermometer and calibrated rectal glass mercury thermometer, *Ann Emerg Med* 28:313-317, 1996.
7. Saper CB, Breder CD: The neurologic basis of fever, *N Engl J Med* 330:1880-1886, 1994.
8. Kluger MJ: The adaptive value of fever. In Mackowiak PA, ed: *Fever: basic mechanisms and management,* New York, 1991, Raven Press, pp 105-124.
9. Knockaert DC, Dujardin KS, Bobbaers HJ: Long-term follow-up of patients with undiagnosed fever of unknown origin, *Arch Intern Med* 156:618-620, 1996.

HEAT STROKE AND HEAT EXHAUSTION

Heat stroke is defined as a core body temperature of at least 40.5° C (105° F). Acute neurological symptoms and signs are associated with heat stroke. Hypotension is the rule, and mortality is at least 10%. In contrast, heat exhaustion is due to volume depletion brought about by heat. Symptoms include sweating, dizziness, headache, nausea, vomiting, and muscle weakness. The body temperature does not have to be elevated. Many patients with heat exhaustion can be adequately treated with oral fluids and cool sponging. The elderly are at increased risk for both conditions.[1]

Drugs may interfere with thermoregulation in a variety of ways. Some act by increasing muscle activity and heat production (amphetamines and cocaine), and some by blocking the parasympathetic system and thus inhibiting sweating (tricyclic antidepressants and phenothiazines). Others decrease blood flow to the skin by decreasing cardiac output (e.g., beta-blockers), by causing vasoconstriction (vasoconstrictors in decongestants), or by inducing volume depletion (diuretics, alcohol).[1]

Heat-related mortality can be decreased by increasing fluid intake, decreasing physical exertion, and spending more time in air-conditioned environments. Fans are not protective at temperatures above 32.3° C (90° F) with a relative humidity greater than 35%. At temperatures above 37.8° C (100° F), fans actually cause heat stress.[2]

In a study of excess deaths in the 1995 Chicago heat wave, increased risk was observed for persons who were confined to bed for known medical problems, who did not have air conditioners, or who were socially isolated.[3] Other risk factors include drugs, such as neuroleptics and anticholinergics, and obesity.[4]

REFERENCES

1. Bross MH, Nash BT, Carlton FB Jr: Heat emergencies, *Am Fam Physician* 50:389-396, 1994.
2. Centers for Disease Control and Prevention: Heat-related mortality—Chicago, July 1995, *JAMA* 274:602, 1995.
3. Semenza JC, Rubin CH, Falter KH, et al: Heat-related deaths during the July 1995 heat wave in Chicago, *N Engl J Med* 335: 84-90, 1996.
4. Centers for Disease Control and Prevention: Heat-wave-related mortality—Milwaukee, Wisconsin, July 1995, *JAMA* 276:275, 1996.

HEMOCHROMATOSIS

Major symptoms of hemochromatosis that lead to medical consultation are abdominal pain, joint pains, and weakness. Eight percent of males with this disease are impotent. Evidence of liver disease (hepatomegaly or abnormal liver enzymes) is found in 84% of cases.[1,2]

Screening asymptomatic white men for hemochromatosis has been suggested by a number of workers.[3] Those who advocate it usually suggest initial screening with transferrin saturation; levels of 62% or higher would lead to further investigations such as repeated measurement of transferrin and ferritin levels and perhaps liver biopsy. In one study of 3977 men 30 or more years of age screened in this way, 40 patients had a transferrin level of at least 62% and 8 patients with hemochromatosis were identified, a frequency of 0.002

(1:497); if only white males were included, the rate was 0.004 (1:282).[3] Whether any of these men would have become symptomatic with time had they not been detected by screening is unknown. There is a huge discrepancy between the prevalence of hemochromatosis detected by biochemical screening, which can be as high as 1:200,[4] and the prevalence rate of cases detected clinically, which is in the range of 1:7000.[5] Screening for hemochromatosis is not discussed in the most recent guidelines published by the Canadian Task Force on the Periodic Health Examination[6] or by the U.S. Preventive Services Task Force.[7]

REFERENCES

1. Desforges JF: Screening for hemochromatosis, *N Engl J Med* 328:1616-1620, 1993.
2. Adams PC: Uncovering the symptoms of hemochromatosis, *Can J Diagn,* September 1993, 10:127-134.
3. Baer DM, Simons JL, Staples RL, et al: Hemochromatosis screening in asymptomatic ambulatory men 30 years of age and older, *Am J Med* 98:464-468, 1995.
4. Edwards CQ, Griffen LM, Goldgar D, et al: Prevalence of hemochromatosis among 11,065 presumably healthy blood donors, *N Engl J Med* 318:1355-1362, 1988.
5. Finch SC, Finch CA: Idiopathic hemochromatosis, an iron storage disease. A. Iron metabolism in hemochromatosis, *Medicine (Baltimore)* 34:381-430, 1955.
6. Canadian Task Force on the Periodic Health Examination: *Canadian guide to clinical preventive health care,* Ottawa, 1994, Canada Communication Group—Publishing.
7. US Preventive Services Task Force: *Guide to clinical preventive services,* ed 2, Baltimore, 1996, Williams & Wilkins.

INFORMED CONSENT

(See also attitudes; cardiopulmonary resuscitation; follow-up of cancer patients who have had curative treatments; investigations; labeling; maternal serum screening; patient education; prevention; screening; prostate cancer; uncertainty)

Informed consent implies that the patient has a right to consent to or refuse a medical intervention. Consent may be implicit or explicit. Explicit consent, which can be oral or written, should be obtained for any intervention that involves risk or more than mild discomfort. A recognized exception is a medical emergency in which the patient is not able to give consent.[1]

Consent has three important components[1]:

1. Disclosure. This is the provision by the physician, in a comprehensible fashion, of the essential information required for the patient to make a decision.
2. Capacity. This is the ability of the patient to understand the information given and to appreciate the consequences of his or her decision.
3. Voluntariness. This means the patient is allowed to make a decision free of coercion or manipulation.

A number of myths have arisen about informed consent.[2] One is that physicians are obliged to present alternatives in an unbiased fashion without ever stating their own opinions. This is false. Physicians should indeed present the alternatives but are free to volunteer their own opinions or to give them if requested. Informed consent is an ongoing dialogue between physician and patient. A second myth is that patients must be given complete information about any proposed interventions. This too is false. Patients should be given *reasonable* amounts of information. A third myth is that patients cannot give informed consent because the data are too complex for them to comprehend. It does not follow that because patients are unable to recall the data after the physician-patient interview, they were unable to make a rational decision at the time. The main points about informed consent are that patients be given the important relevant information and be allowed to ask questions about it, mull over the options, and make their decisions either on their own or on the advice of their physicians. A fourth myth is that physicians are compelled to inform patients of relevant medical data even if they specifically ask not to be given such information. Respect for patient autonomy in this situation (not telling them) is legally acceptable and is termed a waiver.[2]

Informed Consent for Screening Procedures

Why should patients be required to give informed consent for screening tests? The answer in brief is that the benefits are not always great,[3,4] that significant adverse consequences may be produced,[5,6] that many screening programs are experimental (if they were not, there would be no controversy),[7] and, most important, that patients, not physicians, should be the ones to determine the interventions to which they will be subjected.[7,8]

When a screening test is abnormal, further diagnostic tests, often invasive, are indicated, as are therapeutic interventions with their attendant risks (screening cascade).[4] All patients with positive tests are immediately subjected to these risks, while the benefits, which accrue to only a few, will be realized only in the future.[4] Even when benefits are conclusively proved, individual patients may not be healthy enough or live long enough to enjoy them. When presented with all the facts of a screening program, some patients may not wish to risk the immediate risks of morbidity or mortality even if the overall statistics favor a particular intervention.[7]

No matter what the screening program, the vast majority of abnormal tests turn out to be false positives. However, all patients with positive tests, be they true positives or false positives, are subject to the anxiety of knowing that their test is abnormal and the adverse physical consequences of further investigative procedures.[4]

For the preceding and other reasons, a patient should never be subjected to a case finding or screening procedure without giving informed consent.[7,8] Unfortunately, this is almost impossible to implement in daily practice for several reasons. Some of the more immediate are lack of time and knowledge on the part of the physician and lack of understanding of complex data on the part of the patient.[6-9] Skrabanek[10] suggests another reason that physicians may be reluctant to mention the harm of screening: if they did, patients might not participate in the programs.

Despite the difficulties, informed consent for cancer screening can make a difference. This has been documented by Wolf and associates,[11] who randomly divided a group of men of predominantly lower socioeconomic status to receive either a scripted informational intervention about prostate specific antigen (PSA) screening or a single sentence about PSA. Those who received the informational intervention were much less likely to want PSA screening.[11]

In practice, physicians often resolve the dilemma of obtaining informed consent for preventive programs by following their own inclinations without fully discussing the issues with the patients. In some cases this is because they are overconfident about their medical recommendations even though no such certainty exists in the medical literature. Such "micro-certainty" in the face of "macro-uncertainty" may adversely affect the ability of patients to participate actively in decision making and to give truly informed consent.[12]

Patient Preconceptions and Informed Consent

Physicians are often astounded to learn the error of some patients' preconceptions that may influence their decisions in giving informed consent. For example, most elderly patients grossly overestimate the success rate of cardiopulmonary resuscitation and may opt for it under the illusion that they would have an 80% or better chance of surviving to discharge when the actual figure is between zero and 15%.[13] Similar findings have been reported in younger individuals. In one study women between the ages of 40 and 50 were found to overestimate their risk of dying of breast cancer 20 fold and to overestimate the benefit of screening 6 fold.[14]

Patient Preferences and Informed Consent

Learning a patient's preferences is essential before any medical action is taken.[15] Patients' viewpoints may surprise or even dismay their physicians. For example, a patient who has had a transient ischemic attack and has significant carotid artery stenosis may be unwilling to accept a small risk of a catastrophic adverse effect from surgical intervention (such as a stroke or death) even if the intervention has been conclusively shown to benefit many more people than it harms.[15,16]

An important concern for some physicians may be whether patients can adequately understand medical concepts and weigh cost-benefit issues rationally (as judged by physicians). This hypothesis was tested on a group of parents of young children who were asked hypothetical questions about their choices for managing fever of undetermined origin in very young children. The parents were given the kind of background data that physicians require to make these choices; they made rational, logical choices, which in the majority of cases were for minimal investigation and careful follow-up.[17]

Language and Informed Consent

The language used in obtaining informed consent may play a pivotal role in determining what option the patient chooses. This was demonstrated in a 1982 study in which subjects were asked to imagine that they had lung cancer and then to choose between surgery and radiation therapy as the two optional therapeutic modalities.[18] If the data were presented in terms of dying, using a statement such as, "Among those operated on for lung cancer, 10% will die from the operation, a third will have died by 1 year, and two thirds by 5 years. On the other hand, among those given radiation therapy, no one will die from the treatment, a quarter will be dead after 1 year, and more than three quarters by 5 years," the vast majority of subjects chose radiation therapy. On the other hand, if the data were presented in terms of living, expressed as something like, "Among those operated on for lung cancer, 90% will be alive right after surgery, two thirds at 1 year, and one third by 5 years," most people chose surgery even though the same perioperative death rate of 10% was given to them. This difference probably reflects the fact that perioperative death rates loom larger in the context of cumulative death rates than they do in the context of cumulative survival rates. This is an illusion with wide ethical ramifications.

A less subtle issue is whether information is given in a fashion the patient can understand. As Surbone[19] aptly put it, if information is given in abstruse or technical terms that patients cannot comprehend, they do not have the knowledge, or the autonomy that goes with such knowledge, to make informed decisions.

Cultural Values and Informed Consent

Should all patients be told the truth about their medical conditions? In the North American context the answer is yes in most instances for these reasons: patients must be given autonomy and have a "right to know," medical decisions cannot be made by a patient who is ignorant of his or her diagnosis, a conspiracy of silence by the physician and the patient's family may lead the patient to die in lonely isolation, and ignorance may prevent the patient from completing "unfinished business."[20] In a number of other cultures, however, the answer is no. For example, Mediterranean countries such as Italy, Greece, and Morocco have a strong tradition that family members and not the patient should be informed of bad news.[19,20] The rationale is that the sick patient would be overwhelmed by frightening and complicated information and unable to make decisions on the basis of what he or she heard, and therefore that telling the patient would do more harm than good.[19] Similar attitudes are found among Koreans and Mexican Americans, and it has been recommended that patients in these groups be asked whether they prefer to receive information and make their own medical decisions or to have their families handle the matter.[21] Among traditional Navajo peoples, receiving negative information, as is often necessary when issues of informed consent arise, conflicts with the concept of hózhó,which in over-simplified terms is a belief in beauty, harmony, and a positive outlook on life.[22]

What are North American physicians to do when faced with families who do not want the patient informed of his or her condition? They could of course ignore the family and inform the patient anyway, but a more humane alternative is probably to ask the patient what he or she wants to know. Freedman[20] calls this "offering truth." Patients are asked a series of questions that allow the physicians to determine whether the patients want to know everything, a little bit, or nothing at all. Patients have every right to choose to be uninformed, and such a waiver has been supported in law.[23,24] However, if the correct course of action remains uncertain, physicians may decide to ask for a formal ethical review.[25]

REFERENCES

1. Etchells E, Sharpe G, Walsh P, et al: Bioethics for clinicians. I. Consent, *Can Med Assoc J* 155:177-180, 1996.
2. Meisel A, Kuczewski M: Legal and ethical myths about informed consent, *Arch Intern Med* 156:2521-2526, 1996.
3. Marshall KG: Prevention. How much harm? How much benefit? I. Influence of reporting methods on perception of benefits, *Can Med Assoc J* 154:1493-1499, 1996.
4. Marshall KG: Prevention. How much harm? How much benefit? II. Ten potential pitfalls in determining the clinical significance of benefits, *Can Med Assoc J* 154:1837-1843, 1996.
5. Marshall KG: Prevention. How much harm? How much benefit? III. Physical, psychological and social harm, *Can Med Assoc J* 155:169-176, 1996.
6. Marshall KG: Screening for prostate cancer: how can patients give informed consent? *Can Fam Physician* 39:2385-2390, 1993.
7. Marshall KG: Prevention. How much harm? How much benefit? IV. The ethics of informed consent for preventive screening programs, *Can Med Assoc J* 155:377-383, 1996.
8. Lee JM: Screening and informed consent, *N Engl J Med* 328:438-440, 1993.
9. Hofman KJ, Tambor ES, Chase GA, et al: Physicians' knowledge of genetics and genetic tests, *Acad Med* 68:625-631, 1993.
10. Skrabanek P: The physician's responsibility to the patient, *Lancet* 1:1155-1157, 1988.
11. Wolf A, Nasser JF, Wolf AM, et al: The impact of informed consent on patient interest in prostate-specific antigen screening, *Arch Intern Med* 156:1333-1336, 1996.
12. Baumann AO, Deber RB, Thompson GG: Overconfidence among physicians and nurses: the "micro-certainty, macro-uncertainty" phenomenon, *Soc Sci Med* 32:167-174, 1991.
13. Murphy DJ, Burrows D, Santilli S, et al: The influence of the probability of survival on patients' preferences regarding cardiopulmonary resuscitation, *N Engl J Med* 330:545-549, 1994.
14. Black WC, Nease RF, Tosteson A: Perceptions of breast cancer risk and screening effectiveness in women under 50, *J Natl Cancer Inst* 87:720-731, 1995.
15. Kassirer JP: Incorporating patients' preferences into medical decisions (editorial), *N Engl J Med* 330:1895-1896, 1994.
16. O'Meara JJ III, McNutt RA, Evans AT, et al: A decision analysis of streptokinase plus heparin as compared with heparin alone for deep-vein thrombosis, *N Engl J Med* 330:1864-1869, 1994.
17. Oppenheim PI, Sotiropoulos G, Baraff LJ: Incorporating patient preferences into practice guidelines: management of children with fever without source, *Ann Emerg Med* 24:836-841, 1994.
18. McNeil BJ, Pauker SG, Sox HC Jr, et al: On the elicitation of preferences for alternative therapies, *N Engl J Med* 306:1259-1262, 1982.
19. Surbone A: Letter from Italy: truth telling to the patient, *JAMA* 268:1661-1662, 1992.
20. Freedman B: Offering truth: one ethical approach to the uninformed cancer patient, *Arch Intern Med* 153:572-576, 1993.
21. Blackhall LJ, Murphy ST, Frank G, et al: Ethnicity and attitudes toward patient autonomy, *JAMA* 274:820-825, 1995.
22. Carrese J, Rhodes LA: Western bioethics on the Navajo reservation: benefit or harm? *JAMA* 274:826-829, 1995.
23. Hébert PC: Truth-telling in clinical practice, *Can Fam Physician* 40:2105-2113, 1994.
24. Greenlaw J: Talk about not talking (editorial), *Arch Intern Med* 153:557-558, 1993.
25. Gostin LO: Informed consent, cultural sensitivity, and respect for persons (editorial), *JAMA* 274:844-845, 1995.

INVESTIGATIONS

(See also attitudes, physician; informed consent; labeling as ill person; periodic health examination; positive predictive value; screening; statistics; uncertainty)

Multiple Tests

Multiple tests compound the problem of false-positive results. Because of the norms of the bell-shaped curve, the odds that a single test will be abnormal by chance alone are 5%. This increases to 26% for six tests, 46% for 12 tests, and 64% for 20 tests, assuming that each test is independent of the others.[1] This is one reason that ignoring borderline abnormal results is often good practice.[2]

"Routine" Laboratory Tests

Are routine laboratory investigations a helpful form of case finding in well person care? A prospective study from the Mayo Clinic analyzed the yield of selected case-finding blood and urine tests among patients with a mean age of 63. Overall, 36% of the tests were positive (see discussion of multiple tests above), but in only 4.8% were new diagnoses (diagnostic yield) made and in only 4% was a therapeutic intervention started (therapeutic yield) as a result of the testing. The majority of therapeutic yields came from the lipid profiles (16.5%). Therapeutic yields for the chemistry panel were 2.8%, complete blood count 0.9%, urinalysis 0.8%, and thyroid tests 0.7%.[3] Almost identical results were previously reported in a study from Basel, Switzerland.[4]

Detrimental Effects of Investigation

Both false-positive and false-negative results of tests may have adverse consequences.[4] False-negative results may erroneously reassure both the patient and the physician and unnecessarily delay treatment. False-positive results not only cause considerable mental distress, but also lead to a cascade of further investigations and interventions, some of which, such as angiograms, colonoscopies, and breast biopsies, involve significant morbidity and in rare instances death. Although true-negative results often reassure patients, this is not always the case (see discussion of screening).[6-8]

Even a true-positive test may have more detrimental than beneficial effects. The individual concerned has now been labeled as an ill person,[9] and this is particularly harmful if the abnormality detected is untreatable or there is no reliable evidence that treatment does any good. In the United States the rate of testing has increased sharply in the past few years, and since a clear relationship exists between number of tests ordered and number of therapeutic interventions undertaken, the latter have also increased at a striking rate.[10-12] Examples are cardiac catheterization and cardiac revascularization,[10-12] mammography and breast surgery,[10,11] imaging of the spine and back surgery,[10,11] prostate biopsy and prostatectomy,[10,11] and oral glucose challenge test in pregnancy and Cesarean section.[13] Although it is possible that the increased testing and treatment are a result of increased disease and therefore clinically justified, it is more probable that many patients will not benefit from treatment of the disorders being detected. In other words, testing drives therapy. If this is so, patient care would be improved (and costs decreased) by programs directed at decreasing testing rather than decreasing therapeutic interventions, since physicians have more difficulty withholding therapy once a precise diagnosis has been made.[10]

Excessive Investigations

Feldman[14] and Woolf and Kamerow[5] have concluded that lack of awareness of the significance of sensitivity, specificity, and, particularly, positive predictive value is one cause of excessive testing (see later discussion). Other causes include pressure from peers and supervisors, demands of patients or families, and fear of litigation.[15] Woolf and Kamerow[5] suggest that physicians' attitudes are an even more important cause of excessive testing than is lack of statistical knowledge. They point out that much of medical school training is done in tertiary care hospitals where students learn that errors of omission are more serious than errors of commission. In other words, failure to detect a disease is worse than any adverse effects that might result from the testing procedure itself or the consequences of false-positive or false-negative results. Physicians' discomfort with uncertainty probably underlies this kind of rationalization.[5,15] As Kassirer[15] points out, such discomfort is often illogical, since high diagnostic certainty is necessary only for diseases in which treatment is not very effective and morbidity is significant. If a disease is easily treated with a therapy that has few adverse effects, it can reasonably be initiated even if the diagnosis is not absolutely certain.

Positive Predictive Value and Disease Prevalence

The positive predictive value of a test is the percentage of positive results that are true positives, and this varies directly with the prevalence of the disease in the community. Family physicians must understand the concept of positive predictive value if they want to avoid harming their patients through screening procedures. If the prevalence of a disease is low, the vast majority of patients with "positive" results have false-positive tests and do not have the disease[5]; these unfortunate patients go through agony until or even beyond the time that the diagnosis is clarified.[16-18]

To illustrate the clinical importance of the relationship between disease prevalence and positive predictive value, Woolf and Kamerow[5] give two examples. The first involves testing for a disease with a known prevalence of 10%, and the second is testing for a disease with a known prevalence of 0.1%. If both these diseases could be detected by tests that had sensitivities of 90% and specificities of 90%, half of all the positive tests would be false positives in the group with a disease prevalence of 10% (positive predictive value of 50%), whereas more than 99% of the positive tests in the group with a disease prevalence of 0.1% would be false positives (positive predictive value of 0.9%).[4] A test with a positive predictive value of 50% probably does more good than harm, but it would be extraordinary indeed if a test with a positive predictive value of 0.9% did not cause much more harm than good.

Once the relationship between disease prevalence and positive predictive value is understood, it can be seen that the positive predictive values of tests performed on "sick" hospitalized patients are likely to be much higher than the positive predictive values of tests performed on ambulatory patients in the office setting. This is perhaps another reason that physicians trained primarily in hospitals are enthusiastic about tests.

REFERENCES

1. Cebul RD, Beck JR: Biochemical profiles: applications in ambulatory screening and preadmission testing of adults, *Ann Intern Med* 106:403-413, 1987.
2. Cnanji AA: Misleading biochemical laboratory test results, *Can Med Assoc J* 130:1435-1441, 1984.
3. Boland BJ, Wollan PC, Silverstein MD: Yield of laboratory tests for case-finding in the ambulatory general medical examination, *Am J Med* 101:142-152, 1996.
4. Ruttimann S, Dreifuss M, Clemençon D, et al: Multiple biochemical blood testing as a case-finding tool in ambulatory medical patients, *Am J Med* 94:141-148, 1993.
5. Woolf SH, Kamerow DB: Testing for uncommon conditions: the heroic search for positive test results, *Arch Intern Med* 150:2451-2458, 1990.
6. Huggins M, Bloch M, Wiggins S, et al: Predictive testing for Huntington disease in Canada: adverse effects and unexpected results in those receiving a decreased risk, *Am J Med Genet* 42: 508-515, 1992.

Miscellaneous 251

7. King M, Rowell S, Love SM: Inherited breast and ovarian cancer: what are the risks? what are the choices? *JAMA* 269:1975-1980, 1993.
8. McDonald IG, Jelinek VM, Panetta F, et al: Opening Pandora's box: the unpredictability of reassurance by a normal test result, *BMJ* 313:329-332, 1996.
9. Meador CK: The last well person, *N Engl J Med* 330:440-441, 1994.
10. Verrilli D, Welch G: The impact of diagnostic testing on therapeutic interventions, *JAMA* 275:1189-1191, 1996.
11. Epstein AM: Use of diagnostic tests and therapeutic procedures in a changing health care environment (editorial), *JAMA* 275: 1197-1198, 1996.
12. Wennberg DE, Kellett MA, Dickens JD Jr, et al: The association between local diagnostic testing intensity and invasive cardiac procedures, *JAMA* 275:1161-1164, 1996.
13. Naylor CD, Sermer M, Chen E, et al (Toronto Trihospital Gestational Diabetes Investigators): Cesarean delivery in relation to birth weight and gestational glucose tolerance: pathophysiology or practice style? *JAMA* 275:1165-1170, 1996.
14. Feldman W: On ordering tests (editorial), *Ann RCPSC* 26:269-270, 1993.
15. Kassirer JP: Our stubborn quest for diagnostic certainty: a cause of excessive testing, *N Engl J Med* 320:1489-1491, 1989.
16. Lerman C, Trock B, Rimer BK, et al: Psychological and behavioral implications of abnormal mammograms, *Ann Intern Med* 114:657-661, 1991.
17. Lerman C, Rimer BK, Engstrom PF: Cancer risk notification: psychosocial and ethical implications, *J Clin Oncol* 9:1275-1282, 1991.
18. Wardle J, Pope R: The psychological costs of screening for cancer, *J Psychosom Res* 36:609-624, 1992.

LEG CRAMPS

Although a number of studies have concluded that quinine is no more effective than a placebo for controlling nocturnal leg cramps,[1-3] others have shown some benefit. In one such trial quinine reduced by 50% the frequency of cramps experienced by the patients, although it did not reduce their severity.[4] Another small, nonblinded evaluation from England found quinine to be more effective than going to bed with three corks tied in a sock.[5] A metaanalysis of six randomized controlled crossover studies of elderly patients taking 200, 300, or 500 mg of quinine at bedtime concluded that the drug decreased the number of nights with cramps by 27% but not the intensity or duration of the cramps. The effect of quinine is cumulative, so a 4-week trial should be given before deciding whether the drug is beneficial.[6] The usual dose is 200 to 300 mg qhs.

Several nonpharmacological treatments of leg cramps have been recommended. Daniell[7] reported successful prevention of cramps within a week when the 44 patients tested performed stretching exercises three times a day. While barefoot, patients stood 2 to 3 feet from a wall and faced it. They placed their hands on the wall and, keeping their heels on the ground, leaned forward to the point that they felt the stretch in their calf muscles. This position was maintained for 10 seconds, and the maneuver was then repeated once after a 5-second rest.[7] Another recommendation is to place a pillow at the bottom of the bed to keep the feet dorsiflexed; if cramps still occur, the patient should passively dorsiflex the ankle and massage the calf.[8]

REFERENCES

1. Lim SH: Randomised double-blind trial of quinine sulphate for nocturnal leg cramp, *Br J Clin Pharmacol* 11:462, 1986.
2. Smith C, Jee R, O'Neill C, Dobbs SM: Double-blind, placebo-controlled cross-over study of maintenance treatment with quinine bisulphate for night cramps, *Br J Clin Pharmacol* 21:108, 1986.
3. Warburton A, Royston JP, O'Neill CJ, et al: A quinine a day keeps the leg cramps away? *Br J Clin Pharmacol* 23:459-465, 1987.
4. Connolly PS, Shirley EA, Wasson JH, et al: Treatment of nocturnal leg cramps: a crossover trial of quinine vs. vitamin E, *Arch Intern Med* 152:1877-1880, 1992.
5. Maule B: Nocturnal cramp: quinine versus folklore, *Practitioner* 234:420-421, 1990.
6. Man-Son-Hing M, Wells G: Meta-analysis of efficacy of quinine for treatment of nocturnal leg cramps in elderly people, *BMJ* 310:13-17, 1995.
7. Daniell HW: Simple cure for nocturnal leg cramps (letter), *N Engl J Med* 301:216, 1979.
8. Weiner IH, Weiner HL: Nocturnal leg muscle cramps, *JAMA* 244:2332-2333, 1980.

MEDICAL EDUCATION

(See also investigations; skepticism; uncertainty)

Career Choice

Physician career changes appear to be the rule rather than the exception. An 11-year prospective study in Great Britain found that 30% of physicians changed careers once and 39% two or more times.[1] By their third year of medicine, 60% of Saskatchewan physicians were not following the career path they had planned and 40% had made career changes after starting internship or residency.[2] At present it is almost impossible for licensed physicians to enter a postgraduate program in Canada.[2] Among the probable consequences of this are that some physicians will find themselves stuck in fields they dislike, which may have negative consequences for their patients as well as themselves, training programs will probably have more unsuitable residents, undergraduates will use electives to try and make career choices rather than to broaden their education, and the absence of practice-experienced physicians in residency programs will narrow the scope of the training experience.[3]

Medical Journal Proliferation

Approximately 30,000 biomedical journals are published in the world. It has been estimated that only 1% of articles in medical journals are scientifically sound.[4,5]

Systematic Reviews

Quickly finding up-to-date high-quality information about clinical interventions is a never-ending frustration for physicians. An ongoing attempt to alleviate this problem is the development of high-quality peer-reviewed systematic reviews by a group of international experts working together as the Cochrane Collaboration (named after the late British epidemiologist Archie Cochrane). The Cochrane Reviews are published in an electronic journal, the *Cochrane Database of Systematic Reviews,* which is updated quarterly. So far only a few subjects have been covered, but the long-range goal is to include a wide range of clinical topics. Subscription to the *Cochrane Database* is available through the Cochrane Collaboration Reviews, American College of Physicians, P.O. Box 7777, Philadelphia, PA 19175-0980; telephone (800) 523-1546 or (215) 351-2600.[6]

Undergraduate Medical Education

By the mid-1990s women constituted 40% of the U.S. undergraduate student body in medicine. This contrasts with a less than 10% representation two decades earlier.[7]

Women in Academic Medicine

In the United States women physicians on medical school faculties are promoted more slowly than men, even taking into account productivity and differential attrition rates from academic medicine.[8] One reason women may not advance as rapidly is that those who have children at home tend to spend fewer hours in professional activities and far more hours in domestic activities than do male physicians. A Canadian study found that women family physicians with children at home spent a mean of 90.5 hours a week in combined professional and domestic work, whereas male family physicians with children at home spent a mean of 68.6 hours.[9] A cross-sectional survey of salaried academic pediatricians in 126 centers in the United States found that women devoted somewhat fewer hours than men to professional activities and that relatively few were "academically productive" (meaning obtained grants and published extensively) in comparison with men. The women surveyed spent more time than men in patient care and teaching.[10]

At Johns Hopkins, institutional reforms within the department of medicine without any changes in promotion criteria resulted in a marked increase in promotion and retention of female academic staff.[11]

REFERENCES

1. Parkhouse J, Ellin DJ: Reasons for doctors' career choice and change of choice, *BMJ* 296:1651-1653, 1988.
2. Shaw S, Goplen G, Houston DS: Career changes among Saskatchewan physicians, *Can Med Assoc J* 154:1035-1038, 1996.
3. Houston S: Postgraduate training: unfair to students and recent graduates (editorial), *Ann RCPSC* 29:136-137, 1996.
4. Smith R: Where is the wisdom . . .? The poverty of medical evidence (editorial), *BMJ* 303:798-799, 1991.
5. Lock S: Introduction. In Lock S, ed: The future of medical journals, London, 1991, British Medical Journal, pp 1-8.
6. Bero L, Rennie D: The Cochrane Collaboration: preparing, maintaining, and disseminating systematic reviews of the effects of health care, *JAMA* 274:1935-1938, 1995.
7. Women in Medical Services Office: *Leading change, women in medicine,* Chicago, 1995, American Medical Association.
8. Tesch BJ, Wood HM, Helwig AL, et al: Promotion of women physicians in academic medicine: glass ceiling or sticky floor? *JAMA* 273:1022-1025, 1995.
9. Woodward CA, Williams AP, Ferrier B, et al: Time spent on professional activities and unwaged domestic work: is it different for male and female primary care physicians who have children at home? *Can Fam Physician* 42:1928-1935, 1996.
10. Kaplan SH, Sullivan LM, Dukes DA, et al: Sex differences in academic advancement: results of a national study of pediatricians, *N Engl J Med* 335:1282-1289, 1996.
11. Fried LP, Francomano CA, MacDonald SM, et al: Career development for women in academic medicine: multiple interventions in a department of medicine, *JAMA* 276:898-905, 1996.

MULTIPLE CHEMICAL SENSITIVITIES

(See also chronic fatigue syndrome; fibromyalgia)

Multiple chemical sensitivities, chronic fatigue syndrome, and fibromyalgia are three conditions whose existence is controversial. Believers search ever more intensely for organic causes, while unbelievers attribute the symptoms to psychiatric disorders such as depression or personality disorders. The symptoms and epidemiology of the three conditions overlap.[1] There is substantial evidence that multiple chemical sensitivities does not exist as a specific disease entity.[1-7]

Agents reputed to cause the patient's illness are protean, including everything from formaldehyde and ammonia to hospitals, office machines, airplanes, and certain brands of tampons.[5] Most of the patients in whom the condition is diagnosed are middle-aged women. Symptoms vary tremendously. Some of the more common complaints are fatigue, headaches, nausea, pain, and sleep disturbances.[1,5] Physical and laboratory investigations, including immunological testing, show no specific abnormalities.[2] A recently popular hypothesis is that abnormalities of porphyrin metabolism might account for the disorder. According to Hahn and Bonkovsky,[8] the scientific evidence for this is nonexistent.

The main investigative tool used by clinical ecologists is the provocation-neutralization test, in which the patient is administered a series of suspect agents by the subcutaneous, sublingual, oral, or inhalation route. The patient reports symptoms after 10 minutes. Neutralization is accomplished by injecting or applying sublingually a lower dose of the original test substance.[5] Standardization and quality control of this procedure are questionable.[4]

When psychiatric evaluation of patients with multiple chemical sensitivities has been undertaken, between 40% and 100% have been found to have psychiatric disorders. The most common psychiatric diagnoses have been somatization disorder, hypochondriasis, affective disorder, and anxiety disorders. Other recorded psychiatric diagnoses include personality disorders and schizophrenia.[3,6]

In some regions a fairly effective political lobby represents persons claiming to have multiple chemical sensitivities. For example, despite severe budget restraints the Province of Nova Scotia pledged 1 million dollars to help establish an environmental health clinic in 1995[9] and subsequently funded an environmental health center that cost 2.4 million dollars and was opened in 1997.[10]

What are skeptical physicians to do when faced with patients claiming to have multiple chemical sensitivities? After sighing, they must take careful histories and perform punctilious physical examinations to rule out recognized specific physical and mental illnesses. At that point, in my opinion, they should politely but unequivocally give the patients their opinions about "multiple chemical sensitivities," outline the ways in which they may be able to help the patients, and specify the limits to what they are willing to undertake.

REFERENCES

1. Buchwald D, Garrity D: Comparison of patients with chronic fatigue syndrome, fibromyalgia, and multiple chemical sensitivities, *Arch Intern Med* 154:2049-2053, 1994.
2. Simon GE, Daniell W, Stockbridge H, et al: Immunologic, psychological, and neuropsychological factors in multiple chemical sensitivity, *Ann Intern Med* 119:97-103, 1993.
3. Black DW, Rathe A, Goldstein R: Environmental illness: a controlled study of 26 subjects with "20th century disease," *JAMA* 264:3166-3170, 1990.
4. American College of Physicians: Clinical ecology (position paper), *Ann Intern Med* 111:168-178, 1989.
5. Terr AI: Environmental illness: a clinical review of 50 cases, *Arch Intern Med* 146:145-149, 1986.
6. Stewart DE: Psychiatric assessment of patients with "20th-century disease" ("total allergy syndrome"), *Can Med Assoc J* 133:1001-1006, 1985.
7. Council on Scientific Affairs, American Medical Association: Clinical ecology, *JAMA* 268:3465-3467, 1992.
8. Hahn M, Bonkovsky HL: Multiple chemical sensitivity syndrome and porphyria: a note of caution and concern, *Arch Intern Med* 157:281-285, 1997.
9. Moulton D: The enigma of environmental illness, *Med Post* 31: 19, 1995.
10. N.S. unveils health-research centre: Canada's first specially designed high-tech facility to study environment-related illnesses, *Toronto Globe and Mail,* May 3, 1997.

PATIENT EDUCATION

(See also informed consent; prevention)

According to one survey the average reading level of adults in the United States is grade 8 or 9 and 47% of the American population has deficient literacy skills.[1] This has enormous implications for patient care because patients with inadequate reading ability are less compliant with medical regimens.[2] Suggested solutions are to combine written and oral instructions, present illustrations in the latter, use simple language in both, and give only essential information.[2]

REFERENCES

1. *Adult literacy in America: a first look at the results of the National Adult Literacy Survey,* ed 2, Washington, DC, 1993, Office of Educational Research and Improvement, Department of Education.
2. Mayeaux EJ Jr, Murphy PW, Arnold C, et al: Improving patient education for patients with low literacy skills, *Am Fam Physician* 53:205-211, 1996.

PERFORMANCE REPORTS

(See also coronary artery bypass grafting and angioplasty; practice patterns)

Because outcomes for a variety of procedures vary from one center to another and from one operator to another, publication of consumer guides of performance data has been proposed. This has been done for outcomes of coronary bypass surgery in Pennsylvania. A survey of both cardiologists and cardiac surgeons revealed considerable concern about this approach. The most important criticism was a failure of the guide to adjust adequately for risk (high-risk patients have poorer outcomes) and a fear that such a publication might cause surgeons to refuse to operate on high-risk patients. Other criticisms were a failure to measure quality by anything but mortality and a perception that the data provided by hospitals and surgeons were unreliable.[1]

When performance outcomes of individual physicians are correlated with the volume of procedures performed, interpretation of data becomes even more complex. Although a higher rate of adverse effects is generally correlated with performance of fewer procedures, there are exceptions to this rule. Greater experience (the learning curve) does not always lead to better results; some physicians are simply less competent than others, and this shows up in their statistics no matter how many cases they handle.[2]

REFERENCES

1. Schneider EC, Epstein AM: Influence of cardiac-surgery performance reports on referral practices and access to care: a survey of cardiovascular specialists, *N Engl J Med* 335:251-256, 1996.
2. Hannan EL, Racz M, Ryan T, et al: Coronary angioplasty volume-outcome relationships for hospitals and cardiologists, *JAMA* 279:892-898, 1997.

PETS

Specially trained dogs (service dogs) can perform a multitude of tasks to help physically disabled persons who have ambulatory difficulties. Among other things they can turn on switches, open and close doors, pull a person up from a sitting or lying position, pick up objects, pull on clothing, help a person get into or out of the bath, and pull a wheelchair. In one study of their efficacy for patients with spinal cord injuries, muscular dystrophy, multiple sclerosis, and traumatic brain injury, they significantly decreased the need for other helping resources and thus the overall cost of the disability. Having such dogs increased the self-esteem of the owners.[1]

Some pet tarantulas have urticarious hairs that if accidentally rubbed on the cornea (by hands or fingers that had previously been handling the spider) can penetrate it and seriously compromise visual acuity.[2]

REFERENCES

1. Allen K, Blascovich J: The value of service dogs for people with severe ambulatory disabilities, *JAMA* 275:1001-1006, 1996.
2. Blaikie AJ, Ellis J, Sanders R, et al: Eye disease associated with handling pet tarantulas: three case reports, *BMJ* 314:1524-1525, 1997.

PHARMACEUTICALS

Drug Expiration Dates

Dry formulation drugs (e.g., tablets and capsules) stored in unopened containers generally maintain 70% to 80% of their potency for up to 10 years. Even drugs in opened containers maintain 70% to 80% of their potency for up to 2 years, especially if stored in locations that are not excessively humid. Except for tetracycline, outdated drugs are unlikely to be harmful.[1] Liquid formulations of drugs are less stable and should not be used after the expiration dates. Epinephrine is particularly unstable and must be stored in the dark. It is oxidized when exposed to air.[2]

Pharmaceutical Representatives

There is about 1 pharmaceutical representative for every 15 to 30 physicians in the United States, and estimates are that the industry spent more than $13,000 per physician on advertising in 1993.[3] Most physicians find the information given by the representatives useful.[4] Evidence indicates that pharmaceutical representatives influence the prescribing habits of physicians.[5] In one study a third of residents and a quarter of faculty said that they changed their prescribing habits as a result of information gleaned from the representatives.[6] About half of U.S. residency training programs permit representatives to give presentations, and the majority allow them to provide food for conferences. In one survey 11% of the statements made by the representatives about drugs were considered inaccurate by an assessing team, but few physicians in the audience recognized these errors.[4] It should be noted that there were no controls to determine how often physicians' statements about drugs were considered inaccurate.

Direct Consumer Advertising

Direct advertising of drugs to consumers is becoming more prevalent, and the effect of this on the health of the population is unknown. Since studies of physicians have shown that the more they depend on information obtained from the pharmaceutical industry, the less appropriate are their prescribing practices, it is reasonable to assume that inappropriate expectations raised by drug advertising will be even greater in the general population. These expectations will probably pressure some physicians into writing unwarranted prescriptions.[7]

REFERENCES

1. Drugs past their expiration date, *Med Lett* 38:65-66, 1996.
2. Stability of drugs in solution, *Med Lett* 38:90, 1996.
3. Drake D, Uhlman M: *Making medicine, making money,* Kansas City, Mo, 1993, Andrews & McMeel.
4. Ziegler MG, Lew P, Singer BC: The accuracy of drug information from pharmaceutical sales representatives, *JAMA* 273:1296-1298, 1995.
5. Lexchin J: Interactions between physicians and the pharmaceutical industry: what does the literature say? *Can Med Assoc J* 149:1401-1407, 1993.
6. Lurie N, Rich EC, Simpson DE, et al: Pharmaceutical representatives in academic medical centers: interaction with faculty and house staff, *J Gen Intern Med* 5:240-243, 1990.
7. Lexchin J: Consequences of direct-to-consumer advertising of prescription drugs (editorial), *Can Fam Physician* 43:594-596, 1997.

PHYSICIAN-PATIENT COMMUNICATIONS

(See also appeal of alternative medicine)

A review of 21 randomized controlled studies of physician-patient communication showed that effective communication correlated with improved patient outcomes. In order of frequency the reported improvements were in emotional health, symptom resolution, function, blood pressure control, blood sugar levels, and pain control.[1]

In the United States the quality of physician-patient interviews correlates with the likelihood that physicians will be sued. In an audiotape analysis comparing interviewing styles between primary care physicians who had been subject to malpractice claims and those who had not, physicians who had never been sued seemed to have a warmer relationship with patients as expressed by humor and laughter. They also used more orienting comments, such as "First I'll examine you, and then we will talk," and more facilitative comments, such as "Go on, tell me more about that." The actual content of the interview in terms of biopsychosocial balance or the provision of information was the same for both groups.[2]

REFERENCES

1. Stewart MA: Effective physician-patient communication and health outcomes: a review, *Can Med Assoc J* 152:1423-1433, 1995.
2. Levinson W, Roter DL, Mullooly JP, et al: Physician-patient communication: the relationship with malpractice claims among primary care physicians and surgeons, *JAMA* 277:553-559, 1997.

PRESCRIBING HABITS

(See also prescribing habits and the elderly)

Prescription and over-the-counter drugs are the fastest growing health care expenditure in Canada. In 1993 they accounted for 15% of money spent on health care, and the annual rate of increase is 8.2%.[1] Probably many of the drugs prescribed are inappropriate.[2] On the other hand, there is evidence that drugs are underused for some important conditions, including hypertension, myocardial infarction, and depression.[3] Properly used drugs can actually save the system money.[4]

Poor prescribing habits are of particular concern for the elderly. This subject is discussed in the section on geriatrics under "Prescribing Habits and the Elderly."

An occasional problem with drug prescriptions is the substitution of one drug for another with a similar name. For example, after two patients who were prescribed Losec (the original trade name of omeprazole in the United States) were given Lasix,[5] Merck Sharp & Dohme changed the name in the United States to Prilosec.[6] You just can't win; a patient for whom Prilosec was prescribed was given Prozac.[7]

REFERENCES

1. *National health expenditures in Canada, 1975-1993,* Ottawa, 1994, Health Canada, pp 3-4.
2. Anis AH, Carruthers G, Carter AO, Kierulf J: Variability in prescription drug utilization: issues for research, *Can Med Assoc J* 154:635-640, 1996.
3. MacLeod SM: Improving physician prescribing practices: bridge over troubled waters (editorial), *Can Med Assoc J* 154: 675-677, 1996.
4. McIsaac W, Naylor CD, Anderson GM, et al: Reflections on a month in the life of the Ontario Drug Benefit Plan (editorial), *Can Med Assoc J* 150:473-477, 1994.
5. Fine SN, Isdorfer RM, Miskovitz PF, et al: Losec or Lasix (letter)? *N Engl J Med* 322:1674, 1990.
6. Hoffman JP: More on "Losec or Lasix?" (letter), *N Engl J Med* 323:1428, 1990.
7. Costable JM Jr, McKinley MJ: Prozac or Prilosec for gastric ulcer? (letter), *N Engl J Med* 335:600, 1996.

RISK ANALYSIS

(See also attitudes, physician; investigations; labeling; positive predictive value; risk assessment in pregnancy; screening; uncertainty)

Risk and uncertainty are inextricably linked. In medicine one way of attempting to diminish the degree of uncertainty is to develop systems for placing patients in different risk categories. For example, scoring systems may be applied to pregnant women to categorize their pregnancies as "high risk" or "low risk." Various terms used to encompass risk-categorizing systems include risk approach, risk analysis, risk scoring, risk screening systems, and risk management.[1]

Three important assumptions underlie risk analysis:

1. Risk factors that will allow an accurate determination of which cohort of patients is at high risk are well established.
2. One or more interventions are available to improve the outcome of patients identified as being at high risk.
3. Above all else the physician must look for, identify, and manage the worst case scenario. This is an attitudinal issue and reflects the "maximalist" approach of "If in doubt, do something" (see discussion of physician attitudes).

Risk analysis tends to ameliorate a physician's anxiety in an ambiguous situation by reformulating the problem in a numerical fashion. High numbers equal high risk and the need to do something, whereas low numbers equal low risk about which the physician need not worry. Numbers give magical and often false reassurance because they appear to represent certainty.[2]

Developing a risk analysis protocol is extremely complex[3] and is seldom well done. Even a carefully prepared analysis in which cohorts at high risk are clearly distinguished from cohorts at low risk often does little to help the individual patient. This is because in situations in which the prevalence rate of adverse outcomes is low, the positive predictive value of any screening system is low. As a result, many persons who will not have adverse outcomes are labeled as at "high risk" and may suffer both the psychological adverse effects of being so labeled (see discussion of labeling) and the physical adverse effects of unwarranted investigations or interventions.[4] For example, when risk evaluation is performed in pregnancy, the "high-risk" label is applied to 16% to 55% of pregnant women.[5] However, a large percentage of adverse outcomes occur in persons who have no identifiable risk factors and so are categorized as being at "low risk." Half of all perinatal morbidity and mortality occurs in "low-risk" pregnancies.[5,6]

The conclusion of one thoughtful analyst of this subject is that pregnancy risk scoring has not been proved to cause more benefit than harm to the women and infants who have been subject to it.[1] This view is echoed in an editorial by Klein,[7] who points out that labeling pregnant women as at high risk may itself lead to consultations and unnecessary interventions.[7]

REFERENCES

1. Hall PF: Rethinking risk (editorial), *Can Fam Physician* 40: 1239-1244, 1994.
2. Postman N: *Technopoly: the surrender of culture to technology,* Mississauga, Ontario, 1992, Vintage Books.
3. Morgan MG: Risk analysis and management, *Sci Am* 269:32-41, 1993.
4. Woolf SH, Kameron DB: Testing for uncommon conditions—the heroic search for positive test results, *Arch Intern Med* 150: 2451-2458, 1990.
5. Wall EM: Assessing obstetric risk: a review of obstetric risk-scoring systems, *J Fam Pract* 27:153-163, 1988.
6. Hall PF: Obstetric risk scoring: a Trojan horse, *Manitoba Med* 63:43-45, 1993.
7. Klein M: Family physician maternity care: outcomes when family physicians provide most community-based care (editorial), *Can Fam Physician* 41:546-548, 1995.

SKEPTICISM

(See also attitudes, physician; medical education; periodic health examination; screening)

Good physicians are skeptical about much of what they do and most of what they read, including this text. Being skeptical helps keep physicians attuned to new evidence and will probably keep them from harming patients by either prematurely endorsing new investigative or therapeutic procedures or rigidly staying with outmoded interventions. Skepticism is one of the driving forces behind "evidence-based medicine" and is well exemplified by the critical approaches of the Canadian Task Force on the Periodic Health Examination[1] and the U.S. Preventive Services Task Force.[2] However, skepticism carried to extremes leads to diagnostic and therapeutic paralysis.

Evidence-based data are only part of what physicians require to care adequately for their patients. They need easy access to accurate information that is relevant to everyday practice; as Slawson and Shaghnessy[3] put it, they are looking for "patient oriented evidence that matters (POEM)."

Expert opinion, whether expressed orally or in the form of a review article, is a common and sometimes unreliable source of information for generalists. Antman and associates[4] compared current written reviews of "experts" in the specific content area of myocardial infarction with current meta-analyses on the subject. The reviews of the "experts" often contained potentially harmful recommendations and omitted newer beneficial therapeutic modalities.[4] (On the other hand, metaanalyses themselves may lead to erroneous conclusions when comparing large randomized controlled trials.[5,6]) Oxman and Guyatt[7] analyzed the methodological rigor of a number of review articles and concluded that the greater the expertise of the authors, the poorer the quality of the reviews. One possible reason for this is that some "experts" are consciously or unconsciously biased because they have a vested interest in certain viewpoints.[7] Put more bluntly, many hold the attitude that because they believe one approach was successful, they will continue with it regardless of the evidence.[3] Another explanation is that the databases from which specialists draw their conclusions are often derived from selected populations that do not reflect the problems seen in family practice.[3]

It has often been stated that only 10% to 20% of medical interventions are evidence based. When this hypothesis was tested on inpatients in a general medical service in Oxford, England, 82% of treatments were found to be evidence based (53% by randomized controlled trials and 29% by "convincing nonexperimental evidence").[8]

REFERENCES

1. Canadian Task Force on the Periodic Health Examination: *Canadian guide to clinical preventive health care,* Ottawa, 1994, Canada Communication Group—Publishing.
2. US Preventive Services Task Force: *Guide to clinical preventive services,* ed 2, Baltimore, 1996, Williams & Wilkins.
3. Slawson DC, Shaughnessy AF: Obtaining useful information from expert based sources, *BMJ* 314:947-949, 1997.
4. Antman EM, Lau J, Kupelnick B, et al: A comparison of results of meta-analyses of randomized control trials and recommendations of clinical experts: treatments for myocardial infarction, *JAMA* 268:240-248, 1992.
5. LeLorier J, Grégoire G, Benhaddad A, et al: Discrepancies between meta-analyses and subsequent large randomized, controlled trials, *N Engl J Med* 337:536-542, 1997.
6. Bailar JC III: The promise and problems of meta-analysis (editorial), *N Engl J Med* 337:559-561, 1997.
7. Oxman AD, Guyatt GH: The science of reviewing research, *Ann NY Acad Sci* 703:125-133, 1993.
8. Ellis J, Mulligan I, Rowe J, Sackett DL (A-Team, Nuffield Department of Clinical Medicine): Inpatient general medicine is evidence based, *Lancet* 346:407-410, 1995.

SLEEP

(See also motor vehicle accidents)

Insomnia

(See also hip fractures; jet lag; narcolepsy; restless legs syndrome; prescribing habits and the elderly; seasonal affective disorder; sleep apnea)

Etiology

About 60% of cases of chronic insomnia are due to major psychiatric disorders, most commonly depression.[1] Anxiety disorders and sleep apnea are also relatively common causes of insomnia and must be ruled out (snoring is a clue for sleep apnea).[2] Another common cause of insomnia is the intake of various chemical agents such as alcohol, nicotine, caffeine, or a variety of prescription or nonprescription drugs.[2-4] Even one or two glasses of wine in the evening can cause awakening around 2 AM as the sedative effect wears off. The half-life of coffee is 3 to 7 hours, so some people should avoid drinking it in the afternoon or evening if they want to sleep.

Epidemiology

Complaints of insomnia are more common in women than men, in the divorced, widowed, or separated, in lower socioeconomic groups, and in the elderly.[2] Polygraph studies of sleep in the elderly show it to be shallower, shorter, and more fragmented. However, older people do not have a decline in the subjective need for sleep; for some the poorer quality of nighttime sleep may lead to daytime somnolence.[3]

Nonpharmacological management

Aside from elimination of precipitating causes of insomnia such as those listed above, the following behavioral approach may be helpful[2-5]:

1. Go to bed only when sleepy.
2. Do not read, eat, or watch television in bed. Bed is for sleeping and sex.
3. If you are in bed and can't sleep, get up, go to another room, and stay up until you are really sleepy and then go back to bed. Do not watch television because the bright-

ness of its light has an arousing effect; instead read with as dim a light as possible. If after returning to bed you still can't sleep, get up again and repeat the cycle.
4. Set the alarm for the same time every morning, and get up when it rings regardless of how little sleep you have had.
5. Never sleep during the day.

An additional approach is to document the number of hours the patient sleeps and to make bedtime that number of hours (or that number of hours plus 30 minutes) before the fixed morning wakeup time. If, for example, an insomniac sleeps only 5 hours and the morning wakeup time is to be 7 AM, bedtime should be 1:30 or 2 AM. This will probably cause the patient to accumulate a sleep deficit and fall asleep more easily. After a week the bedtime can be made earlier by 15 minutes, and further 15-minute weekly increments of time spent in bed can be added provided that at least 85% of the time in bed is spent sleeping.[2]

A study from Stanford University compared sleep hygiene alone (fixed wakeup times and bedtimes, no alcohol after 4 PM, caffeine at breakfast only, fixed eating times, and leaving the bedroom to sit in an armchair at night if sleep did not resume within 10 minutes after awakening), sleep hygiene plus late afternoon exercise, or sleep hygiene plus early morning exposure to bright light for 45 minutes. After 4 weeks of treatment all groups improved, but only the group exposed to early morning light showed a statistically significant improvement compared with the others (see discussion of seasonal affective disorders).[6]

A 16-week randomized trial of moderate-intensity aerobic exercises for elderly patients with sleep disturbances showed a significant improvement in self-rated sleep quality. Each subject performed low-impact aerobics, brisk walking, or stationary cycling four times a week for 30 to 40 minutes before the evening meal.[7]

Hypnotics

Serious side effects from taking hypnotic drugs are common, especially in the elderly, whose elimination of many of these drugs is greatly delayed. A good example is benzodiazepine ingestion, which is a risk factor for hip fracture (see discussion of hip fractures). According to Kupfer and Reynolds[2] no data from randomized trials have shown taking hypnotic drugs for more than 35 days provides sustained benefits.

The following are basic principles of the pharmacotherapy of insomnia[2]:

1. Use the lowest dose possible.
2. Prescribe for a limited period (no more than 4 weeks on a regular basis).
3. Prescribe intermittent doses (two to four times a week).
4. Discontinue hypnotics gradually.

Standard hypnotics are the benzodiazepines (intermediate- or short-acting compounds preferred), zolpidem (Ambien), and chloral hydrate (Noctec). Zolpidem is not a benzodiazepine but has a similar therapeutic profile. How habituating it is has not been determined.[2] A nonbenzodiazepine available in Canada is zopiclone (Imovane). Amnestic reactions with triazolam (Halcion) are common, and like other benzodiazepines, it is addictive.[8] I never prescribe it.

Antidepressants, especially those that are serotonin specific, have been widely used as hypnotics. No systematic studies of the efficacy of these agents for this purpose have been published. The tricyclic drugs such as amitriptyline (Elavil) or doxepin (Sinequan) have significant anticholinergic side effects. More promising are trazodone (Desyrel), nefazodone (Serzone), and paroxetine (Paxil).[2] Trazodone 100 mg hs has been used successfully as a hypnotic in depressed patients who had persistent, exacerbated, or new-onset insomnia when being treated with fluoxetine or bupropion.[9]

Alcohol is not a good sedative because the initial central nervous system depression is followed by rebound excitation that disturbs sleep.[2,8]

Melatonin may turn out to be a useful clinical hypnotic.[2,8] So far, adequate trials have not been published and the purity of some of the products available is questionable.[10] Doses of 5 mg hs may assist shift workers in adjusting to their schedules[11,12] and help blind people sleep, since they often have a disturbed circadian rhythm. The drug may also counter some of the effects of jet lag (see discussion of jet lag).[11,12]

Table 46 lists a few of the drugs that are approved or used as hypnotics. In prescribing them the physician should remember that except with the antidepressants, efficacy usually dissipates in a few weeks and dependency is a major risk.[2,8]

Table 46 Hypnotics

Drug	Usual doses
Aldehydes and Derivatives	
Chloral hydrate	500-1000 mg qhs
Benzodiazepine Derivatives	
Short acting	
Triazolam (Halcion)	0.125 mg qhs
Intermediate acting	
Oxazepam (Serax)	15-30 mg qhs
Lorazepam (Ativan)	0.5-2 mg qhs
Temazepam (Restoril)	5-30 mg qhs
Long acting	
Diazepam (Valium)	2-10 mg qhs
Flurazepam (Dalmane)	15-30 mg qhs
Cyclopyrrolones	
Zopiclone (Imovane)	3.75-14 mg qhs
Imidazopyridines	
Zolpidem (Ambien)	10 mg qhs
Tricyclics	
Amitriptyline (Elavil)	10-75 mg qhs
Doxepin (Sinequan)	10-75 mg qhs
Modified Cyclic Derivatives	
Trazodone (Desyrel)	150-300 mg qhs
Phenylpiperazine Compounds	
Nefazodone (Serzone)	100-250 mg hs
Selective Serotonin Reuptake Inhibitors	
Paroxetine (Paxil)	20 mg qhs

REFERENCES

1. Ford DE, Kamerow MD: Epidemiologic study of sleep disturbances and psychiatric disorders: an opportunity for prevention? *JAMA* 262:1479-1484, 1989.
2. Kupfer DJ, Reynolds CF III: Management of insomnia, *N Engl J Med* 336:341-346, 1997.
3. Mendelson W: A 96-year-old woman with insomnia, *JAMA* 277:990-996, 1997.
4. Mamelak M, Lipsitz J: When your patient can't sleep, *Patient Care Can* 5:32-44, 1994.
5. Bootzin RR, Perlis ML: Nonpharmacologic treatments of insomnia, *J Clin Psychiatry* 53(suppl 6):37-41, 1992.
6. Guilleminault C, Clerk A, Black J, et al: Nondrug treatment trials in psychophysiologic insomnia, *Arch Intern Med* 155:838-844, 1995.
7. King AC, Oman RF, Brassington GS, et al: Moderate-intensity exercise and self-rated quality of sleep in older adults: a randomized controlled trial, *JAMA* 277:32-37, 1997.
8. Hypnotic drugs, *Med Lett* 38:59-61, 1996.
9. Nierenberg AA, Adler LA, Peselow E, et al: Trazodone for antidepressant-associated insomnia, *Am J Psychiatry* 151:1069-1072, 1994.
10. Epstein FH: Melatonin in humans, *N Engl J Med* 336:186-195, 1997.
11. Arendt J: Melatonin (editorial), *BMJ* 312:1242-1243, 1996.
12. Folkard S, Arendt J, Clark M: Can melatonin improve shift workers' tolerance of the night shift? Some preliminary findings, *Chronobiol Int* 10:315-320, 1993.

Narcolepsy

(See also insomnia)

The usual sequence of symptom development in narcolepsy is as follows:

1. Hypersomnia
2. Cataplexy
3. Sleep paralysis
4. Hypnagogic/hypnopompic hallucinations

Pharmacological treatment is with methylphenidate (Ritalin). The usual dosage for adults is 10 to 30 mg/day in two or three divided doses. The maximum dose is 60 mg/day.

Sleep Apnea

(See also insomnia)

The prevalence of sleep apnea has been estimated to be 2% to 4% among middle-aged adults. The condition is most common in middle-aged obese men. Important symptoms are loud snoring and fatigue, while gasping, snorting, or observed apnea during sleep is highly suggestive. Patients with obstructive sleep apnea are said to have an increased incidence of hypertension, ischemic heart disease, cerebrovascular disease, and motor vehicle accidents.[1-3] A systematic review of the literature was unable to confirm an association between sleep apnea and any of these outcomes except possibly motor vehicle accidents. The authors of this review believe that many of the reputed adverse affects are explained by confounding variables such as obesity and smoking.[3]

Primary medical treatment of sleep apnea consists of weight loss and avoidance of alcohol. Sleeping in the lateral position may give some relief. In some mild cases protriptyline (Triptil) or fluoxetine (Prozac) or oral appliances are helpful, but the prime medical therapeutic modality is positive airway pressure. Surgical procedures include palatal surgery and tracheostomy.[1] Even the efficacy of positive airway pressure is questionable when the evidence is systematically reviewed.[3] Possibly patients with severe symptoms benefit while others do not, but this is unproved at present.[3]

REFERENCES

1. Strollo PJ Jr, Rogers RM: Obstructive sleep apnea, *N Engl J Med* 334:99-104, 1996.
2. Kingman P, Strohl KP, Redline S: Recognition of obstructive sleep apnea, *Am J Respir Crit Care Med* 154:279-289, 1996.
3. Wright J, Johns R, Watt I, et al: Health effects of obstructive sleep apnoea and the effectivenss of continuous positive airways pressure: a systematic review of the research evidence, *BMJ* 314:851-860, 1997.

Sleep Walking

About 10% to 15% of children between the ages of 5 and 12 have at least one episode of sleep walking. Between one fourth and one third of children who are sleep walkers have enuresis, and a fair number also have night terrors. The incidence is increased in patients with Tourette's syndrome. Somnambulism generally occurs in the first 3 to 4 hours of sleep during stages 3 and 4 of non-rapid-eye-movement (NREM) sleep. Injuries during the episodes are common, especially in adults. In children the condition is generally self-limited.[1]

REFERENCES

1. Masand P, Popli AP, Weilburg JB: Sleepwalking, *Am Fam Physician* 649-653, 1995.

Snoring

A study of snoring overweight men found that sleeping on one side or using nasal decongestants had little effect. However, weight loss was effective. Men who lost 3 kg or more cut their hourly snoring rates in half, and three subjects who lost an average of 7.6 kg stopped snoring entirely.[1]

Protriptyline 5 to 20 mg qhs is reputed to reduce snoring.

REFERENCES

1. Braver HM, Block AJ, Perri MG: Treatment for snoring—combined weight loss, sleeping on side, and nasal spray, *Chest* 107:1283-1288, 1995.

SPORTS MEDICINE

(See also acute exertional rhabdomyolysis; concussion; diagnosis of seizures; exercise; exercise in pregnancy; urinalysis-blood)

Bicycle Seats

Bicycle seats have been associated with a number of clinical conditions. Skin problems include chafing of the inner thighs or groins, pain over the ischial tuberosities, skin ulceration, and furunculosis in the seat area. Less common but of more concern is pudendal neuropathy characterized by numbness of the scrotum and penile shaft. This is thought to be caused by compression of the dorsal branch of the pudendal nerve between the bicycle seat and the symphysis pubis; in many cases it results from an upward tilting of the bicycle seat. In a few case reports temporary impotence has been associated with biking, but whether a causal relationship exists is uncertain.[1]

REFERENCES

1. Weiss BD: Clinical syndromes associated with bicycle seats, *Clin Sports Med* 13:175-186, 1994.

Diarrhea and Hematochezia in Runners

(See also exercise-induced hematuria)

Diarrhea occurs in 20% to 25% of marathon runners.[1-3] Symptoms vary from loose stools to frank diarrhea and are associated with increased mileage or a particularly strenuous effort. They occur during or right after the training. About half the patients have fecal urgency and often have to stop the workout to go to the bathroom.[2]

Hematochezia may also occur in runners. Occult blood in the stool has been found in 20% of runners immediately after a marathon, and 6% had frank rectal bleeding.[4] Gastrointestinal blood loss has been proposed as a cause of runners' anemia.[5]

REFERENCES

1. Butcher JD: Runner's diarrhea and other intestinal problems of athletes, *Am Fam Physician* 48:623-627, 1993.
2. Keeffe EB, Lowe DK, Goss JR, Wayne R: Gastrointestinal symptoms of marathon runners, *West J Med* 141:481-484, 1984.
3. Worobetz LF, Gerrard DF: Gastrointestinal symptoms during exercise in endurance athletes: relevance and speculations on the aetiology, *NZ Med J* 98:644-646, 1985.
4. McCabe ME 3d, Peura DA, Kadakia SC, et al: Gastrointestinal blood loss associated with running a marathon, *Dig Dis Sci* 31:1229-1232, 1986.
5. Stewart JG, Ahlquist DA, McGill DB, et al: Gastrointestinal blood loss and anemia in runners, *Ann Intern Med* 100:843-845, 1984.

Drugs and Sports

Banned substances

A large number of drugs are banned for Olympic competitors. Even if prescription or nonprescription drugs are not banned, competitors must declare their use before Olympic meets. Banned substances include the following[1,2]:

1. Stimulants (epinephrine, amphetamines, cocaine, and decongestants such as pseudoephedrine, phenylephrine, and phenylpropanolamine). Many cold remedies contain these agents.
2. Narcotics (except codeine)
3. Beta-blockers for specific sports such as archery, diving, or shooting
4. Diuretics
5. Probenecid (because it affects urine samples)
6. Anabolic steroids
7. Peptide hormones and analogues (growth hormone, adrenocorticotropic hormone, human chorionic gonadotropin, erythropoietin)
8. Tetracaine (because of the cocaine)
9. Corticosteroids by the IV, intramuscular, or oral route. Intraarticular and inhaled corticosteroids are allowed but must be reported.
10. Autologous blood transfusions ("blood doping")

Natural and herbal remedies should be avoided because some contain unlabeled banned substances. Many banned agents can be detected by toxicological analysis, but this is more difficult or even impossible for some, particularly the peptide analogues.

Anabolic steroids. Illicit use of anabolic steroids is common. One U.S. survey found that 7% of male high school students had taken these drugs.[3]

Anabolic steroids increase muscle mass and strength but not aerobic capacity. There is no convincing evidence that they increase performance. A variety of anabolic steroids are used, often concomitantly and in doses up to 100 times those required for replacement therapy. Common adverse effects are acne, decreased testicular volume, and azoospermia. Other documented complications are cholestasis, peliosis hepatis (liver cysts), and hepatocellular adenomas and carcinomas. The high-density lipoprotein level is lowered and the low-density lipoprotein level elevated, the erythrocyte count is increased, and platelet numbers and platelet aggregation are augmented. Increased or decreased libido, increased aggression, psychosis, and withdrawal symptoms have been reported.[4]

REFERENCES

1. Olson R: Drugs, athletes, and family physicians: when to withhold medications and when to document prescriptions, *Can Fam Physician* 42:1953-1960, 1996.
2. MacAuley D: Drugs in sport, *BMJ* 313:211-215, 1996.
3. Buckley WE, Yesalis CE III, Friedl KE, et al: Estimated prevalence of anabolic steroid use among male high school seniors, *JAMA* 260:3441-3445, 1988.
4. Bagateli CJ, Bremner WJ: Androgens in men—uses and abuses, *N Engl J Med* 334:707-714, 1996.

Female Athletes

(See also risks of exercise)

A serious problem for some female athletes is the combination of an eating disorder, amenorrhea, and osteoporosis. The incidence of the so-called female athlete triad[1,2] in top women athletes has been reported to be between 15% and 62%.[2] In amenorrheic athletes bone density has been shown to be decreased not only in the spine and proximal femur, but in many other sites, including cortical weight-bearing bone.[3]

In a small retrospective study of amenorrheic runners, hormone replacement therapy with either conjugated estrogen

(Premarin) 0.625 mg/day or an estradiol transdermal patch of 50 μg/day plus medroxyprogesterone acetate 10 mg/day for 14 days a month resulted in greater bone density in the treated than in the untreated cohort.[4]

REFERENCES

1. Nattiv A, Agostini R, Drinkwater B, et al: The female athlete triad: the inter-relatedness of disordered eating, amenorrhea, and osteoporosis, *Clin Sports Med* 13:405-418, 1994.
2. Tofler IR, Stryer BK, Micheli LJ, et al: Physical and emotional problems of elite female gymnasts, *N Engl J Med* 335:281-283, 1996.
3. Rencken ML, Chesnut CH III, Drinkwater BL: Bone density at multiple skeletal sites in amenorrheic athletes, *JAMA* 276:238-240, 1996.
4. Cumming DC: Exercise-associated amenorrhea, low bone density, and estrogen replacement therapy, *Arch Intern Med* 156: 2193-2195, 1996.

Preparticipation Medical Examinations

(See also cardiac arrest; cardiac arrest during exercise; cardiopulmonary resuscitation)

The purpose of preparticipation medical examinations is to prevent illness or injuries during athletic activities. Such examinations rarely result in interventions,[1] and when they do, treatment is mainly on the basis of history.[2]

A study of 100 cardiac deaths that occurred during or within an hour of exercise in young athletes found that over 50% were due to hypertrophic cardiomyopathy and 11% to coronary artery anomalies.[3] Another study of sudden deaths in young competitive athletes reported that one third were due to hypertrophic cardiomyopathy and 13% to anomalous origins of the coronary arteries. Preparticipation medical examinations identified only 3% of those who died as having possible cardiovascular disease.[4] If preparticipation examinations fail to detect cardiac disease, especially hypertrophic cardiomyopathy, would screening echocardiograms be indicated? Five studies involving a total of 5458 students failed to find any case of cardiac disease.[5]

Preparticipation medical examinations also seem to have little value for marathon runners, since in a tabulation of 215,413 runners in a variety of marathons only four sudden cardiac deaths occurred, for a prevalence rate of 0.002%.[6] Exercise testing is not indicated for prospective marathon runners because it is neither sensitive nor specific.[5]

Although preparticipation medical examinations do not appear to be cost effective, some authors rationalize continuing them as a way to capture adolescent patients for general preventive health counseling.[7]

REFERENCES

1. Risser Wl, Hoffman HM, Bellah GG Jr, et al: A cost-benefit analysis of preparticipation sports examinations of adolescent athletes, *J Sch Health* 55:270-273, 1985.
2. Goldberg B, Saraniti A, Witman P, et al: Pre-participation sports assessment—an objective evaluation, *Pediatrics* 66:736-745, 1980.
3. Van Camp SP, Bloor CM, Mueller FO, et al: Nontraumatic sports death in high school and college athletes, *Med Sci Sports Exerc* 27:641-647, 1995.
4. Maron BJ, Shirani J, Poliac LC, et al: Sudden death in young competitive athletes: clinical, demographic, and pathological profiles, *JAMA* 276:199-204, 1996.
5. Thompson PD: The cardiovascular complications of vigorous physical activity, *Arch Intern Med* 156:2297-2302, 1996.
6. Maron BJ, Poliac LC, Roberts WO: Risk for sudden cardiac death associated with marathon running, *J Am Coll Cardiol* 28: 428-431, 1996.
7. Briner WW Jr: Getting more out of athletic examinations (editorial), *Am Fam Physician* 48:225, 1993.

Pyschological Morbidity Among Olympic-Level Athletes

An assessment of Olympic-level gymnastic training programs found that training often begins between the ages of 5 and 7 years and that some children leave home by the age of 12 to obtain specialized instruction. At this point in their development they may be training for 30 to 45 hours a week and become socially isolated.[1] Tofler and associates[1] suggest that one of the driving forces behind this phenomenon is pressure from parents and coaches motivated by their need for vicarious achievement. This could be considered a form of child abuse.[1] Allowing Kerri Strug to perform a second vault during the 1996 Olympics after she had sustained a major injury to her ankle is an example of this phenomenon.[2]

REFERENCES

1. Tofler IR, Stryer BK, Micheli LJ, et al: Physical and emotional problems of elite female gymnasts, *N Engl J Med* 335:281-283, 1996.
2. O'Connor PJ, Lewis RD: Physical and emotional problems of elite female gymnasts (letter), *N Engl J Med* 336:140-141, 1997.

Scuba Diving

A number of medical problems result from scuba diving. One of the most serious is decompression sickness, which usually manifests itself within 8 hours of the dive but may not become obvious for up to 24 hours. This disorder is usually seen in divers who have exceeded the time limits set out in standard dive tables for the depth attained. The most common symptoms are joint pains, especially in the shoulder or elbow. Skin rash, skin marbling (cutis marmorata), and pruritus are also frequent. Central nervous symptoms often involve the spinal cord and cause numbness, paresthesias, and weakness. Mentation may be altered. Pulmonary symptoms are relatively rare and consist of substernal pain, dyspnea, and coughing ("the chokes"), which usually develop immediately after surfacing. If inert gas bubbles form in the inner ear, the patient will experience vertigo, tinnitus, and sensorineural hearing loss (inner ear decompression syndrome). Treatment of decompression sickness is recompression; this may be beneficial for patients with neurological symptoms even after several days.[1]

Other serious or even fatal consequences of scuba diving are pulmonary barotrauma and arterial gas embolism. If a diver fails to exhale while ascending (which is most likely to occur in an uncontrolled ascent), the expanding air may rupture the alveoli. Subcutaneous emphysema and pneumothorax may occur, and if air bubbles enter the pulmonary vasculature and from there the arterial circulation, cerebrovascular accidents or myocardial infarction may ensue. Symptoms of arterial gas embolism usually come on immediately after the ascent, whereas those of decompression sickness develop gradually.[1] Hyperbaric oxygen is the treatment of choice for both arterial gas embolism and decompression sickness.[2]

The most common form of barotrauma from scuba diving is barotitis media or "middle ear squeeze." It is caused by a failure of the eustachian tube to open, often because of an upper respiratory tract infection. In severe cases patients may have hemotympanum or even perforation. In some cases barotrauma also affects the inner ear (inner ear barotrauma). If the diver is unable to clear the ears in the presence of a blocked eustachian tube, the high intracranial pressure associated with diving may be transmitted through the internal auditory canal to the inner ear and cause a round window tear or a rupture of the membranous labyrinth. In either case a sudden onset of vertigo, tinnitus, and hearing loss will occur. As stated previously, similar symptoms may occur in decompression sickness involving the inner ear, but in that case symptoms usually appear later and more gradually.[1]

REFERENCES

1. Clenney TL, Lassen LF: Recreational scuba diving injuries, *Am Fam Physician* 53:1761-1766, 1996.
2. Tibbles PM, Edelsberg JS: Hyperbaric-oxygen therapy, *N Engl J Med* 334:1642-1648, 1996.

SURGERY

Many references to surgery are made throughout the text and may be found by searching the index for specific topics such as coronary artery bypass grafting, prostate cancer, lung cancer, and breast cancer. This section deals with only a few selected areas.

Anesthesia

(See also coronary artery bypass grafting and angioplasty)

Whether general anesthesia causes permanent cognitive deficits is controversial. In a randomized controlled trial elderly patients who were having total knee replacements were assigned to receive either general or epidural anesthesia. After 6 months 5% of each group showed a significant deterioration in cognitive function. Whether a similar group of patients who had no surgery or anesthesia would have had a similar rate of cognitive decline is unknown.[1] However, cognitive functioning is diminished in about 3% of patients subjected to coronary artery bypass grafting.[2] Whether this is related to anesthesia or other aspects of the surgery is uncertain.

REFERENCES

1. Williams-Russo P, Sharrock NRE, Mattis S, et al: Cognitive effects after epidural vs general anesthesia in older adults: a randomized trial, *JAMA* 274:44-50, 1995.
2. Roach GW, Kanchuger M, Mangano M, et al: Adverse cerebral outcomes after coronary bypass surgery, *N Engl J Med* 335: 1857-1863, 1996.

Appendicitis

The most effective way of diagnosing appendicitis is through the history and physical examination. Important points in the history favoring the diagnosis are migration of the pain from the periumbilical region to the right lower quadrant and presence of pain before vomiting. Previous episodes of similar pain argue against the diagnosis. Most patients with appendicitis have right lower quadrant tenderness, guarding, or rigidity.[1]

Although ultrasound is reasonably effective in detecting a distended appendix, no studies have shown it to be superior to clinical examination in making the diagnosis of appendicitis. Plain x-ray views of the abdomen are neither sensitive nor specific.[1]

REFERENCES

1. Wagner JM, McKinney WP, Carpenter JL: Does this patient have appendicitis? *JAMA* 276:1589-1594, 1996.

Burns

Burns are classified according to the depth of the burn and the percentage of body surface covered (rule of nines).

Depth of burn

Depth of burns is determined clinically according to the following criteria.[1]

First-degree burns. First-degree burns involve only the epidermis. They are erythematous and blanch with pressure. Sensation is intact, and they are mildly painful.

Second-degree burns. Superficial second-degree burns involve the epidermis and superficial dermis, but the epithelial appendages are intact. These occur as blanching erythema with superficial blisters. Sensation is intact, and they are mildly painful. Deep second-degree burns involve the epidermis, most of the dermis, and most of the skin appendages. They appear dry, waxy, and whitish with red elements. The skin does not blanch with pressure. Sensation is present but diminished, and the burn is only slightly painful. Scarring usually occurs.

Third-degree burns. Third-degree burns involve the epidermis, all of the dermis, and all of the skin appendages. They appear white, red, tan, or charred. The skin is dry and leathery and does not blanch with pressure. It is anesthetic, and the burn is not painful. Scarring occurs.

Fourth-degree burns. Fourth-degree burns involve the same structures as third-degree burns but also underlying structures such as tendons, muscle, or bone. Their appearance is the same as that of third-degree burns. They are anesthetic.

Rule of nines

The extent of burns according to the rule of nines is as follows[1]:

Head and neck	9%
Each upper limb	9%
Each lower limb	18%
Back and buttocks	18%
Chest and abdomen	18%

REFERENCES

1. Waitzman AA, Neligan PC: How to manage burns in primary care, *Can Fam Physician* 39:2394-2400, 1993.

Hernias

The prevalence of groin hernias is 3% to 4%. The incidence and the risk of strangulation increase with age. Once a groin hernia develops, it never spontaneously resolves and over the years it gradually enlarges. The risk of strangulation is highest for femoral hernias but still significant for inguinal hernias with rates of 2.8% within 3 months of discovery and 4.5% within 2 years. The risk of strangulation is greatest in the 3 months after onset.[1]

There is a strong familial predisposition for groin hernias. Physical activities such as weight lifting do not cause hernias but may aggravate a hernia that has already developed.[1]

If not strangulated, most groin hernias can be repaired in outpatient surgery using a local anesthetic; if a laparoscopic technique is used, regional or general anesthesia is required. The classic way of repairing hernias is to close the defect with sutures (Shouldice hernioplasty). Tension-free hernioplasties are now generally preferred, and these require the placement of a prosthesis over the defect. Adverse effects, including postoperative pain, are minimal. Normal activities of daily living may commence immediately; jogging, golf, and similar activities within 10 to 14 days; and heavy lifting as soon as it can be done without pain. Recurrence rates are usually less than 1%.[1]

Tension-free hernioplasties performed with the laparoscope have excellent results.[2]

REFERENCES

1. Wantz GE: A 65-year-old man with an inguinal hernia, *JAMA* 277:663-669, 1997.
2. Liem MS, van der Graaf Y, van Steensel CJ, et al: Comparison of conventional anterior surgery and laparoscopic surgery for inguinal-hernia repair, *N Engl J Med* 336:1541-1547, 1997.

Ingrown Toenails

A conservative way of managing ingrown toenails is to have the patient soak the affected foot for 20 to 30 minutes daily and then clean the "gutter" between the nail and the skin with a swab or a blunt object such as a butter knife.[1]

REFERENCES

1. Scherger JE: Successful technique for treating ingrown toenails (letter), *Am Fam Physician* 53:499, 1996.

Skin Excisions

One of the goals of skin excision is to avoid unsightly scars. Among the ways of achieving this are avoidance of elective excisions during the prepubertal growth spurt and early teens, since at this time the chance of hypertrophic scar formation is greater, and avoidance of incisions in the presternal area, deltoid region, or back, since poor scar formation is common in these regions.[1] The patient should be told that complete healing takes about 1 year and that scars are often most noticeable 2 to 3 months after the initial wound.

REFERENCES

1. Wilkes GH: Office excision and suture techniques for the family physician, *Can J CME,* July 1994, 6:49-53.

Lacerations

(See also bites)

Lacerations of the face may be sutured up to 24 hours after injury provided aggressive irrigation and debridement are used. In most cases the patient can remove the outer dressing of the wound and take a shower after a day or so. Swimming and tub baths should be avoided until healing is complete. Nonabsorbable sutures should be removed from the face in 4 to 5 days, the trunk and extremities in 7 to 10 days, and the palms and soles in 12 to 15 days. If traumatic tattooing is found, the area should be scrubbed with a brush before closure. The flap of flap-type lacerations of the anterior tibia in the elderly should be debrided of subcutaneous tissues with sharp curved scissors before being sutured. A pressure dressing should be applied.[1]

Tissue adhesives

A new cyanoacrylate tissue adhesive, octylcyanoacrylate (Dermabond), has been developed that is stronger and less brittle than previous products. It can be used on long or short facial lacerations and selected lacerations elsewhere. It should not be used on the hands or feet, over joints, in wounds crossing mucocutaneous junctions, in bite wounds, or in heavily soiled or crushed wounds. In one randomized trial the cosmetic results equaled those of sutures.[2]

Octylcyanoacrylate is used as a topical closure. The skin edges are carefully juxtaposed, and the agent is painted over the apposed edges, which are held together for another 30 seconds to allow complete polymerization to take place. The adhesive should not be permitted to seep into the wound edges because this would inhibit healing. Patients may take showers but should not soak or scrub the area. The adhesive sloughs off in 1 to 2 weeks.[2]

REFERENCES

1. Martin S: Triage and care of wounds, *Can J CME,* November 1995, 7:29-47.
2. Quinn J, Wells G, Sutcliffe T, et al: A randomized trial comparing octylcyanoacrylate tissue adhesive and sutures in the management of lacerations, *JAMA* 277:1527-1530, 1997.

TOXICOLOGY

(See also lead poisoning; screening)

Acetaminophen

Acetaminophen carries little risk of toxicity for an otherwise healthy child if the dose is less than 200 mg/kg.

In a study of acetaminophen overdose in children 1 to 6 years of age, ipecac decreased serum acetaminophen concentrations by 50% if vomiting was induced within 30 minutes of ingestion compared with control subjects who did not vomit. No beneficial effect was noted if the ipecac was taken more than 90 minutes after the acetaminophen ingestion.[1] The usual dose is 5 to 10 ml for children aged 6 to 12 months and 15 ml for those aged 1 to 12 years. The dose is followed by 2 glasses of water. If vomiting has not occurred within 20 minutes, the dose is repeated once.

REFERENCES

1. Bond GR, Requa RK, Krenzelok EP, et al: Influence of time until emesis on the efficacy of decontamination using acetaminophen as a marker in a pediatric population, *Ann Emerg Med* 22: 1403-1407, 1993.

TROPICAL MEDICINE

(See also aviation medicine; cyclosporiasis; diarrhea; diarrhea and dehydration in infants; hepatitis A; hepatitis B; immunizations)

Information for Travelers

General information about traveling in tropical regions, including a directory of physicians who speak English, immunization requirements, and maps showing areas of risk for malaria and yellow fever, is available from the International Association for Medical Assistance to Travelers (IAMAT), 40 Regal Road, Guelph, Ontario, Canada N1K 1B5; 417 Center Street, Lewiston, NY 14092, USA; or 57 Voirets, 2112 Grand-Lancy-Geneva, Switzerland.

Immunizations for Travelers

All travelers to tropical or developing countries should have up-to-date vaccinations against tetanus and diphtheria, and those born after 1956 need up-to-date measles vaccinations. Travelers to developing or tropical countries outside the Western Hemisphere also require up-to-date polio vaccinations. Typhoid and hepatitis A vaccines are recommended primarily for those traveling beyond the usual tourist routes, and hepatitis B vaccination is needed for medical personnel, those who expect to be at risk through sexual contact, or those planning to spend more than 6 months in endemic areas such as sub-Saharan Africa or Southeast Asia. Japanese encephalitis vaccine is advised for those visiting rice-growing rural areas in Southeast Asia; the attack rate in short-term travelers to urban areas is extremely low. Meningococcal vaccines should be given to persons visiting areas where epidemics are in progress (often sub-Saharan Africa or northern India and Nepal). Yellow fever vaccine is indicated for those traveling to rural areas of South America or much of sub-Saharan Africa, excluding South Africa and adjoining countries. Rabies vaccine is advised for travelers with occupational risk or those staying in endemic areas for prolonged periods. Tourists are at low risk of acquiring cholera; the cholera vaccines are not very effective.[1]

Malaria

The four species of *Plasmodium* that infect humans are *vivax, ovale, malariae,* and *falciparum. P. falciparum* is the most lethal species. All the types are spread by bite of the female *Anopheles* mosquito. The incubation period of malaria varies with the species of *Plasmodium* and depends on how long the parasite spends in the human liver in the schizont phase before being released into the bloodstream as merozoites. *P. falciparum* has the shortest incubation period, varying between 2 and 8 weeks. The incubation period of the other species may be months or occasionally years. In the majority of cases the initial symptoms manifest themselves within 1 year of exposure.

Protection against mosquito bites is a key element in malaria prophylaxis. This involves avoiding evening or night-time strolls, wearing clothing that covers most of the body, and using screens and insect repellents containing up to 35% diethyltoluamide (Deet).[1] A mosquito-proof netting to cover the bed at night might be considered; portable types with frames are available through IAMAT. International travelers may need to apply mosquito repellents just before landing at their destination, since waiting lines for customs and immigration in India (and presumably elsewhere) are sometimes in mosquito-infested areas. Hotels in tropical regions may not be screened or fully enclosed and may not have facilities for hanging mosquito netting over beds.[2]

Chloroquine (Aralen) is the drug of choice for the few areas of the world where non-chloroquine-resistant malaria is still extant: Central America west of the Panama Canal Zone, Mexico, Haiti, the Dominican Republic, and parts of the Middle East, including Egypt, Syria, and Iraq. Cases of chloroquine-resistant malaria have been reported in Iran, Oman, and Yemen. The map of chloroquine-resistant malaria is ever changing, and travelers must consult up-to-date sources of information.[1]

The usual dose of chloroquine for malaria prophylaxis is 2 tablets or 500 mg (300 mg of base) weekly starting 2 weeks before departure and continuing until 8 weeks after return. For infants and children the prophylactic dose is 5 mg/kg of the base. If there is insufficient time to start prophylaxis 2 weeks before departure, a loading dose may be given. Adults should take 500 mg (300 mg base) as soon as possible and a second dose of 500 mg in 6 hours; for children the loading dose is chloroquine base 5 mg/kg as soon as possible with a second dose of 5 mg/kg in 6 hours.

Treatment of malaria in adults using chloroquine is 4 tablets (1 g) as a loading dose followed in 6 to 8 hours by 2 tablets (500 mg), followed by a single dose of 2 tablets (500 mg) on each of the next 2 consecutive days. The dose intervals for children with malaria are identical, but the first dose is calculated on the basis of 10 mg/kg of base (maximum 600 mg of base) and the subsequent three doses on the basis of 5 mg/kg of base.

The drug of choice for malaria prophylaxis in areas with chloroquine-resistant malaria is mefloquine (Lariam) except in regions where mefloquine-resistant malaria is present, such as the Thai-Cambodian and Thai-Burmese borders. In these places doxycycline 100 mg/day is recommended.[1] The usual dose of mefloquine for malaria prophylaxis is 250 mg weekly starting 1 week before departure and continuing for 4 weeks after return. The prophylactic dose for children weighing 15 to 19 kg is 1/4 tablet (62.5 mg) weekly, for those weighing 20 to 30 kg is 1/2 tablet (125 mg) weekly, and for those weighing 31 to 45 kg is 3/4 tablet (187.5 mg) weekly. Mefloquine should be taken with food, and adults should drink at least 240 ml (1 glass) of water with it. Caution should be used in prescribing mefloquine to patients with cardiac conduction defects or taking medications such as quinine, chloroquine, beta-blockers, or calcium channel blockers. If quinine or chloroquine has been used for the initial treatment of malaria, 12 hours should elapse from the last dose of either of these drugs before mefloquine is begun. Seizures and psychoses have been reported as rare complications of mefloquine, and minor neuropsychiatric reactions such as irritability, depression, and nightmares occur in about 0.5% of patients.[3] If time is critical, loading doses of 250 mg/day for 3 consecutive days may be given.[4]

Patients taking mefloquine prophylactically should carry a therapeutic dose of sulfadoxine-pyrimethamine (Fansidar) so they can treat themselves if high fever develops and they cannot obtain medical care.[1] The usual adult dosage of Fansidar for treatment of malaria is 3 tablets as a single dose. For children over 2 months of age the dosage is 1 tablet as a single dose for those weighing 11 to 29 kg and 2 tablets as a single dose for those weighing 30 to 45 kg. Fansidar is contraindicated in patients allergic to sulfonamides.

An alternative prophylactic regimen for persons who do not tolerate mefloquine and are traveling to West Africa or the Indian subcontinent may be a combination of 300 mg of chloroquine base weekly plus proguanil (Paludrine) 200 mg/day.[3]

In about 90% of travelers who acquire malaria the disease develops after they return home. The standard treatment of severe falciparum malaria, including cerebral malaria, is IV quinidine or, if that is not available, intramuscular quinine. Unfortunately, many hospital pharmacies in North America do not stock either of these drugs, which has resulted in some deaths.[5] An effective alternative treatment not yet available in North America is intramuscular artemether, a drug derived from the Chinese quinghao plant.[6-8]

Travelers' Diarrhea

The incidence of travelers' diarrhea during the first 2 weeks of stay has been reported to be between 30% to 40%.[9] In a study from Nepal 64% of tourists who had been in the country for 1 month or less reported at least one episode of diarrhea.[10] Risk factors for travelers' diarrhea are younger age, eating in restaurants, and short duration of stay.[10] The Nepal study was unable to confirm that drinking untreated water, using ice in drinks, or eating unpeeled fruit or leafy vegetables was an independent risk factor, but this may be the result of inadequate power of the study. (Even if these findings are confirmed by future studies, avoiding untreated water remains an essential measure for preventing cholera.) The authors point out that to their knowledge no studies have shown that dietary education before travel decreases the risk of diarrhea. Despite this, common sense dictates that dietary discretion be practiced even if the evidence for its efficacy has not yet been demonstrated.[10]

Travelers' diarrhea lasts longer than 1 week in 10% of cases and longer than 1 month in 2% of cases. In the majority of cases it is due to enterotoxigenic *Escherichia coli, Campylobacter, Shigella,* and *Salmonella*. Viruses and parasites are less common causes.[1,11]

Prophylaxis of travelers' diarrhea is generally not recommended.[11] There are several reasons for this. From the public health perspective, widespread use of antibiotics is likely to foster antibiotic resistance. Complications of antibiotic prophylaxis include allergic reactions, photosensitivity reactions, and antibiotic-associated vaginal candidiasis and diarrhea. Since only a small percentage of people acquire travelers' diarrhea, a large number of individuals would be treated unnecessarily. Finally, the treatment of the disorder is simple and efficacious, so prophylaxis is rarely needed. However, even though antibiotic prophylaxis for travelers' diarrhea has not been proved necessary for medical conditions such as achlorhydria or AIDS, it may be recommended in the following circumstances[9-11]:

1. A necessary brief trip during which illness is not acceptable
2. AIDS or other immunodeficiency states
3. Active inflammatory bowel disease
4. Insulin-dependent diabetes
5. Heart disease in elderly patients
6. Chronic renal failure
7. Achlorhydria, gastrectomy, or omeprazole (Losec, Prilosec) use

Table 47 Prophylaxis of Travelers' Diarrhea

Drug	Usual dose
Trimethoprim-sulfamethoxazole DS (TMP-SMX, Bactrim, Septra)	1 tablet daily
Doxycycline (Vibra-Tabs)	100 mg/day
Bismuth subsalicylate (Pepto-Bismol)	Two 262-mg tablets qid with meals and hs
Norfloxacin (Noroxin)	400 mg/day
Ciprofloxacin (Cipro)	500 mg/day
Ofloxacin (Floxin)	300 mg/day

Table 48 Pharmacological Management of Travelers' Diarrhea

Drug	Dose
Symptomatic Control	
Loperamide (Imodium)	4 mg stat, then 2 mg after each loose stool; maximum 16 mg/day
Diphenoxylate 2.5 mg, atropine 0.025 mg (Lomotil)	2 tablets stat, then 1 tablet after each loose stool; maximum 8 tablets daily
Antibacterial	
Bismuth subsalicylate (Pepto-Bismol)	30 ml or two 262-mg tablets q30min for 5 doses; regimen may be repeated on day 2
Norfloxacin (Noroxin)	400 bid for 3 days*
Ciprofloxacin (Cipro)	500 bid for 3 days*
Ofloxacin (Floxin)	300 bid for 3 days*
Trimethoprim-sulfamethoxazole (TMP-SMX) (Bactrim, Septra)	1 double-strength tablet as single dose or 1 double-strength tablet bid for 3 days; for children, trimethoprim 6 mg/kg/day and sulfamethoxazole 30 mg/kg/day in 2 divided doses

*For mild cases a single or double dose of one of the quinolones may be effective. Severe cases should be treated for 3 days.

Drugs that have been effective for prophylaxis are shown in Table 47.[1]

The mainstay of treatment of travelers' diarrhea is adequate fluid replacement,[1,11] which can be supplied with commercial or homemade oral solutions. Commercial oral replacement fluids are available in either a liquid form (Pedialyte, Lytren) or a powder form that has to be reconstituted with water (Gastrolyte and many other brands). For travelers the powder form is most convenient.

A variety of homemade oral replacement fluid recipes are used. The main ingredients are water, sugar, sodium, and potassium. If orange juice is available, it can supply both sugar and potassium. A rough guide is to make up a solution totaling 1 L (a little less than a quart) that contains one third orange juice, two thirds water, and 1/2 teaspoon (2 to 2.5 ml) table salt. Since water, sugar, and sodium are the key initial requirements, an alternative is the World Health Organization rehydration solution, which is 1 L of water to which are added 1 teaspoon (5 ml) of salt and 4 level tablespoons (40 ml) of sugar.[11]

Pharmacotherapy for travelers' diarrhea may be directed at the symptoms with use of loperamide (Imodium) or diphenoxylate-atropine (Lomotil) or may be antibacterial (Table 48). Loperamide may be given concurrently with antibacterial therapy, but diphenoxylate is not recommended for this purpose because it has been associated with toxic megacolon when given to patients with bacillary dysentery.[11] Antibacterial treatment is required only if the diarrhea is severe or the person has fever or associated hematochezia. The only drug suitable for children is trimethoprim-sulfamethoxazole even though many strains of *E. coli* are resistant to this drug, especially in Mexico. Specific antibacterial regimens are shown in Table 48.[1,11]

REFERENCES

1. Advice for travelers, *Med Lett* 38:17-20, 1996.
2. Porter-Steele N: India's hungry mosquitoes, *Can Med Assoc J* 156:1121, 1997.
3. Barrett PJ, Emmins PD, Clarke PD, et al: Comparison of adverse events associated with use of mefloquine and combination of chloroquine and proguanil as antimalarial prophylaxis: postal and telephone survey of travellers, *BMJ* 313:525-528, 1996.
4. Jaspers CA, Hopperus Buma AP, van Thiel PP, et al: Tolerance of mefloquine chemoprophylaxis in Dutch military personnel, *Am J Trop Med Hyg* 55:230-234, 1996.
5. Humar A, Sharma S, Zoutman D, et al: Fatal falciparum malaria in Canadian travellers, *Can Med Assoc J* 156:1165-1167, 1997.
6. Van Hensbroek MB, Onyiorah E, Jaffar S, et al: A trial of artemether or quinine in children with cerebral malaria, *N Engl J Med* 335:69-75, 1996.
7. Hien TT, Day NP, Phu N, et al: A controlled trial of artemether or quinine in Vietnamese adults with severe falciparum malaria, *N Engl J Med* 335:76-83, 1996.
8. Hoffman SL: Artemether in severe malaria—still too many deaths (editorial), *N Engl J Med* 335:124-125, 1996.
9. Steffen R: Epidemiologic studies of travelers' diarrhea, severe gastrointestinal infections, and cholera, *Rev Infect Dis* 8(suppl 2):S122-S130, 1986.
10. Hoge CW, Shlim DR, Echeverria P, et al: Epidemiology of diarrhea among expatriate residents living in a highly endemic environment, *JAMA* 275:533-538, 1996.
11. Canadian Communicable Disease Report: Statement on travellers' diarrhea, *Can Med Assoc J* 152:205-208, 1995.

UNCERTAINTY

(See also attitudes, physician; informed consent; investigations; labeling; positive predictive value; risk analysis; risk assessment in pregnancy; screening)

The ability not only to live with uncertainty, but also to make rapid and effective clinical decisions in the face of uncertainty, is a fundamental attribute of a good family physician. If a physician is unable to live with uncertainty, one of the more nefarious consequences is a propensity to overinvestigate (see discussion of investigations).

Over a decade ago Biehn[1] from the University of Western Ontario wrote about some of the methods of dealing with uncertainty in family medicine. He pointed out that family physicians probably see more patients with undifferentiated diseases than do any other groups of physicians and that this necessarily leads to uncertainty. He suggested that one of the first ways of dealing with this issue is to ensure that the presenting complaint is the patient's real reason for coming to the office and not just a ticket of admission for a hidden agenda. If the patient has a hidden agenda and the physician brings it out and deals with it, the anxiety of both the patient and the physician will drop dramatically and the vague presenting complaint is likely to resolve spontaneously. Another tactic is for the physician to be open and explain to the patient that he or she is uncertain of the diagnosis and that it may take some time for the basis of the symptoms to become clear. This approach is much easier if a trusting physician-patient relationship has already been established, and it has to be accompanied by a satisfactory management plan. The essence of such a plan is a defined schedule for reassessing the situation within a reasonable time, along with assurance that if the problem is still not clarified, further investigations (if appropriate) or consultations will be initiated.[1]

A specific situation in which the physician must deal with uncertainty is that of the critically ill patient.[2] A common strategy is to paint a black prognosis to the family. On the face of it this is a "can't lose" approach for the physician. If the patient dies, the family has been forewarned, but if the patient survives, the family will be doubly grateful for the almost miraculous skills of the physician. However, as Siegler[2] has pointed out, not only is this intellectually dishonest, but psychologically it is analogous to walking the condemned prisoner to the gallows itself before announcing a reprieve. The more honest approach is to admit the uncertainty and give as truthful a prognosis as possible.[2]

One way for health professionals to deal with uncertainty is to deny it. For example, breast surgeons may be quite certain that the treatment they recommend is correct even though no consensus exists in the literature. Baumann and associates[3] label this the "micro-certainty, macro-uncertainty" phenomenon.

Patients probably have even more difficulty living with uncertainty than physicians.[4,5] As Wardle and Pope[4] point out, shades of gray and risk spectrum are not part of most people's conception of illness.[4] Angell[5] makes the same point and adds that many people believe it is possible to avoid all health risks.

REFERENCES

1. Biehn J: Managing uncertainty in family practice, *Can Med Assoc J* 126:915-917, 1982.
2. Siegler M: Pascal's wager and the hanging of crepe, *N Engl J Med* 293:853-857, 1975.
3. Baumann AO, Deber RB, Thompson GG: Overconfidence among physicians and nurses: the "micro-certainty, macro-uncertainty" phenomenon, *Soc Sci Med* 32:167-174, 1991.
4. Wardle J, Pope R: The psychological costs of screening for cancer, *J Psychosom Res* 36:609-624, 1992.
5. Angell M: Shattuck Lecture—evaluating the health risks of breast implants: the interplay of medical science, the law, and public opinion, *N Engl J Med* 334:1513-1518, 1996.

NEPHROLOGY

Topics covered in this section

CHRONIC RENAL FAILURE

(See also diabetes mellitus and hypertension; diabetic nephropathy; diabetic microalbuminuria; microalbuminuria; restless legs syndrome)

Over one third of patients with end-stage renal failure have diabetes. The second most common cause of end-stage renal failure is hypertension. Diabetic patients requiring dialysis have a poor prognosis; only 20% survive 5 years.[1] End-stage renal failure is more common in black than in white men, and this correlates with an increased incidence of hypertension and lower socioeconomic status.[2]

A large 2-year prospective randomized trial of hypertension control and low-protein diet in patients with chronic renal disease demonstrated only a slight positive effect on renal function.[3] However, a metaanalysis of low-protein diets in both diabetic and nondiabetic renal disease found that such diets slowed the progression of the disease.[4]

It has long been known that phenacetin could cause chronic tubulointerstitial nephritis and ultimately chronic renal failure. The evidence is becoming clear that other analgesics, including acetaminophen and nonsteroidal antiinflammatory drugs (except for aspirin), can also induce this disorder.[5,6]

A multicenter European study has shown that the angiotensin-converting enzyme (ACE) inhibitor benazepril (Lotensin) slows the progression of chronic renal failure of various causes. Of some concern is that the death rate in the benazepril cohort was significantly greater than in the placebo group.[7]

REFERENCES

1. Lafayette RA: Preventing disease progression in chronic renal failure, *Am Fam Physician* 52:1783-1791, 1995.

2. Klag MJ, Whelton PK, Randall BL, et al: End-stage renal disease in African-American and white men, *JAMA* 277:1293-1298, 1997.
3. Klahr S, Levey AS, Beck GJ, et al: The effects of dietary protein restriction and blood-pressure control on the progression of chronic renal disease, *N Engl J Med* 330:877-884, 1994.
4. Pedrini MT, Levey AS, Lau J, et al: The effect of dietary protein restriction on the progression of diabetic and nondiabetic renal diseases—a meta-analysis, *Ann Intern Med* 124:627-632, 1996.
5. Perneger TV, Whelton PK, Klag J: Risk of kidney failure associated with the use of acetaminophen, aspirin, and nonsteroidal antiinflammatory drugs, *N Engl J Med* 331:1675-1679, 1994.
6. Ronco PM, Flahault A: Drug-induced end-stage renal disease (editorial), *N Engl J Med* 331:1711-1712, 1994.
7. Maschio G, Alberti D, Janin G, et al: Effect of the angiotensin-converting-enzyme inhibitor benazepril on the progression of chronic renal insufficiency, *N Engl J Med* 334:939-945, 1996.

IgA NEPHROPATHY

(See also fish oil and coronary artery disease; hematuria; urinalysis)

IgA nephropathy is the most common form of glomerulonephritis in industrialized countries.[1] End-stage renal disease develops in 15% to 20% of patients with this disorder within 10 years of the diagnosis, but in most patients the condition is innocuous. Remissions occur in some cases. IgA nephropathy is often detected when red blood cell (RBC) casts are found in a person with asymptomatic microscopic hematuria. No specific treatment is known. However, in one study 12 g of fish oil per day over 2 years retarded deterioration of renal function in patients who had IgA nephropathy with marked proteinuria.[2] As an editorial accompanying the report pointed out, this is interesting but probably not something to be embraced without further studies.[3] In the meantime the mainstay of therapy for IgA nephropathy, as well as many other chronic renal diseases, is rigorous control of blood pressure, preferably with an ACE inhibitor.[3]

REFERENCES

1. IgA nephropathy: the 25th year, *Contrib Nephrol* 1-219, 1993.
2. Donadio JV Jr, Bergstralh EJ, Offord KP, et al (Mayo Nephrology Collaborative Group): A controlled trial of fish oil in IgA nephropathy, *N Engl J Med* 331:1194-1199, 1994.
3. van Ypersele C: Fish oil for IgA nephropathy? *N Engl J Med* 331:1227-1228, 1994.

MICROALBUMINURIA

(See also diabetes mellitus and hypertension; diabetic nephropathy)

Microalbuminuria is a concentration of albumin in the urine of between 30 and 300 mg/dl. The gold standard is a 24-hour urine measurement, but because this may be difficult to obtain, a dipstick specific for microalbuminuria may be used instead. If the dipstick is used on a first morning specimen and the patient does not have a febrile illness, it is reasonably accurate. A second dipstick reading should be performed within a few months to verify the results. Microalbuminuria is an important abnormality in a number of renal conditions, but particularly diabetic nephropathy. Its detection and subsequent treatment with ACE inhibitors slow the progression of diabetic nephropathy.[1]

REFERENCES

1. Cattran DC: Microalbuminuria urine dip tests: recognize limits, *Patient Care Can,* March 1996, 7:8-9.

POSTURAL PROTEINURIA

Patients with postural proteinuria have proteinuria only in the erect position. The diagnosis can be easily made by collecting urine samples immediately on arising in the morning and after being erect for a few hours. In some patients with postural proteinuria, protein excretion is present whenever the patient is erect, and in others it is intermittent.[1,2]

REFERENCES

1. Trempe D: L'analyse d'urine: bandelettes réactives ou sédiment urinaire? *Med Quebec* 29:25-31, 1994.
2. Rapoport A, Richardson RMA: How to tell it's proteinuria, *Patient Care Can* 5:13-18, 1994.

RENAL TRANSPLANTATION

The 3-year survival rate for transplanted cadaveric kidneys in the United States is 70%. It is higher with kidneys from living unrelated donors; for wife-to-husband grafts it is 87%, and it is the same for husband-to-wife grafts if the wife has never been pregnant. If she has been pregnant, the kidney survival rate is 76%. Good survival despite relatively poor histocompatibility is attributed to healthier kidneys.[1] In the United States 27% of transplanted kidneys come from living related donors, whereas in France the figure is only 4%.[2]

REFERENCES

1. Terasaki PI, Cecka JM, Gjertson DW, et al: High survival rates of kidney transplants from spousal and living unrelated donors, *N Engl J Med* 333:333-336, 1995.
2. Soulillou J-P: Kidney transplantation from spousal donors (editorial), *N Engl J Med* 333:379-380, 1995.

URINALYSIS

(See also acute exertional rhabdomyolysis; bacteriuria and pyuria in the elderly; bladder cancer; diabetic nephropathy; exercise-induced hematuria; IgA nephropathy; fever without source; hematuria)

Little is gained by a microscopic examination of urine that is dipstick negative provided the dipstick is capable of detecting leukocytes.[1] Some important features of the urinalysis are described in the following paragraphs.

Specific Gravity

The usual specific gravity of an early morning urine sample is 1014 to 1028. Heavy proteinuria or glucosuria can elevate the specific gravity.

Glucose

False-negative glucose readings may occur if the patient has taken large quantities of aspirin or vitamin C.

Blood

Dipsticks can detect as few as 2 or 3 RBCs per high-power field.[1] If the dipstick is positive for blood but RBCs are not seen on microscopic examination, the explanation might be myoglobinuria or hemolysis of RBCs.[2,3] False-negative readings may result if the patient has ingested large quantities of vitamin C[2,3] or sometimes as a result of captopril (Capoten) therapy.[3] Healthy people have up to 3 RBCs per high-power field in a centrifuged specimen.[3]

If the dipstick reading is positive, microscopy to look for RBC casts is necessary. If such casts are found, the origin of the hematuria is the kidney and in the majority of cases there is underlying glomerular disease. RBC casts lyse quickly, so the urine should be examined by an experienced observer within 2 hours. The casts are better preserved in acid urine.[2,3]

Intermittent microscopic or even gross hematuria may be a result of vigorous exercise. In asymptomatic persons under the age of 40 with microscopic hematuria, the diagnosis can be safely made if microscopy shows RBCs but no RBC casts and if the hematuria clears within 72 hours of the precipitating physical activity.[4,5] If after vigorous exercise the urine is positive for blood, no RBCs are found with microscopy, and the patient is complaining of muscle pain or swelling, acute exercise-induced rhabdomyolysis should be considered. If the patient has this condition, the creatine kinase level is very high.[6]

Whether the incidental finding of microscopic hematuria in asymptomatic individuals merits a complete urological and nephrological workup is controversial.[3] A fairly high incidence of significant disease has been reported from referral clinics where most of the patients were over 40 years of age,[3] but in a population survey the incidence of serious disease was only 2.3%.[7]

Both the Canadian Task Force on the Periodic Health Examination[8] and the U.S. Preventive Services Task Force[9] give a "D" recommendation for dipstick assessment of urine as a screening tool for bladder cancer in the general population.

Leukocytes

The dipstick detects neutrophils by reacting to some of the esterases these cells possess. This reaction takes place even if the white cells have lysed and are therefore not visible on microscopy.[1,3] The test is sensitive and can detect as few as 3 to 5 white blood cells (WBCs) per high-power field.[1] If both the leukocyte esterase test and the nitrite test (see below) are negative, the chance of a positive urine culture is less than 3%.[1]

In microscopy, pyuria is usually defined as 5 or more WBCs per high-power field in a centrifuged specimen.[3] The presence of WBC casts suggests pyelonephritis or an autoimmune disease such as lupus.[1]

Asymptomatic pyuria and asymptomatic bacteriuria are common in elderly women and usually resolve spontaneously.[10]

Nitrites

The presence of nitrites in the urine occurs when certain bacteria convert nitrates to nitrites. This requires time, so a first voided morning specimen is the ideal specimen for testing. Ascorbic acid may cause false-negative readings.[3] If both the leukocyte esterase test and the nitrite test are negative, the chance of a positive urine culture is less than 3%.[1]

Protein

The comments that follow should not be construed as implicitly advocating routine urinalysis of asymptomatic persons. The Canadian Task Force on the Periodic Health Examination recommends against routine protein dipstick analysis of the adult population as a screen for chronic renal disease ("D" recommendation).[11] The reason behind this is that no effective treatment is known for the majority of serious conditions that may cause proteinuria. An exception is diabetic nephropathy in persons with insulin-dependent diabetes. For this group of patients the Canadian Task Force on the Periodic Health Examination recommends screening for microalbuminuria ("A" recommendation) if this test is locally available.[11] The 1996 guidelines of the U.S. Preventive Services Task Force do not give any recommendations about screening for chronic renal disease or about screening for microalbuminuria in diabetic patients.[12] However, in 1989 this body gave a "D" recommendation to screening the general population for proteinuria.[13]

The Ames dipstick is sensitive primarily for albumin and can detect 15 to 20 mg/dl of protein. Results are classified as negative, trace (10 to 20 mg/dl), 1+ (30 mg/dl), 2+ (100 mg/dl), 3+ (300 mg/dl), and 4+ (1000 mg/dl).[4] Healthy persons may excrete a trace of protein, particularly if the urine is concentrated. False-positive tests may be seen with highly alkaline urine (pH 7.5 to 8.0), with very concentrated urine, and in patients with gross hematuria.[3,14,15] False-negative findings occur with dilute urine.[3,14,15] Further investigations are probably unnecessary in a clinically healthy person whose only abnormality on more than one urinalysis is proteinuria of 30 mg/dl or less. Anyone with 100 mg/dl or more has significant proteinuria and needs further tests.[3,15] The dipstick will not detect Bence Jones protein or microalbuminuria.[15] Detection of the latter is important in follow-up of diabetic patients and is discussed under "Diabetic Nephropathy."

Aside from tests for blood urea nitrogen and creatinine and a complete blood count, an important investigation for a patient with proteinuria is a 24-hour urine protein excretion. Creatinine excretion should be measured at the same time to ensure adequacy of the sample. Normal values of 24-hour urine creatinine excretion are 1.3 to 2.2 mmol/kg (15 to 25 mg/kg) for men and 0.9 to 1.9 mmol/kg (10 to 22 mg/kg) for women. The average excretion of protein in the urine is 40 to

80 mg/day, and the upper limit of normal is 150 mg/day or 8 to 10 mg/dl (0.08 to 0.10 g/L) . Proteinuria of 3 g/day or more is always the result of glomerular disease, and patients with this test result often have the nephrotic syndrome. (Patients with the nephrotic syndrome usually excrete more than 3.5 g of protein in the urine per day.) Patients with lesser degrees of proteinuria may have glomerular or tubular disease. If urinary protein is less than 1 g/day in an otherwise healthy person and urinalysis shows no other abnormalities, serious disease is unlikely and the patient simply requires follow-up at intervals of 3 to 6 months.[3,15]

Whether the proteinuria is persistent or intermittent is an important determination. Intermittent or transient proteinuria is generally benign and may be induced by fever, exercise, emotional stress, or posture.[15] Postural proteinuria may be diagnosed if a voiding first thing in the morning is negative for protein whereas voidings in the erect position later in the day are positive.[15]

REFERENCES

1. Kiel DP, Moskowitz MA: The urinalysis: a critical appraisal, *Med Clin North Am* 71:607-624, 1987.
2. Sommerville P: How to investigate for renal disease, *Can J CME,* November-December 1991, 3:45-58.
3. Misdraji J, Nguyen PL: Urinalysis: when—and when not—to order, *Postgrad Med* 100:173-192, 1996.
4. Gambrell RC, Blount BW: Exercise-induced hematuria, *Am Fam Physician* 53:905-911, 1996.
5. Cianflocco AJ: Renal complications of exercise, *Clin Sports Med* 11:437-451, 1992.
6. Line RL, Rust GS: Acute exertional rhabdomyolysis, *Am Fam Physician* 52:502-506, 1995.
7. Mohr DN, Offord KP, Owen RA, et al: Asymptomatic microhematuria and urologic disease: a population-based study, *JAMA* 256:224-229, 1986.
8. Canadian Task Force on the Periodic Health Examination: *Canadian guide to clinical preventive health care,* Ottawa, 1994, Canada Communication Group—Publishing, pp 826-836.
9. US Preventive Services Task Force: *Guide to clinical preventive services,* ed 2, Baltimore, 1996, Williams & Wilkins, pp 181-186.
10. Monane M, Gurwitz JH, Lipsitz LA, et al: Epidemiologic and diagnostic aspects of bacteriuria: a longitudinal study in older women, *J Am Geriatr Soc* 43:618-622, 1995.
11. Canadian Task Force on the Periodic Health Examination: *Canadian guide to clinical preventive health care,* Ottawa, 1994, Canada Communication Group—Publishing, pp 436-445.
12. US Preventive Services Task Force: *Guide to clinical preventive services,* ed 2, Baltimore, 1996, Williams & Wilkins.
13. Woolhandler S, Pels RJ, Bor DH, et al: Dipstick urinalysis screening of asymptomatic adults for urinary tract disorders. I. Hematuria and proteinuria, *JAMA* 262:1214-1219, 1989.
14. Larson TS: Evaluation of proteinuria, *Mayo Clin Proc* 69:1154-1158, 1994.
15. Rapaport A, Richardson RM: How to tell it's proteinuria, *Patient Care Can,* September 1994, 5:13-18.

NUTRITION

(See also alternative medicine; formulas)

Topics covered in this section

ELDERLY AND NUTRITION

(See also exercise)

In one study of very elderly nursing home residents, resistance exercises of the knee and hip extensors significantly increased mobility, whereas liquid nutritional supplements had no effect.[1]

REFERENCES

1. Fiatarone MA, O'Neill EF, Ryan ND, et al: Exercise training and nutritional supplementation for physical frailty in very elderly people, *N Engl J Med* 330:1769-1775, 1994.

FISH OIL AND CORONARY ARTERY DISEASE

(See also IgA nephropathy)

Although a number of studies have shown an inverse correlation between fish consumption and coronary artery disease or total mortality, numerous others have failed to do so.[1]

REFERENCES

1. Ascherio A, Rimm EB, Stampfer MJ, et al: Dietary intake of marine n-3 fatty acids, fish intake, and the risk of coronary disease among men, *N Engl J Med* 332:977-982, 1995.

OBESITY

(See also endometrial carcinoma)

The inclusion of obesity under the general heading "nutrition" is questionable, since it might better be placed under "exercise" or be given its own heading. It is placed here mainly because that is the convention.

Definition

There is no universally accepted definition of obesity. The U.S. National Center for Health Statistics has defined "overweight" as a body mass index (BMI) of 27.8 or more for men and 27.3 or more for women. Severe overweight was defined as a BMI of 31.1 or more in men and 32.3 or more in women.[1,2] (BMI = weight in kg/height in meters^2.) In Canada obesity is defined as a BMI equal to or greater than 27 for both men and women and morbid obesity is defined as a BMI equal to or greater than 35.[3]

Anther parameter of clinically significant obesity is the waist/hip ratio; health risks are significant if the values are above 0.95 for men and 0.80 for women.[4] A simple measurement of abdominal girth also seems a good index of the health risks of obesity.[4-6] Values of ≥102 cm (50 inches) for men and ≥88 cm (35 inches) for women are considered dangerous and indications for weight loss, and values of 94 to 102 cm (38 to 41 inches) in men and 80 to 88 cm (32 to 35 inches) in women are warnings not to gain weight.[4]

REFERENCES

1. Van Itallie TB: Health implications of overweight and obesity in the United States, *Ann Intern Med* 103:983-988, 1985.
2. Najjar MF, Rowland M: *Anthropometric reference data and prevalence of overweight, United States, 1976-80,* Vital and Health Statistics, Ser 11, No 238, DHHS Pub No (PHSS) 87-1688, Washington, DC, 1987, Public Health Service, US Government Printing Office.
3. Health and Welfare Canada: *Canadian guidelines for healthy weight,* Ottawa, 1988, Ministry of National Health and Welfare.
4. Lean MEJ, Han TS, Morrison CE: Waist circumference as a measure for indicating need for weight management, *BMJ* 311: 158-161, 1995.
5. Ledoux M, Lambert J, Reeder BA, et al: A comparative analysis of weight to height and waist to hip circumference indices as indicators of the presence of cardiovascular disease risk factors, *Can Med Assoc J* 157(1 suppl):S32-S38, 1997.
6. Reeder BA, Senthilselvan A, Després J-P, et al: The association of cardiovascular disease risk factors with abdominal obesity in Canada, *Can Med Assoc J* 157(suppl 1):S39-S45, 1997.

Epidemiology of Obesity

(See also obesity in childhood)

In 1993 Williamson[1] estimated that about one fourth of American adults were overweight. However, the results of a 1994 U.S. study indicate that the incidence of obesity, defined as a BMI ≥27.8 for men and ≥27.3 for women, has increased 8% in one decade.[2] The new estimate of the incidence of obesity in the U.S. population over the age of 20 is 33.4%.[2] When subgroups were analyzed in this study, the highest incidence of obesity was found among women and minority groups (black and Hispanic). One of the postulated explanations for the epidemic of obesity is an increasingly sedentary life-style.[1] Foreyt and Goodrick[3] from Baylor College of Medicine in Houston calculated that if the U.S. population continues to gain weight at the same rate as at present, the entire adult population will meet the criteria of obesity by the year 2230.[3] They also point out that Americans spend $33 billion a year on weight control without any benefit at a population level.[3]

Using a BMI of 27 as a cutoff point, a little over one third of Canadian men and a little over one fourth of Canadian women are estimated to be obese. Morbid obesity affects about 3% of Canadian men and 5% of Canadian women.[4] A questionnaire survey done in Ontario found that 33.6% of the men and 22.8% of the women had a BMI greater than 27. Positive correlates were older age and lower socioeconomic status. Persons of Asian origin have a much lower incidence of obesity.[5]

Childhood obesity is a risk factor for adult obesity (see discussion of obesity in childhood).

REFERENCES

1. Williamson DF: Descriptive epidemiology of body weight and weight change in U.S. adults, *Ann Intern Med* 119(7 pt 2):646-649, 1993.
2. Kuczmarski RJ, Flegal KM, Campbell S, et al: Increasing prevalence of overweight among US adults: the National Health and Nutrition Examination Surveys, 1960-1991, *JAMA* 272:205-211, 1994.
3. Foreyt J, Goodrick K: The ultimate triumph of obesity (editorial), *Lancet* 346:134-135. 1995.
4. Reeder BA, Angel A, Ledoux M, et al: Obesity and its relation to cardiovascular disease risk factors in Canadian adults, *Can Med Assoc J* 146:2009-2019, 1992.
5. Ostbye T, Pomerieau J, Speechley M, et al: Correlates of body mass index in the 1990 Ontario Health Survey, *Can Med Assoc J* 152:1811-1817, 1995.

Pathophysiology of Obesity

(See also dietary advice for overweight patients; exercise)

Obesity results from an imbalance between energy input and energy expenditure. A very small imbalance that persists over many years can result in significant weight changes. Most people gradually gain weight with age. Bennett[1] points out that if a 70-kg man gains 10 kg over 20 years, the excess energy intake is equivalent to about one carrot stick a day.

It is usually assumed that overeating causes obesity. The evidence supporting this is far from definitive; more likely the increasing incidence of obesity in our society is due largely to decreased exercise.[1] This is supported by surveys showing that as Americans have become fatter, they have been eating less fat and fewer calories. Although they may also be participating in more leisure time exercise programs, they appear to have decreased household and occupational activity so that total energy expenditure is decreased.[2]

An important finding about weight changes is documentation that the body adjusts its energy output when weight change takes place. Persons who have purposely lost weight have a decreased resting energy output, and those who have purposely gained weight have an increased resting energy output.[3] This "set point" for body fat is a powerful mechanism of homeostasis and undoubtedly explains why dieting so often fails. The only good news about the "set point" is that its level may gradually change as a result of the type of food ingested or the amount of energy expended on a regular basis. In the long run both a sedentary life-style (decreased exercise) and the sustained consumption of high-fat diets shift the set point to promote fat retention. Conversely, regular exercise and a persistent decrease in the fat content of the diet may shift it to promote a leaner body structure.[1]

One theory to explain the weight gain of populations is the optimal foraging theory. Animals are programmed to expend a minimum amount of energy to take in a maximum amount of food. This was beneficial when food was scarce but is harmful when no activity is required to obtain meals.[4]

Does a high fat intake in itself predispose to obesity? Evidence suggests that it does by overriding the normal sensation of satiety. Supporting this is the observation that obese persons tend to have a higher fat content in their diets than do normal weight individuals (see discussion of dietary advice for overweight patients).[5]

REFERENCES

1. Bennett WI: Beyond overeating (editorial), *N Engl J Med* 332: 673-674, 1995.
2. Heini AF, Weinsier RL: Divergent trends in obesity and fat intake patterns: the American paradox, *Am J Med* 102:259-264, 1997.
3. Leibel RL, Rosenbaum M, Hirsch J: Changes in energy expenditure resulting from altered body weight, *N Engl J Med* 332: 621-628, 1995.
4. Foreyt J, Goodrick K: The ultimate triumph of obesity (editorial), *Lancet* 346:134-135, 1995.
5. Toubro S, Astrup A: Randomised comparison of diets for maintaining obese subjects' weight after major weight loss: ad lib, low fat, high carbohydrate diet v fixed energy intake, *BMJ* 314: 29-34, 1997.

Adverse Medical Consequences of Obesity

(See also exercise as a means of weight control; poverty)

A number of medical conditions are associated with obesity. These include the following:

1. Hypertension[1,2]
2. Coronary heart disease[1,3,4]
3. Diabetes mellitus[1,4,5]
4. Gallbladder disease[1]
5. Sleep apnea[1]
6. Snoring[1,6]
7. Some cancers (breast, endometrial, gallbladder, colorectal[7])[1]
8. Osteoarthritis[1]
9. Increased total mortality[1,4,8,9]
10. Complications of pregnancy[1,10]

In the Western world an estimated one third of cases of hypertension are due to obesity.[2]

The relationship between obesity and coronary heart disease was recently evaluated in the Nurses' Health Study.[3] In this study a progressive relationship was found between increasing BMI and coronary artery disease (CAD). The relative risk was lowest for women with a BMI less than 21 and was 3.5 for women whose BMI was greater than 29. Weight gain after the age of 18 was also a risk factor, even if the weight remained well within the "normal" limits.[3] A progressive increase in CAD risk with a BMI over 20 has also been demonstrated in British men.[4]

Total cohort mortality was increased sharply in the Nurses' Health Study among women with a BMI over 27; it was also increased among women who gained more than 10 kg after the age of 18. Although cardiovascular disease accounted for most of the excess mortality, cancers were also contributing factors.[8] Among British men total cohort mortality was increased with a BMI of 30 or more.[4]

An accurate estimate of the nutritional habits of the general population and a correlation of these with mortality statistics are difficult to make. One assessment that attempted to do this concluded that poor dietary habits and sedentary lifestyle accounted for 14% of deaths in the United States.[9]

Perinatal mortality and incidence of neural tube defects are both elevated among the offspring of obese women.[10]

REFERENCES

1. Pi-Sunyer FX: Medical hazards of obesity, *Ann Intern Med* 119 (7 pt 2):655-660, 1993.
2. MacMahon SW, Blacket RB, Macdonald GJ, et al: Obesity, alcohol consumption and blood pressure in Australian men and women: the National Heart Foundation of Australia Risk Factor Prevalence Study, *J Hypertens* 2:85-91, 1984.
3. Willett WC, Manson JE, Stampfer MJ, et al: Weight, weight change, and coronary heart disease in women: risk within the "normal" weight range, *JAMA* 273:461-465, 1995.
4. Shaper AG, Wannamethee G, Walker M: Body weight: implications for the prevention of coronary heart disease, stroke, and diabetes mellitus in a cohort study of middle aged men, *BMJ* 314:1311-1317, 1997.
5. Colditz GA, Willett WC, Rotnitzky A, et al: Weight gain as a risk factor for clinical diabetes mellitus in women, *Ann Intern Med* 122:481-486, 1995.
6. Braver HM, Block AJ, Perri MG: Treatment for snoring—combined weight loss, sleeping on side, and nasal spray, *Chest* 107: 1283-1288, 1995.
7. Giovannucci E, Ascherio A, Rimm EB, et al: Physical activity, obesity, and risk for colon cancer and adenoma in men, *Ann Intern Med* 122:327-334, 1995.
8. Manson JE, Willett WC, Stampfer MJ, et al: Body weight and mortality among women, *N Engl J Med* 333:677-685, 1995.
9. McGinnis JM, Foege WH: Actual causes of death in the United States, *JAMA* 270:2207-2211, 1993.
10. Goldenberg RL, Tamura T: Prepregnancy weight and pregnancy outcome (editorial), *JAMA* 275:1127-1128, 1996.

Dietary Advice for Overweight Patients

(See also pathophysiology of obesity)

Dieting does not lead to long-term weight loss in most patients. However, since other weight loss programs are equally ineffective or, in the case of pharmacological interventions, uncertain and possibly dangerous, many patients ask for and receive dietary advice. Some of the traditional suggestions are that patients eat three reasonably sized meals a day, try to avoid snacking, and decrease fat intake.

High-fat versus high-carbohydrate diets

There is evidence that a high-fat intake contributes to obesity (see discussion of pathophysiology of obesity) and therefore that low-fat, high-carbohydrate diets may be beneficial. This was tested in a two-stage Danish study of the management of obesity in women. In the initial stage one group was treated with an extremely low-calorie diet in the form of a prepared liquid formulation (2 MJ/day) for 8 weeks while the other was treated with a standard, ordinary food, low-calorie diet (5 MJ/day) for 17 weeks. Both cohorts were also treated with an ephedrine-caffeine anorexiant. Both groups had lost an average of 12.6 kg (28 lb) at the completion of the initial diet. At this point anorexiant therapy was discontinued for all patients who were then randomly assigned to either a fixed energy intake diet or an ad lib, low-fat, high-carbohydrate diet. At the end of 1 year those on the fixed energy diet had regained 11.3 kg, whereas those on the ad lib high-carbohydrate diet had regained only 5.4 kg. Weight gain in the maintenance phase did not correlate with the form of the initial diet (low calorie versus extremely low calorie).[1]

Quantity of food

Patients should be made aware of the size of average servings. They should know the difference between a 4-ounce steak and a 16-ounce steak. They should know that milk with a meal means one glass, not four glasses, and that thirst is quenched with water and not glass after glass of juice or soft drinks. It is quite amazing how people can fool themselves. I had one diabetic patient who was so careful of his diet that he made carrot sandwich snacks without butter, margarine, mayonnaise, or other condiments. The only problem was that he would eat 10 such sandwiches at a sitting. As he told me later, "I finally figured out that even rabbits get fat on carrots."

Calorie content of food types

A concept that patients who are serious about weight loss should grasp is the caloric content of various food classes:

Proteins	4 kcal/g
Carbohydrates	4 kcal/g
Fats	9 kcal/g
Alcohol	7 kcal/g

Once patients understand these principles, they can recognize and try to avoid or cut down on alcohol and high-calorie foods with a high fat content. Ways of avoiding excessive fat are to cut off (and avoid eating) all visible fat from meat, to avoid high-calorie fast foods and most fried foods, and to avoid or use sparingly margarine, butter, oils such as salad dressings, delicatessen salads drenched in oil, nuts, mayonnaise, sauces, and rich desserts such as pies, cakes, cookies, Danish pastries, and ice cream. Complex carbohydrates should make up a significant proportion of the diet.

Most vegetables are low in calories and can be eaten in large quantities. Exceptions that have moderate numbers of calories (approximating the numbers in fruit) are potatoes, lima beans, sweet corn, and green peas.

Fruit should be eaten in moderation. Fruit juices, especially apple juice, have more calories than the whole fruit. Raisins are dehydrated and so have a relatively high caloric content.

One way for a family physician to help patients with diet is to have them keep a diet diary in which they record everything they eat or drink for 3 days. The physician can go over the diary with the patient at a subsequent visit.

REFERENCES

1. Toubro S, Astrup A: Randomised comparison of diets for maintaining obese subjects' weight after major weight loss: ad lib, low fat, high carbohydrate diet v fixed energy intake, *BMJ* 314: 29-34, 1997.

Efficacy of Dieting

(See also drug treatment of obesity; exercise as a means of weight control; pathophysiology of obesity; weight cycling)

Dieting is a national U.S. (and Canadian) pastime. U.S. studies have shown that at any one time 40% of women and 20% of men are dieting.[1,2] Since less than 5% to 10% of people maintain weight loss,[3] very low-calorie dieting seems a largely futile and perhaps even dangerous activity (see discussion of weight cycling). In most studies one third to two thirds of any initial weight loss is regained within a year and almost all of it within 5 years.[4] For those who initially lose weight, the best predictor of the maintenance of weight loss is the frequency of exercise after the completion of dieting and a good predictor for regaining weight is the amount of television watched.[5]

Patients who have succeeded in losing weight, whether through dieting, exercise, drugs, or a combination of these modalities, must realize that because of a change in their set point their caloric requirements for maintaining this "normal" weight will be about 15% less than are required by someone of the same weight who was never obese (see discussion of pathophysiology of obesity).[6]

Although obesity is associated with significant morbidity and mortality, conclusive studies are not yet available to show that weight loss rectifies the situation.[4] Furthermore, dieting may be associated with increased morbidity and mortality.[1,7,8] In terms of morbidity, dieting may be associated with decreased psychosocial functioning and sometimes leads to binge eating and even bulimia.[8,9] Wooley and Garner[8] conclude that the detrimental effects of dieting outweigh the advantages and recommend that physicians stop prescribing a treatment that is risky and ineffective.

REFERENCES

1. Serdula M, Collins ME, Williamson DF, et al: Weight control practices of US adolescents and adults: Youth Risk Behavior Survey and Behavioral Risk Factor Surveillance System, *Ann Intern Med* 119:667-671, 1993.
2. Horm J, Anderson K: Who in America is trying to lose weight? *Ann Intern Med* 119:672-676, 1993.
3. Garner DM, Wooley SC: Confronting the failure of behavioral and dietary treatments of obesity, *Clin Psychol Rev* 11:729-780, 1991.
4. NIH Technology Assessment Conference Panel: Methods for voluntary weight loss and control, *Ann Intern Med* 119(7 pt 2): 764-770, 1993.

5. Grodstein F, Levine R, Troy L, et al: Three-year follow-up of participants in a commercial weight loss program, *Arch Intern Med* 156:1302-1306, 1996.
6. Rosenbaum M, Leibel RL, Hirsch J: Obesity, *N Engl J Med* 337:396-407, 1997.
7. Anders R, Muller DC, Sorkin JD: Long-term effects of change in body weight on all-cause mortality, *Ann Intern Med* 19:737-743, 1993.
8. Wooley SC, Garner DM: Dietary treatments for obesity are ineffective, *BMJ* 309:655-656, 1994.
9. Wadden AT, Stunkard AJ: Psychosocial consequences of obesity and dieting: research and clinical findings. In Stunkard AJ, Wadden TA, eds: *Obesity theory and therapy,* ed 2, New York, 1993, Raven Press, pp 163-177.

Weight Cycling

(See also efficacy of dieting; exercise as a means of weight control)

The literature on weight cycling can be summed up in one word: controversial.[1] Some studies have found that with repeated cycles of dieting the body becomes more metabolically efficient (burns less energy) and so inhibits weight loss, but most have refuted this. There is some evidence that individuals who diet in cycles develop a preference for fats. Weight cycling appears to be related to psychopathological conditions and decreased satisfaction with life, and it may be a factor predisposing to bulimia. Some of the epidemiological literature suggests an increased all-cause mortality in weight cyclers. On the other hand, severe obesity is a major risk factor for premature mortality. In the view of some expert organizations, this far outweighs the possible risks of weight cycling and should not inhibit the obese from trying to lose weight.[2]

REFERENCES

1. Brownell KD, Rodin J: Medical, metabolic, and psychological effects of weight cycling, *Arch Intern Med* 154:1325-1330, 1994.
2. National Task Force on the Prevention and Treatment of Obesity: Weight cycling, *JAMA* 272:1196-1202, 1994.

Exercise as a Means of Weight Control

(See also efficacy of dieting; exercise; pathophysiology of obesity; weight cycling)

Exercise is a logical technique for inducing weight loss in the obese, since overweight persons generally do not take in more calories than lean persons but usually expend fewer calories (see discussion of pathophysiology of obesity). Exercise does not lead to as much initial weight loss as dieting, but when dieting and exercise are combined, the total initial weight loss is greater. Weight loss induced by exercise is almost all from body fat, particularly central abdominal fat, whereas much of the weight loss of dieting is from lean body mass. Exercise has been found to be particularly helpful in maintaining weight loss.[1] Perhaps the most important reason to make exercise part of a weight control program is that active obese individuals have lower morbidity rates than do the sedentary obese.[2]

REFERENCES

1. Grodstein F, Levine R, Troy L, et al: Three-year follow-up of participants in a commercial weight loss program, *Arch Intern Med* 156:1302-1306, 1996.
2. Blair SN: Evidence for success of exercise in weight loss and control, *Ann Intern Med* 119(7 pt 2):702-706, 1993.

Drug Treatment of Obesity

(See also efficacy of dieting; exercise as a means of weight control; informed consent; prevention; weight cycling)

A 1996 in-depth analysis of the literature on the pharmacotherapy of obesity noted that few studies have had follow-up periods longer than 6 months and many have not been blinded, randomized, or placebo controlled. According to this article, follow-up reports have been published on fewer than 200 patients taking anorexiant drugs of any sort for a duration of 2 or more years.[1]

When reading reports of the efficacy of anorexiants, the physician should bear in mind not only that almost all studies are short term, but also that behavioral treatment alone has been reported to lead to an average weight loss of 8.5 kg (19 lb) by 21 weeks and 5.6 kg (12 lb) by 1 year.[1] Clearly the benefits of drugs must be measured against behaviorally obtained weight loss, not baseline weight.

The benefits of fenfluramine (Pondimin, Ponderal) in the treatment of obesity are uncertain. Fenfluramine is a serotonin uptake inhibitor that has been on the world market for 24 years, but only five studies of 1 year's duration have been reported and only two have been double blind and placebo controlled. The drug is effective in causing initial weight loss over the short term, but in some studies this effect was less than that of dietary therapy. Furthermore, after discontinuation of the drug more weight was regained in the fenfluramine group than in the behavioral therapy group.[1]

An anorexiant that is related to fenfluramine is dexfenfluramine (Redux). It is effective in short-term trials, but long-term benefits have not yet been established. In one randomized placebo-controlled double-blind study the treated patients received dexfenfluramine 15 mg bid. At the end of 6 months the mean weight loss among those receiving dexfenfluramine was close to 10 kg (22 lb) whereas that of the placebo group was 5 kg (11 lb). However, 5 months after cessation of treatment (11 months after the start of the study) the dexfenfluramine group had regained the extra weight lost so that the total average weight loss in both the treated and control groups was 6 kg (13 lb).[2]

A rare adverse reaction to appetite suppressant drugs, particularly fenfluramine and its derivatives, is primary pulmonary hypertension. Among patients taking these drugs for more than 3 months the risk of acquiring this disorder is increased more than 20 fold.[3,4] However, because the disorder is so uncommon, the absolute risk is only 28 cases per million person-years of exposure.[5] The pathogenesis of this disorder is probably excessive circulating serotonin causing massive intimal and medial proliferation of the pulmonary arterioles.[6] Since long-term studies of these drug types have not been done, the degree of risk to those taking them over many months or years is unknown. According to one editorialist, even if the risk is high, long-term use may still be indicated in the severely obese (if the patient is fully informed of the risks of this experimental treatment program and consents) because of the high morbidity and mortality associated with obesity itself.[5]

A major concern about both fenfluramine and dexfenfluramine is the possibility that they are neurotoxic. When given to a variety of experimental animals both these drugs cause long-lasting depletion of serotonin in the brain, and some studies of fenfluramine have described long-lasting reductions in serotonin axones. Despite case reports of an association between fenfluramine and depression, psychoses, and sleep disturbances, no proof of neurotoxicity in humans has been presented.[4]

Combinations of anorexiants have been used for weight control. In 1992 Weintraub and associates published a series of nine articles on the use of a combination of fenfluramine and phentermine (e.g., Ionamin, Phentrol), popularly known as Fen/Phen. These papers were reviewed and summarized by the National Task Force on the Prevention and Treatment of Obesity in 1996.[1] A total of 121 patients were assigned to behavioral therapy plus either the combined anorexiant regimen or placebo. In the first 6 months weight loss was 14.3 kg (31.5 lb) in the treatment group versus 4.6 kg (10 lb) in the placebo group. After 3.5 years only half the patients in the treatment group were still taking the drug. At that point the weight loss from baseline in the treatment group was 7 kg (15.4 lb) versus 2 kg (4.4 lb) in the placebo group.[1]

In the mid-1990s an advertising blitz for anorexiants was mounted in North America, and this was reflected in an astonishing increase in the sale of drugs such as phentermine and fenfluramine. Many physicians in the United States set up Fen/Phen treatment programs for obesity, and even some of the commercial weight loss chains began hiring medical consultants to prescribe anorexiants.[7] These drugs were often prescribed on a long-term basis.[8] As of July 1997 the U.S. Food and Drug Administration had received 33 reports of significant valvular insufficiency (usually involving multiple valves) that was apparently related to these drugs,[8] and in late August 1997 two articles on this treatment appeared in the *New England Journal of Medicine,* one reporting valvular insufficiencies in 24 women after taking fenfluramine-phentermine therapy[9] and the other reporting a case of fatal pulmonary hypertension in a woman who had taken fenfluramine-phentermine for only 23 days.[6] In September 1997 fenfluramine and dexfenfluramine were voluntarily withdrawn from the market. An important lesson from this sequence of events is that it can take decades before the adverse effects of drugs are recognized and widely publicized.

Fluoxetine (Prozac) has been studied as a possible therapeutic agent for weight control. Over an initial period of 8 weeks a dose-response effect was noted,[10] but when patients were maintained on the drug for more than 4 to 5 months, most regained weight.[11]

Over-the-counter products marketed as weight control agents include the ephedrine-like alkaloid phenylpropanolamine (Acutrim, Control, Dex-A-Diet, Dexatrim Pre-Meal, Prolamine, Phenyldrine, Phenoxine). Serious adverse effects, including stroke and seizures, have been reported with use of these agents.[12]

REFERENCES

1. National Task Force on the Prevention and Treatment of Obesity: Long-term pharmacotherapy in the management of obesity, *JAMA* 276:1907-1915, 1996.
2. O'Connor HT, Richman RM, Steinbeck KS, et al: Dexfenfluramine treatment of obesity: a double blind trial with post trial follow-up, *Int J Obesity* 19:181-189, 1995.
3. Abenhaim L, Moride Y, Brenot F, et al: Appetite-suppressant drugs and the risk of primary pulmonary hypertension, *N Engl J Med* 335:609-616, 1996.
4. McCann UD, Seiden LS, Rubin LJ, et al: Brain serotonin neurotoxicity and primary pulmonary hypertension from fenfluramine and dexfenfluramine, *JAMA* 278:666-672, 1997.
5. Manson JE, Faich G: Pharmacotherapy for obesity—do the benefits outweigh the risks? (editorial), *N Engl J Med* 335:659-660, 1996.
6. Mark EJ, Chang HT, Evans RJ, et al: Fatal pulmonary hypertension associated with short-term use of fenfluramine and phentermine, *N Engl J Med* 337:602-606, 1997.
7. Kushner R: The treatment of obesity: a call for prudence and professionalism (editorial), *Arch Intern Med* 157:602-604, 1997.
8. Food and Drug Administration: Health advisory on concomitant fenfluramine and phentermine use, *JAMA* 278:379, 1997.
9. Connolly HM, Crary JL, McGoon MD, et al: Valvular heart disease associated with fenfluramine-phentermine, *N Engl J Med* 337:581-588, 1997.
10. Levine LR, Enas GG, Thompson WL, et al: Use of fluoxetine, a selective serotonin-uptake inhibitor, in the treatment of obesity: a dose-response study, *Int J Obesity* 3:635-645, 1989.
11. Darga LL, Carroll-Michals L, Botsford SJ, et al: Fluoxetine's effect on weight loss in obese subjects, *Am J Clin Nutr* 54:321-325, 1991.
12. Centers for Disease Control and Prevention: Adverse events associated with ephedrine-containing products—Texas, December 1993–September 1995, *JAMA* 276:1711-1712, 1996.

Olestra

Olestra (Olean), a Procter & Gamble product, is a nonabsorbable fat substitute. It was approved for use in certain snack foods by the FDA on January 24, 1996, the day before Procter & Gamble's patent was due to expire.[1] Olestra may cause abdominal cramps and diarrhea, particularly if large quantities are taken, and it absorbs fat-soluble vitamins. To prevent vitamin deficiencies, Procter & Gamble has added vitamins A, D, E, and K to the snack foods containing olestra. Because no long-term clinical trials of the product have been conducted, the full spectrum of possible adverse effects is unknown.[1]

REFERENCES

1. Blackburn H: Olestra and the FDA, *N Engl J Med* 334:984-986, 1996.

Obesity Screening and Obesity Counseling

(See also screening)

The Canadian Task Force on the Periodic Health Examination gives a "C" recommendation for both calculating the BMI and counseling methods of weight reduction as part of the periodic health examination in adults.[1] The U.S. Preventive Services Task Force gives a "B" recommendation for periodic measurement of height and weight.[2]

REFERENCES

1. Canadian Task Force on the Periodic Health Examination: *Canadian guide to clinical preventive health care,* Ottawa, 1994, Canada Communication Group—Publishing, pp 574-584.
2. US Preventive Services Task Force: *Guide to clinical preventive services,* ed 2, Baltimore, 1996, Williams & Wilkins, pp 219-229.

Obesity in Childhood

(See also cholesterol lowering studies in children; epidemiology of obesity)

In the United States obesity in children has been increasing just as it has in adults.[1] Studies of twins[2] and adopted children[3] suggest that genetic factors are much more important than environmental factors in determining obesity. Children under age 3 who are obese but whose parents are not obese have a very low risk of becoming obese adults. Obesity in the teenage years, particularly if marked, is a greater risk factor for adult obesity. The risk is even greater if one or both parents are obese.[4,5] Another important risk factor is lack of physical exercise. One study of children aged 10 to 15, which defined obesity as a BMI higher than the 85th percentile for age, found that the odds incidence for obesity was 8.3 times greater for those who watched more than 5 hours of television daily than for those watching 2 hours or less daily.[6] Whether preventive interventions for children at high risk are useful is not known. A 1981 review found no evidence that diet and exercise programs alone brought about long-term weight reduction in children,[7] whereas a 1990 study reported that the addition of an intensive behavioral modification program was effective in reducing obesity in the treated group in their early adult years (after a 10-year follow-up).[8] Common sense dictates that all children, not just obese ones, be encouraged to be physically active (with strict limitation of television time) and to eat a balanced diet.

The U.S. Preventive Services Task Force gives a "B" recommendation for the periodic measurement of height and weight for both children and adults.[9] The Canadian Task Force on the Periodic Health Examination gives these strategies a "C" recommendation.[10] The Canadian Task Force also gives a "C" recommendation to exercise and to family-based nutrition and exercise counseling as a means of controlling obesity in children, and it gives a "D" to very low-calorie diets in preadolescents.[10]

REFERENCES

1. Troiano RP, Flegal KM, Kuczmarski RJ, et al: Overweight prevalence and trends for children and adolescents: the National Health and Nutrition Examination Surveys, 1963-91, *Arch Pediatr Adolesc Med* 149:1085-1091, 1995.
2. Stunkard AJ, Foch TT, Hrubvec Z: A twin study of human obesity, *JAMA* 256:51-54, 1986.
3. Stunkard AJ, Sorensen TIA, Hanis C, et al: An adoption study of human obesity, *N Engl J Med* 314:193-198, 1986.
4. Whitaker RC, Wright JA, Pepe MS, et al: Predicting obesity in young adulthood from childhood and parental obesity, *N Engl J Med* 337:869-873, 1997.
5. Bouchard C: Obesity in adulthood—the importance of childhood and parental obesity (editorial), *N Engl J Med* 337:926-927, 1997.
6. Gortmaker SL, Must A, Sobol AM, et al: Television viewing as a cause of increasing obesity among children in the United States, 1986-1990, *Arch Pediatr Adolesc Med* 150:356-362, 1996.
7. Committee on Nutrition: Nutritional aspects of obesity in infancy and childhood, *Pediatrics* 68:880-883, 1981.
8. Epstein LH, Valoski, Wing RR, et al: Ten-year follow-up of behavioural, family-based treatment for obese children, *JAMA* 264:2519-2523, 1990.
9. US Preventive Services Task Force: *Guide to clinical preventive services,* ed 2, Baltimore, 1996, Williams & Wilkins, pp 219-229.
10. Canadian Task Force on the Periodic Health Examination: Periodic health examination, 1994 update. I. Obesity in childhood, *Can Med Assoc J* 150:871-879, 1994.

VEGETARIANS

(See also antioxidants)

Vegetarians can be classified as follows:

Vegans	Eat no animal food except possibly honey
Lactovegetarians	Eat dairy products
Lacto-ovo-vegetarians	Eat dairy products and eggs

VITAMINS

(See also alternative medicine)

In the past the daily requirement of a nutritional element such as a vitamin was called the "recommended daily allowance." The current terminology (or jargon) is "recommended nutrient intake (RNI)."

Antioxidants

(See also vitamin A; vitamin E)

Vitamins A, C, and E have antioxidant properties, as do a variety of other compounds, including the lipid-lowering drug probucol (Lorelco). This characteristic has been claimed to protect not only against coronary artery disease and some cancers, but also against age-related macular degeneration. Many epidemiological studies have shown a lower rate of cardiovascular disease and cancer in individuals who eat a diet containing large amounts of fruits and vegetables.[1-3] One of the postulated mechanisms for this protection is that such diets lead to a high intake of antioxidant vitamins such as A and E and that these are the protective agents.[2] However, as Gaziano[4] points out, this may simply reflect the fact that persons who lead healthy life-styles in general tend to eat more fruits and vegetables. Support for a somewhat skeptical view of the ability of antioxidants to protect against coronary artery disease comes from a comparative review of prospective epidemiological studies versus randomized trials of antioxidant vitamins; benefits were found in the epidemiological studies but not the randomized trials.[5] An intriguing study published in 1997 found that the rate of restenosis after angioplasty was significantly reduced in patients treated with the powerful antioxidant probucol but not in those treated with a combination of beta-carotene, vitamin C, and vitamin E. The weak cholesterol-lowering properties of probucol were insufficient to explain the results.[6]

If antioxidants do indeed decrease the risk of cardiovascular disease, what is their mechanism of action? One hypothesis is that antioxidants inhibit oxidation of low-density lipoprotein and this in turn inhibits foam cell development and the generation of atherosclerotic plaques. In addition, there is evidence that antioxidants are beneficial even in the presence of established atherosclerotic plaques by enhancing plaque stability, inhibiting platelet activation, and protecting the vascular endothelium.[7]

There is the possibility that antioxidant vitamin supplementation may be harmful. The Finnish Alpha-Tocopherol/Beta-Carotene study showed a non–statistically significant trend toward an increased incidence of cardiovascular disease in the beta-carotene arm of the study, as well as an increased incidence of lung cancer in smokers taking supplemental beta-carotene.[8] Similar deleterious effects have been reported from an American multicenter trial of beta-carotene plus vitamin A.[9]

Toxic effects of antioxidant vitamins are rare. A few cases of vitamin A toxicity, generally from ingesting more than 100,000 units per day, are reported annually in the United States. Ascorbic acid seems to be nontoxic in doses under 4 g/day as is vitamin E in doses under 3200 mg/day.[10]

At present the best advice family physicians can give their patients on the subject of vitamins is to eat plenty of fruits and vegetables.[2] Whether supplemental antioxidant vitamins are beneficial remains unknown.

REFERENCES

1. National Research Council, Committee on Diet and Health, Food and Nutrition Board, Commission on Life Sciences: *Diet and health: implications for reducing chronic disease risk*, Washington, DC, 1989, National Academy Press.
2. Greenberg ER, Sporn MB: Antioxidant vitamins, cancer, and cardiovascular disease (editorial), *N Engl J Med* 334:1189-1190, 1996.
3. Key TJ, Thorogood M, Appleby PN, et al: Dietary habits and mortality in 11,000 vegetarians and health conscious people: results of a 17 year follow up, *BMJ* 313:775-779, 1996.
4. Gaziano JM: Antioxidant vitamins and coronary artery disease risk, *Am J Med* 97(suppl 3A):18S-21S, 1994.
5. Jha P, Flather M, Lonn E, et al: The antioxidant vitamins and cardiovascular disease: a critical review of epidemiologic and clinical trial data, *Ann Intern Med* 123:860-872, 1995.
6. Tardif J-C, Coté G, Lespérance J, et al (Multivitamins and Probucol Study Group): Probucol and multivitamins in the prevention of restenosis after coronary angioplasty, *N Engl J Med* 337:365-372, 1997.
7. Diaz MN, Frei B, Vita JA, et al: Antioxidants and atherosclerotic heart disease, *N Engl J Med* 337:408-416, 1997.
8. Alpha-Tocopherol, Beta Carotene Cancer Prevention Study Group: The effect of vitamin E and beta carotene on the incidence of lung cancer and other cancers in male smokers, *N Engl J Med* 330:1029-1035, 1994.
9. Omenn GS, Goodman GE, Thornquist MD, et al: Effects of a combination of beta carotene and vitamin A on lung cancer and cardiovascular disease, *N Engl J Med* 334:1150-1155, 1996.
10. Meyers DG, Maloley PA, Weeks D: Safety of antioxidant vitamins, *Arch Intern Med* 156:925-935, 1996.

Vitamin A

(See also antioxidants; macular degeneration; vitamin A supplements in pregnancy; vitamin E)

Good sources of vitamin A are green and yellow vegetables, cantaloupes, and apricots.

Antioxidants, including carotenoids, have been thought to protect against coronary artery disease. For example, a follow-up study of the Lipid Research Clinics Primary Prevention Trial showed an inverse relationship between serum carotenoid levels and coronary heart disease.[1] Another investigation found that patients whose initial beta-carotene concentrations were in the highest quartile had about half the total and cardiovascular mortality of those whose initial beta-carotene concentrations were in the lowest quartile.[2] However, other studies have failed to confirm any protective effect[3] or have even suggested an increased incidence of cardiovascular disease.[4,5]

Antioxidants have been thought to protect against cancer. Recent evaluations have found either no benefit[3] or in the case of beta-carotene an increased incidence of lung cancer.[4,5] For example, a Finnish study of smokers taking beta-carotene 20 mg/day for 5 to 8 years found that they had a higher incidence of lung cancer than did control subjects,[4] and similar results were reported by the American Beta-Carotene and Retinol Efficacy Trial (CARET), in which smokers, former smokers, and persons exposed to asbestos were treated with a combination of 30 mg of beta-carotene plus 25,000 IU of retinol (vitamin A) daily.[5] A study from Dartmouth failed to demonstrate any benefit of antioxidants in preventing the recurrence of colonic polyps.[6]

A high intake of carotenoids has been shown to be inversely correlated with the incidence of age-related macular degeneration.[7] It is important to realize that beta-carotene derived from vitamin A is only one of many carotenoids. In this study the specific foods associated with the reduction of age-associated macular degeneration were dark green leafy vegetables, especially spinach and collard greens.[7] The specific carotenoids that were thought to be beneficial were lutein and zeaxanthin. Preformed vitamin A did not appear to be beneficial, nor did supplements of vitamin C or vitamin E.

Supplements of vitamin A in excess of 10,000 IU are teratogenic (see discussion of vitamin A supplements in pregnancy).[8]

REFERENCES

1. Morris DL, Kritchevsky SB, Davis CE: Serum carotenoids and coronary heart disease: the lipid research clinics coronary prevention trial and follow-up study, *JAMA* 272:1439-1441, 1994.
2. Greenberg ER, Baron JA, Karagas MR, et al: Mortality associated with low plasma concentration of beta carotene and the effect of oral supplementation, *JAMA* 275:699-703, 1996.
3. Nennekens CH, Buring JE, Manson JE, et al: Lack of effect of long-term supplementation with beta carotene on the incidence of malignant neoplasms and cardiovascular disease, *N Engl J Med* 334:1145-1149, 1996.
4. Alpha-Tocopherol, Beta Carotene Cancer Prevention Study Group: The effect of vitamin E and beta carotene on the incidence of lung cancer and other cancers in male smokers, *N Engl J Med* 330:1029-1035, 1994.
5. Omenn GS, Goodman GE, Thornquist MD, et al: Effects of a combination of beta carotene and vitamin A on lung cancer and cardiovascular disease, *N Engl J Med* 334:1150-1155, 1996.
6. Greenberg ER, Baron JA, Tosteson TD, et al: A clinical trial of antioxidant vitamins to prevent colorectal adenoma, *N Engl J Med* 330:1029-1035, 1994.
7. Seddon JM, Ajani UA, Sperduto RD, et al: Dietary carotenoids, vitamins A, C, and E, and advanced age-related macular degeneration, *JAMA* 272:1413-1420, 1994.
8. Rothman KJ, Moore LL, Singer MR, et al: Teratogenicity of high vitamin A intake, *N Engl J Med* 333:1369-1373, 1995.

Vitamin C

The RNI of vitamin C is 35 mg for infants, 45 to 50 mg for children, and 45 to 60 mg for adults.

Ascorbic acid is essential for collagen formation; it catalyzes the hydroxylation of proline and lysine. In the absence of hydroxylation the collagen is unstable, and this is particularly manifest in blood vessel walls. Clinical manifestations of scurvy are perifollicular hemorrhages, corkscrew hairs, large ecchymoses, and hemorrhagic gingivitis. Those at risk of scurvy in North America are alcoholics, persons following fad diets, institutionalized individuals, and the isolated elderly.[1] In 1844 the British parliament required that seamen be issued lime or lemon juice on a regular basis, hence the term "Limey."

REFERENCES

1. Offinger KC: Scurvy: more than historical relevance, *Am Fam Physician* 48:609-613, 1993.

Vitamin D

The usual daily requirement of vitamin D for the population at large is 400 IU. Those with osteoporosis should probably have 800 IU/day. Almost all multivitamins contain 400 IU of vitamin D.

A study of elderly homebound (sunlight-deprived) patients found that many had inadequate intake and low serum levels of vitamin D.[1]

REFERENCES

1. Gloth FM III, Gundberg CM, Hollis BW, et al: Vitamin D deficiency in homebound elderly persons, *JAMA* 274:1683-1686, 1995.

Vitamin E

(See also antioxidants; coronary artery disease; tardive dyskinesia; vitamin A)

Recommended nutrient intake

The RNI of vitamin E (alpha-tocopherol) is 8 to 15 IU/day. Vitamin E is found mainly in fats. Foods high in vitamin E include vegetable oils, margarine, mayonnaise, sunflower seeds, nuts, avocados, and mangos.

Safety

The long-term safety of vitamin E supplements of 100 IU or more per day has not been studied, but toxicity appears to be low. There are reports that vitamin E can aggravate the coagulation defects of vitamin K deficiency.[1]

Cardiovascular disease

Studies have shown a decreased incidence of coronary artery disease in women and men taking vitamin E supplements at doses of 100 IU/day. There were no greater effect with higher doses and no benefits with lower doses.[2-4] A 1996 study from Finland found that the relative risk of angina in male smokers taking alpha-tocopherol 50 mg/day over 5 years was 0.91 compared with control subjects receiving placebo.[5] The Iowa Women's Health Study showed that postmenopausal women who had a high intake of foods rich in vitamin E, such as dark green leafy vegetables, seeds, nuts, vegetable oils, mayonnaise, and margarine, had a lower risk of death from coronary artery disease than did those with a low intake from dietary sources; no protective effect was noted from vitamin E supplements.[6] A randomized controlled trial in which 400 to 800 mg of vitamin E daily was given to patients with angiographically proven coronary artery disease found that this regimen decreased the incidence of nonfatal myocardial infarctions compared with the placebo-treated control subjects.[7]

Lung cancer

A study of the effect of vitamin E on lung cancer in male smokers given alpha-tocopherol 50 mg/day over 5 to 7 years showed no beneficial effects.[8]

Tardive dyskinesia

A number of studies, many of them double blind, have shown an amelioration of tardive dyskinesia with vitamin E treatment. The usual doses were 1200 to 1600 mg/day.[9-12]

REFERENCES

1. Kappus H, Diplock AT: Tolerance and safety of vitamin E: a toxicological position report, *Free Radical Biol Med* 13:55-74, 1992.
2. Stampfer MJ, Hennekens CH, Manson JE, et al: Vitamin E consumption and the risk of coronary disease in women, *N Engl J Med* 328:1444-1449, 1993.
3. Rimm EB, Stampfer MJ, Ascherio A, et al: Vitamin E consumption and the risk of coronary heart disease in men, *N Engl J Med* 328:1450-1456, 1993.
4. Steinberg D: Antioxidant vitamins and coronary heart disease (editorial), *N Engl J Med* 328:1487-1489, 1993.
5. Rapola JM, Virtamo J, Haukka JK, et al: Effect of vitamin E and beta carotene on the incidence of angina pectoris: a randomized, double-blind, controlled trial, *JAMA* 275:693-698, 1996.
6. Kushi LH, Folsom AR, Prineas RJ, et al: Dietary antioxidant vitamins and death from coronary heart disease in postmenopausal women, *N Engl J Med* 334:1156-1162, 1996.
7. Stephens NG, Parsons A, Schofield PM, et al: Randomised controlled trial of vitamin E in patients with coronary disease: Cambridge Heart Antioxidant Study (CHAOS), *Lancet* 347: 781-786, 1996.
8. Alpha-Tocopherol, Beta Carotene Cancer Prevention Study Group: The effect of vitamin E and beta carotene on the incidence of lung cancer and other cancers in male smokers, *N Engl J Med* 330:1029-1035, 1994.
9. Dabiri LM, Pasta D, Darby JK, et al: Effectiveness of vitamin E for treatment of long-term tardive dyskinesia, *Am J Psychiatry* 151:925-926, 1994.
10. Adler LA, Peselow E, Rotrosen J, et al: Vitamin E treatment of tardive dyskinesia, *Am J Psychiatry* 150:1405-1407, 1993.
11. Laugharne J, Rangarajan N, Reynolds GP: Tardive dyskinesia, lipid peroxidation, and sustained amelioration with vitamin E treatment, *Int Clin Psychopharmacol* 8:151-153, 1993.
12. Egan MF, Hyde TM, Albers GW, et al: Treatment of tardive dyskinesia with vitamin E, *Am J Psychiatry* 149:773-777, 1992.

OBSTETRICS

(See also adverse medical consequences of obesity; diabetic retinopathy; prematurity; smoking in pregnancy)

Topics covered in this section

EPIDEMIOLOGY

Since the 1960s fetal deaths have declined 70% overall in the United States. However, the risk of fetal death is about twice as high among women over 35 as it is among younger women.[1]

REFERENCES

1. Frettis RC, Schmittdiel J, McLean FH, et al: Increased maternal age and the risk of fetal death, *N Engl J Med* 333:953-957, 1995.

ANTENATAL CARE FOR PHYSICIANS WHO DO NOT PRACTICE OBSTETRICS

(See also anemia; risk assessment in pregnancy)

Even physicians who do not practice obstetrics have patients who are pregnant or who want to become pregnant, and the physician should be able to give them some basic counseling. For example, every woman who could become pregnant should be taking at least 0.4 mg of folate daily before conception (see discussion of neural tube defects). The following paragraphs outline some aspects of a typical antenatal protocol.

Frequency of Visits

The schedule of visits should be as follows:

Initial visit	8 weeks
Weeks 8-28	Every 4 weeks
Weeks 28-36	Every 2 weeks
Week 36–term	Every week

Weight Gain

Recommended weight gain in pregnancy for women of normal weight is 11 to 16 kg (25 to 35 lb). Underweight women should gain about 16 to 18 kg (35 to 40 lb) and obese women about 7 to 11 kg (15 to 25 kg). For normal weight women the rate of gain should be about 1.3 to 2.3 kg (3 to 5 lb) per month in the first trimester and 0.5 to 1.0 kg (1 to 2 lb) during the second and third trimesters. Failure to gain adequate weight puts the baby at risk of intrauterine growth retardation.[2]

Uterine Growth in Pregnancy

The uterus has the features below at various stages of pregnancy:

Weeks	Uterine Size
6	Normal
8	Globular; slightly enlarged
12	Symphysis
20	Just below umbilicus
20-38	Ht/cm = weeks of pregnancy

Quickening

Quickening takes place at 16 weeks for multiparas and at 20 weeks for primiparas.

Vaginal Bleeding

About one fifth of pregnant women have vaginal bleeding during the first 20 weeks of pregnancy, and about half of these go on to spontaneous abortion. In one study women who had a spontaneous abortion were not at an increased risk of abortion in subsequent pregnancies.[3]

Initial Visit

The initial visit comprises a complete history, including experience with babies and availability of social supports, an obstetrical risk assessment (controversial; see below), a physical examination including pelvic examination, laboratory investigations, counseling, and a prescription for folic acid and iron. The usual laboratory examinations are a complete blood count, Venereal Disease Research Laboratories (VDRL) test, rubella titer, hepatitis B surface antigen (HBsAg), ABO-Rh typing, urine culture and sensitivity, cervical cultures for gonorrhea and *Chlamydia,* and a Papanicolaou (Pap) smear. Important points to cover in counseling include the avoidance of smoking and secondhand smoke, abstention from alcohol (an occasional single drink is probably not harmful), and eating a balanced diet. This type of counseling is best given before the patient becomes pregnant, and advice at the first prenatal visit should function as a reinforcement of what has already been said. All women who are pregnant should receive supplements containing 0.4 to 0.8 mg of folic acid[4,5] and at least 30 mg of elemental iron.[6] This is most easily done by prescribing a daily multivitamin containing adequate quantities of folic acid and iron. Patients should be referred to prenatal classes.

REFERENCES

1. Williams T, Zaltz A: Deliver effective prenatal care, *Patient Care Can* 5:39-51, 1994.
2. Kolasa K, Weismiller DG: Nutrition during pregnancy, *Am Fam Physician* 56:205-212, 1997.
3. Everett C: Incidence and outcome of bleeding before the 20th week of pregnancy: prospective study from general practice, *BMJ* 315:32-34, 1997.
4. Canadian Task Force on the Periodic Health Examination: Periodic health examination, 1994 update. III. Primary and secondary prevention of neural tube defects, *Can Med Assoc J* 151: 159-166, 1994.
5. US Preventive Services Task Force: *Guide to clinical preventive services,* ed 2, Baltimore, 1996, Williams & Wilkins, pp 467-483.
6. Allen LH: Nutritional supplementation for the pregnant woman, *Clin Obstet Gynecol* 37:587-595, 1994.

CONGENITAL ANOMALIES

(See also drugs and chemicals in pregnancy; informed consent; positive predictive value; screening)

Risk Factors

A mother who has an infant with a congenital anomaly has a 2.5 times increased relative risk of having a second infant with a congenital anomaly. The increase is due primarily to a 7.6 times increase in the same anomaly. In one study the risk decreased significantly if the woman moved to another community before having the second child, which suggests an environmental cause.[1]

Folic Acid

Folic acid supplements taken before conception and during pregnancy decrease the incidence of neural tube defects, as discussed in more detail below in the section on neural tube defects. Less well known is that this form of supplementation also decreases the incidence of congenital heart disease, especially conotruncal malformations, hypertrophic pyloric stenosis, urinary tract abnormalities, and congenital limb deficiencies.[2]

At present individual prescription of folic acid to women in the childbearing age group is the usual way of trying to ensure widespread use of this supplement. Food supplementation is another option that is being debated. One of the arguments against it is the well-established fact that folic acid can prevent or correct the anemia of pernicious anemia, and as a result, subacute degeneration of the cord and peripheral neuropathies might progress without the diagnosis being made. According to one author, this would be a rare event compared with the numerous proven benefits of universal supplementation, and that diagnosis would not be difficult if physicians were aware that the absence of macrocytic anemia does not rule out pernicious anemia as a cause of neurological symptoms.[3]

Amniocentesis

Indications for amniocentesis are numerous and include all women who will have reached their thirty-fifth birthday at the time of delivery, women with a past history of having an infant with chromosomal abnormalities, or women who are at high risk of carrying a fetus with such conditions as Tay-Sachs disease, sickle cell anemia, and thalassemia. Amniocentesis is generally performed between 15 and 20 weeks of gestation, and the estimated pregnancy loss is 0.5 to 1%. If the procedure is performed before 15 weeks, the pregnancy loss is two to three times greater.[4]

Chorionic Villus Sampling

Chorionic villus sampling is best performed between 10 and 12 weeks of gestation. The approach may be transcervical or transabdominal. When this procedure is compared with midtrimester amniocentesis, an excess of pregnancy loss between 0.5% and 4.5% is reported. However, fetal loss with chorionic villus sampling is less than that with early (before 15 weeks) amniocentesis. The indications for chorionic villus sampling are similar to those for amniocentesis except that a few conditions such as osteogenesis imperfecta are better assessed by chorionic villus sampling.[4]

Maternal Serum Screening

An elevated maternal alpha-fetoprotein (AFP) level at 16 to 18 weeks suggests an elevated relative risk of a neural tube defect. A low AFP level in conjunction with a low unconjugated estriol (uE_3) and an elevated human chorionic gonadotropin (hCG) level suggests an elevated relative risk of Down syndrome (see below).

The pros and cons of maternal serum screening with AFP, uE_3, and hCG are well reviewed by Carroll,[5] and the problems of informed consent for these procedures are described by Summers.[6] Maternal serum screening of all pregnancies would detect an estimated 60% to 70% of infants with Down syndrome and 80% of those with open neural tube defects. However, the positive predictive value (percentage of patients with positive tests who actually have the disorder) is very low. About 8% of women undergoing maternal serum screening would have an initial positive test (6% for Down syndrome, 1.6% for neural tube defect, and the remainder for other rare fetal anomalies), but only 1% to 2% of this 8% would actually have an abnormal baby; a negative test would not guarantee the absence of the anomalies being sought. The Canadian Task Force on the Periodic Health Examination estimates that if all women were screened for Down syndrome, 58% of cases would be detected. Of women screened, 0.1% (1:1000) would have true-positive results and 3.7% would have false-positive results.[7] Put another way, the positive predictive value would be a little less than 3%.

The recommendations of the Canadian Task Force on the Periodic Health Examination and the U.S. Preventive Services Task Force for the secondary prevention of Down syndrome and neural tube defects are discussed below.

The principal factor motivating parents to seek prenatal diagnosis is reassurance that the baby is normal.[8] In view of the very low positive predictive value of maternal serum screening (and for that matter the low sensitivity of ultrasound for detecting fetal abnormalities at 18 to 20 weeks[9]), these wishes can never be fully met and can be partially met only at the cost of many false-positive results. These tests should be ordered only if the patient is aware of the implications of positive and negative tests and has given informed consent. In most situations maternal serum screening would probably do more harm than good if the patient would not consider having an abortion should defects be detected.[10]

Down Syndrome

Between 70% and 80% of children with Down syndrome are born to women younger than 35 years of age. In the last 5 years a significant number of Down syndrome babies have been detected antenatally by blood tests performed at 16 weeks. In the typical case the serum AFP and uE_3 levels are low and the hCG level is high.[11] This is discussed in more detail under "Maternal Serum Screening." In a study of maternal serum screening in women 35 years of age or older, 89% of Down syndrome cases were detected (11% false-negative rate) but the false-positive rate was 25%.[12] Both the Canadian Task Force on the Periodic Health Examination[7] and the U.S. Preventive Services Task Force[13] give a "B" recommendation to maternal serum screening of women under the age of 35, within the context of a comprehensive program, and they also give a "B" recommendation for chorionic villus sampling or amniocentesis in pregnant women over the age of 35. Amniocentesis results in a 1% increase in pregnancy loss and chorionic villus sampling a slightly higher rate of loss.[7] An alternative for women over 35 could be triple marker maternal serum screening.[7,13]

Average life expectancy of persons with Down syndrome is 56,[14] but at least one has lived as long as 83 years.[15]

Neural Tube Defects

The incidence of neural tube defects varies from one geographical area to another. The highest incidence is in Britain and Ireland where it is 8 or 9 per 1000 births. In Canada the rate is 1 or 2 per 1000 live births; the lowest incidence is in British Columbia and Ontario with rates of 1.6 per 1000 live births, and the highest is in Quebec and Newfoundland at 4 per 1000 live births. Between 90% and 95% of neural tube defects occur in families with no history of the disorder. However, the risk is much higher if there is a family history of neural tube defects. If a woman has had one affected infant, the chance of having a second affected infant is increased 10 fold for an absolute rate of 2% to 3%.[16] Maternal obesity is also an independent risk factor for neural tube defects.[17-19]

Primary prevention of neural tube defects has been shown to be effective by the administration of folic acid for the month before conception and for the first trimester.[20-22] Secondary prevention is based on screening maternal serum for AFP. If it is elevated, a confirmatory repeat examination is performed followed by high-resolution ultrasonography and, if the latter is not definitive, amniocentesis with assessment of amniotic fluid AFP. In low-risk women, ultrasonography alone may be an adequate screening technique.[16,23]

Both the U.S. Preventive Services Task Force[23] and the Canadian Task Force on the Periodic Health Examination[16] give an "A" recommendation for prescribing folic acid 4 mg/day to women with a family or personal history of having an infant with a neural tube defect and for prescribing 0.4 mg/day[16] or 0.4 to 0.8 mg/day[23] to all women capable of becoming pregnant. (Most multivitamins contain at least 0.4 mg of folic acid, but a few contain less. Patients should be instructed to check the label carefully before purchasing a particular brand.) Maternal serum screening for AFP at 16 to 18 weeks gets a "B" recommendation from both task forces provided it is part of a quality-controlled program.

The Canadian Task Force states that ultrasonography may be adequate for low-risk women if performed between 16 and 18 weeks ("B" recommendation),[16] whereas the U.S. Preventive Services Task Force gives midtrimester ultrasound screening for this purpose a "C" recommendation.[23] Aside from dramatically decreasing the incidence of neural tube defects, folic acid supplements have been shown to decrease the incidence of other congenital anomalies.

Congenital Heart Disease

A case-control study found that women who took multivitamins around the time of conception had a 43% lower risk of having babies with conotruncal defects of the heart. The major defects involved were tetralogy of Fallot, transposition of the great vessels, and truncus arteriosus.[24]

REFERENCES

1. Lie RT, Wilcox AJ, Skærven R: A population-based study of the risk of recurrence of birth defects, *N Engl J Med* 331:1-4, 1994.
2. Czeizel AE: Nutritional supplementation and prevention of congenital abnormalities, *Curr Opin Obstet Gynecol* 7:88-94, 1995.
3. Dickinson CJ: Does folic acid harm people with vitamin B12 deficiency? *QJM* 88:357-364, 1995.
4. Kuller JA, Laifer SA: Contemporary approaches to prenatal diagnosis, *Am Fam Physician* 52:2277-2281, 1995.
5. Carroll JC: Maternal serum screening, *Can Fam Physician* 40: 1756-1764, 1994.
6. Summers AM: Informed choice in prenatal screening: current issues (editorial), *Can Fam Physician* 40:1688-1690, 1994.
7. Dick PT (Canadian Task Force on the Periodic Health Examination): Periodic health examination, 1996 update. I. Prenatal screening for and diagnosis of Down syndrome, *Can Med Assoc J* 154:465-479, 1996.
8. Green JM: Women's experiences of prenatal diagnosis and screening. In Abramsky L, Chapple J, eds: *Prenatal diagnosis: the human side,* New York, 1994, Chapman & Hall.
9. Ewigman BG, Crane JP, Frigoletto FD, et al (RADIUS Study Group): Effect of prenatal ultrasound screening on perinatal outcome, *N Engl J Med* 329:821-827, 1993.
10. Zamorski MA: Prenatal diagnosis: more than meets the eye (editorial), *Am Fam Physician* 52:2173-2177, 1995.
11. Pauker SP, Pauker SG: Prenatal diagnosis—why is 35 a magic number? *N Engl J Med* 330:1151-1152, 1994.
12. Haddow JE, Palomaki GE, Knight GJ, et al: Reducing the need for amniocentesis in women 35 years of age or older with serum markers for screening, *N Engl J Med* 330:1114-1118, 1994.
13. US Preventive Services Task Force: *Guide to clinical preventive services,* ed 2, Baltimore, 1996, Williams & Wilkins, pp 449-465.
14. Demissie A, Aryes RC, Briggs R: Old age in Down's syndrome, *J R Soc Med* 81:740, 1988.
15. Chicoine BA: Down Syndrome and longevity (letter), *Am Fam Physician* 52:775, 1995.
16. Canadian Task Force on the Periodic Health Examination: Periodic health examination, 1994 update. III. Primary and secondary prevention of neural tube defects, *Can Med Assoc J* 151:159-166, 1994.
17. Werler MM, Louik C, Shapiro S, et al: Prepregnant weight in relation to risk of neural tube defects, *JAMA* 275:1089-1092, 1996.
18. Shaw GM, Velie EM, Schaffer D: Risk of neural tube defect—affected pregnancies among obese women, *JAMA* 275:1093-1096, 1996.
19. Goldenberg RL, Tamura T: Prepregnancy weight and pregnancy outcome (editorial), *JAMA* 275:1127-1128, 1996.
20. MRC Vitamin Study Research Group: Prevention of neural tube defects: results of the Medical Research Council vitamin study, *Lancet* 338:131-137, 1991.
21. Cziezel AE, Duadas I: Prevention of the first occurrence of neural-tube defects by periconceptional vitamin supplementation, *N Engl J Med* 327:1832-1835, 1992.
22. Werler MM, Shapiro S, Metchel AA: Periconceptional folic acid exposure and risk of occurrence of neural tube defects, *JAMA* 269:1257-1261, 1993.
23. US Preventive Services Task Force: *Guide to clinical preventive services,* ed 2, Baltimore, 1996, Williams & Wilkins, pp 467-483.
24. Botto LD, Khoury MJ, Mulinare J, et al: Periconceptional multivitamin use and the occurrence of conotruncal heart defects—results from a population-based, case-control study, *Pediatrics* 98:911-917, 1996.

DRUGS AND CHEMICALS IN PREGNANCY

(See also hypertensive disorders of pregnancy; nausea and vomiting in pregnancy)

Acetaminophen

Acetaminophen is the nonnarcotic analgesic of choice in pregnancy.[1]

REFERENCES

1. Zuber C, Hom M, Vought L, Donnenfeld AE: Common chemical exposures in pregnancy: cosmetics, paint fumes, and cold medications, *Postgrad Obstet Gynecol* 12:1-6, 1992.

Alcohol

Epidemiological evidence suggests that the incidence of the fetal alcohol syndrome is 10% in pregnant women who drink fewer than 8 drinks a week and up to 30% to 40% in women who drink more than that. It also seems likely that binge drinking is particularly likely to cause the syndrome. Although no reliable evidence has shown that mild social drinking in pregnancy is detrimental, many women who have had a few social drinks before they were aware they were pregnant become panic stricken at the thought they may have harmed their infant.[1] The main characteristics of the fetal alcohol syndrome are prenatal and postnatal growth retardation, microcephaly, hypotonia, mental retardation, microphthalmia and short palpebral fissures (distance from inner to outer canthi), thin upper lip, and poorly developed philtrum (groove on upper lip). Some of the facial abnormalities are difficult to discern in the newborn but become more obvious as the child develops.[2]

REFERENCES

1. Koren G: Alcohol consumption in early pregnancy: how much will harm a fetus? *Can Fam Physician* 42:2141-2143, 1996.
2. Lewis DD, Woods SE: Fetal alcohol syndrome, *Am Fam Physician* 50:1025-1032, 1994.

Antibacterials and Antiviral Agents

Acyclovir

Acyclovir (Zovirax) is not approved for use in pregnant women, but no evidence has shown that it is teratogenic.[1]

Clindamycin

Vaginal clindamycin is probably safe in pregnancy.[1]

Erythromycin estolate

Erythromycin estolate is contraindicated in pregnancy.[1]

Metronidazole

Oral metronidazole (Flagyl) is considered to be contraindicated in the first trimester, but vaginal metronidazole is probably safe.[1] Six prospective studies and one retrospective study of oral metronidazole use during the first trimester of pregnancy, as well as a metaanalysis of all seven of these studies, showed no increased incidence of teratogenesis.[2]

Quinolones

Quinolones such as norfloxacin (Noroxin), ofloxacin (Floxin), and ciprofloxacin (Cipro) are contraindicated in children because they have been shown to cause arthropathy in the weight-bearing joints of immature animals. However, they have not been shown to cause birth defects in experimental animals or in the limited studies that have been done in humans.[3] According to the *Medical Letter*, fluoroquinolones are contraindicated in pregnancy.[1]

Sulfonamides

Sulfonamides may be given in the first two trimesters of pregnancy.

Tetracyclines

Tetracyclines are contraindicated in pregnancy.[1]

REFERENCES

1. Drugs for sexually transmitted diseases, *Med Lett* 37:117-122, 1995.
2. Burtin P, Taddio A, Ariburnu O, et al: Safety of metronidazole in pregnancy: a meta-analysis, *Am J Obstet Gynecol* 172:525-529, 1995.
3. Koren G: Use of the new quinolones during pregnancy, *Can Fam Physician* 42:1097-1099, 1996.

Antidepressants

A follow-up study of children exposed to tricyclic antidepressants or fluoxetine (Prozac) in the first trimester of pregnancy showed no abnormalities of cognitive, language, or behavioral development.[1,2] A 1996 prospective cohort study of 228 women taking fluoxetine during pregnancy did not find any increased rate of anomalies or of pregnancy loss. However, in this study women who took the drug in the third trimester had a higher incidence of premature deliveries and, independent of this, more of their infants required admission to special care nurseries.[3] Five other cohort studies involving a total of 450 women taking fluoxetine during pregnancy also reported no increased teratogenesis, but unlike the one quoted above, they failed to demonstrate increased premature births or other adverse effects from taking the drug in the third trimester.[4] No extensive studies of tricyclic antidepressants in the first trimester are available, but the studies that have been done have not found evidence of teratogenicity.[5]

A critical review of the literature found no adverse effects on the infants of nursing mothers who were taking amitriptyline (Elavil), nortriptyline (Aventyl), desipramine (Norpramin, Pertofrane), clomipramine (Anafranil), dothiepin (Prothiaden), and sertraline (Zoloft). None of these drugs or their metabolites were detectable in the serum of healthy full-term infants. Some adverse effects were reported when the mother was taking doxepin or fluoxetine while breast feeding, and detectable infant serum levels of these two drugs have been reported. The authors suggest that if a nursing mother requires antidepressants and continues to breast feed, serum levels of the drug be measured in infants under 10 weeks of age once a maternal therapeutic dose of the drug has been reached. Measurement of serum levels is needed for infants over 10 weeks only if they display symptoms.[6]

REFERENCES

1. Koren G: First-trimester exposure to fluoxetine (Prozac): does it affect pregnancy outcome? *Can Fam Physician* 42:43-44, 1996.
2. Nulman I, Rovet J, Stewart DE, et al: Neurodevelopment of children exposed in utero to antidepressant drugs, *N Engl J Med* 336:258-262, 1997.
3. Chambers CD, Johnson KA, Dick LM, et al: Birth outcomes in pregnant women taking fluoxetine, *N Engl J Med* 335:1010-1015, 1996.
4. Robert E: Treating depression in pregnancy (editorial), *N Engl J Med* 335:1056-1059, 1996.
5. Altshuler LL, Cohen L, Szuba MP, et al: Pharmacologic management of psychiatric illness during pregnancy; dilemmas and guidelines, *Am J Psychiatry* 153:592-606, 1996.
6. Wisner KL, Perel JM, Findling RL: Antidepressant treatment during breast-feeding, *Am J Psychiatry* 153:1132-1137, 1996.

Anticonvulsants in Pregnancy

(See also seizures)

Pregnant patients with seizure disorders who are not taking medications have an approximate risk of having an infant with congenital anomalies of 3% compared with a rate of 2% in the general population; if they are taking one antiepileptic medication, the rate is also 3%, but it increases to 5% with two, 10% with three, and 20% with four. A common syndrome resulting from a variety of antiepileptic drugs is facial dimorphism, cleft lip, cleft palate, cardiac defects, hypoplasia of the digits, and nail dysplasia. Originally described as a complication of phenytoin (Dilantin), this syndrome is now known to be associated with other antiepileptic drugs, including carbamazepine (Tegretol) and valproate (Depakene, Depakote).[1] There is evidence that phenytoin (Dilantin) is associated with an increased risk of low intelligent quotients.[2,3] This effect is not seen with carbamazepine (Tegretol), which therefore is the anticonvulsant of choice in pregnancy.[3] On the other hand, patients taking carbamazepine[1,2,4,5] or valproic acid have an increased risk of neural tube defects.[1,4] The addition of 5 mg of folate daily before and after conception for patients taking these drugs has been suggested, even though the efficacy of such an approach has not been established.[1]

REFERENCES

1. Brodie MJ, Dichter MA: Antiepileptic drugs, *N Engl J Med* 334:168-175, 1996.
2. Koren G: In utero exposure to phenytoin or carbamazepine, *Can Fam Physician* 41:1862-1863, 1995.
3. Scolnik D, Nulman I, Rovet J, et al: Neurodevelopment of children exposed in utero to phenytoin and carbamazepine monotherapy, *JAMA* 271:767-770, 1994.
4. Drugs for epilepsy, *Med Lett* 37:37-40, 1995.
5. Rosa FW: Spina bifida in infants of women treated with carbamazepine during pregnancy, *N Engl J Med* 324:674-676, 1991.

Antihistamines in Pregnancy

(See also antihistamines)

Tripelennamine (Pyribenzamine), chlorpheniramine (Chlor-Tripolon), dexchlorpheniramine (Polaramine), dimenhydrinate (Gravol, Dramamine), and loratadine (Claritin) are all classified by the U.S. Food and Drug Administration as being in Category B, which means probably safe with no toxicity demonstrated in animal studies or controlled trials in women.[1] A 1997 metaanalysis of over 200,000 women who were exposed to a variety of antihistamines in the first trimester of pregnancy not only found no increase in the risk of congenital anomalies, but actually documented a slight decrease in risk. Possibly the use of antihistamines to control nausea and vomiting in pregnancy actually improves fetal outcomes.[2]

REFERENCES

1. Peggs JF, Shimp SA, Opdycke RAC: Antihistamines: the old and the new, *Am Fam Physician* 52:593-600, 1995.
2. Koren G: Antihistamines are safe during the first trimester, *Can Fam Physician* 43:33-34, 1997.

Antihypertensives

See hypertensive disorders of pregnancy.

Antipsychotics

It appears that the psychotic state itself may adversely affect fetal outcome, and neuroleptics may result in a slight increase in congenital anomalies. Patients taking phenothiazines have a rate of 2.4% compared with a background rate of 2%.[1]

REFERENCES

1. Altshuler LL, Cohen L, Szuba MP, et al: Pharmacologic management of psychiatric illness during pregnancy: dilemmas and guidelines, *Am J Psychiatry* 153:592-606, 1996.

Aspartame

No adverse effects have been reported from the ingestion of aspartame in pregnancy.[1]

REFERENCES

1. Zuber C, Librizzi RJ, Bolognese RJ: Do aspartame and video display terminals pose pregnancy risks? *Postgrad Obstet Gynecol* 9:1-5, 1989.

Aspirin

Low-dose aspirin is safe throughout pregnancy. Whether high doses of aspirin or other nonsteroidal antiinflammatory drugs (NSAIDs) are safe in the second half of pregnancy is unknown.[1]

REFERENCES

1. Theis JG: Acetylsalicylic acid (ASA) and nonsteroidal antiinflammatory drugs (NSAIDs) during pregnancy: are they safe? *Can Fam Physician* 42:2347-2349, 1996.

Benzodiazepines

Reports are conflicting as to whether benzodiazepines increase the risk of cleft palate or cleft lip when taken during pregnancy. One reviewer concluded that if indeed an association exists, the risk is small.[1]

Since many women become pregnant while taking benzodiazepines, considerable anxiety and even some pregnancy terminations have occurred as a result of concern about cleft lip and cleft palate. A recent prospective case-control study of 137 women who took benzodiazepines during their pregnancies found no increased rate of congenital anomalies. Although the power of the study was inadequate to rule out a small teratogenic effect, the results suggest that such an outcome is unlikely.[2]

REFERENCES

1. Altshuler LL, Cohen L, Szuba MP, et al: Pharmacologic management of psychiatric illness during pregnancy; dilemmas and guidelines, *Am J Psychiatry* 153:592-606, 1996.

2. Pastuszak A, Milich V, Chan S, et al: Prospective assessment of pregnancy outcome following first trimester exposure to benzodiazepines, *Can J Clin Pharmacol* 3:167-171, 1996.

Cosmetics and Hair Care Products

Cosmetics and hair care products have not been found to be detrimental during pregnancy.[1,2]

REFERENCES

1. Zuber C, Hom M, Vought L, et al: Common chemical exposures in pregnancy: cosmetics, paint fumes, and cold medications, *Postgrad Obstet Gynecol* 12:1-6, 1992.
2. Koren G: Hair care during pregnancy, *Can Fam Physician* 42: 625-626, 1996.

Inhaled Steroids

No adverse effects of inhaled steroids have been found in pregnancy, labor, or delivery.[1]

REFERENCES

1. Barnes PJ, Pedersen S: Efficacy and safety of inhaled corticosteroids in asthma: report of a workshop held in Eze, France, October 1992, *Am Rev Respir Dis* 148:S1-S26, 1993.

Lithium

The incidence of Ebstein's anomaly is increased in patients taking lithium in the first trimester. Although the relative risk is increased 10 to 20 times, the condition is rare, so the absolute risk is about 1:1000 or 0.1%.[1] Ebstein's anomaly is distal displacement of the tricuspid valve into the right ventricle, and this usually results in inadequate right ventricular outflow, tricuspid regurgitation, and sometimes cyanotic heart disease from a right to left atrial shunt.

REFERENCES

1. Altshuler LL, Cohen L, Szuba MP, et al: Pharmacologic management of psychiatric illness during pregnancy; dilemmas and guidelines, *Am J Psychiatry* 153:592-606, 1996.

Nonsteroidal Antiinflammatory Drugs

There is no evidence of adverse effects of NSAIDs in the first half of pregnancy. Whether NSAIDs are detrimental in the second half of pregnancy is uncertain. There is concern that these drugs may lead to prenatal closure of the ductus arteriosus and persistent pulmonary hypertension.[1]

REFERENCES

1. Theis JG: Acetylsalicylic acid (ASA) and nonsteroidal anti-inflammatory drugs (NSAIDs) during pregnancy: are they safe? *Can Fam Physician* 42:2347-2349, 1996.

Pseudoephedrine

If a decongestant is essential in pregnancy, pseudoephedrine appears to be the drug of choice.[1] The physician should caution the patient not to buy combination products inadvertently.

REFERENCES

1. Niebyl JR, Repke JT: Treatment of the common cold. In Niebyl JR, ed: *Drug use in pregnancy,* ed 2, Philadelphia, 1988, Lea & Febiger, pp 235-238.

Vitamin A Supplements in Pregnancy

(See also vitamin A)

The odds ratio of having a child with a congenital anomaly was 4.8 for women taking vitamin A supplements of 10,000 IU or more compared with those taking 5000 IU or less. Among women taking more than 10,000 units, about 1 in 57 had a baby with congenital malformation attributable to the vitamin. These data do not apply to beta-carotene.

REFERENCES

1. Rothman KJ, Moore LL, Singer MR, et al: Teratogenicity of high vitamin A intake, *N Engl J Med* 333:1369-1373, 1995.

EPISIOTOMY

Midline episiotomies are almost routine procedures for the delivery of primiparous women in many North American obstetrical practices. The rationale for performing them is that they are thought to reduce the mechanical and metabolic morbidity of the infant, prevent perineal relaxation, and decrease the incidence of perineal pain, urinary incontinence, and sexual dysfunction.[1,2] As documented by Klein and associates[2,3] in a randomized controlled trial, there is no substance to these hypotheses and, in fact, patients who had episiotomies not only had more pain and sexual dysfunction, but also had a much higher incidence of third- and fourth-degree tears.[3] Labrecque and co-workers[4] in a retrospective cohort study involving over 4000 women also found a much higher rate of third- and fourth-degree tears in patients who had episiotomies. Family physicians who refer their patients for obstetrical care should determine whether their consultants are believers or nonbelievers in episiotomy because it has been shown that believers have great difficulty staying the knife even when they have agreed ahead of time to try to do so.[5]

REFERENCES

1. Helewa ME: Episiotomy and severe perineal trauma: of science and fiction (editorial), *Can Med Assoc J* 156:811-813, 1997.
2. Klein M, Gauthier R, Robbins, et al: Relation of episiotomy to perineal trauma and morbidity, sexual dysfunction, and pelvic floor relaxation, *Am J Obstet Gynecol* 171:591-598, 1994.
3. Klein MC, Gauthier RC, Jorgensen SH, et al: Does episiotomy prevent perineal trauma and pelvic floor relaxation? *Online J Curr Clin Trials* [serial online], Jul 1, 2 (Doc No 10), 1992.
4. Labrecque M, Baillargeon L, Dallaire M, et al: Association between median episiotomy and severe perineal lacerations in primiparous women, *Can Med Assoc J* 156:797-802, 1997.
5. Klein MC, Kaczorowski J, Robbins JM, et al: Physicians' beliefs and behaviour during a randomized controlled trial of episiotomy: consequences for women in their care, *Can Med Assoc J* 153:769-779, 1995.

EXERCISE IN PREGNANCY

A number of theoretical concerns relate to exercise in normal pregnancies.[1]

Hyperthermia

Exercise can increase body temperature to 39° to 40° C, and in experimental animals elevated temperature in the first trimester is associated with an increase in neural tube defects. No prospective studies have shown an increase in congenital malformations in humans as a result of increased body temperature brought about by exercise.[1]

Redistribution of Splanchnic Blood Flow

Splanchnic blood flow decreases significantly with exercise. No studies have shown that this has significant adverse effects on the fetus. Some have shown a slight increase in neonatal birth weight when the mothers engaged in moderate exercise and others a slight decrease when women exercised five or more times a week in the third trimester.[1]

Fetal Distress

In most cases the fetal heart rate responds to maternal exercise by an increase of about 10 beats/min; in a few cases transient bradycardia occurs. No human studies have demonstrated an increased incidence of fetal distress as a result of exercise.

Abortion

Few studies have considered the relationship of exercise around the time of conception or in the first trimester and the rate of spontaneous abortion. What data there are show no increase in the rate of abortion among those who exercise.[1]

Labor

Exercise is not associated with premature rupture of the membranes or premature labor.[1]

Injury

Even though ligaments are lax in pregnancy, maternal injury rates are not reported to be increased in exercising pregnant women.[1]

Maternal Weight Gain

Normal maternal weight gain is not altered by exercise.[1]

A metaanalysis of moderate exercise in pregnancy (three to six times a week) found no adverse effects from a variety of exercise programs, including weight lifting, jogging, swimming, and biking.[2]

Although the evidence clearly supports moderate exercise in normal pregnancies, this does not necessarily apply to women with a past history of obstetrical problems or current medical or obstetrical conditions that could be adversely affected by exercise. Obstetrical problems that are considered to be relative or absolute contraindications to exercise are two or more previous spontaneous abortions, an incompetent cervix, vaginal bleeding or placenta previa, ruptured membranes or premature labor, preeclampsia or toxemia, multiple pregnancies, and fetal growth retardation.[3] General medical conditions that are relative or absolute contraindications to exercise are eating disorders, very low body fat, some forms of heart disease, anemia, and a number of other serious systemic diseases.[3]

REFERENCES

1. Stevenson L: Exercise in pregnancy. I. Update on pathophysiology, *Can Fam Physician* 43:97-104, 1997.
2. Lokey EA, Tran ZV, Wells CL, et al: Effects of physical exercise on pregnancy outcomes: a meta-analytic review, *Med Sci Sports Exerc* 23:1234-1239, 1991.
3. Stevenson L: Exercise in pregnancy. II. Recommendations for individuals, *Can Fam Physician* 43:107-111, 1997.

GESTATIONAL DIABETES MELLITUS

(See also attitudes, physician; screening; surrogate outcomes)

Risk Factors

Gestational diabetes is said to affect from 3% to 10% of pregnancies. The following are classic risk factors:

1. Family history of diabetes
2. Age older than 30
3. Obesity
4. Excessive weight gain during pregnancy
5. History of glucose intolerance
6. Previous macrosomatic infant or stillbirth

Up to 50% of women with gestational diabetes have none of these risk factors.[1]

Pros and Cons of Screening

Patients with gestational diabetes mellitus tend to have macrosomatic infants, and treatment of patients with the disorder decreases birth weight. It has generally been assumed that identifying and treating patients with this condition would decrease the morbidity of both infant and mother, as well as infant mortality. However, such a relationship has not been established, as is clearly acknowledged by an expert committee of the Society of Obstetricians and Gynecologists of Canada.[2] Despite this the committee recommends the continued screening of all pregnant women for gestational diabetes.[2] Both the U.S. Preventive Services Task Force[3] and the Canadian Task Force on the Periodic Health Examination[4] have concluded that the evidence is insufficient to recommend universal screening, and they give this procedure a "C" recommendation.

How can one explain the recommendations of the Society of Obstetricians and Gynecologists of Canada and many similar organizations that screening for gestational diabetes should be continued in the absence of evidence of its efficacy? The answer, as eloquently stated by Stephenson,[5] is twofold. First, the members of these organizations accept "surrogate outcomes," which are sometimes called "intermediate outcomes," as acceptable substitutes for real outcomes.[6] In this case the surrogate outcome of greatest significance is the prevention of macrosomia, which stands in place of perinatal morbidity and mortality. Second and more important, proponents of screening in the absence of high-quality evidence of its efficacy hold the attitude that if in doubt, action is better than inaction. Stephenson[5] labels such individuals "maximalists"—as opposed to "minimalists," while Sackett and Holland[7] would call them "evangelists"—as opposed to "snails" (see section on physician attitudes).

Even though the identification and treatment of gestational diabetes mellitus are often effective in preventing macrosomia, they have not resulted in an overall decrease in the Cesarean delivery rate.[8] This is probably because of the "practice style" of the attending obstetricians, which in this case is a propensity to perform Cesarean sections on patients with gestational diabetes even in the absence of specific clinical indications.[8,9]

Method of Screening for Gestational Diabetes

Screening methods for gestational diabetes have not been well standardized, and the actual methods of performing the tests and the criteria for positive results vary from one center to another.[10] One set of guidelines recommends initial screening between the 24th and 28th weeks because this is the time of expected increased insulin resistance. The test can be done at any time with respect to meals and consists of the oral ingestion of 50 g of glucose followed by a 1-hour blood sugar determination. If the result is ≥7.8 mmol/L (140 mg/dl), a 3-hour 100-g glucose tolerance test (GTT) should be performed.[11]

If a 3-hour GTT is performed, four blood samples are drawn, one fasting and three at hourly intervals after the ingestion of 100 g of glucose. Gestational diabetes is diagnosed if any two glucose levels are at or above the upper limits of normal for that time period. If only one reading is elevated, a diagnosis of impaired glucose tolerance may be made. Generally accepted upper limit values are fasting—5.8 mmol/L (105 mg/dl), 1 hour—10.6 mmol/L (190 mg/dl), 2 hours—9.2 mmol/L (165 mg/dl), and 3 hours—8.1 mmol/L (145 mg/dl).[11]

Management

Management of gestational diabetes consists first of diet, exercise, and careful home glucose monitoring. If the glucose levels cannot be maintained below 5 mmol/L (90 mg/dl) before meals or the bedtime snack, insulin therapy should be started.[11] If insulin is required, fasting and postprandial glucose level monitoring would seem to give better results than fasting and preprandial monitoring.[12]

REFERENCES

1. Lavin JP Jr: Screening of high risk and general population for gestational diabetes: clinical application and cost analysis, *Diabetes* 34(suppl 2):24-27, 1985.
2. SOGC Committee opinion: routine screening for gestational diabetes mellitus in pregnancy, *J Soc Obstet Gynecol Can,* December 1992, pp 35-86.
3. US Preventive Services Task Force: *Guide to clinical preventive services,* ed 2, Baltimore, 1996, Williams & Wilkins, pp 193-208.
4. Canadian Task Force on the Periodic Health Examination: *Clinical preventive health care,* Ottawa, 1994, Canadian Communication Group—Publishing, pp 16-23.
5. Stephenson MJ: Gestational diabetes mellitus (editorial), *Can Fam Physician* 39:745-748, 1993.
6. Scrabenek P, McCormick J: *Follies and fallacies in medicine,* Glasgow, 1989, Tarragon Press.
7. Sackett DL, Holland WW: Controversy in the detection of disease, *Lancet* 2:357-359, 1975.
8. Naylor CD, Sermer M, Chen E, et al (Toronto Trihospital Gestational Diabetes Investigators): Cesarean delivery in relation to birth weight and gestational glucose tolerance: pathophysiology or practice style? *JAMA* 275:1165-1170, 1996.
9. Coustan DR: Management of gestational diabetes mellitus: a self-fulfilling prophecy? (editorial), *JAMA* 275:1199-1200, 1996.
10. Okun N, Verma A, Demianczuk N: Gestational diabetes mellitus: unresolved issues and future research directions, *Can Fam Physician* 43:88-93, 1997.
11. Blair MM, Noc A-M: Detecting and managing gestational diabetes, *Can Fam Physician* 39:810-814, 1993.
12. de Veciana M, Major CA, Morgan MA, et al: Postprandial versus preprandial blood glucose monitoring in women with gestational diabetes mellitus requiring insulin therapy, *N Engl J Med* 33:1237-1241, 1995.

GROUP B STREPTOCOCCAL DISEASE

(See also clinical practice guidelines; prevention; screening)

Group B *Streptococcus (Streptococcus agalactiae)* is known to be an important cause of neonatal infections, and in high-risk circumstances, which are outlined below, the administration of intrapartum antibiotics decreases the incidence of this disorder in neonates.[1,2] Early prenatal screening of women for group B *Streptococcus* does not predict whether colonization will exist at the time of delivery,[1] and treatment of women carrying group B *Streptococcus* before delivery does not decrease the incidence of neonatal sepsis.[1,3,4] The efficacy of detecting *Streptococcus* B by cultures increases if swabs are taken from both the lower third of the vagina and the anorectal canal and if the microbiology laboratory uses selective rather than nonselective growth medium.[1,5]

An estimated 15% to 40% of pregnant women will have a positive vaginal or rectal culture for group B *Streptococcus,* and vertical transmission of the organism to the neonate occurs in 40% to 73% of women who carry the organism. However, infection develops in only 1% to 2% of infants who are colonized.[2] Risk factors during labor for neonatal infection with group B *Streptococcus* include preterm labor, premature rupture of membranes, prolonged rupture of membranes, and fever.[2,3]

With the preceding information, what should be the guidelines for screening and treating pregnant women for group B *Streptococcus?* Unfortunately, this is an area beset by controversy. Various proposals and some of the problems of implementing them follow.[1-9]

A program for screening all women in late pregnancy and treating during labor all women who are carriers has been suggested.[4,6,9] This would involve screening and treating large numbers of individuals in order that a few would benefit. The universal screening approach was taken in an Australian trial. The incidence of group B streptococcal infections in the neonates whose mother were in the screening and treatment protocol was 0.5:1000 compared with a rate of 1:1000 among neonates whose mothers were not screened or treated. Failure of the program has been attributed to a number of causes, including delivery before obtaining a culture, failure to obtain a culture, becoming a carrier after a negative culture, and failure to give antibiotics during labor.[6] A major problem with implementing this approach in regions where antenatal care takes place in private offices is ensuring that the antenatal culture results are available in the hospital at the time of delivery.[4]

Another proposal is to screen all women in late pregnancy and treat carriers during labor if they also have other risk factors such as premature or prolonged rupture of membranes, premature labor, fever, or multiple births.[1-3,7] This is the approach suggested in guidelines published by the American Academy of Pediatrics[7] and is close to the recommendations of the American College of Obstetricians and Gynecologists.[8] Surveys of obstetricians found that compliance with these guidelines was poor. Not all women were screened,[1-3] and if they were screened, cultures were often taken from the vagina only and not the vagina and rectum.[1,3] Perhaps most important, the majority of obstetricians treated detected carriers as soon as the culture reports were received (during the antepartum period) even though the literature clearly indicates that this is not an efficacious practice.[1-4]

A third approach is not to screen for *Streptococcus* B at all but to treat all women who have risk factors during labor such as premature or prolonged rupture of membranes, premature labor, fever, or multiple births.[1,4,9] In one study only 15% of surveyed obstetricians actually used antibiotics when these conditions were met.[1]

The latest clinical practice guidelines from the U.S. Centers for Disease Control and Prevention offer two of the preventive options outlined above.[9] These are[9]:

1. Screen all women between 35 and 37 weeks and treat all who are positive during the intrapartum period. If the results are not known at the time of delivery, treat the women.

2. Do not screen for *Streptococcus* B at all but during the intrapartum period treat women with risk factors such as labor at less than 37 weeks of gestation, duration of rupture of the membranes of 18 hours or more, and a temperature of 38° C (100.4° F) or more.

A special category is women who have previously delivered a child in whom group B streptococcal disease developed. These women do not require screening for the organism because all of them should be treated during the intrapartum period anyway.[9]

The optimal approach to this problem is not clear. Family physicians will have to read the literature, consult with their colleagues, and decide for themselves what they consider best for their patients.

REFERENCES

1. Jafari HS, Schuchat A, Hilsdon R, et al: Barriers to prevention of perinatal group B streptococcal disease, *Pediatr Infect Dis J* 14: 662-667, 1995.
2. Gigante J, Hickson GB, Entman SS, et al: Universal screening for group B *Streptococcus:* recommendations and obstetricians' practice decisions, *Obstet Gynecol* 85:440-443, 1995.
3. Mercer BM, Ramsey RD, Sibai BM: Prenatal screening for group B *Streptococcus*. I. Impact of antepartum screening on antenatal prophylaxis and intrapartum care, *Am J Obstet Gynecol* 173:837-841, 1995.
4. Larsen JW, Dooley SL: Group B streptococcal infections: an obstetrical viewpoint, *Pediatrics* 91:148-149, 1993.
5. Mercer BM, Briggs R: Group B *Streptococcus* and pregnancy, *Pediatr Ann* 25:206-214, 1996.
6. Garland SM, Fliegner JR: Group B *Streptococcus* (GBS) and neonatal infections: the case for intrapartum chemoprophylaxis, *Aust NZ J Obstet Gynaecol* 31:119-122, 1991.
7. Committee on Infectious Diseases and Committee on Fetus and Newborn: Guidelines for prevention of group B streptococcal (GBS) infection by chemoprophylaxis, *Pediatrics* 90:775-778, 1992.
8. American College of Obstetricians and Gynecologists: *Group B streptococcal infections in pregnancy,* ACOG Tech Bull No 170, Washington, DC, 1992, The College.
9. Prevention of preinatal group B streptococcal disease: a public health perspective, *MMWR* 45(RR-7):1-24, 1996.

HIV AND AIDS IN PREGNANCY

(See also HIV and AIDS)

Vertical transmission of HIV occurs in between 14% and 39% of pregnancies in HIV-positive women. It is thought to take place in one of three ways: intrauterine during the second and third trimesters, probably through placental infection; intrapartum through exposure to maternal secretions; and breast feeding. Breast feeding accounts for only a small percentage, and HIV-positive mothers should be advised not to breast feed. In theory Cesarean section might decrease the incidence, but this has not been borne out in practice.[1]

In one study zidovudine (Retrovir) given to pregnant women in the second and third trimesters decreased the number of HIV-positive neonates by two thirds while causing few adverse effects in mothers or babies.[2]

REFERENCES

1. Saglio SD, Kurtzman JT, Radner AB: HIV infection in women: an escalating health concern, *Am Fam Physician* 54:1541-1548, 1996.

2. Connor EM, Sperling RS, Gelber R, et al (Pediatric AIDS Clinical Trials Group Protocol 076 Study Group): Reduction of maternal-infant transmission of human immunodeficiency virus type I with zidovudine treatment, *N Engl J Med* 331: 1173-1180, 1994.

HYPERTENSIVE DISORDERS OF PREGNANCY

(See also hypertension)

Classification

Hypertensive disorders of pregnancy may be divided into three categories: chronic hypertension, gestational hypertension, and preeclampsia.[1]

Definition

Hypertension in pregnancy is defined as any reading over 140/90 mm Hg or an increase of the systolic level by 30 mm Hg compared with average readings before 20 weeks' gestation or an increase of the diastolic level by 15 mm Hg compared with average readings before 20 weeks' gestation.[2,3]

Choice of Drugs

Many antihypertensive drugs are either contraindicated in pregnancy or inadequately studied (which is the case with calcium channel blockers). Angiotensin-converting enzyme (ACE) inhibitors and beta-blockers are generally contraindicated. Some beta-blockers have been shown to have an adverse effect on the hemodynamics of the fetus and the uteroplacental circulation, while ACE inhibitors are associated with fetal growth retardation, congenital malformations, oligohydramnios, and fetal death. Diuretics have not been shown to be harmful, but in theory the induced decrease in plasma volume may inhibit fetal growth. Methyldopa (Aldomet) is the drug generally used when outpatient pharmacotherapy of hypertension is indicated.[1]

Chronic Hypertension

The diagnosis of chronic hypertension is made when patients have a history of hypertension before pregnancy or when the blood pressure is 140/90 mm Hg or higher before 20 weeks of gestation. The latter criterion results in many missed cases because blood pressure normally drops during the second trimester.[1]

Maternal and fetal morbidity are increased in women with severe hypertension (diastolic >110 mm Hg), mainly because of an increased risk of preeclampsia and abruptio placentae. Patients in this category require pharmacotherapy; the drug of first choice is methyldopa (Aldomet), and if it is contraindicated, nifedipine (Adalat, Procardia) or labetalol (Trandate) may be tried.[1]

Mild chronic hypertension is a different story. In the majority of trials of antihypertensive treatment for mildly hypertensive women no beneficial effects for mother or fetus have been noted in the treatment groups compared with the placebo or the no medication groups. In most cases women with chronic hypertension who have systolic levels below 170 or diastolic levels below 110 mm Hg do not require pharmacotherapy.[1]

Gestational Hypertension

Gestational hypertension is the new onset of hypertension after 20 weeks' gestation without associated symptoms or signs of preeclampsia. In general, drug treatment is not required and pregnancy outcome is good.[1]

Preeclampsia

A working clinical definition of preeclampsia is hypertension plus hyperuricemia or proteinuria. (Proteinuria is defined as ≥1+ on dipstick on two or more occasions, or ≥300 mg in a 24-hour urine collection.) The severity of preeclampsia is measured by the degree of hypertension and proteinuria. Edema is common but is not necessary for the diagnosis.[1,2] The problem with this or any other clinical definition is that patients may have the disorder without hypertension or proteinuria. For example, 20% of women in whom seizures (eclampsia) later develop have diastolic blood pressure readings below 90 mm Hg or no proteinuria. Even when the HELLP (hemolysis, elevated liver enzyme levels, and low platelet counts) syndrome develops with resulting acute renal failure and pulmonary edema, the woman may have had no preceding hypertension or proteinuria.[1]

A probable explanation for the lack of hypertension or proteinuria in some women who later have serious disease is that one of the basic pathophysiological abnormalities is reduced vascular perfusion, which is often localized. If decreased perfusion does not involve the glomeruli, proteinuria will not occur; if it involves the central nervous system, the woman may have diplopia or blurred vision; if it involves the gastrointestinal tract, there may be nausea and vomiting. Another basic abnormality in preeclampsia is endothelial cell dysfunction, which can cause increased vascular permeability with edema, thromboses, and low platelet counts.[1,2]

Risk factors for preeclampsia include first pregnancy, family history of preeclampsia, previous personal history of preeclampsia, older age, preexisting hypertension, diabetes, multiple pregnancies, hydatidiform mole, and hydrops fetalis.[2] The clinical significance of preeclampsia is that women with this condition are at greater risk for seizures, cerebral hemorrhage, liver and renal failure, disseminated intravascular coagulation, abruptio placentae, and fetal growth retardation.[1]

Management of mild preeclampsia is controversial. Whether bed rest, hospitalization, antihypertensive therapy, or prophylactic anticonvulsants are beneficial is unknown, but it is generally agreed that if the woman is at 34 weeks or more and the cervix is favorable for induction, immediate delivery should be undertaken. In all cases close monitoring (weight, fetal status, blood pressure, proteinuria, and platelet count) is needed because the disorder may progress rapidly.[1]

Women with severe preeclampsia who are at 34 or more weeks of gestation require immediate delivery, as do many who are at an earlier stage. For those with a diastolic pressure of 110 mm Hg or more, the usual medical treatment is IV hydralazine (Apresoline) or, if it is contraindicated, IV labetalol or oral nifedipine.[1]

In North America the common practice has been administration of prophylactic magnesium sulfate to prevent seizures in patients with severe preeclampsia, whereas in Europe the more common practice has been antihypertensive therapy with or without phenytoin (Dilantin).[1] A recent trial comparing the prophylactic use of magnesium sulfate with phenytoin in women with preeclampsia demonstrated a small benefit for the magnesium sulfate–treated group.[4] Magnesium sulfate is also the anticonvulsant of choice for women with eclampsia.[5]

REFERENCES

1. Sibai BM: Treatment of hypertension in pregnant women, *N Engl J Med* 335:257-265, 1996.
2. Zamorski MA, Green LA: Preeclampsia and hypertensive disorders of pregnancy, *Am Fam Physician* 53:1595-1604, 1996.
3. National High Blood Pressure Education Program Working Group report on high blood pressure in pregnancy, *Am J Obstet Gynecol* 163(5 Pt 1):1691-1712, 1990.
4. Lucas MJ, Leveno KJ Cunningham FG: A comparison of magnesium sulfate with phenytoin for the prevention of preeclampsia, *N Engl J Med* 333:201-205, 1995.
5. Eclampsia Trial Collaborative Group: Which anticonvulsant for women with eclampsia? Evidence from the Collaborative Eclampsia Trial, *Lancet* 242:1455-1463, 1995.

NAUSEA AND VOMITING IN PREGNANCY

(See also nausea and vomiting)

Diet

Meals should be frequent and small with increased carbohydrate and decreased fat. Suggested nutrients for severe nausea are crackers, unbuttered toast, broth, pretzels, and non-diet ginger ale.[1] Iron may have to be omitted until symptoms improve.

Medications

Doxylamine succinate 10 mg in combination with pyridoxine HCl 10 mg is marketed in Canada under the trade name Diclectin. It is an effective and safe antiemetic during pregnancy and was approved for use in pregnancy by the Health Protection Branch of Health and Welfare Canada in 1990. Many studies have shown that it is not teratogenic.[2-4] A similar formulation in the United States called Bendectin was voluntarily withdrawn by the manufacturer in 1983 because of a profusion of legal suits stemming largely from the claims of an Australian obstetrician and gynecologist that his studies had indicated that the drug was teratogenic. It turned out that these claims were fraudulent, since there is no substantiated evidence that such studies were ever performed. In 1989 the Medical Tribunal of New South Wales in Australia revoked this physician's license to practice. Unfortunately, U.S. patients are still deprived of the medication.[4] Pyridoxine is used in this formulation not only to prevent vitamin B_6 deficiency in pregnancy, but also because it has some independent antinauseant effect.[5]

Although doxylamine combined with pyridoxine is not available in the United States, doxylamine alone as 25-mg tablets may be obtained for insomnia under the trade name Unisom Nighttime Sleep-Aid.

An alternative drug for nausea and vomiting of pregnancy is dimenhydrinate (Dramamine, Gravol). The usual dose is 50 to 100 mg qid prn.

REFERENCES

1. Kolasa K, Weismiller DG: Nutrition during pregnancy, *Am Fam Physician* 56:205-212, 1997.
2. Jewell MD: Debendox (Bendectin) for nausea in pregnancy. In Enkin MW, Keirse MJN, Renfrew MJ, Neilson JP, eds: *Pregnancy and childbirth module,* Cochrane Database of Systematic Reviews, Review No 07703, April 30, 1993, Oxford, Eng, Update Software.
3. Caddick R, Colliton IE, Dushinski B, et al: Guidelines for the management of nausea and vomiting in pregnancy, *SOGC Clin Pract Guidelines* No 12, November 1995.
4. Fortin CA, Lalonde AB: The Bendectin Affair (of legal and general interest), *J SOGC* 17:61-63, 1995.
5. Vutyavanich T, Supreeya W, Ruangsri R: Pyridoxine for nausea and vomiting of pregnancy—a randomized double-blind, placebo-controlled trial, *Am J Obstet Gynecol* 173:881-884, 1995.

RISK ASSESSMENT IN PREGNANCY

(See also prevention; risk analysis)

Numerous systems are used to assess risk in pregnancy. On the basis of these, 16% to 55% of pregnancies are labeled high risk, yet half of perinatal mortality and morbidity occurs in "low-risk" pregnancies.[1-3] The conclusion of one thoughtful analyst of this subject is that pregnancy risk scoring has not been proved to do more good than harm.[1] In an editorial on this subject, Klein[4] raises the question of whether categorizing women as being at high risk is in itself a factor leading to increased consultations and interventions. He wonders whether risk scoring may not actually make women sick.

REFERENCES

1. Hall PF: Rethinking risk (editorial), *Can Fam Physician* 40: 1239-1244, 1994.
2. Wall EM: Assessing obstetric risk: a review of obstetric risk-scoring systems, *J Fam Pract* 27:153-163, 1988.
3. Hall PF: Obstetric risk scoring: a Trojan horse, *Manitoba Med* 63:43-45, 1993.
4. Klein M: Family physician maternity care: outcomes when family physicians provide most community-based care (editorial), *Can Fam Physician* 41:546-548, 1995.

SMOKING IN PREGNANCY

(See also poverty)

Known detrimental effects of smoking in pregnancy include increased risks of the following[1]:

1. Intrauterine growth retardation
2. Low-birth-weight babies
3. Preterm birth
4. Spontaneous abortion
5. Placenta previa
6. Abruptio placentae

REFERENCES

1. Brosky G: Why do pregnant women smoke and can we help them quit? (editorial), *Can Med Assoc J* 152:163-166, 1995.

ULTRASOUND IN PREGNANCY

If routine ultrasound is performed, it is usually scheduled at 18 weeks. A number of fetal abnormalities may be detected at this stage of gestation.[1-5] However, the sensitivity is low (17%[1] to 40%[2]), as is the positive predictive value.[5] Gestational age can be assessed and multiple pregnancies detected,[3,4] and in many cases fetal sex can be determined.[1] Studies comparing patients undergoing routine antenatal ultrasound with those having selective ultrasound (when clinically indicated) have shown that those in the routine ultrasound group had twin pregnancies accurately diagnosed in all cases, a lower frequency of induction for apparent post-term pregnancy, fewer low-weight babies, and more induced abortions for fetal abnormalities.[3,4]

Whether a single routine ultrasound screening during the second trimester of pregnancy actually improves perinatal morbidity and mortality is another question. Probably it does not, but this is still an area of heated controversy. Evidence-based reviews of numerous trials addressing this issue[4,6,7] have concluded that except in one study, the Helsinki Ultrasound Trial,[2] no decreased perinatal morbidity or mortality has been documented. The Helsinki study,[2] which has been updated since these reviews were published,[8] reported a decrease in perinatal mortality in the screened group. This turned out to be the result of more children with severe congenital malformation being born and dying in the control group, and the difference disappeared if the induced abortions for congenital anomalies in the screened group were categorized as deaths.[7] A South African trial that was reported in 1996 found no differences in perinatal outcome between the ultrasound-screened and the control groups.[9]

The U.S. Preventive Services Task Force[6] gives a single routine midtrimester ultrasound screening a "C" recommendation, while the Canadian Task Force on the Periodic Health Examination[7] gives it a "B."

REFERENCES

1. Ewigman BG, Crane JP, Frigoletto FD, et al (RADIUS Study Group): Effect of prenatal ultrasound screening on perinatal outcome, *N Engl J Med* 329:821-827, 1993.
2. Saari-Kemppainen A, Karjalainen O, Ylostalo P, et al: Ultrasound screening and perinatal mortality: controlled trial of systematic one-stage screening in pregnancy: the Helsinki Ultrasound Trial, *Lancet* 336:387-391, 1990.
3. Enkin M, Keirse MJ, Renfrew M, et al, eds: *A guide to effective care in pregnancy and childbirth,* ed 2, Oxford, Eng, 1995, Oxford University Press, pp 41-42.
4. Neilson JP: Routine ultrasound in early pregnancy. In Enkin MW, Keirse MJNC, Renfrew MJ, Neilson JP, eds: *Pregnancy and childbirth module,* Cochrane Database of Systematic Reviews, Review No 03872, June 9, 1993, Oxford, Eng, 1994, Update Software.
5. Buskens E, Grobbee DE, Frohn-Mulder IM, et al: Efficacy of routine fetal ultrasound screening for congenital heart disease in normal pregnancy, *Circulation* 94:67-72, 1996.
6. US Preventive Services Task Force: *Guide to clinical preventive services,* ed 2, Baltimore, 1996, Williams & Wilkins, pp 407-417.
7. Canadian Task Force on the Periodic Health Examination: *Canadian guide to clinical preventive health care,* Ottawa, 1994, Canada Communication Group—Publishing, pp 4-14.
8. Leivo T, Tuominen R, Saarikemppainen A, et al: Cost-effectiveness of one-stage ultrasound screening in pregnancy—a report from the Helsinki Ultrasound Trial, *Ultrasound Obstet Gynecol* 7:309-314, 1996.
9. Geerts LT, Brand EJ, Theron GB: Routine obstetric ultrasound examinations in South Africa—cost and effect on perinatal outcome—a prospective randomised controlled trial, *Br J Obstet Gynaecol* 103:501-507, 1996.

VIDEO DISPLAY TERMINALS

There is no good evidence that video display terminals lead to adverse effects in pregnancy.[1]

REFERENCES

1. Zuber C, Librizzi RJ, Bolognese RJ: Do aspartame and video display terminals pose pregnancy risks? *Postgrad Obstet Gynecol* 9:1-5, 1989.

VIRAL DISEASES IN PREGNANCY

Erythema infectiosum

Erythema infectiosum is caused by parvovirus B19. It is contagious before the onset of the rash, but not once the rash has appeared. In pregnant women who are infected with parvovirus B19 a nonimmune hydrops fetalis may develop, with the highest risk between 10 and 20 weeks of gestation.[1,2] The pathogenesis is infection and hemolysis of the fetal red blood cells. Although some cases have been treated with intrauterine exchange transfusions, others, diagnosed and followed by ultrasound, have resolved spontaneously.[3,4] A woman who has been exposed to the disease during the infectious period should have serial ultrasound examinations at 2-week intervals.[5] In addition, maternal serological tests for IgG and IgM antibodies to the virus should be performed.

Herpes Simplex

The risk of transmitting herpes simplex virus (HSV) to the neonate is up to 50% in cases of primary herpes, whereas for women with recurrent episodes it is only 2% to 3% with vaginal birth even in the presence of lesions. In part this is because in recurrent herpes the quantity of virus is less and in part because the baby has developed protective IgG. Serial cultures of HSV during the last weeks of pregnancy are no longer advised, and current recommendations of both the Society of Obstetricians and Gynecologists of Canada and the American College of Obstetricians and Gynecologists are to examine the vulva, buttocks, and thighs for lesions and, if they are present, offer Cesarean section.[6]

Mumps

Mumps is rare in pregnancy. It is not known to be teratogenic. The rate of spontaneous abortions is higher among women who have the disease in the first trimester.[5]

Rubella

An estimated 10% of women in the reproductive age group are susceptible to rubella infection. Rubella is contagious from 1 week before the appearance of the rash until 5 days after its development.[5]

The congenital rubella syndrome is characterized by a number of anomalies. The major ones are congenital heart disease, microcephaly, mental retardation, microphthalmia, cataracts, and deafness. The risk for congenital rubella syndrome among infected pregnant women depends on the gestational age. It is about 50% in the first trimester, 35% in the second trimester, and virtually zero thereafter.[7]

If women have, or fear that they have, been exposed to rubella, the physician should determine whether the exposure was during the contagious phase. If so, the gestational age should be determined. If it is 24 weeks or less, the pregnant woman's antibody status should be determined. If it is negative, maternal serum should be drawn immediately and in 2 weeks for antibody determinations. If IgM antibodies develop or if there is a fourfold increase in IgG levels, the risk of the congenital rubella syndrome is significant.[5]

Rubeola

Rubeola is rare in pregnancy. Teratogenesis or spontaneous abortion in infected women has not been shown. The risk of premature labor, spontaneous abortion, and neonatal mortality is slightly increased.[8]

Varicella

The risk of acquiring varicella in pregnancy is low, about 1 to 7:10,000 pregnancies. The disease is infectious from 1 day before the onset of the eruption until all the crusts have dried.[5,9] The absolute risk that varicella infection of the mother in the first 20 weeks of pregnancy will cause congenital anomalies is about 2%.[9]

REFERENCES

1. Yaegashi N, Okamura K, Yajima A, et al: The frequency of human parvovirus B19 infection in nonimmune hydrops fetalis, *J Perinat Med* 22:159-163, 1994.
2. Torok TJ, Wang QY, Gary GW Jr, et al: Prenatal diagnosis of intrauterine infection with parvovirus B19 by the polymerase chain reaction technique, *Clin Infect Dis* 14:149-155, 1992.
3. Sheikh AU, Ernest JM, O'Shea M: Long-term outcome in fetal hydrops from parvovirus B19 infection, *Am J Obstet Gynecol* 167:337-34, 1992.
4. Pryde PG, Nugent CE, Pridjian G, et al: Spontaneous resolution of nonimmune hydrops fetalis secondary to human parvovirus B19 infection, *Obstet Gynecol* 79:859-861, 1992.
5. Boucher M: Les maladies virales de l'enfance et de la grossesse: petit guide pratico-pratique, *Clinicien,* March 1995, 10:55-70.
6. Sanderson F: Perinatal viral infections: 5 scenarios to manage, *Patient Care Can,* January 1996, 7:43-60.
7. Horstmann DM: Surveillance for rubella, *Contemp Ob Gyn* 34: 43-61, 1989.
8. Stein SJ, Greenspoon JS: Rubeola during pregnancy, *Obstet Gynecol* 78:925-929, 1991.
9. Pastuszak AL, Levy M, Schick B, et al: Outcome after maternal varicella infection in the first 20 weeks of pregnancy, *N Engl J Med* 330:901-905, 1994.

ONCOLOGY, PAIN, PALLIATIVE CARE, NAUSEA, AND VOMITING

Topics covered in this section

NAUSEA AND VOMITING

(See also cachexia; motion sickness; nausea and vomiting in pregnancy; oncology; palliative care)

Pathophysiology

The causes of nausea and vomiting include the following:

1. Direct irritation of visceral afferents from the gut (vagal), often from distention of portions of gut that are not usually distended such as the antrum of the stomach
2. Stimulation of the chemoreceptor trigger zone in the medulla via the circulation by toxins, drugs, or metabolic disorders. The chemoreceptor trigger zone is outside of the blood-brain barrier and thus accessible to humeral stimuli from either the blood or the cerebrospinal fluid.
3. Stimulation of the medullary vomiting center via the vestibular system as occurs in motion sickness and labyrinthitis

Oncology, Pain, Palliative Care, Nausea, and Vomiting

4. Stimulation of the medullary vomiting center via cortical input such as fear and pain

Neuroreceptors Mediating Vomiting

Neuroreceptors mediating vomiting include dopaminic (D_2), HT_3 (serotonin), histaminic (H_1), and muscarinic cholinergic. I doubt that many readers will remember this esoterica of neuropharmacology, but I include it because it is the basis of the theory that the drug selected should be specific for the neurotransmitters that have been activated in any particular situation. This is why recommendations for specific antiemetics vary depending on the clinical circumstances. The all-purpose antiemetics are the phenothiazines, which act on dopaminic, histaminic, and muscarinic receptors, but none is as potent as the more selective drugs (see later discussion).

Specific Disorders and the Choice of Antiemetic Drugs

Table 49 lists some of the common indications for antiemetics, the choice of drugs, and in most cases the usual adult doses. One of the better drugs for nausea and vomiting in pregnancy is the combination of doxylamine succinate and pyridoxine. This drug is available in Canada but is no longer marketed in the United States. The reasons for this are discussed in more detail in the section on nausea and vomiting in pregnancy. Two other drugs that are available in Canada but not in the United States are betahistine (Serc) and nabilone (Cesamet). Betahistine is used for Ménière's disease. It is an H_1 agonist that is thought to inhibit neuronal impulses in the lateral vestibular nucleus. Nabilone is a synthetic cannabinoid that is sometimes used for chemotherapy-induced nausea and vomiting. The use of antiemetics for chemotherapy is discussed in the following paragraphs.

Antiemetics for Chemotherapy

Although in urban areas chemotherapy is usually administered by oncologists, family physicians still must discuss the pros and cons of such treatment with their patients and help them deal with the side effects induced by such treatments. In rural areas family physicians do everything.

Two types of nausea and vomiting may occur with chemotherapy: immediate, which is within the first 24 hours, and delayed, which is from days 2 to 5. Drugs that are effective for ameliorating immediate nausea and vomiting may be different from drugs effective for the delayed form. This is one reason for the use of combination. To complicate matters, for a number of patients vomiting tends to be better controlled than nausea.[1]

Emetic Potential of Chemotherapeutic Drugs

The degree of nausea and vomiting induced by a chemotherapeutic agent is called its emetogenic potential. The choice of an antiemetic in chemotherapy is determined in part by the emetogenic potential of the chemotherapeutic agents being used.[2-4] This correlation is shown in Table 50. The emetogenic potential of some commonly used chemotherapeutic agents is given in Table 51.[2-4]

Table 49 Antiemetics

Indications and drugs	Usual doses
Pregnancy	
Doxylamine succinate 10 mg, pyridoxine 10 mg (Diclectin)	2 tablets hs and 1 tablet qam prn
Dimenhydrinate (Gravol, Dramamine)	50-100 mg qid
Motion Sickness	
Dimenhydrinate (Gravol, Dramamine)	50-100 mg qid
Scopolamine (Transderm-Scop, Transderm V)	Apply patch to postauricular area 12 hours before onset of motion; change every 72 hours prn
Ménière's Disease	
Betahistine (Serc)	4-8 mg q8h
Dimenhydrinate (Gravol, Dramamine)	50-100 mg qid
Diphenhydramine (Benadryl)	25-50 mg tid-qid
Narcotic Induced	
Prochlorperazine (Compazine, Stemetil)	5-10 mg po or rectally tid or qid
Haloperidol (Haldol)	1-2 mg daily or bid
Pseudoobstruction	
Metoclopramide (Maxeran)	5-10 mg tid qid
Domperidone (Motilium)	10 mg qid
Cisapride (Prepulsid)	5-10 mg tid-qid
Chemotherapy	
Dexamethasone (Decadron)	See text for doses
Prochlorperazine (Compazine, Stemetil)	See text for doses
Haloperidol (Haldol)	See text for doses
Domperidone (Motilium)	See text for doses
Nabilone (Cesamet)	See text for doses
Granisetron (Kytril)	See text for doses
Odansetron (Zofran)	See text for doses
Metoclopramide (Maxeran)	See text for doses

Single Versus Combination Antiemetic Drugs for Chemotherapy

Single antiemetic drugs are generally used for mild or moderately emetogenic chemotherapy and combination drugs for moderate or highly emetogenic chemotherapy. Examples of initial single dose or multiple dose regimens are given in Tables 52 and 53.

The literature on the use of antiemetics for patients undergoing chemotherapy is vast, and only selected examples are given here. Some of the combined regimens can be very effective. In an Italian study using dexamethasone and granisetron (initial doses shown in Example 3 in Table 53), a combination of dexamethasone (Decadron) 8 mg IV before chemotherapy followed by 4 mg po q6h for four doses afterward, with 3 mg of granisetron (Kytril), a serotonin

Table 50 Choice of Antiemetics Based on Emetogenic Potential of Chemotherapeutic Agents

Drugs	Emetogenic potential
Steroids	
Dexamethasone (Decadron)	Mild, moderate, marked
Phenothiazines	
Prochlorperazine (Compazine, Stemetil)	Mild, moderate
Butyrophenones	
Haloperidol (Haldol)	Mild, moderate
Domperidone (Motilium)	Mild, moderate
Cannabinoids	
Nabilone (Cesamet)	Mild, moderate
5-HT_3 Receptor Antagonists	
Odansetron (Zofran)	Mild, moderate, marked
Substituted Benzamides	
Metoclopramide (Maxeran)	Mild, moderate, marked

Table 51 Emetic Potential of Chemotherapeutic Drugs

Mild	Moderate	High
Fluorouracil	Cyclophosphamide	Cisplatin
Methotrexate	Doxorubicin	Mechlorethamine hydrochloride (nitrogen mustard)
Etoposide	Carboplatin	Streptozocin
Vincristine	Mitomycin	Dacarbazine
Bleomycin	Asparaginase	Carmustine
	Azacitidine	Dactinomycin

Table 52 Initial Doses of Antiemetic Drugs in Selected Single-Dose Regimens

Drug	Initial dose
Example 1	
Prochlorperazine (Compazine, Stemetil)	5-10 mg po, or IV or a 25-mg rectal suppository
Example 2	
Dexamethasone (Decadron)	10-20 mg IV
Example 3	
Ondansetron (Zofran)	8 mg po or 10 mg IV
Example 4	
Nabilone (Cesamet)	1-2 mg the night before chemotherapy and 1-2 mg 1-3 hours before chemotherapy

(5-hydroxytryptamine$_3$ [5-HT_3]) antagonist, given IV before chemotherapy, resulted in excellent (93%) control of both immediate and delayed nausea and vomiting in patients receiving moderately emetogenic chemotherapy. This two-drug combination gave better results for immediate nausea and vomiting than either drug alone. Dexamethasone alone was as effective as the two-drug combination in controlling delayed nausea and vomiting.[1] Granisetron is closely related to another 5-HT_3 receptor antagonist, odansetron HCl dihydrate (Zofran).

Table 53 Initial Doses of Antiemetic Drugs in Selected Combined Regimens

Drug	Initial dose
Example 1	
Dexamethasone (Decadron)	20 mg IV plus
Metoclopramide (Maxeran)	3 mg/kg IV q 2 h × 2 plus
Diphenhydramine (Benadryl)	25-50 mg IV q 2 h × 2 plus
Lorazepam (Ativan)	1-2 mg IV
Example 2	
Dexamethasone (Decadron)	20 mg IV plus
Ondansetron (Zofran)	8-10 mg IV
Example 3	
Dexamethasone (Decadron)	8 mg IV plus
Granisetron (Kytril)	3 mg IV

REFERENCES

1. Italian Group for Antiemetic Research: Dexamethasone, granisetron, or both for the prevention of nausea and vomiting during chemotherapy for cancer, *N Engl J Med* 332:1-5, 1995.
2. Grunberg SM, Hesketh PJ: Control of chemotherapy-induced emesis, *N Engl J Med* 329:1790-1796, 1993.
3. *Le traitement des nausées et vomissements causés par la radiothérapie et la chimiothérapie,* Québec, 1993, Le Lorier J Redacteur, Gouvernement du Québec.
4. Drugs for vomiting caused by cancer chemotherapy, *Med Lett* 35:14-26, 1993.

ONCOLOGY

(See also antiemetics for chemotherapy; informed consent; nausea and vomiting; palliative care; pain)

Most oncology topics are covered in the discussions of specific neoplasms, palliative care, pain, and nausea and vomiting.

Cachexia

(See also nausea and vomiting)

Appetite and food intake can be increased in patients with cancer cachexia with doses of megestrol acetate (Megace). In one recent study a dose of 1600 mg/day (ten 160-mg tablets taken throughout the day) was effective and the patients also reported less nausea and vomiting. Other studies have shown good results with 800 or even 480 mg/day.[1]

REFERENCES

1. Tchekmedyian NS, Hickman M, Siau J, et al: Megestrol acetate in cancer anorexia and weight loss, *Cancer* 69:1268-1274, 1992.

Clinical Trials

Evidence to date suggests that cancer patients participating in clinical trials have a longer survival than patients treated outside of such trials.[1-4]

REFERENCES

1. Stiller CA: Survival of patients with cancer: those included in clinical trials do better, *BMJ* 99:1058-1059, 1989.
2. Stiller CA, Draper GJ: Treatment centre size, entry to trials, and survival in acute lymphoblastic leukemia, *Arch Dis Child* 64: 657-661, 1989.
3. Karjalainen S, Palva I: Do treatment protocols improve end results: a study of survival of patients with multiple myeloma in Finland, *BMJ* 299:1069-1072, 1989.
4. Weijer C: The breast cancer research scandal: addressing the issues (editorial), *Can Med Assoc J* 152:1195-1197, 1995.

Chemotherapy

(See also antiemetic drugs for chemotherapy; nausea and vomiting)

A relatively new chemotherapeutic agent is paclitaxel (Taxol). It is derived from the bark of the Pacific yew tree and has been found to be effective in a number of patients who no longer responded to conventional chemotherapy. It is commonly used for tumors of the ovaries, lung, breast, and head and neck.[1]

REFERENCES

1. Rowinsky EK, Donehower RC: Paclitaxel (Taxol), *N Engl J Med* 332:1004-1014, 1995.

Follow-Up of Patients with Cancer Who Have Had Curative Treatments

(See also informed consent)

Traditional medical practice involves extensive follow-up investigations of patients who have had curative surgery for cancer; the usual argument for this policy is that early recurrences that could be resected will be detected. Studies of such protocols for patients with breast cancer,[1,2] melanoma,[3] and colon cancer[4,5] have shown no or little survival advantage from their use. Among patients with Hodgkin's disease, only 11% of relapses were detected by physical examination or routine investigation whereas 89% were found through the investigation of newly developed symptoms.[6] Aside from cost, the disadvantage of intensive follow-up investigations is a possible decrease in the patient's quality of life. In a study of patients with breast cancer, twice as many preferred reducing rather than increasing the frequency of follow-up visits.[7] Tests are time consuming and sometimes uncomfortable. False-positive tests may take weeks to be clarified, and true positives that detect incurable disease in otherwise asymptomatic patients do not seem to be beneficial.[8] At present few patients are given these data, so they do not have the opportunity to exercise informed consent.

An additional argument for intensive follow-up is that it is an educational tool for both novice and experienced oncologists. Careful follow-up may lead to observations and research that will improve management in the future.[9]

Oncology, Pain, Palliative Care, Nausea, and Vomiting

REFERENCES

1. GIVIO Investigators: Impact of follow-up testing on survival and health-related quality of life in breast cancer patients: a multicenter randomized controlled trial, *JAMA* 271:1587-1592, 1994.
2. Del Turco MR, Palli D, Cariddi A, et al: Intensive diagnostic follow-up after treatment of primary breast cancer: a randomized trial; National Research Council Project on Breast Cancer Follow-up, *JAMA* 271:1593-1997, 1994.
3. Weiss M, Loprinzi CL, Creagan ET, et al: Utility of follow-up tests for detecting disease recurrence of surgically resected primary malignant melanoma. In *Proceedings of the Annual Meeting of the American Society of Clinical Oncology,* March 1995, Los Angeles, Abstract 893.
4. Virgo KS, Vernava AM, Longo WE, et al: Cost of patient follow-up after potentially curative colorectal cancer treatment, *JAMA* 273:1837-1841, 1995.
5. Makela JT, Laitinen SO, Kairaluoma MI: Five-year follow-up after radical surgery for colorectal cancer—results of a prospective-randomized trial, *Arch Surg* 130:1062-1067, 1995.
6. Radford JA, Eardley A, Woodman C, et al: Follow up policy after treatment for Hodgkin's disease: too many clinic visits and routine tests? A review of hospital records, *BMJ* 314:343-346, 1997.
7. Gulliford T, Opomu M, Wilson E, et al: Popularity of less frequent follow up for breast cancer in randomised study—initial findings from the Hotline Study, *BMJ* 314:174-177, 1997.
8. Loprinzi CL: Follow-up testing for curatively treated cancer survivors: what to do? (editorial), *JAMA* 273:1877-1878, 1995.
9. Rodger A: Routine follow up of breast cancer in primary care (letter), *BMJ* 314:1129-1130, 1997.

Paraneoplastic Syndromes

Some of the paraneoplastic syndromes are listed in Table 54.

Table 54 Paraneoplastic Syndromes

Hypercalcemia (hormonally mediated)
Cushing's syndrome (ectopic production of adrenocorticotropic hormone)
Hyponatremia (ectopic production of antidiuretic hormone)
Clubbing
Hypertrophic osteoarthropathy
Peripheral neuropathies
Cerebellar degeneration
Myasthenia gravis
Lambert-Eaton myasthenic syndrome (more severe in lower limbs and proximal muscles and improves temporarily with exercise)
Polymyositis
Dermatomyositis
Sudden appearance of seborrheic keratoses (Leser-Trélat sign)
Acanthosis nigricans
Migratory thrombophlebitis (Trousseau's syndrome)

PAIN, CHRONIC

(See also constipation; metastatic breast cancer; multiple myeloma; nausea and vomiting; palliative care)

Pain and Cancer

An estimated 65% to 85% of patients with advanced cancer suffer from pain, but this can be effectively controlled in 85% to 95% of cases.[1] In assessing chronic pain, it is important to realize that health care workers often underestimate its severity.[2]

Categories of Pain Control Drugs

Classes of pain control drugs include the following[1,2]:

Nonopioids	Acetaminophen, acetylsalicylic acid (ASA), nonsteroidal antiinflammatory drugs (NSAIDs), tramadol
Weak opioids	Codeine
Strong opioids	Morphine, hydromorphone, oxycodone, fentanyl
Adjuvants	Steroids, psychotropic drugs, anticonvulsants

Analgesic Ladder

A standard stepwise protocol for chronic pain control (analgesic ladder) based on the World Health Organization guidelines is to start with nonopioids, add a mild opioid such as orally administered codeine to a maximum of 120 mg q4h, and end up replacing the mild opioid with a potent opioid such as oral morphine. Adjuvants should be used at each step if indicated.[1,2]

Nonopioids

Standard nonopioids that may be used alone for the treatment of mild cancer pain are acetaminophen, aspirin, NSAIDs, and perhaps tramadol. Doses should be titrated upward to their maximal levels, and if one agent in this class is ineffective, another may be tried. However, if pain is moderate or severe, narcotics should be started immediately.[1,2] Tramadol (Ultram) is a nonopioid approved by the U.S. Food and Drug Administration in 1995. The usual dose is 50 to 100 mg q4-6h. It has the equivalent analgesic effect of 60 mg of codeine or 30 mg of codeine plus 650 mg of acetaminophen. Its role in the management of chronic cancer pain is uncertain, but it may be useful for patients who have mild to moderate chronic pain that is not relieved by acetaminophen and who cannot tolerate NSAIDs.[1]

Weak Opioids

The standard "weak" opioid for chronic pain is codeine. The equivalency of oral codeine to oral morphine is approximately 10:1. That is, 60 mg of codeine phosphate po is roughly equivalent to 6 mg of morphine sulfate po.

Codeine comes in three basic forms: short-acting codeine phosphate, long-acting codeine preparations (Codeine Contin), and short-acting codeine phosphate in combination with another analgesic such as acetaminophen or ASA plus or minus caffeine (e.g., Tylenol 3 or 4, Empirin 30 or 60, Empracet 30 or 60). A major limitation of dosage in the combination forms is the adjuvant drugs (acetaminophen, ASA, caffeine). The numbers 8, 15, and 30 following a trade name (e.g., Empirin 30) refer to the milligrams of codeine in the product. In the case of Tylenol the numbers 1, 2, 3, and 4 refer to 8, 15, 30, and 60 mg of codeine, respectively.

Sorting out the available preparations becomes even more difficult when products with the same names in Canada and the United States are compared. In the United States Tylenol 2 and Tylenol 3 contain acetaminophen 300 mg plus codeine 15 and 30 mg, respectively. In Canada the same ingredients are present but with the addition of 15 mg of caffeine. Tylenol 1 is available only in Canada and contains 300 mg of acetaminophen, 8 mg of codeine, and 15 mg of caffeine. In both countries Tylenol 4 contains 300 mg of acetaminophen and 60 mg of codeine.

Since these various combinations have many brand names, physicians have to check the specific ingredients carefully before prescribing them. One way to avoid mistakes is to write out the generic names of the combinations desired such as "acetaminophen 325 mg plus codeine 30 mg."

A long-acting formulation of codeine, Codeine Contin, has recently been released on the market in Canada. It is supplied as scored 100-, 150-, and 200-mg tablets. The total daily dosage is about 25% less than the total daily dosage of codeine phosphate, and it is given in two equal doses q12h.

Strong Opioids

Strong opioids include morphine, hydromorphone (Dilaudid), oxycodone (Roxicodone, Percodan, Percocet), and fentanyl (Duragesic).

Morphine

The usual strong opioid that is used for chronic pain is morphine. A significant first-pass effect occurs with oral morphine. When it is given as a single dose at the initiation of treatment, the potency ratio of oral to subcutaneous or IV morphine is 1:6 or 1:8. With repeated oral doses the ratio becomes 1:2 or 1:3. That is, the parenteral dose is only two to three times as potent as the oral dose.

For control of chronic pain, medications are given by the oral route if possible because this results in more even blood levels. The next best alternative is the rectal route, and the least desirable is the parenteral route. Initially, short-acting preparations such as solutions or tablets of morphine sulfate should be used. Dosage intervals should be close enough to prevent recurrence of pain (q3-4h for morphine sulfate). If pain does recur, the next dose should be increased by 25% to 50%. Half of the regular dose should be kept available to be given as needed (q1-2h for morphine) in case of breakthrough pain. Initially the patient should be awakened at regular intervals during the night to receive the analgesic doses, but when the patient's condition becomes stable, this can be avoided by giving 1.5 to 2 times the usual dose at bedtime. Once pain is controlled by short-acting oral or rectal opioids, patients may be switched to longer acting oral preparations (e.g., Kadian, MS Contin, Oramorph SR). In the case of morphine the total daily dose of the long-acting preparations is equal to the total daily dose of short-acting morphine but is given in 2 divided doses at 12-hour intervals. Short-acting formulations of the long-acting narcotics should be available to the patient in case of breakthrough pain.[1,2]

Hydromorphone

Hydromorphone (Dilaudid) may be taken orally, rectally, or by injection. Oral formulations are available as solutions, short-acting tablets, and in Canada slow release tablets (Hydromorph Contin). Hydromorphone is four to five times as potent as morphine and it is also more soluble than that drug. The increased solubility means that if high-dose parenteral injections are required, the volume required for equipotent doses is less for hydromorphone than for morphine.

Oxycodone

Although their names sound similar, oxycodone is a narcotic that is 10 times more potent than codeine.[3,4] Its analgesic effect[3,4] and potential for abuse[3] are comparable to morphine. For example, in one study of cancer patients with chronic pain controlled by oral oxycodone, it was possible to change to the same dosage of oral morphine with no loss of pain control.[4]

In Canada the only formulations of short-acting oxycodone available for oral use are in combination with acetaminophen (Percocet) or ASA (Percodan), which limit the dosage. In the United States short-acting oxycodone is available alone (Roxicodone) or, as in Canada, in combination with acetaminophen (Percocet, Roxicet) or ASA (Percodan, Roxiprin). A controlled release formulation of oxycodone (OxyContin) has recently become available; in one study of cancer pain control it was found to be as effective as controlled release hydromorphone.[5]

Although oxycodone may be a useful drug for patients with chronic cancer pain, physicians should be aware that it is a popular drug of abuse and should therefore avoid prescribing it for short-duration musculoskeletal pain.[6]

Fentanyl

Fentanyl (Duragesic) is available as transdermal patches that come in various strengths and are applied to the arms or torso for 72 hours (some patients, especially smokers, may metabolize the drug more rapidly and have to change the patches every 48 hours). The patches do not become fully effective until in place for at least 12 hours. In general, chronic pain should first be controlled by oral narcotics and then the patient can be switched to fentanyl using the conversion figures on the package insert.[7]

Switching Opioids

Patients with chronic pain may require a change of narcotic medications. Sometimes this is done because pain relief is inadequate and for some reason an equivalent dose of another narcotic is more effective and sometimes because the original narcotic has adverse effects. The dose of the new narcotic is usually determined by reference to equivalency tables. When these are used, it is important to remember that they are only rough approximations and that individual patients may require higher or lower doses than those listed.[8]

Supplementary Drugs

All patients taking narcotics should be given laxatives preventively (see discussion of constipation), antiemetics as necessary (see section on nausea and vomiting), and in most cases, adjuvants.[1,2]

Psychomotor Function

Long-term use of narcotics does not appear to impair psychomotor functions such as those required to drive a car.[9]

Opioids To Avoid in the Treatment of Chronic Pain

In general, physicians should avoid prescribing meperidine or pethidine (Demerol) for chronic pain. Meperidine has a short duration of action (1 to 3 hours) and poor oral absorption (oral/parenteral ratio is 4:1), and repeated doses lead to risk of central nervous system toxicity.

Pentazocine (Talwin) has poor bioavailability by the oral route, a short duration of action, and many neuropsychiatric side effects. It is an opioid agonist-antagonist and may induce withdrawal symptoms in opioid-dependent patients.

Propoxyphene (Darvon) is an opioid with the potency of about 600 mg of aspirin.[1,2] Its value for relief of chronic pain is questionable.[2]

Adjuvant Analgesic Drugs

The main classes of adjuvant analgesic drugs for the management of chronic pain are NSAIDs, tricyclic antidepressants, anticonvulsants, corticosteroids, and bisphosphonates.

Nonsteroidal antiinflammatory drugs

NSAIDs are particularly useful as adjunct treatment for bony metastases. A metaanalysis of NSAIDs in the treatment of cancer pain came to the conclusion that the analgesic effect of this class of drugs in standard doses was roughly equivalent to 5 to 10 mg of intramuscular morphine. Increasing the dosage of the NSAID or adding a weak opioid such as codeine did not augment the analgesic effect but did result in more adverse reactions.[10]

Tricyclic antidepressants

Tricyclic antidepressants are highly valuable for neuropathic pain. The usual symptoms of neuropathic pain are hyperalgesia and constant burning pain. Severe pain is experienced from even slight pressure such as clothes. Paresthesias are often present. Neuropathic pain should be distinguished from the lancinating pain of neuralgia such as tic douloureux. Neuralgia does not usually respond to tricyclics or to steroids but is often helped by anticonvulsants such as carbamazepine (Tegretol).[11]

 Oncology, Pain, Palliative Care, Nausea, and Vomiting

5-HT (serotonergic) reuptake inhibitors such as imipramine (Tofranil) and amitriptyline (Elavil) are more effective in controlling pain that are norepinephrine reuptake inhibitors such as desipramine (Norpramin, Pertofrane) and doxepin (Sinequan). However, both groups are effective and desipramine often causes fewer side effects. Usual analgesic doses are 75 to 100 mg/day.

Steroids

Steroids are extremely useful adjuvant drugs. They have antiinflammatory and antiemetic activity, stimulate the appetite, and often elevate the mood. Some of the indications for their use in chronic pain control are as follows:

1. Increased intracranial pressure
2. Spinal cord compression
3. Nerve compression
4. Visceral distention
5. Lymphedema
6. Osseous metastases unresponsive to NSAIDs
7. Soft tissue infiltration
8. Intractable pain not responsive to opioids

In critical situations treatment should start with large IV doses followed by oral doses of a drug such as dexamethasone (Decadron) in the ranges listed below:

Increased intracranial pressure	4-12 mg tid-qid
Nerve compression	4-8 mg bid-tid
Intractable pain	4-8 mg tid-qid
Soft tissue infiltration	2-4 mg bid

Bisphosphonates

The bisphosphonate pamidronate (Aredia) given IV may lead to significant pain relief in some cases of metastatic bone disease[11,12] or in multiple myeloma[13] (see sections on metastatic breast cancer and multiple myeloma).

Opioids for Nonmalignant Pain

Most physicians find it difficult to prescribe narcotics for chronic pain that is not caused by cancer. However, in selected cases this may be an appropriate therapeutic strategy.[14] In one reported series this approach proved very successful. The patients had a variety of conditions causing long-standing chronic pain, the main ones being neuropathy and low back pain. They responded well to narcotics and showed no evidence of addiction.[15] This confirms a much quoted letter to the editor reporting that addiction does not seem to be a problem when narcotics are used for non-malignancy-related pain.[16]

REFERENCES

1. Levy MH: Pharmacologic treatment of cancer pain, *N Engl J Med* 335:1124-1132, 1996.
2. Montauk SL, Martin J: Treating chronic pain, *Am Fam Physician* 55:1151-1160, 1997.
3. Poyhia R, Vainio A, Kalso E: A review of oxycodone's clinical pharmacokinetics and pharmacodynamics, *J Pain Symptom Manage* 8:63-67, 1993.
4. Glare PA, Walsh TD: Dose-ranging study of oxycodone for chronic pain in advanced cancer, *J Clin Oncol* 11:973-978, 1993.
5. Hagen NA, Babul N: Comparative clinical efficacy and safety of a novel controlled-release oxycodone formulation and controlled-release hydromorphone in the treatment of cancer pain, *Cancer* 79:1428-1437, 1997.
6. Hess, H: Police probe ring selling popular painkillers: computers used to produce forged prescriptions in narcotics for growing black market, *Toronto Globe and Mail,* Jan 14, 1997, p. A6.
7. Woodroffe MA, Hays H: Fentanyl transdermal system: pain management at home, *Can Fam Physician* 43:268-272, 1997.
8. Moulin DE: Relative potency estimates of analgesics—are they perceived or real? *Pain Res Manage* 1:195-196, 1996.
9. Vainio A, Ollila J, Matikainen E, et al: Driving ability in cancer patients receiving long-term morphine analgesia, *Lancet* 346: 667-670, 1995.
10. Eisenberg E, Berdey CS, Carr DB, et al: Efficacy and safety of nonsteroidal antiinflammatory drugs for cancer pain: a meta-analysis, *J Clin Oncol* 12:2756-2765, 1994.
11. Davis CL, Hardy JR: Palliative care, *BMJ* 308:1359-1362, 1994.
12. Hortobagyl GN, Theriault RL, Porter L, et al: Efficacy of pamidronate in reducing skeletal complications in patients with breast cancer and lytic bone metastases, *N Engl J Med* 335: 1785-1791, 1996.
13. Berenson JR, Lichtenstein A, Porter L, et al (Myeloma Aredia Study Group): Efficacy of pamidronate in reducing skeletal events in patients with advanced multiple myeloma, *N Engl J Med* 334:529-530, 1996.
14. Hagen N, Flynne P, Hays H, et al: Guidelines for managing chronic non-malignant pain, *Can Fam Physician* 41:49-53, 1995.
15. Zenz M, Strumpf M, Tryba M: Long-term oral opioid therapy in patients with chronic nonmalignant pain, *J Pain Symptom Manage* 7:69-77, 1992.
16. Porter J, Jick H: Addiction rare in patients treated with narcotics (letter), *N Engl J Med* 302:123, 1980.

PALLIATIVE CARE

(See also nausea and vomiting; pain)

Cachexia

The progestogen megestrol acetate (Megace) has been reported to increase appetite and weight in cancer patients.[1]

REFERENCES

1. Tchekmedyian NS, Hickman M, Siau J, et al: Megestrol acetate in cancer anorexia and weight loss, *Cancer* 69:1268-1274, 1992.

Dehydration and Fluid Replacement

Patients dying in hospices rarely receive parenteral fluids and do not appear to suffer as a result. Patients dying in hospitals often receive parenteral fluids until the time of death. Does dehydration decrease the quality of life in the terminally ill? There are no definitive data indicating whether at the end of life parenteral fluids decrease thirst, dry mouth sensation, or nausea, increase cognitive functioning, or prolong survival. By the same token there are no reliable data substantiating serious adverse effects of giving parenteral fluids such as pain from venipunctures, fluid overload and congestive failure, or increased nausea and vomiting in the presence of intestinal obstruction.[1] However, a growing body of literature suggests that dying or seriously ill patients do not suffer from the withdrawal of parenteral nutrition, tube feedings, or IV fluids. In these circumstances thirst is rare, and the discomfort of a dry mouth can be controlled by avoiding drugs that aggravate the condition and by using glycerine swabs, ice chips, and sips of water.[2]

REFERENCES

1. Burge FI: Dehydration and provision of fluids in palliative care: what is the evidence? *Can Fam Physician* 42:2383-2388, 1996.
2. Brody H, Campbell ML, Faber-Langendoen K, et al: Withdrawing intensive life-sustaining treatment—recommendations for compassionate clinical management, *N Engl J Med* 336:652-657, 1997.

Dyspnea

A fan blowing on the patient along with humidification often provides symptomatic relief of dyspnea.[1]

If the patient is already taking morphine for pain, the dose can be increased by 50%. Otherwise, the dosage should start at 5 mg q4h and be titrated rapidly upward until control of dyspnea is achieved. The drug may also be delivered by inhalation through a nebulizer.

If extrinsic obstruction by tumor is the cause of dyspnea, dexamethasone (Decadron) 4 mg q6h po is often effective. In urgent situations 25 to 40 or even 100 mg may be given IV. Radiation therapy may give more definitive palliation.

Chlorpromazine (Largactil, Thorazine) or a benzodiazepine (midazolam [Versed], lorazepam [Ativan]) may be given IV or orally until the patient is sedated and comfortable. One recommended regimen is midazolam 5 mg IV as a bolus followed by 1 mg/min IV until the patient is sedated.[1]

REFERENCES

1. Synnott C, Farley F: Quelques urgences aux soins palliatifs, *Med Quebec,* February 1994, pp 97-103.

Intestinal Obstruction

(See also antiemetics for pseudoobstruction)

Bowel obstruction occurs in close to one half of patients with advanced ovarian cancer and in about one fourth of patients with advanced colorectal cancers.[1]

Limited literature and no randomized controlled trials are available on the medical management of bowel obstruction in terminally ill patients. However, a number of studies have shown effective palliation lasting several months by means of a variety of drugs, usually in combination.[1]

Colicky pain can be controlled with scopolamine (also called hyoscine), atropine, or loperamide (Imodium). Scopolamine may be given subcutaneously, often in large doses, or as two skin patches (Transderm-Scop, Transderm-V) that should be changed every 3 days. Patches take 12 to 24 hours to become effective.[2] The more continuous pain of distended bowel, tumor masses, or hepatic distention is managed with narcotics. Nausea and vomiting are often controlled with a phenothiazine such as chlorpromazine (Largactil, Thorazine) or prochlorperazine (Stemetil) or with butyrophenones such as haloperidol (Haldol). In a few cases obstruction can be alleviated by giving steroids such as dexamethasone (Decadron). If the obstruction is partial, metoclopramide (Maxeran) may be beneficial.[1,2]

REFERENCES

1. Frank C: Medical management of intestinal obstruction in terminal care, *Can Fam Physician* 43:259-265, 1997.
2. Miron S: Occlusion intestinale traitement palliatif, *Med Quebec,* February 1994, pp 89-94.

Superior Vena Cava Syndrome

In 80% of cases the superior vena cava syndrome is due to small cell carcinoma of the lung and in 15% to lymphoma. Treatment is corticosteroids and radiation therapy.[1]

REFERENCES

1. Synnott C, Farley F: Quelques urgences aux soins palliatifs, *Med Quebec,* February 1994, pp 97-103.

OPHTHALMOLOGY

Topics covered in this section

CATARACTS

(See also macular degeneration)

Epidemiology

The incidence of cataracts is increased in patients with diabetes and also probably in smokers.[1] Both oral steroids and inhaled steroids are risk factors in adults,[2,3] and associations have been reported between excessive exposure to ultraviolet B light and cataracts.[3]

Symptoms and Signs

Several symptoms suggest cataracts as the cause of visual changes. One of the early ones is "second sight." The presence of an early cataract may change the refractive index of the lens so that the patient can begin to read without glasses. However, vision dims progressively, which is particularly noticeable at night; the patient needs very bright lights to read or to perform fine work. Another suggestive symptom is the presence of haloes around street lights or the headlights of approaching cars. This and the associated glare make many patients spontaneously stop driving at night. Monocular diplopia is still another symptom of cataracts.[4,5] Most cataracts can be detected with direct ophthalmoscopy. The examiner should set the lens wheel to +4 diopters and examine the red reflex with the ophthalmoscope 15 to 20 cm from the patient's eye. Cataracts are usually seen as dark specks or a haze against the red reflex.[3]

Both cataracts and age-related macular degeneration are common causes of visual loss in the elderly. Clues that the cause is macular degeneration rather than cataracts are loss of color discrimination and spontaneous use of a magnifying glass by the patient.[4]

Treatment

Before cataract surgery it is important to try to predict the degree of visual recovery that can be expected. Such surgery is pointless if macular degeneration will prevent visual acuity from being improved by the procedure. Ophthalmologists use two techniques for assessment: potential acuity measurement (PAM) and laser interferometry. Both procedures are painless and test macular function through small "windows" in the cataracts.[4]

Cataracts can be removed at any stage of their development; it is a myth that surgery must wait until the cataract is "ripe."[4,5] In fact, even in the presence of nearly normal visual acuity, cataract removal is indicated if glare results in significant disability.[5]

Current techniques of cataract removal by extraction or phacoemulsification use an extracapsular approach. This means that the cataract is extracted from within the lens capsule, leaving the capsule behind to support the implant. In about one third of patients the capsule becomes cloudy in the first few weeks or months after surgery. Clear vision is instantly reestablished by use of a laser beam (yttrium aluminum garnet [YAG]), which cuts a hole in the capsule.[4,5]

REFERENCES

1. West S: Does smoke get in your eyes? (editorial), *JAMA* 268: 1025-1026, 1992.
2. Cumming RG, Mitchell P, Leeder SR: Use of inhaled corticosteroids and the risk of cataracts, *N Engl J Med* 337:8-14, 1997.
3. Chylack LT Jr: Cataracts and inhaled corticosteroids (editorial), *N Engl J Med* 337:46-48, 1997.
4. Fowler JH: Investigating cataracts—unveiling vision loss, *Can J Diagn*, February 1994, 11:64-77.
5. Obstbaum SA: An 82-year-old woman with cataracts, *JAMA* 275:1675-1680, 1996.

CONGENITAL LACRIMAL OBSTRUCTION

Congenital lacrimal duct obstruction is common and results in symptoms in 6% to 20% of neonates. Eighty percent of cases are unilateral. In 90% of cases the obstruction spontaneously resolves within a year, and spontaneous resolution is usually seen in the remaining children during the second year of life. Symptoms are watering of the eye and crusting of the lids so that they are stuck together in the morning, but unless the child has a secondary infection, the globe remains white. The only necessary treatment is reassurance and explanation to the parents, cleaning of the lids on a regular basis, and therapy for obvious secondary conjunctivitis (red eye and increased exudate) if it arises. Probing of the lacrimal system is often performed in the first year but is probably unnecessary and may cause strictures. One study has shown that massaging the lacrimal sac while occluding the canaliculi opens the canal in a number of cases.[1]

REFERENCES

1. Young JD, MacEwen CJ: Managing congenital lacrimal obstruction in general practice, *BMJ* 315:293-296, 1997.

CORNEAL ABRASIONS

(See also topical ophthalmic medications)

Care should be taken not to misdiagnose a corneal herpetic infection as a corneal abrasion. Aside from the typical dendritic appearance of the herpetic lesions, there is often decreased corneal sensitivity that can be detected by testing the corneal reflex.

According to a Canadian study antibiotic ointment is not necessary in the routine treatment of corneal abrasions, and there is no published evidence supporting its use. Instead the physician may patch the eye (if that is the physician's practice; see next paragraph) and use a topical mydriatic such as homatropine or cyclopentolate (Cyclogyl) for pain relief (see discussion of topical ophthalmic medications).[1]

Simple corneal abrasions may be treated without eye patches. Healing rates are as rapid as when patches are used, and furthermore, patches may actually increase discomfort.[2-4] Effective pain relief is often achieved with cold compresses and oral nonsteroidal antiinflammatory drugs (NSAIDs).[5] A number of ophthalmic topical NSAIDs are available (see discussion of topical ophthalmic medications). They have been used to relieve the pain of corneal abrasions but are not yet approved for this purpose.[6]

If a corneal abrasion is associated with the wearing of contact lenses, patching is contraindicated. This is because *Pseudomonas* species are frequent pathogenic organisms in this type of corneal abrasion; patching promotes bacterial replication and prevents mechanical clearing of organisms through blinking. Corneal abrasions in contact lens wearers are managed by instilling an antibiotic that is active against

Pseudomonas such as an aminoglycoside (gentamicin [Garamycin Ophthalmic] or tobramycin [Tobrex]) or a quinolone (ciprofloxacin [Ciloxan], norfloxacin [Chibroxin], or ofloxacin [Ocuflox]) and following up within 24 hours (see section on topical ophthalmic medications). Steroid drops should never be used.[7]

REFERENCES

1. King JW, Brison RJ: Do topical antibiotics help corneal epithelial trauma? *Can Fam Physician* 39:2349-2352, 1993.
2. Hulbert MFG: Efficacy of eye pad in corneal healing after corneal foreign body removal, *Lancet* 337:643, 1991.
3. Kirkpatrick JN, Hoh HB, Cook SD: No eye pad for corneal abrasion, *Eye* 7:468-471, 1993.
4. Kaiser PK (Corneal Abrasion Patching Study Group): A comparison of pressure patching versus no patching for corneal abrasions due to trauma or foreign body removal, *Ophthalmology* 102:1936-1942, 1995.
5. Mindlin AM: Treatment of corneal abrasions (letter), *JAMA* 275: 837, 1996.
6. Torok PG, Mader TH: Corneal abrasions: diagnosis and management, *Am Fam Physician* 53:2521-2529, 1996.
7. Jampel HD: Patching for corneal abrasions, *JAMA* 274:1504, 1995.

CORNEAL TRANSPLANTS

The most common indication for corneal transplantation is corneal edema developing as a complication of cataract surgery. Human lymphocyte antigen tissue typing is unnecessary. Success, as measured by a clear cornea, is greater than 90%, but many patients are left with significant astigmatism requiring thick lenses for correction. Risk of graft rejection is lifelong but greatest in the first year; it is controlled primarily by prophylactic or therapeutic topical steroids.[1]

REFERENCES

1. Weston BC, White GL Jr: Corneal transplantation, *Am Fam Physician* 54:1945-1948, 1996.

GLAUCOMA, ACUTE ANGLE CLOSURE

(See also glaucoma, open angle)

Epidemiology

Acute angle closure glaucoma has its peak incidence in the sixth and seventh decades. It occurs more frequently in hypermetropic eyes (long-sighted eyes) because the globe in such an eye is smaller than normal and therefore more crowded internally. It is possible to tell whether someone is hypermetropic by checking their glasses; the lenses are positive and act like magnifying glasses.[1]

Prodromal Symptoms

Patients with acute angle closure glaucoma usually have had prodromal symptoms resulting from temporary increases in intraocular pressure. Such preliminary symptoms include slight blurring of vision, mild headaches, and occasionally seeing haloes around objects. Precipitating factors are those causing pupillary dilation such as the dim light of a movie theater, the adrenergic response to anger or anxiety, and anticholinergic medications such as tricyclic antidepressants.[1]

Sometimes a narrow angle can be detected in patients at risk of angle closure glaucoma by shining a penlight on the temporal side of the iris while checking to see whether the nasal side of the iris remains in shadow because of forward tenting of the iris.

Symptoms and Signs

A patient with fully developed angle closure glaucoma complains of agonizing eye pain, blurred vision, and often headache. Nausea and vomiting are common, and sometimes the patient has abdominal and chest pain. The eye is red with a ciliary flush, the cornea is steamy, and the pupil is dilated, fixed, and usually vertically oval. Ballottement of the globe often reveals a stony hard consistency, although failure to detect this sign does not rule out acute glaucoma. Visual acuity is markedly diminished.[1]

Management

Immediate management of acute angle closure glaucoma is directed toward lowering the intraocular pressure with medication. One three-stage protocol is as follows[1]:

1. Instill 2 drops of a topical beta-blocker such as timolol (Timoptic 0.5%) plus 2 drops of pilocarpine 2%.
2. If the attack is not stopped in 15 minutes, give acetazolamide (Diamox) 200 to 500 mg plus an osmotic diuretic, such as glycerol solution in orange juice, 1.5 to 2 g/kg, or mannitol 1 g/kg IV over a 20-minute period. This step may be repeated twice at 2-hour intervals.
3. Perform surgery, usually in the form of laser iridotomy.

REFERENCES

1. Balazsi AG: Looking into the signs of glaucoma, *Can J Diagn*, October 1993, 10:65-85.

GLAUCOMA, OPEN ANGLE

(See also asthma—inhaled steroids; glaucoma, acute angle closure; screening; surrogate endpoint)

Epidemiology

Open angle glaucoma affects 2% of the population. The prevalence increases with age and is about 1% in the fifth decade and more than 4% in the eighth decade. The prevalence of increased intraocular pressure without evidence of glaucoma is 6% to 8%. Glaucoma later develops in an estimated 1% per year of persons with elevated intraocular pressure.[1,2] In the United States blacks have a higher incidence of open angle glaucoma than whites.[2]

Risk Factors

Recognized risk factors for open angle glaucoma include the following:

1. Age over 65
2. Family history of glaucoma

3. Black race
4. Severe myopia
5. Diabetes
6. Elevated intraocular pressure
7. Previous eye trauma
8. Previous eye surgery
9. Long-term use of ocular adrenocorticosteroids
10. High-dose continuous inhaled steroids (see discussion of asthma)[3]

Screening

Ocular hypertension is the presence of an intraocular pressure above the generally accepted norm of 21 mm Hg without evidence of optic nerve or visual field changes. Many ophthalmologists believe that ocular hypertension leads to glaucoma and should be treated. The American Academy of Ophthalmology recommended in 1993 that everyone over the age of 35 be screened annually for glaucoma. This is controversial because there is no evidence of the efficacy of such a process.[1] Furthermore, in over 70% of patients with intraocular pressures consistently between 21 and 35 mm Hg, no glaucomatous changes develop.[4] Both the Canadian Task Force on the Periodic Health Examination[5] and the U.S. Preventive Services Task Force[6] give a "C" recommendation to screening maneuvers such as measuring elevated intraocular pressure, assessing the optic disc by funduscopy, or looking for peripheral field abnormalities.

An alternative strategy is to limit screening to those at high risk. At particularly high risk are persons over the age of 65 (especially those over the age of 75), those with a sibling who has glaucoma, and blacks.[7] The efficacy of such an approach is unknown.

Most available screening techniques are not sensitive or specific. Tonometry is the oldest technique. Problems with tonometry are that considerable diurnal variation occurs in intraocular pressure, less than 50% of patients with proven glaucoma have randomly measured pressures greater then 21 mm Hg, and glaucoma will never develop in over 70% of individuals with pressures between 21 and 34 mm Hg. Pallor and cupping of the disc and a cup/disc ratio greater than 0.5 are not sensitive or specific signs. Only about half of patients with glaucoma have glaucomatous changes in the optic nerve head, while 20% of normal individuals manifest one or more of these changes. Perimetry is not a practical screening tool.[4]

Clinical Signs

As noted in the section on screening, the sensitivity and specificity of the various signs of open angle glaucoma are low. These signs include[8]:

1. Afferent pupillary defect (Marcus Gunn pupil)
2. Elevated intraocular pressure measured with Schiötz or applanation tonometry
3. Cup/disc ratio greater than 0.7
4. Difference of more than 0.2 in the cup/disc ratio between the two eyes
5. Oval cup with the vertical diameter greater than the horizontal diameter
6. Notching of the cup
7. Occasionally splinter hemorrhages at the disc margins
8. Visual field defects, especially in the nasal quadrants

Treatment

The principle underlying both the medical and surgical treatments of glaucoma is that lowering intraocular pressure will arrest the progression of the disease. Unfortunately, there are no conclusive data confirming this hypothesis. Clear evidence has shown that all modalities of treatment can lower intraocular pressure by varying degrees (a surrogate endpoint), but no reliable randomized placebo-controlled trials have shown that treatment arrests the deterioration of visual fields (a clinically important endpoint).[9]

A wide variety of topical drugs are available for lowering intraocular pressure (Table 55). Beta-blockers are the drugs of first choice, but unfortunately, they have significant adverse effects on both the respiratory and cardiovascular systems. Because they are absorbed directly into the systemic circulation through the nasolacrimal duct and nasal mucosa, no first-pass liver metabolism occurs; it has been calculated that 1 drop of 0.5% timolol solution in each eye is equivalent to a 10-mg oral dose. Specific adverse effects include diminished pulmonary function in about one fourth of patients and a significantly increased incidence of falls, which can be devastating in the elderly. Pilocarpine, the traditional alternative drug, must be taken four times a day, has local side effects, and can cause confusion. Other effective alternatives include the alpha$_2$-adrenergic agonist brimonidine (Allergan),[10] the topical carbonic anhydrase inhibitor dorzolamide (Trusopt),[10,11] and the prostaglandin analogue latanoprost (Xalatan).[10,12] A 12-month study of Trusopt found it to be as effective at lowering intraocular pressure as timolol

Table 55 Topical Medications for Chronic Open Angle Glaucoma

Drugs	Usual dose
Topical Nonselective Beta-Blockers	
Levobunolol (Betagan) 0.25% and 0.5%	1 drop bid or 1 drop 0.5% daily
Metipranolol (OptiPranolol) 0.3%	1 drop bid
Timolol (Timoptic) 0.25% and 0.5%	1 drop bid
Topical Cardioselective Beta-Blockers	
Betaxolol (Betoptic) 0.25% and 0.5%	1 drop bid
Topical Alpha$_2$-Adrenergic Receptor Agonists	
Brimonidine tartrate (Alphagan) 0.2%	1 drop tid
Topical Cholinergic Myopics	
Pilocarpine 1%, 2%, 4%, and 6%	1-2 drops bid
Topical Carbonic Anhydrase Inhibitors	
Dorzolamide (Trusopt) 2%	1 drop tid
Topical Prostaglandin Analogues	
Latanoprost (Xalatan) 0.005% (50 µg/ml)	1 drop qhs

(Timoptic) or betaxolol (Betoptic), and reported side effects were minimal.[11]

While oral carbonic anhydrase inhibitors are usually prescribed for acute angle closure glaucoma, they are occasionally used for patients with chronic open angle glaucoma. Caution is needed because they can cause metabolic acidosis, hypokalemia, paresthesias, altered taste, and, rarely, aplastic anemia. The two most frequently used drugs in this class are acetazolamide (Diamox) 250 mg to 1 g daily in divided doses and methazolamide (Neptazane) 50 to 100 mg bid or tid.

If medical therapy fails or the adverse effects are unacceptable, laser trabeculoplasty, which has about a 50% 5-year success rate in the elderly, or surgical trabeculectomy is the next option.[4,13] In laser trabeculoplasty a low-power argon laser beam is focused on the trabecular meshwork. This usually increases the outflow of aqueous humor with a resultant decrease in the intraocular pressure of about 30%.[4]

REFERENCES

1. Klein BEK, Klein R, Sponsel WE, et al: Prevalence of glaucoma: the Beaver Dam eye study, *Ophthalmology* 99:1499-1504, 1992.
2. Tielsch JM, Sommer A, Katz J: Racial variations in the prevalence of primary open-angle glaucoma: the Baltimore eye survey, *JAMA* 266:369-374, 1991.
3. Garbe E, LeLorier J, Boivin J-F, Suissa S: Inhaled and nasal glucocorticoids and the risks of ocular hypertension or open-angle glaucoma, *JAMA* 277:722-727, 1997.
4. Tucker JB: Screening for open-angle glaucoma, *Am Fam Physician* 148:75-80, 1993.
5. Canadian Task Force on the Periodic Health Examination: Periodic health examination, 1995 update. III. Screening for visual problems among elderly patients, *Can Med Assoc J* 152: 1211-1222, 1995.
6. US Preventive Services Task Force: *Guide to clinical preventive services,* ed 2, Baltimore, 1996, Williams & Wilkins, pp 383-391.
7. Rosenberg LF. Glaucoma: early detection and therapy for prevention of vision loss, *Am Fam Physician* 52:2289-2298, 1995.
8. Balazsi AG: Looking into the signs of glaucoma, *Can J Diagn,* October 1993, 10:65-85.
9. Rossetti L, Marchetti I, Orzalesi N, et al: Randomized clinical trials on medical treatment of glaucoma: are they an appropriate guide to clinical practice? *Arch Ophthalmol* 111:96-103, 1993.
10. Brimonidine—an alpha-2-agonist for glaucoma, *Med Lett* 39: 54-55, 1997.
11. Strahlman E, Tipping R, Vogel R (International Dorzolamide Study Group): A double-masked, randomized 1-year study comparing dorzolamide (Trusopt), timolol, and betaxolol, *Arch Ophthalmol* 113:1009-1016, 1995.
12. Alm A, Widengard I, Kjellgren D, et al: Latanoprost administered once daily caused a maintained reduction of intraocular pressure in glaucoma patients treated concomitantly with timolol, *Br J Ophthalmol* 79:12-16, 1995.
13. Diggory P, Franks W: Medical treatment of glaucoma—reappraisal of the risks, *Br J Ophthalmol* 80:85-89, 1996.

MACULAR DEGENERATION

(See also cataracts; vitamin A)

Both age-related macular degeneration (ARMD) and cataracts are common causes of visual loss in the elderly. Clues that the cause is macular degeneration rather than cataracts are loss of color discrimination and spontaneous use of a magnifying glass by the patient.[1]

Age-related macular degeneration is the most common cause of irreversible blindness among persons over the age of 65. It accounts for 40% to 50% of new cases of blindness in Canada. Its incidence is about 1% in 55-year-olds and rises to 15% by age 80.[2] With funduscopy, drusens and pigment stippling may be seen in the macular area. Smoking is a risk factor for the development of macular degeneration in both men[3] and women,[4] and prolonged exposure to sunlight might also increase risk of the disease.[5]

The U.S. Preventive Services Task Force[6] and the Canadian Task Force on the Periodic Health Examination[2] give a "C" recommendation to funduscopy for the detection of ARMD.[2] However, both these organizations give a "B" recommendation to visual acuity testing in the elderly.[2,6]

Some studies have suggested a protective effect of certain carotenoids, especially lutein and zeaxanthin, which are found in dark green leafy vegetables such as spinach and collard greens. Vitamin A, beta-carotene, and supplements of vitamins C and E have not been found to be protective.[7]

REFERENCES

1. Fowler JH: Investigating cataracts—unveiling vision loss, *Can J Diagn,* February 1994, pp 64-77.
2. Canadian Task Force on the Periodic Health Examination: Periodic health examination, 1995 update. III. Screening for visual problems among elderly patients, *Can Med Assoc J* 152:1211-1222. 1995.
3. Christen WG, Glynn RJ, Manson JE, et al: A prospective study of cigarette smoking and risk of age-related macular degeneration in men, *JAMA* 276:1147-1151, 1996.
4. Seddon JM, Willett WC, Speizer FE, et al: A prospective study of cigarette smoking and age-related macular degeneration in women, *JAMA* 276:1141-1146, 1996.
5. Cruickshanks KJ, Klein R, Klein BE: Sunlight and age-related macular degeneration: the Beaver Dam Eye Study, *Arch Ophthalmol* 111:514-518, 1993.
6. US Preventive Services Task Force: *Guide to clinical preventive services,* ed 2, Baltimore, 1996, Williams & Wilkins, pp 373-391.
7. Seddon JM, Ajani UA, Sperduto RD, et al: Dietary carotenoids, vitamins A, C, and E, and advanced age-related macular degeneration, *JAMA* 272:1413-1420, 1994.

OPTIC NEURITIS

Optic neuritis may be the initial manifestation of multiple sclerosis. In a 1993 study of patients with optic neuritis, only 7.5% of those given methylprednisolone 250 mg q6h IV for 3 days followed by prednisone 1 mg/kg po for 11 days had development of multiple sclerosis within 2 years compared with a rate of 16.7% in the control group. Oral prednisone alone did not give this protective effect.[1]

REFERENCES

1. Beck RW, Cleary PA, Trobe JD: The effect of corticosteroids for acute optic neuritis on the subsequent development of multiple sclerosis, *N Engl J Med* 329:1764-1769, 1993.

REFRACTIVE ERRORS

Surgical Correction

Myopia or short sightedness is associated with a large globe and a relatively excessive convexity of the cornea. This combination causes the image to be focused anterior to the retina. The original procedure for surgical correction of myopia was radial keratotomy. Complications were common, including progressive development of hyperopia. The currently preferred technique is photorefractive keratectomy using excimer lasers. This is an office procedure in which the cornea is sculpted by the laser to decrease its degree of convexity. In most cases the procedure is performed on only one eye at a time. The surgery takes about 15 minutes. In general this procedure is contraindicated in patients less than 18 years of age because of the changing refractive errors in adolescents.[1]

Photorefractive keratectomy was introduced in about 1987. The most reliable results are obtained when patients have a myopia of less than −6 diopters, but it can be used for much higher degrees of myopia. The procedure is also effective in correcting astigmatism, and experimental results suggest it may be useful for hyperopia. A number of patients with corneal scarring can be treated with this technique, thus avoiding corneal transplantation.[1]

Some myopic patients treated with photorefractive keratectomy have a degree of "regression," meaning that during the first few months after surgery the degree of correction of the myopia that had been achieved regresses by a small amount. The degree of regression is usually larger in patients with severe myopia. About 1% to 2% of patients see haloes around lights that make night driving difficult, and infections complicate the procedure in about 1:1000 cases.[1]

REFERENCES

1. Mortimer CB, Sher NA, Trobe JD: New options for vision loss, *Patient Care Can,* March 1996, 7:63-79.

TOPICAL OPHTHALMIC MEDICATIONS

(See also allergic rhinitis; glaucoma)

Eyedrop Instillation in Children

Instilling drops in the eyes of recalcitrant children is difficult. An effective technique is to have the child lie supine with eyes closed while the drops are applied. When the eyes are opened, most of the drops flow onto the conjunctiva. When this technique was tested with pilocarpine and the resultant degree of pupillary dilation was measured, it was calculated that 66% of the drug dose entered the eye.[1]

Anesthetics

A frequently used topical anesthetic is proparacaine (Alcaine, Ophthaine, Ophthetic). The usual dose for removing corneal foreign bodies and other procedures is 1 or 2 drops of a 0.5% solution.

Antibacterials

A variety of topical antibiotics are available, and a number of them are listed in Table 56. These are all available in the form of ophthalmic drops and ointments. Dosages vary slightly among products, but as a general rule for severe conjunctivitis, 1 or 2 drops is instilled every 1 to 2 hours while the patient is awake for the first 1 to 2 days and the dose is then reduced to q4-6h for the next few days. If the infection is mild, drops are applied q4-6h. Ointments may be applied at bedtime. Sulfacetamide sodium (Sodium Sulamyd) comes as a 10% and a 30% solution; most family physicians use the 10% solution. Tobramycin ophthalmic products are safe for children of all ages; the safety of fluoroquinolone ophthalmic preparations for children under 1 year of age has not been established.

Antihistamines, Vasoconstrictors, and Mast Cell Stabilizers

Topical antihistamines or antihistamines combined with vasoconstrictors may give relief to some patients with allergic conjunctivitis. Levocabastine (Livostin) is an example of an ophthalmic antihistamine. The recommended dose is 1 drop in each eye bid.

Many antihistamine-vasoconstrictor combinations are available over the counter. The use of these agents has been associated with induction of both acute and chronic conjunctivitis.[2] Examples of this drug combination are naphazoline plus pheniramine (Naphcon-A) and naphazoline plus antazoline (Vasocon-A). The usual dose is 1 or 2 drops in each eye every 3 to 4 hours.

Topical vasoconstrictors alone decrease redness of the eyes in patients with allergic conjunctivitis, and many of these are available over the counter. Examples are phenyl-

Table 56 Topical Ophthalmic Antibacterials

Generic names	Trade names
Aminoglycosides	
Gentamicin	Garamycin
Tobramycin	Tobrex, AKTob
Fluoroquinolones	
Ciprofloxacin	Ciloxan
Norfloxacin	Chibroxin
Ofloxacin	Ocuflox
Sulfonamides	
Sulfacetamide sodium	Sodium Sulamyd
Other	
Chloramphenicol	Chloroptic

ephrine (Neo-Synephrine), tetrahydrozoline (Visine), and naphazoline (Clear Eyes, Naphcon).

Two mast cell stabilizers that may relieve symptoms of allergic conjunctivitis are cromolyn sodium (Crolom, Opticrom) and lodoxamide (Alomide). The usual dose for each is 1 or 2 drops qid.

Ketorolac (Acular), a topical ophthalmic NSAID, has been used for treatment of allergic conjunctivitis.

Cycloplegic Mydriatics

Drugs that paralyze the ciliary muscle and thus inhibit accommodation are cycloplegics, and of course those that dilate the pupils are mydriatics. Some agents do both. Short-acting cycloplegic mydriatics such as tropicamide (Mydriacyl) 0.5% or 1% are generally used by family physicians for dilating the pupil to facilitate funduscopy. Longer acting drugs such as cyclopentolate (Cyclogyl) 1% or 2% or homatropine 2% or 5% may be used to relieve ciliary spasm (and pain) from corneal abrasions or for the treatment of iritis or uveitis.

Glaucoma Medications

See the earlier section on glaucoma.

Nonsteroidal Antiinflammatory Drugs

Ophthalmic NSAIDs have been used but are not approved for pain relief in cases of corneal abrasion. Some of the available agents are flurbiprofen (Ocufen), diclofenac (Voltaren), and ketorolac (Acular).

Tears and Lubricants

A large number of artificial tear preparations are available without prescription for symptomatic treatment of dry eyes. The usual dose is 1 to 2 drops q1-4h. Some examples are hydroxypropyl methylcellulose (Isopto Tears, Lacril, Tears Naturale), polyvinyl alcohol (Hypotears, Liquifilm, Tears Plus), and polysorbate (Teardrops). Lubricating ointments containing white petrolatum and mineral oil may be applied to dry eyes at bedtime. They are often used in cases of Bell's palsy to prevent the cornea from drying. Examples are DuraTears and Lacri-Lube.

REFERENCES

1. Smith SE: Eyedrop instillation for reluctant children, *Br J Ophthalmol* 75:480-481, 1991.
2. Soparkar CN, Wilhelmus KR, Koch DD, et al: Acute and chronic conjunctivitis due to over-the-counter ophthalmic decongestants, *Arch Ophthalmol* 115:34-48, 1997.

OTOLARYNGOLOGY

(See also dysphagia)

Topics covered in this section

EXTERNAL EAR

Foreign Bodies

Many foreign bodies may be removed from the external auditory canal by syringing. This method should not be used for organic materials (e.g., peas, beans) because they may absorb the water and swell.

A good way of removing a live insect is to put the patient in a darkened room and shine a light on the ear. In many cases the insect will be attracted to the light and crawl out. Alternative methods are to kill the insect by instilling mineral oil or 2% lidocaine into the canal and then gently syringe it out.[1]

Otitis Externa

Seborrheic dermatitis and other skin conditions can affect the ear canal and cause otitis externa. A common treatment for these conditions is steroid drops alone such as betamethasone (Betnesol Otic) or steroid drops combined with other ingredients such as hydrocortisone plus acetic acid and propylene glycol (VoSol HC Otic).

A variety of bacterial organisms, especially *Staphylococcus aureus* and *Pseudomonas aeruginosa,* have been associated with otitis externa, but in many cases an infectious etiology cannot be ascertained. The most consistently observed predisposing factor is frequent water exposure,[2,3] and one reported method of preventing the condition is to instill 2 to 4 drops of an equal mixture of vinegar (5% acetic acid) and rubbing alcohol (70% isopropyl alcohol) into the ear canals immediately after coming out of the water.[3] Outbreaks of *P. aeruginosa* cases have been caused by swimming in freshwater lakes.[4] Fungal infections, whether caused by *Candida* or *Aspergillus niger,* are rare in North America.

Medications for bacterial otitis externa often include aminoglycosides (gentamicin, neomycin, or framycetin). Ototoxicity from the use of gentamicin (Garasone Otic) drops has been reported in patients with perforated drums. In patients with perforations topical drugs containing aminoglycosides should not be used or should be used for as short a time as possible, applied to an ear wick (gauze strip) rather than directly into the canal, and discontinued immediately if tinnitus, hearing loss, vertigo, or imbalance develops.[5]

Most of the topical antibiotics used for otitis externa are combinations of antibiotics and steroids; the steroids are used to diminish inflammation and prevent obstruction of the canal. Combinations of hydrocortisone, neomycin, and polymyxin B are available in both the United States and Canada (e.g., Cortisporin Otic). In Canada combinations of betamethasone and gentamicin (Garasone Otic) or of dexamethasone, framycetin, and gramicidin (Sofracort) are also on the market, and chloramphenicol drops without steroids (Chloromycetin Otic) may be obtained in the United States.

REFERENCES

1. Shulman M: Managing foreign objects in various body orifices, *Can J CME* 6:10-13, 1994.
2. Russell JD, Donnelly M, McShane DP, et al: What causes acute otitis externa? *J Laryngol Otol* 107:898-901, 1993.
3. Larimore WL, Hartman JR, Shupe TB, et al: Diary from a week in practice, *Am Fam Physician* 55:2651, 1997.
4. van Asperen IA, de Rover CM, Schijven JF, et al: Risk of otitis externa after swimming in recreational fresh water lakes containing *Pseudomonas aeruginosa, BMJ* 311:1407-1410, 1995.
5. Canadian Adverse Drug Reaction Newsletter: Aminoglycoside ear drops and ototoxicity, *Can Med Assoc J* 156:1056, 1997.

MIDDLE EAR

(See also aerotitis media)

Otitis Media

(See also middle ear effusion; tonsillectomy)

Symptoms of upper respiratory tract infection such as cough or rhinorrhea are seen in 94% of children with acute otitis media. In the absence of such symptoms the diagnosis of otitis media is unlikely.[1] When these symptoms were present in children, the positive predictive value of ear pain as a symptom of acute otitis media was found to be 83% in one Finnish study; however, 40% of children with otitis media did not have pain.[2]

The major etiological agents causing acute otitis media are viruses (25%, often in conjunction with bacteria), *Streptococcus pneumoniae* (30% to 50%), *Haemophilus influenzae* (20% to 35%), and *Moraxella catarrhalis* (3% to 20%). A few cases are caused by beta-hemolytic streptococci, *Staphylococcus aureus,* and gram-negative rods.[3]

About 30% to 40% of *Haemophilus* and 50% to 90% of *Moraxella* organisms produce beta-lactamase and are resistant to amoxicillin in vitro. In some areas 40% of pneumococci are resistant to trimethoprim-sulfamethoxazole, and a few are resistant to penicillin. However, this in vitro resistance does not usually translate into clinical ineffectiveness if these antibiotics are used.[3] If antibiotics are to be used at all (see below), most authorities recommend amoxicillin as the first choice or trimethoprim-sulfamethoxazole (Septra, Bactrim) as the least expensive alternative.[3] One metaanalysis of acute otitis media in 5400 children found no clinical advantage of using beta-lactamase-stable antibiotics.[4] Suggested indications for using beta-lactamase-stable drugs, such as amoxicillin-clavulanic acid (Augmentin, Clavulin), erythromycin-sulfisoxazole (Pediazole), or a second- or third-generation cephalosporin, are persistent symptoms for more than 48 to 72 hours while the patient is taking the initial antibiotic, development of otitis media while the patient is taking amoxicillin, or an episode of otitis media within the previous 2 months that did not respond to amoxicillin.[5]

No solid guidelines for optimal duration of treatment with antibiotics have been established. Good results have been reported with 2, 3, 5, and 10 days.[6]

Reputed advantages of routinely using antibiotics for acute otitis media are that these drugs decrease the duration of symptoms and the rate of complications. Careful review of the literature does not substantiate this. Some studies found no improvement in outcomes with antibiotics,[6,7] and others reported only a slight advantage with antibiotics.[4,8] One metaanalysis found that 1 in 7 children benefited from antibiotics.[4] Another metaanalysis found that after 24 hours 60% of children were pain free regardless of whether they received antibiotics and that between days 2 and 7 only 14% of the control patients had persistent pain. The incidence of pain at this time in the antibiotic-treated group was slightly lower, but 17 children had to be treated for every one who achieved pain relief. This analysis also found a decreased incidence of contralateral otitis media in the antibiotic-treated group.[8]

If antibiotics are not used, it must not be assumed that persistence of pain is necessarily due to persistent bacterial infection. One study of children treated with antibiotics found that 62% had persistent symptoms even when bacteriological cure was shown by tympanostomy cultures.[9] Viral infection is probably a major cause of this phenomenon.[10]

A cogent reason for avoiding antibiotic use for otitis media is a rising incidence of antibiotic resistance that correlates with increasing use of these drugs in ambulatory children.[6,11] Is it safe not to use antibiotics? In most of the developed world they are prescribed routinely, but a notable exception is the Netherlands. In that country guidelines recommend no initial antibiotics. For children 2 years and over, reevaluation is suggested after 3 days if symptoms persist, and at that time antibiotics may be prescribed. For children 6 months to 2 years, antibiotics are also withheld initially, but mandatory reassessment by visit or phone after 24 hours is required.[6] There have been no controlled trials of this approach, but persistence of symptoms for more than 3 to 4 days has been noted in only 3% of children. Serious complications have been extremely rare.[6]

The first-line management of recurrent otitis media is to make sure that environmental risk factors are eliminated if possible. Important ones are eliminating exposure to tobacco smoke, using small rather than large day care facilities,[12] and possibly taking pacifiers away from the child.[13] (A Finnish prospective study of children under 3 years attending day care found that those who used pacifiers had 25% more episodes of acute otitis media than those who did not use a pacifier.[13])

According to some experts three episodes of otitis media occurring within a 6-month period are an indication for prophylactic antibiotics.[14] These are usually given daily for several months, especially during the winter. Some workers give antibiotics only at the onset of an upper respiratory tract infection, but this does not seem to be as effective. Prophylactic regimens include amoxicillin 20 mg/kg/day given as a single dose or in two divided doses or sulfisoxazole 75 mg/kg/day as a single dose or in two divided doses. Prophylactic antibiotics are at least as effective as ventilation tubes in preventing further infections.[14]

Whether prophylactic antibiotics (or for that matter, ventilation tubes) should be prescribed for every case of recurrent otitis media should be decided in the context of the natural history of the disease. A study in northern Finland followed 222 children with recurrent otitis media, defined as three episodes within 6 months or four episodes within 1 year.[15] None of the children received prophylactic antibiotics or ventilation tubes. During the first 6 months after recurrent otitis media was diagnosed, 38% had no subsequent ear infections, 28% had one more episode, 18% two more episodes, and 12% three or more episodes. In only 4% did chronic otitis media with effusion develop. The major risk factor for recurrent infections was age under 16 months.[15]

There is little evidence that tonsillectomy or adenoidectomy is an effective treatment for recurrent otitis media (see discussion of tonsillectomy). Donnelly and associates[16] submitted a questionnaire on the indications for tonsillectomy to 400 general practitioners and 31 consultant specialists in Ireland. The specialists and general practitioners generally agreed except for the treatment of recurrent otitis media and glue ear; the general practitioners thought these conditions were indications for tonsillectomy but the consultants did not.[16]

REFERENCES

1. Ruuskanen O, Heikkinen T: Otitis media: etiology and diagnosis, *Postgrad Med* 13(suppl 1):S23-S26, 1994.
2. Heikkinen T, Ruuskanen O: Signs and symptoms predicting acute otitis media, *Arch Pediatr Adolesc Med* 149:26-29, 1995.
3. Drugs for treatment of acute otitis media in children, *Med Lett* 36:19-21, 1994.
4. Rosenfeld RM, Vertrees JE, Carr J, et al: Clinical efficacy of antimicrobial drugs for acute otitis media: meta-analysis of 5400 children from thirty-three randomized trials, *J Pediatr* 124:355-367, 1994.
5. Paradise JL: Treatment guidelines for otitis media: the need for breadth and flexibility, *Postgrad Med* 14:429-435, 1995.
6. Froom J, Culpepper L, Jacobs M, et al: Antimicrobials for acute otitis media? A review from the International Primary Care Network, *BMJ* 315:98-102, 1997.
7. Lehnert T: Acute otitis media in children: role of antibiotic therapy, *Can Fam Physician* 39:2157-2162, 1993.
8. Del Mar C, Glasziou P, Hayem M: Are antibiotics indicated as initial treatment for children with acute otitis media? A meta-analysis, *BMJ* 314:1526-1529, 1997.
9. Marchant CD, Carlin SA, Johnson CE, et al: Measuring the comparative efficacy of antibacterial agents for acute otitis media: the "Polyanna phenomenon," *J Pediatr* 120:72-77, 1992.
10. Arola M, Ziegler T, Ruuskanen O: Respiratory virus infection as a cause of prolonged symptoms in acute otitis media, *J Pediatr* 116:697-701, 1990.
11. Aronoff SC: Antimicrobials in children and the problem of drug resistance (editorial), *Am Fam Physician* 54:44-56, 1996.
12. Giebink GS: Preventing otitis media, *Ann Otol Rhinol Laryngol* 163(suppl):20-23, 1994.
13. Niemela M, Uhari M, Mottonen M: A pacifier increases the risk of recurrent acute otitis media in children in day care centers, *Pediatrics* 96:884-888, 1995.
14. Berman S: Otitis media in children, *N Engl J Med* 332:1560-1565, 1995.
15. Alho OP, Laara E, Oja H: What is the natural history of recurrent acute otitis media in infancy, *J Fam Pract* 43:258-264, 1996.
16. Donnelly MJ, Quraishi MS, McShane DP: Indications for paediatric tonsillectomy, GP versus consultant perspective, *J Laryngol Otol* 108:131-134, 1994.

Middle Ear Effusion

(See also otitis media)

The management of otitis media with effusion has traditionally involved the insertion of ventilation tubes. This is the second most common surgical procedure in U.S. children, superseded only by circumcision.[1] The evidence that this is necessary is of poor quality.

Risk factors for otitis media with effusions include bottle feeding, exposure to passive smoke, and attendance at day care or other group infant facilities.[2]

Longitudinal studies of young children with middle ear effusions have shown that by 3 months 50% of effusions have resolved spontaneously and that resolution continues thereafter at a constant rate so that by 1 year few children still have an effusion.[2]

Suggested initial treatment is observation and probably antibiotics. Antibiotics have been shown to increase the resolution rate by 14%.[2] However, expectant watching of these children for 4 to 6 months is quite safe if they do not have significant hearing loss or other symptoms.[3] A cogent reason for avoiding antibiotics whenever possible in the treatment of serous otitis media is to slow the development of antibiotic-resistant organisms.[4]

The rationale for myringotomy with tube insertion is primarily to improve hearing and prevent difficulties in language development. However, no conclusive evidence has been presented to support or reject this hypothesis. In view of this the recommendation of the Otitis Media Panel is that myringotomy with tube insertion be considered for a child who has had bilateral effusions for a total of 3 months and who has a hearing deficit of at least 20 dB in the better hearing ear.[2]

Treatments that are not recommended include antihistamines, decongestants, corticosteroids, and tonsillectomy.[2] Adenoidectomy is a controversial issue. Some experts, as represented by the Otitis Media Panel,[2] believe there is almost no indication for adenoidectomy in the treatment of serous otitis media, others that it has a role in primary treatment with or without ventilation tubes,[5,6] and still others that it is indicated if treatment with ventilation tubes is unsuccessful.[7]

A historical note: During World War II a number of flyers and submariners in the U.S. military were subjected to nasopharyngeal irradiation to shrink nasopharyngeal lymphoid tissue and thus prevent barotrauma to the ear.[8]

REFERENCES

1. Berman S: Otitis media in children, *N Engl J Med* 332:1560-1565, 1995.
2. Otitis Media Guideline Panel: Managing otitis media with effusion in young children, *Am Fam Physician* 50:1003-1010, 1994.
3. Aronoff SC: Antimicrobials in children and the problem of drug resistance (editorial), *Am Fam Physician* 54:44-56, 1996.
4. Paradise JL: Managing otitis media: a time for change (editorial), *Pediatrics* 96:712-715, 1995.
5. Bicknell PG: Role of adenotonsillectomy in the management of pediatric ear, nose and throat infections, *Postgrad Med* 13:S75-S78, 1994.
6. Maw AR: Tonsils and adenoids: their relation to secretory otitis media, *Acta Otorhinolaryngol* 40:81-88, 1988.
7. Paradise JL, Bluestone CD, Rogers KD, et al: Efficacy of adenoidectomy for recurrent otitis media in children previously treated with tympanostomy-tube placement: results of parallel randomized and nonrandomized trials, *JAMA* 263:2066-2073, 1990.
8. Skolnick AA: Discovery of 50-year-old naval logbook may aid follow-up study of radium-exposed veterans, *JAMA* 276:1628-1630, 1996.

INNER EAR

(See also vertigo)

Benign positional vertigo and Ménière's disease are discussed in the section on vertigo.

Hearing Impairment

Cochlear implants

Modern cochlear implants use multielectrode arrays that provide several channels of stimulation. The electrodes are implanted into the cochlea near the auditory nerve. Adults with profound sensorineural hearing loss receive significant benefit. One advantage of the implants is that speech-reading ability is significantly improved because of supplemental information from the implant. Children with severe hearing loss may also benefit. At present 2 years is the lower age limit for implants. Most cochlear implants may be damaged by magnetic resonance imaging.[1]

Hearing aids

Digital hearing aids not only amplify specific frequencies, but also distinguish speech from background noise and suppress the background noise. With this system, amplified sounds are less distorted than with many earlier devices.[2]

Screening for hearing loss in the elderly

A Dutch study found that the sensitivity and specificity of the whispered voice test were excellent compared with formal audiograms for detecting hearing losses greater than 30 dB (a level of loss causing social disability). Overall, this technique had a sensitivity of 90% and a specificity of 80%. Screening audiograms and auriscopes with built-in audiometric devices had high sensitivities for losses greater than 40 dB, but specificities were about 40%. The whispered voice test is much less expensive.[3]

The Canadian Task Force on the Periodic Health Examination[4] and the U.S. Preventive Services Task Force[5] both give "B" recommendations to screening elderly people for hearing impairment.

REFERENCES

1. NIH Consensus Conference: Cochlear implants in adults and children: NIH Consensus Development Panel on Cochlear Implants in Adults and Children, *JAMA* 274:1955-1961, 1995.
2. Werner J, Gottschlich S: Recent advances: otorhinolaryngology, *BMJ* 315:354-357, 1997.
3. Eekhof JA, de Bock GH, de Laat JA, et al: The whispered voice: the best test for screening for hearing impairment in general practice? *Br J Gen Pract* 46:473-474, 1996.
4. Canadian Task Force on the Periodic Health Examination: *Canadian guide to clinical preventive health care,* Ottawa, 1994, Canada Communication Group—Publishing, pp 954-963.
5. US Preventive Services Task Force: *Guide to clinical preventive services,* ed 2, Baltimore, 1996, Williams & Wilkins, pp 393-405.

Tinnitus

Intermittent tinnitus lasting a few minutes is common among healthy persons. Although tinnitus lasting weeks, months, or years may occur in individuals with normal hearing, it is usually associated with hearing loss. The most frequent causes of such hearing loss are sensorineural loss as occurs in presbycusis, noise-induced hearing loss, and Ménière's disease. It may also be induced by middle ear disease such as otitis media, serous otitis media, and otosclerosis, external ear disease such as an occluding wax plug, and certain drugs such as aspirin. With time most people become less bothered by their tinnitus. The most important therapeutic intervention is reassurance. For some patients with both hearing impairment and tinnitus, hearing aids ameliorate both symptoms. A few patients benefit from tinnitus-masking devices that can be worn in or behind the ear.[1]

REFERENCES

1. Vesterager V: Tinnitus—investigation and management, *BMJ* 314:728-732, 1997.

MOTION SICKNESS

The traditional medications for motion sickness are dimenhydrinate (Gravol, Dramamine) 50 to 100 mg qid, preferably given 1 to 2 hours before onset of motion, and scopolamine patches (Transderm-Scop, Transderm-V) applied to the postauricular area 12 hours before onset of motion and changed every 72 hours. There is anecdotal evidence that calcium channel blockers may be effective in motion sickness. Larimore and Hartman[1] recommend the use of a sustained release preparation once a day, beginning 4 days before the trip.

REFERENCES

1. Larimore WL, Hartman JR: Family physician's notebook: diary from a week in practice, *Am Fam Physician* 47:1589-1590, 1993.

MOUTH

Aphthous Ulcers

A number of studies have suggested that thalidomide (Synovir) in doses of 50 to 200 mg/day is effective in treating and preventing aphthous ulcers in both HIV-negative and HIV-positive patients.[1]

A blinded study from Israel found that the application of a solution of sucralfate (Sulcrate) to the ulcers four times a day using an applicator stick not only decreased the duration of pain and the time until healing, but also increased the duration of remissions.[2]

Amlexanox (Aphthasol), an inhibitor of inflammatory mediators, is marketed as a 5% oral paste to be applied to the ulcers four times a day. Controlled trials have shown it to be effective.[3]

REFERENCES

1. New uses of thalidomide, *Med Lett* 38:15-16, 1996.
2. Rattan J, Schneider M, Arber N, et al: Sucralfate suspension as a treatment of recurrent aphthous stomatitis, *J Intern Med* 236: 341-343, 1994.
3. Khandwala A, Vaninwegen RG, Alfano MC: 5-Percent amlexanox oral paste, a new treatment for recurrent minor aphthous ulcers. I. Clinical demonstration of acceleration of healing and resolution of pain, *Oral Surg Oral Med Oral Pathol* 83:222-230, 1997.

NOSE

Allergic and vasomotor rhinitis are discussed in the immunology section.

PHARYNX

Pharyngitis

(See also streptococcal infections)

Symptomatic relief of the symptoms of pharyngitis may be obtained by gargling with 15 ml (1 tbsp) of benzydamine HCl (Tantum) every 1½ to 3 hours and especially before meals.

Tonsillectomy

(See also otitis media; streptococcal infections)

Absolute indications for tonsillectomy are obstructive tonsils causing sleep apnea or obstructive tonsils unresponsive to antibiotics, which cause failure to thrive or progressive weight loss. Elective indications are recurrent acute tonsillitis (with each episode seen and documented by a physician) defined as more than five episodes in 1 year, seven in 2 years, and nine in 3 years; peritonsillar abscess (one episode only is a controversial indication); obstructive tonsils without sleep apnea or cor pulmonale; and chronic bad breath from retention of debris in tonsillar crypts.[1-3]

Recurrent otitis media and glue ear are not recognized indications for tonsillectomy (see discussion of otitis media).

REFERENCES

1. Bluestone CD: Current indications for tonsillectomy adenoidectomy, *Ann Otol Rhinol Laryngol* 101:58-64, 1992.
2. Benjamin B: Guidelines on tonsillectomy and adenoidectomy, *J Paediatr Child Health* 28:136-140, 1992.
3. Fabian MC, Smitheringale A: Tonsillitis—making the right decisions, *Can J Diagn* 11:53-63, 1994.

SINUSES

Sinusitis

Acute sinusitis lasts 1 to 3 weeks. Chronic sinusitis is defined as disease lasting more than 3 months, as three or more recurrent infections annually, or as repeated failures of medical therapy to cure the condition.[1]

Making a clinical diagnosis of acute bacterial sinusitis is difficult. Symptoms and signs of particular value are facial pain, particularly if unilateral, maxillary toothache, purulent nasal secretions, poor response to decongestants, and abnormal transillumination. This last sign is of value only if transillumination is performed by an experienced operator in a completely dark room. If on a clinical basis a patient has either a high or low probability of having sinusitis, x-ray examination adds little. In inconclusive cases or when the patient has frontal pain leading to a concern about frontal sinusitis (which can be complicated by a brain abscess), x-ray studies might be helpful.[1]

In both adults and children, *H. influenzae* and *S. pneumoniae* account for about 70% of cases of bacterial sinusitis. In children most of the remaining cases are due to *M. catarrhalis.* In adults other etiological agents include *Staphylococcus aureus, Streptococcus pyogenes, M. catarrhalis,* anaerobes, and gram-negative organisms.[1]

Antibiotics are considered standard treatment for sinusitis but may not always be necessary. A randomized placebo-controlled trial of amoxicillin for radiologically proven maxillary sinusitis in patients of general practitioners found no benefit from the antibiotic in terms of rapidity of symptom resolution, complications, or recurrences.[2]

Although one trial of children with sinusitis has shown that a 3-day course of trimethoprim-sulfamethoxazole (Septra,

Bactrim) was as effective as a 10-day course,[3] the standard duration of therapy for this disease remains 10 days. Beta-lactamase agents do not offer any significant advantage as first-line therapy for acute bacterial sinusitis. The antibiotics of first choice are amoxicillin 500 mg q8h (40 mg/kg/day in 3 divided doses for children) or trimethoprim-sulfamethoxazole 160/800 mg q12h (8/40 mg/kg/day in 2 divided doses for children). Second-line drugs include cefuroxime axetil (Ceftin), Cefaclor (Ceclor), cefixime (Suprax), clarithromycin (Biaxin), erythromycin-sulfisoxazole (Pediazole), and amoxicillin-clavulanate (Clavulin, Augmentin).[1]

Although no placebo-controlled trials have been published, use of a topical nasal decongestant spray such as oxymetazoline (Dristan Long Lasting Nasal) or xylometazoline (Otrivin) two or three times a day or phenylephrine (Neo-Synephrine) three or four times a day for 3 to 4 days may be helpful.[1]

The organisms causing chronic sinusitis are similar to those causing acute sinusitis except that anaerobes are much more common. An effective regimen for this condition is cefuroxime axetil (Ceftin) 500 mg q12h plus metronidazole (Flagyl) 500 mg q6-8h. An alternative is clindamycin.[4]

REFERENCES

1. Low DE, Desrosiers M, McSherry J, et al: A practical guide for the diagnosis and treatment of acute sinusitis, *Can Med Assoc J* 156(suppl 6):S1-S14, 1997.
2. van Buchem FL, Knottnerus JA, Schrijnemaekers VJ, et al: Primary-care-based randomised placebo-controlled trial of antibiotic treatment in acute maxillary sinusitis, *Lancet* 349:683-687, 1997.
3. Williams JW Jr, Holleman DR Jr, Samsa GP, et al: Randomized controlled trial of 3 vs 10 days of trimethoprim/sulfamethoxazole for acute maxillary sinusitis, *JAMA* 273:1015-1021, 1995.
4. Brook I, Yocum P: Antimicrobial management of chronic sinusitis in children, *J Laryngol Otol* 109:1159-1162, 1995.

VERTIGO

(See also motion sickness)

Benign Positional Vertigo

Benign positional vertigo is thought to be due to the accumulation of particles (probably otoconia) in the endolymph of the posterior semicircular canal. With head movements these strike the crista of the affected semicircular canal, causing vertigo and nystagmus.

The diagnosis of benign positional vertigo is confirmed by performing the Bárány (Hallpike, Dix-Hallpike) maneuver. The examiner helps the patient, who is seated on the examining table, to lie rapidly back so that his or her head, which is rotated to one side by about 45 degrees, hangs down over the upper edge of the examining table by about 45 degrees. Characteristics of a positive test are latency, adaptability, and fatigability, as well as rotary nystagmus toward the dependent ear and the subjective sensation of vertigo. These features are described in any standard textbook dealing with the subject.

Particle repositioning maneuvers

In recent years head maneuvers have been described as a means of permanently controlling the symptoms of benign positional vertigo.[1-3] The theory is that the particles lodged in the posterior semicircular canal can be made to fall into the utricle, where they will do no further harm. The method described below is that described by Epley,[1] who reported a 77% success rate after only one treatment session.

The Epley canalith repositioning procedure is performed as follows.[1-4] The affected ear is first determined by the Bárány or Hallpike maneuver. It is the ear that is dependent when symptoms are produced. Each movement in the particle repositioning maneuver (Epley's maneuver) is performed rapidly and then maintained for at least 30 seconds or until symptoms have subsided. The initial maneuver is identical to the Bárány or Hallpike maneuver. The seated patient is assisted in lying back on the examining table so that the head hangs over the edge of the table with the neck extended about 45 degrees and rotated 45 degrees toward the affected side. The physician helps support the patient's head in this position while reassuring him or her that the vertigo will subside. Next the head is rapidly rotated through 90 degrees to the opposite side. After at least 30 seconds in this position, the physician helps the patient roll over on to his or her side, the direction of the roll being in the direction the face was pointing in the last maneuver. The head rotation of 45 degrees is maintained throughout this roll over. Finally the patient is helped to move from the side to the sitting position, always keeping the head in the same position of rotation. Finally, after another 30 seconds, the head is rotated back to the straight ahead position and flexed 20 degrees. In cases of treatment failure the procedure is repeated. In some patients both ears are affected; in those cases only one side is treated at a time.

The original studies recommended that patients try to keep the head in the vertical position for 48 hours (supine sleeping position with two or three pillows). However, a 1996 study found no benefit from this type of posttreatment protocol.[4]

A patient who still has symptoms after performing Epley's maneuver may perform the positional or habituation exercises of Brandt and Daroff at home; every position is maintained for at least 30 seconds. The patient begins by sitting on the side of the bed with feet on the floor and head turned 45 degrees to one side. The patient then rapidly lies down on the side away from the direction in which he or she is looking so that the portion of the occiput behind the ear touches the bed. The patient sits up, turns the head so it points 45 degrees in the opposite direction, and lies down quickly on the opposite side.[3,5]

REFERENCES

1. Epley JM: The canalith repositioning procedure for treatment of benign paroxysmal positional vertigo, *Otolaryngol Head Neck Surg* 107:399-404, 1992.

2. Parnes LS, Price-Jones RG: Particle repositioning maneuver for benign paroxysmal positional vertigo, *Ann Otol Rhinol Laryngol* 102:325-331, 1993.
3. Lempert T, Gresty MA, Bronstein AM: Benign positional vertigo: recognition and treatment, *BMJ* 489-491, 1995.
4. Massoud EA, Ireland DF: Post-treatment instructions in the nonsurgical management of benign paroxysmal positional vertigo, *J Otolaryngol* 25:121-125, 1996.
5. Brandt T, Daroff RB: Physical therapy for benign paroxysmal positional vertigo, *Arch Otolaryngol* 106:484-485, 1980.

Ménière's Disease

(See also nausea and vomiting)

The four characteristic symptoms of Ménière's disease are episodic vertigo, fluctuating sensorineural hearing loss, tinnitus, and sense of fullness in the ear.[1] At the onset of the disease, not all these symptoms may be present; only in later episodes will the diagnosis become evident. Two of the major conditions to consider in the differential diagnosis are benign positional vertigo and vestibular neuronitis.[1]

Few controlled trials on the treatment of Ménière's disease have been conducted, so as might be expected, there are a variety of unproven management protocols. Medical regimens include prescription of many classes of drugs, including diuretics, benzodiazepines, tricyclic antidepressants, and antihistamines, and limitations on the intake of salt, caffeine, alcohol, and tobacco. Promethazine and the antihistamines, which include meclizine (Antivert, Bonine, Bonamine), promethazine (Phenergan), and dimenhydrinate (Dramamine, Gravol), are used as antinauseants during the acute attack.[1]

Canadian physicians should be aware that in Canada Antivert contains both meclizine and niacin, whereas in the United States Antivert contains no niacin. As far as I can determine, niacin has no beneficial effects on Ménière's disease.

Another drug that is used in Canada and Europe in the treatment of Ménière's disease is betahistine (Serc).[2,3] It is usually prescribed as 4 to 8 mg q8h. Its mode of action is thought to be an inhibition of neuronal impulses to the lateral vestibular nucleus.[3]

The value of most surgical treatments involving decompression of the labyrinth or shunting of endolymph is controversial. Patients with no serviceable hearing may obtain complete relief of symptoms at the cost of total hearing loss through a complete labyrinthectomy.[1]

REFERENCES

1. Knox GW, McPherson A: Meniere's disease: differential diagnosis and treatment, *Am Fam Physician* 55:1185-1190, 1997.
2. Fraysse B, Bebear JP, Dubreuil C, et al: Betahistine dihydrochloride versus flunarizine: a double-blind study on recurrent vertigo with or without cochlear syndrome typical of Meniere's disease, *Acta Otolaryngol* 490(suppl):1-10, 1991.
3. Aantaa E: Treatment of acute vestibular vertigo, *Acta Otolaryngol* 479(suppl):44-47, 1991.

PEDIATRICS

Topics covered in this section

ASTHMA IN CHILDREN

(See also allergic rhinitis–environmental control; asthma)

About half of all children have one or more episodes of wheezing before the age of 3 years, usually in association with respiratory infections, but only one fourth still have wheezing episodes at the age of 6. A history of maternal asthma is associated with an increased risk of the child continuing to wheeze at the age of 6, maternal smoking with an increased incidence of wheezing before the age of 3,[1] and exposure to passive smoke with a delayed resolution of acute asthmatic attacks.[2] The morbidity rate from asthma among poor inner city children is particularly high, almost certainly because of sensitivity and continued exposure to cockroaches.[3]

Between 30% and 70% of children with asthma have marked improvement or resolution of symptoms by the time they become adults. Such resolution is seen more often in patients with milder forms of the disease.[4]

Inhaled medications are the ideal way of controlling asthma in both children and adults. For children who cannot use that method the first choice of an oral agent is usually a beta$_2$-adrenergic agonist such as metaproterenol (Alupent), which has the generic name orciprenaline in Canada. The usual dose of this product is 10 mg tid prn for children aged 4 to 12 years and 20 mg tid prn for children over 12. In some instances a theophylline derivative such as oxtriphylline (Choledyl) is still used. For children under 5 the dosage is 24 to 36 mg/kg/day divided into 3 equal doses given at 8-hour intervals. The usual dose for children over the age of 5 is 22 mg/kg/day divided into 4 equal doses. Both metaproterenol and oxtriphylline can cause hyperactivity, nausea, and vomiting.

The bulk of evidence based on short- and intermediate-duration studies is that standard pediatric doses of inhaled glucocorticoids do not affect a child's growth. Long-term prospective studies and comparisons of specific glucocorticoids are needed.[5]

Asthma is discussed in detail in under "Respirology."

REFERENCES

1. Martinez FD, Wright AL, Taussig LM, et al: Asthma and wheezing in the first six years of life, *N Engl J Med* 332:133-138, 1995.
2. Abulhosn RS, Morray BH, Llewellyn CE, et al: Passive smoke exposure impairs recovery after hospitalization for acute asthma, *Arch Pediatr Adolesc Med* 151:135-139, 1997.
3. Rosenstreich D, Kattan M, Baker D, et al: The role of cockroach allergy and exposure to cockroach allergen in causing morbidity among inner-city children with asthma, *N Engl J Med* 336:1356-1363, 1997.
4. O'Connor GT, Weiss ST, Speizer FE: The epidemiology of asthma. In Gershwin ME, ed: *Bronchial asthma,* ed 2, Orlando, Fla, 1986, Grune & Stratton.
5. Wolthers OD: Long-, intermediate- and short-term growth studies in asthmatic children treated with inhaled glucocorticosteroids, *Eur Respir J* 9:821-827, 1996.

ATTENTION DEFICIT/HYPERACTIVITY DISORDER

(See also antisocial personality disorder)

Common comorbid conditions of attention deficit/hyperactivity disorder (ADHD) are learning disabilities (25% to 35% of children) and oppositional, conduct, and mood disorders. A family history of conversion disorder, sociopathy, and alcoholism may be present.[1,2] ADHD has been diagnosed in about 5% of children in North America and affects boys more often than girls. There is a strong familial tendency; 30% of first-degree relatives of affected children also have the condition. The increased risk for siblings is five fold for boys and three fold for girls.[3] Children with ADHD are at increased risk for antisocial personality disorder or drug abuse disorder when they reach adulthood.[4,5] This risk is particularly marked if the child meets the criteria of both ADHD and conduct disorder.[4]

The diagnosis of ADHD is based on the history.[1,2] DSM IV divides the symptoms into the two major categories of inattention and hyperactivity/impulsivity. Each category contains nine sets of symptoms, and the diagnosis is made if the child has six of the listed symptoms in either category, has had symptoms before the age of 7 years, has symptoms in two or more settings (such as school and home), and suffers impairment in social, academic, or occupational functioning because of the symptoms. The following are examples of symptoms associated with inattention[2]:

1. Fails to pay attention to detail at school and makes careless mistakes
2. Has difficulty sustaining attention when playing or performing tasks
3. May not seem to listen when spoken to directly
4. Is often distracted

These are examples of symptoms of hyperactivity/impulsivity[2]:

1. Often squirms in chair or fidgets with hands or feet
2. Often runs or climbs excessively
3. Often talks excessively
4. May have difficulty waiting his or her turn
5. Often blurts out an answer before a question is completed

The child may not display any symptoms when in a physician's office, so short periods of observation are not sufficient to rule out the diagnosis. Usually the practitioner must question a number of observers from different settings to obtain a diagnostic history. Questionnaires such as the Connors Parent Rating Scales and the Connors Teacher Rating Scales are useful. Not all children "outgrow" the condition, and about half continue to benefit from medications during adulthood.[3]

A 1995 metaanalysis found no correlation between sugar intake and childhood hyperactivity or cognitive functioning [6]

The medication of first choice for ADHD is methylphenidate (Ritalin).[1,3] The dosage is 0.3 to 0.7 mg/kg/dose given two or three times daily. This usually translates to an initial dose of 5 mg bid for children under age 8 and 10 mg bid for those over 8.[3] A dose of 10 mg bid is often sufficient for adults as well as children.[1] The duration of action of methylphenidate tablets is only 3 to 4 hours, so frequent doses may be necessary to control symptoms. For schoolchildren this often means a morning and noon dose with a third dose in the late afternoon or at suppertime if necessary. Such a regimen may be difficult to implement, particularly when the child is at school; in these situations the slow release tablets (20 mg), which have a duration of action of 6 to 8 hours, may be worth trying.[3] However, the slow release formulation is not always effective because the slow rise and lower peak may not give adequate control.[7]

Other drugs that may be used are dextroamphetamine (Dexedrine, Dextrostat), methamphetamine (Desoxyn), and pemoline (Cylert). Clonidine (Catapres) has been reported useful, but according to the *Medical Letter* there are no reliable controlled trials documenting this and a few unexplained sudden deaths have occurred in children who were taking or who had recently taken the drug.[8]

REFERENCES

1. Zametkin AJ: Attention-deficit disorder: born to be hyperactive? *JAMA* 273:1871-1874, 1995.
2. American Psychiatric Association: *Diagnostic and statistical manual of mental disorders,* ed 4, Washington, DC, 1994, The Association, pp 78-85.
3. Taylor ME: Evaluation and management of attention-deficit hyperactivity disorder, *Am Fam Physician* 55:887-901, 1997.
4. Lynam DR: Early identification of chronic offenders: who is the fledgling psychopath? *Psychol Bull* 120:209-234, 1996.
5. Mannuzza S, Klein RG, Bessler A, et al: Adult outcome of hyperactive boys: educational achievement, occupational rank, and psychiatric status, *Arch Gen Psychiatry* 50:565-576, 1993.
6. Wolraich ML, Wilson DB, White W: The effect of sugar on behavior or cognition in children: a meta-analysis, *JAMA* 274: 1617-1621, 1995.
7. Lawrence JD, Carson DS: Optimizing ADHD therapy with sustained-release methylphenidate, *Am Fam Physician* 55:1705-1709, 1997.
8. Clonidine for the treatment of attention-deficit/hyperactivity disorder, *Med Lett* 38:109-110, 1996.

BREAST FEEDING

(See also formulas; neonatal jaundice)

These are signs of successful breast feeding in the neonate[1]:

1. Eight to ten feedings a day
2. Audible swallowing
3. Six to eight wet diapers a day
4. Three to five bowel movements a day
5. Birth weight regained by 2 weeks

REFERENCES

1. Spencer JP: Practical nutrition for the healthy term infant, *Am Fam Physician* 54:138-144, 1996.

BRONCHIOLITIS

Bronchiolitis is a common disease of infants that is usually caused by the respiratory syncytial virus. The peak age is 2 to 6 months, although the condition occurs in children up to 2 years of age. It is more common in premature infants and those from lower socioeconomic environments. The incubation period usually lasts 3 days and is followed by symptoms of an upper respiratory tract infection with rhinorrhea and cough. Between 2 and 3 days after the onset of symptoms, respiratory distress and appetite loss develop. Physical findings are tachycardia, tachypnea, cyanosis, an increase in the anteroposterior diameter of the chest, intercostal and subcostal retractions, hyperresonance, prolonged expiration, wheezes, and fine crackles. Because the diaphragm is depressed by hyperinflation, the liver and spleen are easily palpable. When the diagnosis is suspected, investigations including chest x-ray examination are indicated and in many cases the child requires admission to the hospital.[1]

REFERENCES

1. Jeng M-J, Lemen R: Respiratory syncytial virus bronchiolitis, *Am Fam Physician* 55:1139-1146, 1997.

CIRCUMCISION

Neonatal circumcision without anesthesia is painful. Complications occur in 0.2% to 0.6% of cases and are usually minor episodes of bleeding or local infections. The relative rate of urinary tract infections in boys under 1 year of age is 10 times greater in the uncircumcised than in the circumcised. However, since the overall incidence of urinary tract infections in male infants, including those who have been circumcised, is only 1% to 2%, the absolute risk increase is small.[1,2] For example, in one large U.S. study the incidence of urinary tract infections in uncircumcised boys was 1.03%, whereas that among the circumcised was 0.1% (the rate among female infants was 0.52%).[3] Penile cancer is rare in circumcised males, and epidemiological evidence (primarily cross-sectional studies) suggests that the incidence of sexually transmitted diseases, including HIV infection, is lower in the circumcised than the uncircumcised.[4-6] Uncircumcised children have a higher incidence of balanitis and phimosis.[1,2] Should routine circumcision be recommended? The Canadian Paediatric Society says that it should not,[2] while an editorialist in the *New England Journal of Medicine* makes a good case for doing so.[7]

Applying 1 g of a cream composed of 2.5% lidocaine mixed with 2.5% prilocaine to the penis of the newborn under an occlusive dressing 60 to 80 minutes before circumcision prevents pain from the procedure.[8]

REFERENCES

1. American Academy of Family Physicians: Fact sheet for physicians regarding neonatal circumcision, *Am Fam Physician* 52: 523-526, 1995.
2. Fetus and Newborn Committee, Canadian Paediatric Society: Neonatal circumcision revisited, *Can Med Assoc J* 154:769-780, 1996.
3. Wiswell TE, Enzenauer RW, Holton ME, et al: Declining frequency of circumcision: implications for changes in the absolute incidence and male to female sex ratio of urinary tract infections in early infancy, *Pediatrics* 79:338-403, 1987.
4. Cook LS, Koutsky LA, Holmes KK: Circumcision and sexually transmitted diseases, *Am J Public Health* 84:197-201, 1994.
5. Moses S, Plummer FA, Bradley JE, et al: The association between lack of male circumcision and risk for HIV infection: a review of the epidemiological data, *Sex Transm Dis* 21:201-210, 1994.
6. Royce RA, Sena A, Cates W Jr, et al: Sexual transmission of HIV, *N Engl J Med* 336:1072-1078, 1997.
7. Wiswell TE: Circumcision circumspection (editorial), *N Engl J Med* 336:1244-1245, 1997.
8. Taddio A, Stevens B, Craig K, et al: Efficacy and safety of lidocaine-prilocaine cream for pain during circumcision, *N Engl J Med* 336:1197-1201, 1997.

COLIC

(See also formulas)

Definition

Colic is probably best defined as excessive crying of unknown cause in an otherwise normal infant.[1] The classic definition is excessive crying that occurs in the first 3 months of an otherwise healthy infant's life, lasts longer than 3 hours a day, takes place on more than 3 days a week, and is longer than 3 weeks in duration. According to this definition, about 20% to 30% of infants are colicky.[2] The condition almost always resolves by 4 months.

Symptoms

Crying in colicky babies varies a great deal from day to day, is typically paroxysmal, and, older literature to the contrary, occurs at any time of day.[3] During these episodes the babies are almost impossible to soothe, but in the intervals they are settled and normal.

How much do normal infants cry? In 1962 Brazelton reported on 80 normal infants. The median daily crying time was 1³/₄ hours in the second week of life, 2³/₄ hours at 6 weeks, and less than 1 hour by the 12th week.[4]

Etiology

The etiology of colic is unknown. It has not been shown to have a relationship to the personality of the mother. Lactose intolerance has been proposed, but there is no consistent evidence supporting this. A current popular hypothesis is that the disorder is related to sensitivity to cow's milk protein, either in the formulas of bottle-fed babies or in the diet of the mothers of breast-fed babies. The seminal article supporting this was by Lothe and associates[5] in 1982. They reported a dramatic resolution of symptoms in colicky infants within 48 hours of being switched from cow's milk or soy formulas to casein hydrolysate formulas. Some subsequent studies have had similar results.[6,7] However, such clear-cut improvements have not been duplicated in a number of other studies. Some workers estimate that switching to a hydrolyzed protein formula eliminates colic in about 30% of children and improves it in another 10% to 15% of cases.[8] The Committee on Nutrition of the American Academy of Pediatrics claims that no evidence supports the use of protein hydrolysates for colic.[9]

In the case of breast-fed infants a 1981 study by Evans and associates showed no relationship between the mothers' consumption of cow's milk and colic,[10] whereas 2 years later Jakobsson and associates[11] reported a 70% improvement in colic when cow's milk protein was removed from the mothers' diets.

Management

If the infant is thriving and the physical examination is normal, no investigations are required. The traditional management of colic is reassurance and counseling of the parents. Usual recommendations are that parents change their interventions every 10 minutes or so during crying episodes—carrying, rocking using a mechanical swing, putting the baby down, and so on. Parental relief provided by extended family or other support systems is often critical. In one study a group of volunteer mothers giving behavioral treatment recommendations by phone made a significant difference compared with both an empathy-only phone support system and a no treatment plan.[3] As indicated previously, some workers have proposed trying a dietary change (no cow's milk protein for the nursing mother or a switch to a protein hydrolysate formula for the bottle-fed baby).[5-7,11] Others claim there is little or no evidence to support such an approach.[9,10]

REFERENCES

1. Thiessen P: Colic in infancy, *Can J CME,* May 1994, 6:10-12.
2. Hewson P, Oberklaid F, Menahem S: Infant colic, distress, and crying, *Clin Pediatr* 26:69-76, 1987.
3. Wolke D, Meyer R: Excessive infant crying: a controlled study of mothers helping mothers, *Pediatrics* 94:322-332, 1994.
4. Brazelton TB: Crying in infancy, *Pediatrics* 29:579, 1962.
5. Lothe L, Lindberg T, Jakobsson I: Cow's milk formulas as a cause of infant colic—a double-blind study, *Pediatrics* 70:7-10, 1982.
6. Lothe L, Lindberg T: Cow's milk whey protein elicits symptoms of infantile colic in colicky formula-fed infants: a double-blind crossover study, *Pediatrics* 83:262-266, 1989.
7. Iacono G, Carroccio A, Montalto G, et al: Severe infantile colic and food intolerance: a long-term prospective study, *J Pediatr Gastroenterol Nutr* 12:332-335, 1991.
8. Colon AR, Dipalma JS: Colic, *Am Fam Physician* 40:122-124, 1989.
9. Finberg L, Bell EF, Hatch TF, et al (American Academy of Pediatrics, Committee on Nutrition): Hypoallergenic infant formulas, *Pediatrics* 83:1068-1069, 1989.
10. Evans RW, Fergusson DM, Allardyce RA, et al: Maternal diet and infantile colic in breast-fed infants, *Lancet* 1:1340-1342, 1981.
11. Jakobsson I, Lindberg T: Cow's milk protein causes infantile colic in breast-fed infants: a double-blind crossover study, *Pediatrics* 71:268-271, 1983.

CROUP

Croup is a viral laryngotracheobronchitis usually caused by parainfluenza viruses, although similar clinical pictures may result from infection with the respiratory syncytial virus or rhinovirus or from influenza. Characteristic symptoms, which usually occur at night, are a harsh, barking, seal-like cough, stridor, and hoarse voice. Most cases are in children 6 months to 4 years of age. There is often a preceding upper respiratory tract infection, but fever is rarely above 39° C and toxicity is absent. The major differential diagnoses are epiglottitis, inhalation of a foreign body, and bacterial tracheitis. Children with epiglottitis and bacterial tracheitis are sick, and those with epiglottitis almost never have a barking cough, tend to assume the sitting position, and often drool.

Traditional treatment of croup has been to expose the child to a hot, steamy environment created by running a hot shower with the bathroom door closed, but there are no reliable studies documenting the effectiveness of this regimen.

Inhaled or oral corticosteroids or a combination of the two appears to be beneficial for outpatient children with mild to moderate croup.[1-4] For example, in one British trial a single oral dose of dexamethasone 0.15 mg/kg decreased the number of patients returning for further medical care for the same episode of illness.[2] A Canadian study found that outpatient children with mild to moderate croup who were given 4 ml of a budesonide (Pulmicort) solution (2 mg) by updraft nebulizer with continuous flow oxygen at 5 to 6 L/min had more rapid improvement in croup scores and fewer admissions than in the placebo control group.[1] In a subsequent study by the same authors, inhaled budesonide given as in the first study improved the outcome of children who had been pretreated with dexamethasone 0.6 mg/kg as a single oral dose.[4]

REFERENCES

1. Klassen TP, Feldman ME, Watters LK, et al: Nebulized budesonide for children with mild-to-moderate croup, *N Engl J Med* 331:285-289, 1994.
2. Doull I: Corticosteroids in the management of croup: nebulised corticosteroids are the treatment of choice (editorial), *BMJ* 311: 1244, 1995.
3. Geelhoed GC, Turner J, Macdonald WB: Efficacy of a small single dose of oral dexamethasone for outpatient croup: a double blind placebo controlled clinical trial, *BMJ* 313:140-142, 1996.
4. Klassen TP, Watters LK, Feldman ME, et al: Efficacy of nebulized budesonide in dexamethasone-treated outpatients with croup, *Pediatrics* 97:463-466, 1996.

DEVELOPMENTAL COORDINATION DELAY

Developmental coordination delay is a failure of motor coordination development to a such a degree that it adversely affects the child's activities of daily living or academic performance. The condition can be diagnosed only if other causative medical conditions have been ruled out. Boys are affected more often than girls, and the prevalence rate is probably about 6%. Manifestations may include delays in early milestones such as crawling and walking and difficulty cutting with scissors, tying shoelaces, doing up buttons, riding a bike, or being proficient at sports. These children are often labeled clumsy. The physical deficits tend to persist, and many children do not "grow out of them." Adolescent psychosocial problems are common, possibly because of low self-esteem.[1,2] Treatment results are uncertain, but explanations and organized teaching of specific activities with the assistance of occupational therapists are probably helpful.[2]

REFERENCES

1. American Psychiatric Association: *Diagnostic and statistical manual of mental disorders,* ed 4, Washington, DC, 1994, American Psychiatric Association, pp 53-55.
2. Fox AM, Lent B: Clumsy children: primer on developmental coordination disorder, *Can Fam Physician* 42:1965-1971, 1996.

DIAPER RASH

Diaper rash or diaper dermatitis is a descriptive term for dermatitis occurring in the diaper area. The two most common causes are irritant diaper dermatitis and *Candida* dermatitis. These two conditions can be distinguished by physical examination. Irritant diaper dermatitis tends to spare the creases and is accentuated on convex surfaces such as the lower abdomen, buttocks, thighs, and genitalia. *Candida* dermatitis almost always involves the inguinal creases, and usually the infant has red plaques with white scales and satellite lesions.[1,2] The cause of irritant diaper dermatitis is primarily contact with moisture from urine. Contributing factors are fecal enzymes and irritant chemicals.[1,2]

Treatment and prevention of both irritant and *Candida* diaper dermatitis consist of measures to keep the diaper area dry. This can involve exposure to air for as long as possible, as well as the use of highly absorbent disposable diapers (superabsorbent) and frequent changes of diapers.[1,2] Superabsorbent disposable diapers have been shown to be more effective than cloth diapers in the prevention and treatment of diaper dermatitis.[2] Pharmacological agents include a barrier cream such as a 15% to 20% zinc oxide ointment (Zincofax) to keep the area dry. When the clinical picture suggests candidiasis[1] or there is no response to symptomatic treatment after 3 days,[2] topical antifungal agents such as nystatin (Mycostatin), clotrimazole (Canesten), or miconazole (Monistat Derm Cream) should be gently rubbed into the area several times a day.[1,2] A low-potency steroid such as 1% hydrocortisone may alleviate symptoms in more severe cases[1,2] but is not necessary.[1]

REFERENCES

1. Ipp M: Pediatric dermatology: recognizing, treating what's serious, *Patient Care Can,* October 1996, 7:20-32.
2. Sires UI, Mallory SB: Diaper dermatitis: how to treat and prevent, *Postgrad Med* 98:79-84, 1995.

DIARRHEA AND DEHYDRATION IN INFANTS

(See also formulas; tropical medicine)

In 1996 the American Academy of Pediatrics published guidelines for the management of gastroenteritis in children between the ages of 1 month and 5 years.[1] These were the principal recommendations[1]:

1. Children with mild diarrhea and no dehydration do not require glucose-electrolyte solutions and may be given a regular diet including milk.
2. Oral rehydration therapy is the initial treatment of choice for children with mild or moderate dehydration.
3. Any one of a variety of glucose-electrolyte solutions may be used for oral rehydration therapy. Examples of commercial products are Naturalyte, Pediatric electrolyte, Pedialyte, Infalyte, Rehydralyte, Gastrolyte, and WHO/UNICEF oral rehydration salts.

4. Chicken broth, soft drinks, apple juice, and sports beverages (such as Gatorade) should not be used. Chicken broth has too much salt and no glucose, and the rest have too much glucose and inadequate salt.
5. The replacement volume of glucose-electrolyte replacement fluid for mild diarrhea is 50 ml/kg over a 4-hour period plus replacement of continuing losses. An additional 10 ml/kg should be given after each stool.
6. The replacement volume of glucose-electrolyte replacement fluid for moderate diarrhea is 100 ml/kg over a 4-hour period plus replacement of continuing losses. An additional 10 ml/kg should be given after each stool.
7. The secret of successful oral rehydration therapy in children who are vomiting is to give small amounts at frequent intervals. Every 1 to 2 minutes the child should be given 5 ml (1 teaspoon) of solution; as rehydration occurs and vomiting diminishes, larger amounts may be given at less frequent intervals.
8. Once rehydration is achieved, other fluids, including milk, and, if age appropriate, solid foods should be added.
9. Early refeeding does not worsen diarrhea and may even improve it. The majority of children tolerate full-strength milk and have no need for lactose-free formulations. Any food may be used, but the best tolerated seem to be complex carbohydrates such as bread, potatoes, and rice, lean meats, yogurt, fruits, and vegetables. Fatty foods and high-sucrose foods (dessert-type foods and soft drinks) are less well accepted.
10. IV fluids are indicated for severe dehydration, shock or near shock, or moderate dehydration if the child cannot retain orally administered fluids because of persistent vomiting.
11. Antidiarrheal drugs should not be used.

These guidelines differ from the traditional approach in two important ways. They recommend the rapid reintroduction of whole milk rather than switching to a soy-based or other lactose-free formula for 1 to 2 weeks before going back to milk, and they recommend the rapid introduction of food with only minor concern about what type. A 1994 meta-analysis found that except for infants with severe dehydration, there was no benefit in switching to a lactose-free formula or in diluting the formula.[2] Analysis of the literature has shown no adverse effects from the early introduction of solids[3] and no advantage to using the BRAT diet of bananas, rice, applesauce, and tea.[4]

An inexpensive alternative to commercial electrolyte solutions that was developed at St. Justine's Children's Hospital in Montreal is 360 ml (12 ounces or 1 1/2 cups) of orange juice without added sugar, 600 ml (20 ounces or 2 1/2 cups) of boiled water, and 2 ml (a little less than half a teaspoon) of salt.[5]

Evidence increasingly shows that cereal-based solutions containing complex rather than simple carbohydrates are effective. None is commercially available in North America at present, but one can be made up with 1/2 cup of dry precooked baby rice cereal, 2 cups of water, and 1/4 teaspoon of salt (care should be taken to measure the salt accurately; if the solution tastes salty, too much has been added).[6]

REFERENCES

1. Nazarian LF, Berman JH, Brown G, et al: Practice parameter: the management of acute gastroenteritis in young children, *Pediatrics* 97:424-435, 1996.
2. Brown KH, Peerson JM, Fontaine O: Use of nonhuman milks in the dietary management of young children with acute diarrhea: a meta-analysis of clinical trials, *Pediatrics* 93:17-27, 1994.
3. Brown KH: Dietary management of acute childhood diarrhea: optimal timing of feeding and appropriate use of milks and mixed diets, *J Pediatr* 118:S92-S98, 1991.
4. Meyers A: Modern management of acute diarrhea and dehydration in children, *Am Fam Physician* 51:1103-1115, 1995.
5. Deschênes M, Nazair P: La gaastro-entérite: déshydratation, réhydratation, *Med Quebec,* March 1994, pp 27-101.
6. Meyers A: Modern management of acute diarrhea and dehydration in children, *Am Fam Physician* 51:1103-1115, 1995.

ENURESIS

Most children gain daytime and nighttime bladder control by the age of 5. Enuresis is failure to achieve bladder control by this age. Enuresis is primary (no period of continence) in 90% of cases and secondary (reversion to incontinence after an extended period of dryness) in 10%. Secondary incontinence is often associated with psychological stress. Daytime incontinence is rare and needs a more thorough investigation than nocturnal enuresis.[1]

The overall incidence of nocturnal enuresis is about 10% to 20% among 5-year-olds, 5% to 7% among 10-year-olds, and 2% to 4% among 12- to 14-year-olds. The spontaneous remission rate is 15% per year. Boys are affected twice as often as girls. Enuresis may be familial; if one parent was affected, the incidence among the offspring is 40%, and if both parents were affected, the incidence is 70%.[1,2]

If by history and physical examination (including a careful neurological examination) no abnormalities are detected other than nocturnal enuresis, the only investigations required are a urinalysis and urine culture.[1]

Numerous treatment regimens have been used, and most have a reported success rate of 50% to 70%. Even when treatment is successful, frequent relapses occur when the programs are discontinued. Alarm systems are triggered by sensor pads that detect moisture. The older systems use a pad on which the child sleeps, and the newer ones use a small Velcro pad that is attached to the child's undergarments.[2] Alarm systems are often used initially, since adverse effects are few and the reported success rates are about 70%.[1,2]

Drugs that may be used for primary nocturnal enuresis include imipramine (Tofranil) 25 to 50 mg hs (maximum 2.5 mg/kg/day) and desmopressin (DDAVP) 10 to 40 µg (1 to 4 sprays) intranasally hs. The recurrence rate after discontinuing medication is high, so some workers suggest that use of drugs be restricted to special occasions such as sleepovers.[2]

Charting dry nights with appropriate rewards for success is common to many programs, but its therapeutic efficacy is uncertain. It does serve as a record for the child, parents, and physician. Fluid restriction in the evenings is frequently suggested, but its value also has not been proved.[1] A complex home program called dry-bed training incorporates a wide variety of the nonpharmacological treatments, including alarms, and may have value for children who do not respond to simpler therapeutic modalities.[1]

REFERENCES

1. Ullom-Minnich MR: Diagnosis and management of nocturnal enuresis, *Am Fam Physician* 54:2259-2266, 1996.
2. Tietjen DN, Husmann DA: Nocturnal enuresis: a guide to evaluation and treatment, *Mayo Clin Proc* 71:857-862, 1996.

ERYTHEMA INFECTIOSUM

Erythema infectiosum is also called fifth disease.[1,2] It is caused by human parvovirus B19. Clinical manifestations begin with nonspecific symptoms, including headache, coryza, and mild fever. After a few days the typical pruritic rash appears on the cheeks ("slapped-cheek" appearance). It tends to spread to the trunk and extremities and lasts 2 to 4 days. Infection is thought to be spread by respiratory secretions, but by the time the rash has appeared, the child can no longer spread infection.

Erythema infectiosum or fifth disease is one of six classic childhood exanthems.[1] The others are measles (rubeola), German measles (rubella), scarlet fever, Filatov-Dukes disease, and exanthema subitum (roseola infantum). Filatov-Dukes disease is only of historical interest. It was the fourth exanthem to be recognized, and when it was described at the turn of the last century, it was thought to be a specific infection. In fact it is usually a variant of scarlet fever but may also result from staphylococcal toxins. As might be inferred, erythema infectiosum was the fifth exanthem to be described.

A potentially serious complication of erythema infectiosum is infection of a pregnant woman. Parvovirus B19 is known to cause nonimmune hydrops fetalis.[3] The pathogenesis is infection and hemolysis of the fetal red cells. Although some cases have been treated with intrauterine exchange transfusions, others, diagnosed and followed by ultrasound, have resolved spontaneously.[5,6]

REFERENCES

1. Kirchner JT: Erythema infectiosum and other parvovirus B19 infections, *Am Fam Physician* 50:335-341, 1994.
2. Feder H Jr: Fifth disease (Images in Clinical Medicine), *N Engl J Med* 331:1062, 1994.
3. Yaegashi N, Okamura K, Yajima A, et al: The frequency of human parvovirus B19 infection in nonimmune hydrops fetalis, *J Perinat Med* 22:159-163, 1994.
4. Torok TJ, Wang QY, Gary GW Jr, et al: Prenatal diagnosis of intrauterine infection with parvovirus B19 by the polymerase chain reaction technique, *Clin Infect Dis* 14:149-155, 1992.
5. Sheikh AU, Ernest JM, O'Shea M: Long-term outcome in fetal hydrops from parvovirus B19 infection, *Am J Obstet Gynecol* 167:337-341, 1992.
6. Pryde PG, Nugent CE, Pridjian G, et al: Spontaneous resolution of nonimmune hydrops fetalis secondary to human parvovirus B19 infection, *Obstet Gynecol* 79:859-861, 1992.

FEBRILE SEIZURES

(See also fever in children; seizures)

Are children without evident neurological disorders who have febrile seizures at greater risk for epilepsy than other children? Population studies in both the United States and the United Kingdom show that in most cases the risk increase is very small.[1-4] For example, the background risk for epilepsy in the general population of children is 1.4%, and among children with simple febrile seizures it is about 2.4%. However, the relatively small subgroup of children with "complex" febrile seizures (defined as focal, lasting more than 15 minutes, or recurring during the same febrile illness) are at higher risk for seizure disorders.[1,2] In one study the rate was 6% to 8% among children with only one "complex" feature, 17% to 22% among those with two, and 49% among those with three.[1]

In one study children with a history of febrile seizures were selected at random to receive an initial rectal dose of diazepam followed in 6 hours by diazepam 0.2 mg/kg po tid plus placebo; acetaminophen 10 mg/kg qid plus placebo; a combination of diazepam and acetaminophen; or two different placebos during subsequent febrile episodes. The rate of febrile seizures was identical in all groups.[5] Whether acetaminophen 15 mg/kg would have been more effective is unknown.

REFERENCES

1. Annegars JF, Hauser WA, Shirts SB, et al: Factors prognostic of unprovoked seizures after febrile convulsions, *N Engl J Med* 316:493-498, 1987.
2. Verity CM, Golding J: Risk of epilepsy after febrile convulsions: a national cohort study, *BMJ* 303:1373-1376, 1991.
3. Robinson RJ: Febrile convulsions: further reassuring news about prognosis (editorial), *BMJ* 303:1345-1346, 1991.
4. Shinnar S, Berg AT, Moshe SL, et al: The risk of seizure recurrence after a first unprovoked afebrile seizure in childhood—an extended follow-up, *Pediatrics* 98:216-225, 1996.
5. Uhari M: Effect of acetaminophen and of low intermittent doses of diazepam on prevention of recurrences of febrile seizures, *J Pediatr* 126:991-995, 1995.

FEVER IN CHILDREN

(See also febrile seizures; fever; urinalysis)

Various types of thermometers and the ability of parents to determine whether their children are febrile are discussed under "Fever."

Antipyretics

The traditional symptomatic treatment of fever in children is acetaminophen (Tempra) in doses of 10 to 15 mg/kg q4-6h. A double-blind study of febrile children under 12 years of age compared ibuprofen (Advil, Motrin) 20 mg/kg/day with acetaminophen (Tempra, Tylenol) 50 mg/kg/day. No difference in efficacy or adverse effects was observed.[1]

When acetaminophen is prescribed for children, it is important to remember that drops are more concentrated than syrups and that various strengths of both chewable and regular tablets are available.

Sponging

Sponging is rarely if ever indicated except when temperatures exceed 40° to 41° C. If this technique is used, a single oral dose of an antipyretic should be given first and the sponging fluid should be lukewarm (neutral to the touch). Cold water or alcohol should never be used. Cold water causes shivering and raises body temperature, while alcohol may be inhaled and cause hypoglycemia and coma.[2]

Fever Without Source

The common practice for fever of unknown origin in children under 3 months of age has been to do a complete workup for sepsis and to treat them with antibiotics pending culture results. In some cases this may not be necessary.[3-6] The main reason for an aggressive approach to this problem was that before mass immunization for *Haemophilus influenzae,* meningitis developed in 5% to 10% of children who had fever without source. At present *Streptococcus pneumoniae* is the causative organism in the majority of cases that are found to be bacteremic. This bacterium rarely causes meningitis in young infants, and most cases resolve without treatment.[3,4]

Baraff and associates[3] suggest the following management protocols for children with rectal temperatures of 38° C (100.4° F) or higher and no clinically evident focus of infection.

Infants under 28 days

All infants under 28 days of age, with or without a toxic appearance, should be admitted to the hospital and have a complete workup for sepsis, including blood, urine, and cerebrospinal fluid cultures. Most cases are treated with parenteral antibiotics pending culture results. For selected "low-risk" (criteria listed below) infants who do not appear toxic, acceptable management would be the same sepsis workup with careful observation but no antibiotic therapy pending culture results.

Infants 28 to 90 days

A variety of approaches may be taken for infants between the ages of 28 and 90 days. If they appear toxic, they should be admitted to the hospital, have a complete sepsis workup, including blood, urine, and cerebrospinal fluid cultures, and be treated with parenteral antibiotics pending culture results.

Two options exist for the management of fever in "low-risk" infants in this age range. (Low risk is defined as previously healthy, nontoxic, no evidence of focal infection [excluding otitis media], white blood cell count of 5000 to 15,000/mm^3 [5 to 15 $\times$ 10^9/L], fewer than 1500 band cells/mm^3 [1.5 $\times$ 10^9/L], normal urinalysis findings, and if diarrhea is present, fewer than 5 white blood cells per high-power field in stool.) Both approaches may be followed on an outpatient basis provided the parents are reliable and close follow-up can be ensured. Protocol 1 is a sepsis work-up, including blood, urine, and cerebrospinal fluid cultures. Ceftriaxone 50 mg/kg (maximum 1 g) intramuscularly is given stat, and follow-up takes place within 24 hours. At follow-up a second dose of ceftriaxone may be given. Protocol 2 involves no sepsis workup other than a urine culture, no antibiotics (unless needed to treat otitis media), careful observation by parents, and physician follow-up within 24 hours.

Children aged 3 to 36 months

Toxic-appearing children should be admitted to the hospital, have a complete sepsis workup, including blood, urine, and cerebrospinal fluid cultures, and be treated with parenteral antibiotics pending culture results.

The management of previously healthy, non-toxic-appearing children aged 3 to 36 months depends on the rectal temperature. If it is below 39° C (102.2° F), no diagnostic tests or antibiotics are needed. The child should be treated as an outpatient with acetaminophen 15 mg/kg/dose q4h and should be reassessed if the fever persists for more than 48 hours or if the clinical condition deteriorates. If the temperature is 39° C (102° F) or higher, management may in most cases be on an outpatient basis after the following workup:

1. Urine culture for boys under 6 months of age and girls under 2 years of age or for any child who has a positive urine dipstick test for leukocyte esterase or nitrites. Urine dipsticks may be negative in up to 20% of young children with urinary tract infections, which is why culture is recommended for all young children regardless of the dipstick results.
2. Stool cultures if stool contains blood and mucus or more than 5 white blood cells per high-power field
3. Chest x-ray examination if respiratory symptoms are present
4. Blood cultures for all children in this category or for those with a white blood cell count of 15,000/mm^3 (15 $\times$ 10^9/L) or higher
5. Antibiotics either for all children in this category or for those with a white blood cell count of 15,000/mm^3 (15 $\times$ 10^9/L) or higher
6. Acetaminophen 15 mg/kg per dose q4h
7. Follow-up in 24 to 48 hours

REFERENCES

1. McIntyre J, Hull D: Comparing efficacy and tolerability of ibuprofen and paracetamol in fever, *Arch Dis Child* 74:164-167, 1996.
2. Impicciatore P, Pandolfini C, Casella N, et al: Reliability of health information for the public on the World Wide Web: systematic survey of advice on managing fever in children at home, *BMJ* 314:1875-1881, 1997.
3. Baraff LJ, Bass JW, Fleisher GR, et al: Practice guideline for the management of infants and children 0-36 months of age with fever without source, *Pediatrics* 92:1-12, 1993.
4. Long SS: Antibiotic therapy in febrile children: "best-laid schemes . . .," *J Pediatr* 124:585-588, 1994.
5. Daaleman TP: Fever without source in infants and young children, *Am Fam Physician* 54:2503-2512, 1996.
6. Jaskiewicz JA, McCarthy CA, Richardson AC, et al: Febrile infants at low risk for serious bacterial infection—an appraisal of the Rochester criteria and implications for management, *Pediatrics* 94:390-396, 1994.

FORMULAS

(See also colic; breast feeding; diarrhea and dehydration in infants)

Infant formulas have as their bases cow's milk, soy, or protein hydrolysates (Table 57). The last are the most expensive. Almost all formulas come with and without iron fortification, and almost all are available as ready-to-feed, as liquid concentrates that require dilution, and as powders that require reconstitution. The first are the most expensive and the last the least.[1] With rare exceptions bottle-fed infants should probably receive iron-fortified formulas from birth because otherwise they are at risk for iron deficiency anemia.[1-4] (The iron is not really required until 4 to 6 months, but because parents rarely change the formulas begun in the neonatal period, iron-fortified formulas should be used from the beginning of bottle feeding.) The Canadian Task Force on the Periodic Health Examination gives iron-fortified formulas a "B" rating,[4] and the U.S. Preventive Services Task Force gives it a "C."[5]

Table 57 Selected Examples of Infant Formulas

Formula	Manufacturer and comments
Milk-Based Formulas	
Bonamil	Wyeth, casein dominant
Carnation Goodstart	Carnation, partial protein hydrolysate
Enfamil, Enfalac	Mead Johnson, whey-dominant protein
Lactofree, Enfalac Lactose Free	Mead Johnson, lactose free
SMA	Wyeth, whey dominant
Similac	Ross
Similac LF	Ross, lactose free
Soy-Based Formulas	
Enfalac Soy	Mead Johnson, contains sucrose
Prosobee	Mead Johnson, does not contain sucrose
Gerber Soy Formula	Gerber
Isomil	Ross
Nursoy	Wyeth
Soyalac	Nutricia–Loma Linda
Protein Hydrolysates	
Alimentum	Ross
Nutramigen	Mead Johnson

Most cow's milk–based formulas contain lactose (some are produced as lactose free), whereas soy-based formulas and protein hydrolysates do not. Traditionally infants with diarrhea were switched to non-lactose-containing formulas or to formulas diluted with water. A 1994 metaanalysis of 29 randomized trials found that if infants with severe dehydration were excluded, no benefit was achieved by switching to soy-based formulas or protein hydrolysates or by diluting formulas with water.[6]

A controversial issue is whether infantile colic responds to protein hydrolysates (see discussion of colic). The Committee on Nutrition of the American Academy of Pediatrics claims no evidence supports the use of protein hydrolysates for colic,[7] but papers keep appearing with contrary views.[8]

REFERENCES

1. Spencer JP: Practical nutrition for the healthy term infant, *Am Fam Physician* 54:138-144, 1996.
2. American Academy of Pediatrics, Committee on Nutrition: Iron-fortified infant formulas, *Pediatrics* 84:1114-1155, 1989.
3. National Committee, Canadian Pediatrics Society: Meeting the iron needs of infants and young children: an update, *Can Med Assoc J* 144:1451-1453, 1991.
4. Canadian Task Force on the Periodic Health Examination: *Clinical preventive health care,* Ottawa, 1994, Canadian Communication Group—Publishing, pp 244-255.
5. US Preventive Services Task Force: *Guide to clinical preventive services,* ed 2, Baltimore, 1996, Williams & Wilkins, pp 231-246.
6. Brown KH, Peerson JM, Fontaine O: Use of nonhuman milks in the dietary management of young children with acute diarrhea: a meta-analysis of clinical trials, *Pediatrics* 93:17-27, 1994.
7. American Academy of Pediatrics, Committee on Nutrition: Hypoallergenic infant formulas, *Pediatrics* 83:1068-1069, 1989.
8. Hill DJ, Hudson IL, Sheffield LJ, et al: A low allergen diet is a significant intervention in infantile colic: results of a community-based study, *J Allergy Clin Immunol* 96:886-892, 1995.

INTUSSUSCEPTION

Intussusception occurs most frequently between the ages of 5 and 9 months. Males are affected twice as often as females. The classic triad of vomiting, abdominal pain, and bloody diarrhea is seen in only one third of patients. The most common symptoms are colicky abdominal pain, irritability, and vomiting. Fever, lethargy, and diarrhea may also be presenting symptoms.[1]

REFERENCES

1. Winslow BT, Westfall JM, Nicholas RA: Intussusception, *Am Fam Physician* 54:213-217, 1996.

Pediatrics

LEAD POISONING

In October 1991 the U.S. Centers for Disease Control and Prevention (CDC) redefined lead poisoning by lowering acceptable blood lead levels from 25 µg/dl (1.21 µmol/L) to 10 µg/dl (0.48 µmol/L). Both the CDC and the American Academy of Pediatrics (APA) have recommended universal lead level screening for children younger than 6 years. This recommendation is controversial.[1,2]

REFERENCES

1. Reigart JR: Blood lead screening: the argument for it (editorial), *Am Fam Physician* 48:1369-1371, 1993.
2. Schoen EJ: Blood lead screening: the argument against it, *Am Fam Physician* (editorial), 48:1371-1372, 1377, 1993.

NEONATAL JAUNDICE

(See also breast feeding)

Unconjugated hyperbilirubinemia or physiological jaundice of the newborn is extremely common. It is more frequent and more severe in premature, Asian, and breast-fed infants. The unconjugated bilirubin tends to peak about the fourth day of life and then gradually declines over several weeks. The difference between normal full-term breast-fed and bottle-fed babies is that in most studies both the peaks and the duration of jaundice tend to be higher in the breast-fed babies.[1,2]

Gartner[2] has marshaled considerable evidence that the initial hyperbilirubinemia of the breast-fed infant is a form of starvation jaundice and that when feeding is started early and given frequently, the bilirubin peaks of breast-fed infants are not higher than those of bottle-fed babies. He has suggested that although bottle-fed babies may thrive on six feedings a day, breast-fed infants probably require 10 in the early days and weeks of life. According to him, breast-fed babies should not be given glucose and water supplementation because this decreases their milk intake.

The differential diagnosis of physiological jaundice must consider a wide variety of conditions, including extrahepatic and intrahepatic obstructions, liver disease, various metabolic abnormalities, hemolytic disorders, large hematomas, sepsis, hypothyroidism, and bowel obstruction.[1]

Not all jaundiced babies need extensive investigation. One set of recommendations is that further laboratory evaluations are indicated for jaundiced babies who are premature or sick and for those, even if well, who have a bilirubin level greater than 15 mg/dl (256 µmol/L). Initial tests, aside from total bilirubin, are measurement of direct bilirubin, a complete blood count and blood smear, a reticulocyte count, and for infants of Asian, African, or Mediterranean descent a glucose-6-phosphate dehydrogenase measurement. Elevations of conjugated bilirubin levels are always abnormal.[1]

When should physiological jaundice be treated? The reason for treatment is to prevent the development of kernicterus or bilirubin encephalopathy. Although there is reasonable evidence that moderate bilirubin elevations do not cause neurological sequelae in healthy full-term babies, no definitive data are available to determine the bilirubin level above which treatment is required, and so the physician must depend on "expert opinion." Because doubt exists about the total innocuousness of high bilirubin levels in a healthy full-term baby and phototherapy is relatively harmless, it should be used more frequently than tends to be the current practice.[3] Lasker[1] recommends starting light therapy or phototherapy when the bilirubin is 17 mg/dl (300 µmol/L) or higher and continuing treatments until the level is no higher than 12 mg/dl (200 µmol/L). Treatment is instituted at lower levels for low-weight neonates.[4] In most instances breast feeding may continue during the period of phototherapy, and this may be facilitated by home phototherapy.[5]

REFERENCES

1. Lasker MR, Holzman IR: Neonatal jaundice: when to treat, when to watch and wait, *Postgrad Med* 99:187-193, 197-198, 1996.
2. Gartner LM: On the question of the relationship between breastfeeding and jaundice in the first 5 days of life, *Semin Perinatol* 18:502-509, 1994.
3. Dennery PA, Rhine WD, Stevenson DK: Neonatal jaundice—what now? *Clin Pediatr* 34:103-107, 1995.
4. Bratlid D: Criteria for treatment of neonatal jaundice, *J Perinatol* 16:S83-S88, 1996.
5. James JM, Williams SD, Osborn LM: Discontinuation of breast-feeding infrequent among jaundiced neonates treated at home, *Pediatrics* 92:153-155, 1993.

PNEUMONIA IN CHILDREN

(See also pneumonia)

The incidence of pneumonia in North American children is highest before age 5 and then decreases. Risk factors include prematurity, low socioeconomic status, exposure to passive smoke, and attendance at day care.[1]

The World Health Organization has suggested that tachypnea (>50 breaths/min in infants up to 11 months and >40 breaths/min in children over 11 months) is a reasonably good indicator of pneumonia in children with cough and fever. Ideally, respiratory rate should be measured for 1 minute when the child is awake and not crying. Intercostal, subcostal, or suprasternal notch retraction suggests more severe disease. However, subsequent studies have shown that depending on respiratory rates alone leads to a failure of diagnosis in a number of cases and overdiagnosis in considerably more (sensitivity and specificity are not ideal). However, pneumonia can be excluded with confidence if the child lacks all the following signs: respiratory distress, tachypnea, crackles, and decreased breath sounds.[1]

The causative organisms of pneumonia in children are determined largely by age. Under the age of 2 years, viruses are predominant, but *Chlamydia trachomatis, Mycoplasma pneumoniae, Streptococcus pneumoniae, Haemophilus influenzae* type b, and nontypable *H. influenzae* cause some infections. Among children aged 2 or older, *S. pneumoniae, M. pneumoniae,* and *C. trachomatis* become the predominant pathogens, although the organisms primarily responsible for infections in infants and toddlers still account for a number of infections in this age group. *Staphylococcus aureus* is a cause of severe pneumonia necessitating admission to an intensive care unit in all age groups.[1]

Management varies with age and severity of infection. In general, children under the age of 3 months are admitted, as are those who are toxic, in severe respiratory distress, vomiting, or dehydrated or have not responded to oral antibiotics as outpatients. The recommended antibiotics for outpatient treatment of pneumonia in children, as outlined by a Canadian Consensus Panel of Pediatric Infectious Disease specialists and a microbiologist, are[1]:

1. For children 3 months to 5 years: amoxicillin 40 mg/kg/day in 3 divided doses, erythromycin 40 mg/kg/day in 4 divided doses, or clarithromycin (Biaxin) 15 mg/kg/day in 2 divided doses. Treatment duration for all regimens is 7 to 10 days.
2. For children 5 to 18 years: erythromycin 40 mg/kg/day in 4 divided doses or clarithromycin (Biaxin) 15 mg/kg/day in 2 divided doses. Treatment duration for both regimens is 7 days.

REFERENCES

1. Jadavji T, Law B, Lebel MG, et al: A practical guide for the diagnosis and treatment of pediatric pneumonia, *Can Med Assoc J* 156(suppl):S703-S711, 1997.

PREMATURITY

A follow-up study of surviving premature infants weighing less than 750 g at birth found that these children were at high risk for neurobehavioral dysfunction and poor school performance.[1] The rate of mental retardation (intelligence quotient below 70) was 21% versus 2% in the control group of full-term children, the rate of cerebral palsy was 9% versus none, and the rate of severe visual disability was 25.5% versus 2%. Children weighing between 750 and 1499 g at birth also had higher disability rates in all categories but to a lesser degree than the children under 750 g at birth.[1]

A prospective evaluation of premature births in northern England found that one fourth of those born at less than 26 weeks of gestation and surviving past 1 year had severe disabilities. Ten percent were incapable of meaningful communication or independent mobility.[2]

A study from McMaster University of adolescents who had been extremely low-birth-weight infants (less than 1000 g) found that these children had significantly more limitations in the areas of cognition, sensation, self-care, and pain compared with the control group. Despite this the majority viewed their health-related quality of life as quite satisfactory.[3]

REFERENCES

1. Hack M, Taylor G, Klein N, et al: School-age outcomes in children with birth weights under 750g, *N Engl J Med* 331:753-759, 1994.
2. Tin W, Wariyar U, Hey E (Northern Neonatal Network): Changing prognosis for babies of less than 28 weeks' gestation in the north of England between 1983 and 1994, *BMJ* 314:107-111, 1997.
3. Saigal S, Feeny D, Rosenbaum P, et al: Self-perceived health status and health-related quality of life of extremely low-birth-weight-infants at adolescence, *JAMA* 276:453-459, 1996.

PUBERTY

Normally puberty begins in girls between the ages of 8 and 13 and in boys between the ages of 9 and 14. The initial manifestation of puberty is breast development or thelarche in 85% of girls and the growth of pubic hair in 15%. Acceleration in growth occurs at this stage. Pubic hair growth or pubarche usually begins 6 months after thelarche, and axillary hair appears 2 years after the development of pubic hair. Menarche follows thelarche by about 2 years. For boys the initial manifestation of puberty is almost always testicular enlargement, followed in about 6 months by the development of pubic hair. The penis enlarges 12 to 18 months after testicular enlargement, and facial and axillary hair appears 2 years after the development of pubic hair.[1]

Precocious puberty is defined as the development of secondary sexual characteristics before the age of 8 in girls and before the age of 9½ in boys. The most important differential diagnoses are isolated premature thelarche and isolated premature pubarche, since neither of these conditions is of clinical significance and neither requires treatment.[1,2] Diagnosing true precocious puberty is important because a few cases are caused by virilizing tumors and in other cases premature closure of the epiphyses leads to abnormally short adult stature.[1,2]

REFERENCES

1. Lee PA: Advances in the management of precocious puberty, *Clin Pediatr* 33:54-61, 1994.
2. Merke DP, Cutler GB Jr: Evaluation and management of precocious puberty, *Arch Dis Child* 75:269-271, 1996.

REYE'S SYNDROME

Reye's syndrome was first described in 1963. The major abnormalities are a fatty liver and encephalopathy. The disorder usually develops 5 to 7 days after the onset of a viral illness, and the major clinical manifestations are progressive vomiting, mental status changes, and eventually coma.[1] In the 1980s most cases were associated with aspirin use and the worst offenders among viral illnesses were influenza and chickenpox. Since the decreased use of aspirin among children, the incidence of Reye's syndrome has dropped remarkably, but cases still occur.[2] In the United States most cases of Reye's syndrome occur in children aged 4 to 12 with a peak incidence at age 6.[3] However, cases may occur into the late teens. Therefore children and adolescents of any age should avoid using aspirin if possible.

REFERENCES

1. Quam DA: Recognizing a case of Reye's syndrome, *Am Fam Physician* 50:1491-1496, 1994.
2. Baird RE, Foley C, Bresee J, et al: Reye's syndrome: lessons for family physicians (editorial), *Am Fam Physician* 50:1454-1461, 1994.
3. Reye syndrome surveillance—United States, 1989, *MMWR* 40: 88-90, 1991.

ROSEOLA INFANTUM

Roseola infantum is thought to be caused by human herpesvirus type 6 (HHV-6). The incubation period is 7 to 17 days with a mean of 10 days. Most cases occur between 6 and 18 months of age, and the disorder is rare over the age of 3.

SINGLE-PARENT FAMILIES

(See also abuse; antisocial personality disorder; poverty)

Approximately 24% of American children live with only one parent and another 15% live in melded families. About half of American children have or will have lived with one parent. Mothers head 86% of single-parent families, and 63% are white. Most single parents are in their twenties and thirties, and the situation is usually a result of separation or divorce.[1]

Births to unwed women increased in the United States from 18% in 1980 to 31% in 1995.[2] Part of this increase may be explained by a decrease in the birth rate among married women, and it must be also realized that 25% of single mothers are living in a common-law relationship. Although the out-of-wedlock birth rate has increased in teenagers, it has increased more sharply in women aged 20 to 29. The illegitimacy rate among blacks is about 2.5 times that among whites, but over the last decade there has been a decrease among blacks and an increase among whites. The most striking correlates of out-of-wedlock births are failure to graduate from high school and poverty.[2] Children, especially boys, who are subject to high-conflict divorce have a two to four times greater frequency of emotional and behavioral problems than is the norm in the community. Girls are particularly prone to respond poorly to court-ordered joint custody or frequent visitations.[3]

There is little evidence that welfare fosters single motherhood; a more likely explanation for the high rate of single parenthood among the poor is that disadvantaged young men and women do not feel that marriage is a realistic possibility.[2] While pregnancies and births among single teenagers have been increasing in the United States so that they are now among the highest in the developed world,[4] they have been decreasing in Sweden.[1] This may be related to a much higher level of contraceptive use and sex education in Sweden.[2]

One fact about adolescent pregnancies is that without intensive follow-up one third of these young women become pregnant again within the first year and nearly one half do so by the end of the second year.[5] Interventions to alter this pattern of behavior, such as peer support groups, are often failures.[6]

Children from single-parent families are at double the risk for behavioral problems, dropping out of high school, failing a grade, being out of work, and in the case of girls becoming teenage mothers. This applies across all economic levels, but the rates are halved in the better off.[1]

REFERENCES

1. McLanahan S, Sandefur G: *Growing up with a single parent: what hurts, what helps,* Cambridge, Mass, 1994, Harvard University Press.
2. Usdansky ML: Single motherhood: stereotypes vs. statistics, *New York Times,* February 11, 1996, Sect 4, p 4.
3. Meurer JR, Meurer LN, Holloway RL: Clinical problems and counseling for single-parent families, *Am Fam Physician* 54: 864-870, 1996.
4. Spitz AM, Velebil P, Koonin LM, et al: Pregnancy, abortion, and birth rates among US adolescents—1980, 1985, and 1990, *JAMA* 275:989-994, 1996.
5. Stevens-Simon C, White M: Adolescent pregnancy, *Pediatr Ann* 20:322-331, 1991.
6. Stevens-Simon C, Dolgan JI, Kelly L, et al: The effect of monetary incentives and peer support groups on repeat adolescent pregnancies: a randomized trial of the Dollar-a-Day program, *JAMA* 277:977-982, 1997.

SUDDEN INFANT DEATH SYNDROME

(See also cardiopulmonary resuscitation)

Important risk factors for sudden infant death syndrome (SIDS) include the following:

1. Sleeping in the prone position[1-3]
2. Sleeping on the side[1,2]
3. Sleeping in the mother's bed all night,[1,2] especially if she smokes[1]
4. Maternal smoking during pregnancy and postnatally[4,5]
5. Passive exposure to smoke[1,4,5]
6. Poverty[1]
7. Young maternal age[1]

Although not all studies agree,[6] the bulk of evidence suggests that an important preventive measure is to avoid sleeping in the prone position[1-3] and to ban cigarettes from the environment both antenatally and postnatally.[1,4,5]

REFERENCES

1. Brooke H, Gibson A, Tappin D, et al: Case-control study of sudden infant death syndrome in Scotland, 1992-95, *BMJ* 314: 1516-1520, 1997.
2. Fleming PJ, Blair PS, Bacon C, et al: Environment of infants during sleep and risk of the sudden infant death syndrome: results of 1993-5 case-control study for confidential inquiry into stillbirths and deaths in infancy, *BMJ* 313:191-195, 1996.
3. Hiley CM, Morley C: Risk factors for sudden infant death syndrome: further change in 1992-93, *BMJ* 312:1397-1398, 1996.

4. Blair PS, Fleming PJ, Bensley D, et al: Smoking and the sudden infant death syndrome: results from 1993-5 case-control study for confidential inquiry into stillbirths and deaths in infancy, *BMJ* 313:195-198, 1996.
5. Klonoff-Cohen HS, Edelstein SL, Lefkowitz ES, et al: The effect of passive smoking and tobacco exposure through breast milk on sudden infant death syndrome, *JAMA* 273:795-798, 1995.
6. Klonoff-Cohen HS, Edelstein SL: A case-control study of routine and death scene sleep position and sudden infant death syndrome in southern California, *JAMA* 273:790-794, 1995.

URINARY TRACT INFECTIONS IN CHILDREN

An ongoing controversy is whether one uncomplicated urinary tract infection without fever in a female child under 5 years necessitates a urological workup. One urologist's view is that it does not but that if she acquires a second infection, the workup should be done.[1]

REFERENCES

1. Charendoff M: Work-ups for UTI in young girls revisited, *Patient Care Can* 5:7, 10, 1994.

VARICELLA IN CHILDREN

(See also varicella; varicella vaccines)

Treatment of varicella in otherwise healthy children with acyclovir (Zovirax) is of questionable value. Defervescence may occur 1 to 2 days earlier than in untreated patients, and there may be fewer skin lesions. However, treatment does not appear to decrease the rate of transmission of the infection, reduce complications, or cause less scarring.[1] Immunization against varicella is discussed in the section on varicella vaccines.

REFERENCES

1. Balfour HH JR, Kelly JM, Suarez CS, et al: Acyclovir treatment of varicella in otherwise healthy children, *J Pediatr* 116:633-639, 1990.

PSYCHIATRY

Topics covered in this section

ABUSE

(See also adverse effects associated with low cholesterol levels; aggression; false memories; guns; homicide; psychological morbidity among Olympic-level athletes; single-parent families; suicide)

Childhood Abuse

Aside from the obvious types of childhood abuse, a more subtle form may be parental pressure for, or even compliance with, activities that lead to prestige and high income but at the risk of significant psychological or physical harm. Fashion modeling is one example. The winner of Ford Models Inc.'s Supermodel for the World in 1997 was a 15-year-old girl who, according to the *Toronto Globe and Mail,* lost 11 kg (22 lb) in the 2 years before winning.[1] With a height of 180 cm (5 feet 11 inches) and a weight of 55 kg (123 lb) she had a body mass index (BMI) of 17. According to the *Diagnostic and Statistical Manual of Mental Disorders,* edition 4 (DSM-IV), the diagnosis of anorexia nervosa should be considered in any adolescent with a BMI less than 17.5.[2]

One clue to child abuse is a history of running away.[3] Childhood abuse and neglect are associated with an increased rate of arrests for criminal behavior, including violent crimes.[4]

The Canadian Task Force on the Periodic Health Examination has given screening parents for risk of child abuse a "D" recommendation. This is because a high false-positive rate is associated with this type of screening and many parents who would never abuse their children would be labeled as at risk of doing so.[5] The U.S. Preventive Services Task Force does not deal with this issue.[6]

Domestic Violence

The lifetime prevalence of domestic violence is extraordinarily high.[7,8] According to one study, which defined domestic violence as an assault, threat, or intimidation by a male partner, the cumulative incidence was 54.2%.[8] Victims of domestic violence who go to emergency rooms for care are rarely questioned about it,[7,8] even though it is known that up to 20% of women seen in emergency rooms have been abused.[7] Part of the reason for this may be the reluctance of physicians to become involved with such issues.[9] In one study 3% of women seen in an emergency room and 11% of injured women were battered.[10] Although the injuries of abused women tended to be concentrated in the head, face, neck, thorax, and abdomen, the sensitivity and specificity of such injuries for abuse were low. The authors recommended universal screening for domestic violence among injured women.[10] In one emergency room study a single question asking patients whether anyone had punched, kicked, hit, or hurt them in some other way in the past year detected over two thirds of abused patients as established by a standardized 19-item questionnaire.[11]

Pregnant women appear to be more subject to both physical and sexual abuse than nonpregnant women.[12]

Elderly Abuse

Elderly abuse has been divided into the following categories[13]:

1. Physical violence
2. Psychological or emotional abuse
3. Material or financial exploitation
4. Neglect (intentional or unintentional)

The incidence of elderly abuse in the general population as determined by epidemiological surveys in the United States,[14] Canada,[15] and Great Britain is about 3%.[16] Two thirds of abuse cases are perpetrated by spouses and one third by adult offspring.[13] The degree of frailty of the older person has been considered a major risk for abuse, but this has not been substantiated by recent studies. Specific risk factors that have been identified among caregivers are a history of mental illness or substance abuse, a history of violent or antisocial behavior, and significant financial dependence on the elderly person.[13]

Although elderly abuse is obviously a serious issue, there does not seem to be evidence that physician screening for this problem is useful. Both the U.S. Preventive Services Task Force[17] and the Canadian Task Force on the Periodic Health Examination[18,19] give case finding for elderly abuse a "C" rating.

Sexual Abuse

A statewide anonymous survey of adolescent schoolchildren in a Midwestern state found a 10% prevalence of sexual abuse. The female/male ratio was 4:1, and the rate was twice as high among blacks and Native Americans as among whites. Girls who had been sexually abused as children were six times as likely to report later sexual victimization as were nonabused girls, while boys who had been sexually abused were twice as likely to report sexual aggression as were nonabused boys.[20]

A seven-page questionnaire on sexual abuse was administered to 1193 adolescents of both sexes in 17 schools in Geneva, Switzerland. Overall reported abuse rates were 33.8% for the girls and 10.9% for the boys. Abuse with physical contact occurred in 20.4% of the girls and 3.3% of the boys, and penetration was reported by 5.6% of the girls and 1.1% of the boys. Perpetrators were known to the children in two thirds of the cases, and family members were responsible for 20.5% of events against girls and 6.3% of events against boys. A little less than half the events were experienced before the age of 12.[21]

The lifetime risk of suicide attempts is increased in persons who have been sexually abused. This is particularly so for women who have been assaulted before the age of 16.[22]

Genital examination of girls who had been subject to penetration was normal in 44% of cases; an intact hymen did not rule out penetration.[23]

REFERENCES

1. Appleby T, Milner B: Fashion serves up girls as women, *Toronto Globe and Mail,* February 1, 1997, pp A1, A8.
2. American Psychiatric Association: *Diagnostic and statistical manual of mental disorders,* ed 4, Washington, DC, 1994, American Psychiatric Association, pp 539-545.
3. Lawrenson F: Runaway children: whose problem? A history of running away should be taken seriously: it may indicate abuse (editorial), *BMJ* 314:1064, 1997.
4. Maxfield MG, Widom CS: The cycle of violence—revisited 6 years later, *Arch Pediatr Adolesc Med* 150:390-395, 1996.
5. Canadian Task Force on the Periodic Health Examination: *Canadian guide to clinical preventive health care,* Ottawa, 1994, Canada Communication Group—Publishing, pp 320-332.
6. US Preventive Services Task Force: *Guide to clinical preventive services,* ed 2, Baltimore, 1996, Williams & Wilkins.
7. Council on Scientific Affairs, American Medical Association: Violence against women: relevance for medical practitioners, *JAMA* 267:3194-3195, 1992.
8. Abbott J, Johnson R, Koziol-McLain J, Lowenstein SR: Domestic violence against women: incidence and prevalence in an emergency department population, *JAMA* 273:1763-1767, 1995.
9. Sugg NK, Inui T: Primary care physicians' response to domestic violence: opening Pandora's box, *JAMA* 267:3157-3160, 1992.
10. Muelleman RL, Lenaghan PA, Pakieser RA: Battered women: injury locations and types, *Ann Emerg Med* 28:486-492, 1996.
11. Feldhaus KM, Koziol-Mclain J, Amsbury HL, et al: Accuracy of 3 brief screening questions for detecting partner violence in the emergency department, *JAMA* 277:1357-1361, 1997.
12. Mezey GC, Bewley S: Domestic violence and pregnancy: risk is greatest after delivery (editorial), *BMJ* 314:1295, 1997.
13. Lachs MS, Pillemer K: Abuse and neglect of elderly persons, *N Engl J Med* 332:437-443, 1995.
14. Pillemer K, Finkelhor D: The prevalence of elder abuse: a random sample survey, *Gerontologist* 28:51-57, 1988.
15. Podkieks I: National survey on abuse of the elderly in Canada, *J Elder Abuse Neglect* 4:5-58, 1992.
16. Ogg J, Bennett G: Elder abuse in Britain, *BMJ* 305:988-989, 1992.
17. US Preventive Services Task Force: *Guide to clinical preventive services,* ed 2, Baltimore, 1996, Williams & Wilkins, pp 555-565.
18. Canadian Task Force on the Periodic Health Examination: Periodic health examination, 1994 update. IV. Secondary prevention of elder abuse and mistreatment, *Can Med Assoc J* 151: 1413-1420, 1994.
19. Canadian Task Force on the Periodic Health Examination: *Canadian guide to clinical preventive health care,* Ottawa, 1994, Canada Communication Group—Publishing, pp 921-929.
20. Lodico MA, Gruber E, Diclemente RJ: Childhood sexual abuse and coercive sex among school-based adolescents in a Midwestern state, *J Adolesc Health* 18:211-217, 1996.
21. Halpérin DS, Bouvier P, Jaffé PD, et al: Prevalence of child sexual abuse among adolescents in Geneva: results of a cross sectional survey, *BMJ* 312:1326-1329, 1996.

22. Davidson JR, Hughes DC, George LK, Blazer DG: The association of sexual assault and attempted suicide within the community, *Arch Gen Psychiatry* 53:550-555, 1996.
23. Adams JA, Knudson S: Genital findings in adolescent girls referred for suspected sexual abuse, *Arch Pediatr Adolesc Med* 150:850-857, 1996

AGGRESSION

(See also abuse; guns; homicide; suicide)

On the basis of a literature search, the optimal drugs for short-term management of aggression seem to be high-potency antipsychotics or short-acting benzodiazepines. A variety of drugs have been used to treat chronic aggressive behavior. For adults without other psychiatric disorders lithium and propranolol (Inderal) are probably the first-line drugs.[1] Relatively high doses of propranolol also appear to be effective for pathological aggression in children.[2]

REFERENCES

1. Pabis DJ, Stanislav SW: Pharmacotherapy of aggressive behavior, *Ann Pharmacother* 30:278-287, 1996.
2. Simeon JG: Propranolol in aggressive children and adolescents, *Child Adolesc Psychopharmacol News* 2:11-12, 1997.

ANXIETY DISORDERS

(See also chest pain; depression; fibromyalgia; insomnia; palpitations; serotonin syndrome)

Classification

The following conditions are included under the rubric of anxiety disorders:

1. Generalized anxiety disorder
2. Panic disorder
3. Phobias (simple, social, agoraphobia)
4. Obsessive-compulsive disorder
5. Posttraumatic stress disorder

Nonpharmacological Therapy

Nonpharmacological therapy is an essential element of therapy for all the anxiety disorders. Discontinuing or at least diminishing central nervous system stimulants and depressants such as caffeine, alcohol, and hypnotic drugs is step one.[1] Step two is to initiate a regular aerobic exercise program because this has been shown to decrease anxiety.[2] For disorders such as panic attacks, phobic disorders, and obsessive-compulsive disorder, behavioral therapy is an effective element of therapy and medications should be considered important adjuncts.

Medications

Probably the most important principle for the family physician to remember about the pharmacotherapy of anxiety disorders is that benzodiazepines are not the drugs of first choice. Various classes of antidepressants (tricyclics, selective serotonin reuptake inhibitors [SSRIs], and monoamine oxidase [MAO] inhibitors) and buspirone (Table 58), all of which are nonaddictive, have proved to be at least as effective as benzodiazepines.[1,3-6]

Table 58 Pharmacotherapy of Anxiety Disorders

Drugs	Usual doses and comments
Benzodiazepines	Addictive; lead to rebound anxiety as blood levels drop; antidepressants usually preferable
Alprazolam (Xanax)	0.125-0.25 mg tid or qid
Clonazepam (Rivotril)	0.5 mg bid or tid
Diazepam (Valium)	2-10 mg bid-qid
Lorazepam (Ativan)	2-3 mg/day in 3 divided doses
Azapirones	
Buspirone (Buspar)	20-30 mg/day in 2 or 3 divided doses
Tricyclics	
Imipramine (Tofranil)	Panic and phobic disorder (low doses)
Desipramine (Norpramin, Pertofrane)	Panic and phobic disorder (low doses)
Nortriptyline (Aventyl)	Panic and phobic disorder (low doses)
Clomipramine (Anafranil)	Obsessive-compulsive disorder (high doses)
Selective Serotonin Reuptake Inhibitors	Panic and phobic disorder (low doses); obsessive-compulsive disorder (high doses)
Fluoxetine (Prozac)	
Fluvoxamine (Luvox)	
Paroxetine (Paxil)	
Sertraline (Zoloft)	
Monoamine Oxidase Inhibitors	Panic and phobic disorders
Phenelzine (Nardil)	30 mg qam and 15-30 mg at noon
Tranylcypromine (Parnate)	20 mg qam and 10 mg in the afternoon
Beta-Blockers	Focused social phobias (performance anxiety)
Atenolol (Tenormin)	Single dose, start low and increase prn
Nadolol (Corgard)	Single dose, start low and increase prn
Oxprenolol (Trasicor)	Single dose, start low and increase prn
Propranolol (Inderal)	Single dose, start low and increase prn

Buspirone (Buspar) is a member of a class of antianxiety agents that is not sedative, has little potential for abuse, and is not associated with withdrawal symptoms. Its primary use is for chronic anxiety states, particularly generalized anxiety disorder,[5,6] but it also has some antidepressant effects and has been used for augmentation therapy of SSRIs in the treatment of depression.[6] Other reported benefits are a reduction in irritability and aggressiveness in dementia or other organic brain disorders[6] and a reduction of anxiety in alcoholics.[6,7] It has no value in panic attacks. A period of 2 or 3 weeks is required for full therapeutic effect, and the drug has to be taken three times a day. Adverse effects are relatively mild; short periods of lightheadedness may occur half an hour after ingesting the medication.[6]

The tricyclic antidepressants imipramine (Tofranil), desipramine (Norpramin, Pertofrane), and nortriptyline (Aventyl) have all been shown to be effective in panic disorders.

For this condition low doses should be used. Starting with 10 mg/day and raising the dose slowly is often advisable.[8] For obsessive-compulsive disorder clomipramine (Anafranil) is the tricyclic of choice.[9,10] Many patients require high doses, with a reported effective range of 100 to 250 mg/day.[11]

SSRIs are effective agents for panic attacks,[12-16] phobic disorders,[16-19] and obsessive-compulsive disorder.[9-11,20,21] In general, doses are low for phobic disorders and panic attacks and high for obsessive-compulsive disorder. A metaanalysis of the pharmacotherapy of panic disorder found that not only were SSRIs more effective than placebo, but also they were more effective than imipramine (Tofranil) or alprazolam (Xanax).[3]

Although rarely used now, the MAO inhibitors phenelzine (Nardil) and tranylcypromine (Parnate) are effective in panic disorders[22,23] and phobic disorders.[16,17]

Beta-blockers are often useful for limited or focused social phobias (performance anxiety) such as may occur before making a speech, performing on a musical instrument, or taking an examination.[16,17] Positive results have been reported with single doses of atenolol (Tenormin) 100 mg, nadolol (Corgard) 40 mg, oxprenolol (Trasicor) 40 mg, and propranolol (Inderal) 40 mg.[16] Patients should take a test dose before any important performance to ensure that no unexpected adverse effects occur.[17]

Phobias may be a symptom of underlying depression. Treatment of the depression by the usual means often leads to resolution of the phobias.[17]

Obsessive-compulsive disorder

The lifetime prevalence of obsessive-compulsive disorder is 2% to 3%. It is the fourth most common psychiatric disorder after substance abuse, phobias, and affective disorders. It has a higher prevalence rate than panic disorders or schizophrenia. Obsessive-compulsive disorder often begins in childhood. It is rare for the onset to occur over the age of 40. Slightly more females than males are affected.[24]

Behavioral therapy is almost always an essential component of the therapy of obsessive-compulsive disorder, but medications play an important role. Patients with obsessive-compulsive disorder are often slow to respond to medications and often require larger doses of antidepressants than are necessary for depression. Once they respond, they will probably require long-term or indefinite therapy because of the high relapse rate with discontinuation of medications.[24]

The tricyclic antidepressant clomipramine (Anafranil) has long been known to be effective in the treatment of obsessive-compulsive disorder. For some it is still the drug of choice.[9,10] The dosage range for obsessive-compulsive disorder is 100 to 250 mg.[11] SSRIs are effective drugs for obsessive-compulsive disorder. Fluoxetine (Prozac),[9,20,21] fluvoxamine (Luvox),[9,10] and sertraline (Zoloft)[9] are all effective if given long enough and in high enough doses. In a recent metaanalysis of drugs used for the treatment of obsessive-compulsive disorder, clomipramine (Anafranil), fluoxetine, fluvoxamine, and sertraline were all more effective than placebo, but of the four, clomipramine appeared to be the most effective.[9] In a comparison of clomipramine (100 to 250 mg/day) and fluvoxamine (100 to 250 mg/day), both were equally effective. Fluvoxamine caused more headaches and insomnia, and clomipramine produced more anticholinergic side effects and sexual dysfunction.[10]

The dosage range for fluoxetine in obsessive-compulsive disorder is 20 to 80 mg/day, and that for fluvoxamine is 100 to 300 mg/day.[11]

REFERENCES

1. Antony MM, Swinson RP: *Anxiety disorders and their treatment: a critical review of the evidence-based literature,* Ottawa, 1996, Publications Health Canada, pp 1-101.
2. Petruzello SJ, Landers DM, Hatfield BD, et al: A meta-analysis on the anxiety-reducing effects of acute and chronic exercise, *Sports Med* 11:143-182, 1991.
3. Boyer W: Serotonin uptake inhibitors are superior to imipramine and alprazolam in alleviating panic attacks: a meta-analysis, *Int Clin Psychopharmacol* 10:45-49, 1995.
4. Piccinelli M, Pini S, Bellantuono C, et al: Efficacy of drug treatment in obsessive-compulsive disorder: a meta-analytic review, *Br J Psychol* 166:424-443, 1995.
5. Gammans RE, Stringfellow JC, Hvizdos AJ, et al: Use of buspirone in patients with generalized anxiety disorder and coexisting depressive symptoms: a meta-analysis of eight randomised controlled trials, *Neuropsychobiology* 25:193-201, 1992.
6. Cadieux RJ: Azapirones: an alternative to benzodiazepines for anxiety, *Am Fam Physician* 53:2349-2353, 1996.
7. Kranzler HR, Burleson JA, Del Boca FK, et al: Buspirone treatment of anxious alcoholics: a placebo-controlled trial, *Arch Gen Psychiatry* 51:720-731, 1994.
8. Bakish D, Swinson RP: Panic disorder: strategies that work, *Patient Care Can,* April 1994, 5:23-32.
9. Greist JH, Jefferson JW, Kobak KA, et al: Efficacy and tolerability of serotonin transport inhibitors in obsessive-compulsive disorder—a meta-analysis, *Arch Gen Psychiatry* 52:53-56, 1995.
10. Freeman CP, Trimble MR, Deakin JF, et al: Fluvoxamine versus clomipramine in the treatment of obsessive-compulsive disorder: a multicenter, randomized, double-blind, parallel group comparison, *J Clin Psychiatry* 55:301-305, 1994.
11. Fluvoxamine for obsessive-compulsive disorder, *Med Lett* 37: 13-14, 1995.
12. Louie AK, Lewis TB, Lannon RA: Use of low-dose fluoxetine in major depression and panic disorder, *J Clin Psychiatry* 54: 435-438, 1993.
13. Black DW, Wesner RB, Gabel J, et al: Predictors of short-term treatment response in 66 patients with panic disorder, *J Affect Dis* 30:233-241, 1994.
14. Hoehn-Saric R, McLeaod DR, Hipsley PA: Effect of fluvoxamine on panic disorder, *J Clin Psychopharmacol* 13:321-326, 1993.
15. Oehrberg S, Christiansen PE, Behnke K, et al: Paroxetine in the treatment of panic disorder: a randomised, double-blind, placebo-controlled study, *Br J Psychiatry* 167:374-379, 1995.
16. Jefferson JW: Social phobia: everyone's disorder? *J Clin Psychiatry* 57(suppl 6):28-32, 1996.

17. Jefferson JW: Social phobia: a pharmacologic treatment overview, *J Clin Psychiatry* 56(suppl 5):18-24, 1995.
18. Van Ameringen M, Mancini C, Streiner DL: Fluoxetine efficacy in social phobia, *J Clin Psychiatry* 54:27-32, 1993.
19. Mancini C, Van Ameringen M: Paroxetine in social phobia, *J Clin Psychiatry* 57:519-522, 1996.
20. Pigott TA, Pato MT, Bernstein SE, et al: Controlled comparisons of clomipramine and fluoxetine in the treatment of obsessive-compulsive disorder: behavioral and biological results, *Arch Gen Psychiatry* 47:926-932, 1990.
21. Montgomery SA, McIntyre A, Osterheider M, et al (Lilly European OCD Study Group): A double-blind, placebo-controlled study of fluoxetine in patients with DSM-III R obsessive-compulsive disorder, *Eur Neuropsychopharmacol* 3:143-152, 1993.
22. Klerman GL: Treatments for panic disorder, *J Clin Psychiatry* 53(suppl):14-19, 1992.
23. Bowden CL: Psychopharmacological treatment of panic disorder, *Bull Menninger Clin* 56(2 suppl A):A29-A41, 1992.
24. Warneke L: Anxiety disorders: focus on obsessive-compulsive disorder, *Can Fam Physician* 39:1612-1621, 1993.

CREATIVITY

A popular belief is that creative artists are more prone to psychopathology than is the general population. To elucidate this issue, Post[1] read 350 biographies of world-famous creative persons in an attempt to measure the presence or absence of psychiatric disorders. He found that personality deviations were increased among visual artists and writers. Alcoholism was common among writers, artists, and composers, and depression was frequent among writers. Scientists were, as a group, mentally stable.[1] (And boring?)

REFERENCES

1. Post F: Creativity and psychopathology: a study of 291 world-famous men, *Br J Psychiatry* 165:22-34, 1994.

EATING DISORDERS

(See also diabetic retinopathy)

The incidence of eating disorders is increased among women with insulin-dependent diabetes mellitus (IDDM). The disorder may be bulimia or anorexia. Some women skip or reduce insulin doses in an attempt to lose weight.[1] Persons who have IDDM with eating disorders are at increased risk of retinopathy (see section on diabetic retinopathy).

A school survey of thousands of adolescents in Minnesota found that those who had unhealthy weight loss behaviors as manifested by induced vomiting or the use of diet pills, laxatives, or diuretics had a higher incidence of other maladjusted behavior patterns such as suicide attempts, alcohol, tobacco, and drug use, unprotected sexual intercourse, and multiple sex partners.[2]

REFERENCES

1. Jacobson AM: The psychological care of patients with insulin-dependent diabetes mellitus, *N Engl J Med* 334:1249-1253, 1996.
2. Neumark-Sztainer D, Story M, French SA: Covariations of unhealthy weight loss behaviors and other high-risk behaviors among adolescents, *Arch Pediatr Adolesc Med* 150:304-308, 1996.

Anorexia Nervosa

(See also Addison's disease; amenorrhea; bulimia; female athletes)

Along with the behavior patterns described in DSM-IV, anorexia nervosa should be seriously considered in any adolescent or young adult with a BMI (weight in kilograms/height in square meters) of less than 17.5.[1]

Epidemiology

Anorexia nervosa can be a fatal disease, and crude mortality rates as high as 18% have been reported.[2] The cause of death is usually an arrhythmia, often during sleep. One criterion for an urgent medical admission is a daytime pulse below 50 or a blood pressure of 90/50 mm Hg or less.

The prevalence rate of anorexia nervosa is approximately 1%, whereas that of bulimia is 2% to 4%.[3] Some authors have reported a doubling of the incidence of eating disorders in the last two decades.[3] The ratio of women to men for anorexia nervosa is 10 to 20:1. Anorexia is rare in prepubertal children, particularly in boys. Tumors affecting the hypothalamus or brainstem may be the cause of an anorexia-like symptom complex, and sometimes repeated neuroradiological examinations are necessary to detect them.[4]

The cultural pressures fostering anorexia are symbolized by the everlastingly popular Barbie dolls, which were introduced in 1959. Apparently the doll was in part modeled on a German streetwalker doll named Lilli. One of the cofounders of the company that manufactures Barbie had designers take Lilli and make her look more "wholesome."[5] A recent backlash against the gender stereotyping manifested by Barbie has been a form of creative vandalism under the auspices of the "Barbie Liberation Organization." Members of the group buy talking GI Joe action figures and talking Barbies, exchange the computerized voice chips, repackage the dolls, and surreptitiously put them back on store shelves. As a result, GI Joe issues the war cry "Wanna go shopping?" while Barbie commands "Eat lead, Cobra."[6]

Physical findings

Aside from emaciation, other features of starvation may be seen in patients with advanced anorexia. These include muscle weakness, dry skin with desquamation, yellow palms and soles, thinning of scalp or pubic hair, lanugo hair, bradycardia, hypotension, arrhythmias, and edema of the lower extremities.[3,7]

Differential diagnosis

The differential diagnosis of anorexia nervosa includes panhypopituitarism, Addison's disease, hyperthyroidism, hypothyroidism, diabetes mellitus, and malabsorption syndromes. A pituitary or hypothalamic tumor may be the most difficult condition to differentiate from anorexia nervosa.

Unacknowledged bulimia is often associated with anorexia nervosa. This is sometimes suspected if the serum amylase level is elevated. In patients with anorexia nervosa, amenorrhea secondary to hypothalamic-pituitary dysfunction is common with associated reductions in follicle-stimulating hormone (FSH) and luteinizing hormone (LH).

Investigations

Many laboratory abnormalities have been described in patients with anorexia nervosa, and these are discussed below. However, it is imperative to realize that the "routine" tests usually done in an emergency room setting may be entirely normal even though the patient is in imminent danger of death from a cardiac arrhythmia.

The most common laboratory abnormality in anorexia nervosa is probably anemia, which may be associated with leukopenia and thrombocytopenia. The cause of the anemia may be iron, folate, or vitamin B_{12} deficiency. As stated previously, FSH and LH levels are often reduced, the growth hormone level is elevated in half of the cases, and elevated prolactin and cortisol levels are common. Antidiuretic hormone may be suppressed with resultant polyuria. Some patients manifest the euthyroid sick syndrome. Hepatic enzyme concentrations may be slightly elevated, probably as a result of a fatty liver, and the blood urea nitrogen (BUN) and creatinine levels may be elevated from volume depletion. Hypocalcemia, hypomagnesemia, and hypophosphatemia occur. The last is a particularly ominous sign. Electrolyte abnormalities may result from vomiting or diuretic abuse. The cholesterol level is sometimes elevated.

Laboratory investigations for patients with suspected anorexia nervosa should include a complete blood count (and if that patient is anemic, ferritin and iron studies, folate, and vitamin B_{12}), electrolytes, BUN and creatinine, fasting glucose, calcium, phosphorus, magnesium, amylase (as a screen for associated bulimia), thyroid-stimulating hormone (TSH), prolactin, FSH, LH, and growth hormone.[3,7]

Bone density evaluations often show marked osteoporosis, particularly in amenorrheic patients. This test may be worth performing as a therapeutic maneuver because a low result sometimes acts as an effective stimulus to the patient to start eating again. Computed tomography of the brain may be necessary to rule out a hypothalamic or pituitary tumor.

Management

Weight gain to prevent death or severe morbidity from osteoporosis is the immediate goal of treatment. For preventing osteoporosis it is important that amenorrheic women regain sufficient weight to permit functioning of the hypothalamic-pituitary-ovarian axis. In one study menses returned within 6 months in most women whose body weight returned to within 90% of "standard body weight" charts. The actual weight for return of menses was 2 kg (4.4 lb) more than the weight at which menses ceased. Rise of serum estradiol to levels of 110 pmol/L (30 pg/ml) showed a good correlation with return of menses. Other indicators of improvement are an increase in ovarian size or the presence of a dominant ovarian follicle on ultrasonography.[8] Although weight gain is the ideal way of preventing osteoporosis, oral contraceptives have been shown to increase bone density in some patients with anorexia nervosa and amenorrhea (see amenorrhea).[9]

The consensus in the literature is that unlike bulimia, antidepressants of any type are ineffective for anorexia nervosa.[10-12] A few small open trials have shown a positive effect on anorexia with the use of fluoxetine (Prozac).[12,13] Until placebo-controlled trials confirming these results are reported, this drug should probably not be used for the treatment of anorexia.

REFERENCES

1. American Psychiatric Association: *Diagnostic and statistical manual of mental disorders,* ed 4, Washington, DC, 1994, American Psychiatric Association, pp 539-545.
2. Theander S: Outcome and prognosis in anorexia nervosa and bulimia: some results of previous investigations, compared with those of a Swedish long-term study, *J Psychiatr Res* 19: 493-508, 1985.
3. Comerci GD: Medical complications of anorexia nervosa and bulimia nervosa, *Med Clin North Am* 74:1293-1310, 1990.
4. DeVile CJ, Sufraz R, Lask BD, et al: Occult intracranial tumours masquerading as early onset anorexia nervosa, *BMJ* 311:1359-1360, 1995.
5. Kesterton M: Social studies, *Toronto Globe and Mail,* November 24, 1994, p A26.
6. Strauss S: Barbie seeks vengeance, *Toronto Globe and Mail,* December 22, 1994, p A12.
7. Sharp CW, Freeman CPL: The medical complications of anorexia nervosa, *Br J Psychiatry* 162:452-462, 1993.
8. Golden NH, Jacobson MS, Schebendach J, et al: Resumption of menses in anorexia nervosa, *Arch Pediatr Adolesc Med* 151: 16-21, 1997.
9. Hergenroeder AC, O'Brian Smith E, Shypailo R, et al: Bone mineral changes in young women with hypothalamic amenorrhea treated with oral contraceptives, medroxyprogesterone, or placebo over 12 months, *Am J Obstet Gynecol* 176:1017-1025, 1997.
10. Leach AM: The psychopharmacotherapy of eating disorders, *Psychiatr Ann* 25:628-633, 1995.
11. Crow SJ, Mitchell JE: Rational therapy of eating disorders, *Drugs* 48:372-379, 1994.
12. Advokat C, Kutlesic V: Pharmacotherapy of the eating disorders: a commentary, *Neurosci Biobehav Rev* 19:59-66, 1995.
13. Kaye WH, Weltzin TE, Hsu LG, et al: An open trial of fluoxetine in patients with anorexia nervosa, *J Clin Psychiatry* 52: 464-471, 1991.

Bulimia

(See also Addison's disease; anorexia nervosa)

The incidence of bulimia is estimated to be between 2% and 4%, and some workers in the field believe that the incidence has doubled in the past two decades.[1] Over half of bulimic patients have a past history of anorexia, usually of the milder form. One worker has estimated that in time twice as many persons with restrictive anorexia become bulimic as bulimics become restrictive anorectics.[2]

Characteristic physical findings in bulimia include the following[1,3]:

1. Parotid swelling ("chipmunk cheeks") seen in about 25% of patients
2. Calluses or red marks on the backs of the hands (Russell sign) as a result of trauma from teeth during induced vomiting
3. Damaged teeth from acid erosion of enamel. This is usually on the lingual surfaces in contrast to erosions from excessive intake of soft drinks or from sucking lemons, which are usually on the facial surfaces.

A number of laboratory tests may be abnormal in patients with bulimia. About 50% have an elevated amylase level. Other common abnormalities reflect a hypokalemic hypochloremic alkalosis induced by vomiting; a urine pH greater than 8 (25% of cases), decreased potassium and chloride levels, and an increased bicarbonate level. The sodium concentration is usually normal. Electrolyte abnormalities may persist for 2 to 7 days after the last binge.

The natural history of bulimia has not been well defined. According to one review of 88 studies in which follow-up took place, about half of bulimic women fully recovered by 5 to 10 years, 20% still met the criteria for bulimia, and the remainder experienced relapses. Relapses were most common in the first 4 years after diagnosis.[4]

In short-term studies fluoxetine (Prozac) has been shown effective in bulimia at a dose of 60 mg/day, whereas lower doses had little effect.[5] Tricyclics and MAO inhibitors are also effective.[6] Whether treatment alters the long-term prognosis is not known.[4]

REFERENCES

1. Comerci GD: Medical complications of anorexia nervosa and bulimia nervosa, *Med Clin North Am* 74:1293-1310, 1990.
2. Hsu LKG: The outcome of anorexia nervosa: a reappraisal, *Psychol Med* 18:807-812, 1988.
3. Sharp CW, Freeman CPL: The medical complications of anorexia nervosa, *Br J Psychiatry* 162:452-462, 1993.
4. Keel PK, Mitchell JE: Outcome in bulimia nervosa, *Am J Psychiatry* 154:313-321, 1997.
5. Fluoxetine Bulimia Nervosa Collaborative Study Group: Fluoxetine in the treatment of bulimia nervosa: a multicenter, placebo-controlled, double-blind trial, *Arch Gen Psychiatry* 49:139-147, 1992.
6. Walsh BT: Fluoxetine treatment of bulimia nervosa, *J Psychosomat Res* 35(suppl 1):33-40, 1991.

FALSE MEMORIES

(See also childhood abuse, sexual abuse)

The issue of whether repressed memories of childhood sexual abuse exist and can be recovered through psychotherapy is an emotionally heated one. Supporting the existence of repressed memories is a study by Williams[1] of 129 women with previously documented histories of sexual abuse in childhood; 38% did not recall the abuse that had occurred more than 17 years previously. The younger they were, the less likely they were to remember. In commenting on this paper, Loftus[2] stated that the study proves that some children may forget an abusive sexual experience in the past, but it does not prove that this is a standard response to such trauma or that such memories can be recovered through therapy. A more radical view is that of Ofshe and Watters[3] who consider the recovery of false memories to be pseudoscience that causes considerable harm to patients and their families. Frankel took a more measured approach but found little evidence supporting the validity of recovered memories of abuse.[4,5] A comprehensive review of the topic by Penfold[6] concluded that both true and fabricated memories may be recovered. The clinician has to be both open minded and skeptical.

Closely related to the issue of recovered memories and childhood sexual abuse is the question of multiple personality disorders, which is called dissociative identity disorder in DSM-IV. This is because those who believe in multiple personalities think that childhood sexual abuse is a common basis for them. According to Merskey,[7] the number of diagnosed cases has increased remarkably in recent years and this is due to a few psychiatrists making large numbers of such diagnoses. In his view it seems likely that large numbers of cases are iatrogenically produced.[8]

REFERENCES

1. Williams SM: Recall of childhood trauma: a prospective study of women's memories of child sexual abuse, *J Consult Clin Psychol* 62:1167-1176, 1994.
2. Loftus EF, Maryanne G, Feldman J: Forgetting sexual trauma: what does I mean when 38% forget? *J Consult Clin Psychol* 1177-1181, 1994.
3. Ofshe R, Watters E: *Making monsters: false memories, psychotherapy, and sexual hysteria,* New York, 1994, Scribner's.
4. Frankel FH: Discovering new memories in psychotherapy—childhood revisited, fantasy, or both? *N Engl J Med* 333:591-594, 1995.
5. Frankel FH: Adult reconstruction of childhood events in the multiple personality literature, *Am J Psychiatry* 150:954-958, 1993.
6. Penfold PS: The repressed memory controversy: is there middle ground? *Can Med Assoc J* 155:647-653, 1996.
7. Merskey H: Multiple personality disorder and false memory syndrome, *Br J Psychiatry* 166:281-283, 1995.
8. Merskey H: The manufacture of personalities: the production of multiple personality disorder, *Br J Psychiatry* 160:327-340, 1992.

MOOD DISORDERS

Bipolar Affective Disorder

(See also depression; electroconvulsive therapy; hypothyroidism; subclinical hypothyroidism; seizures; serotonin syndrome)

About half of all patients with bipolar disorder have a parent with an affective disorder. About one fourth of the children of one parent with a bipolar disorder have an affective disorder.[1]

A diagnosis of bipolar I disorder requires the patient to have had at least one full-blown manic episode; there may or may not have been a depressive episode. The diagnosis of bipolar II disorder can be made if the patient has had one or more major depressions, as well as one or more hypomanic episodes, provided that no true manic attacks have occurred.[2]

Management

Recent evidence suggests that either lithium or valproate may be the drug of first choice for classic mania or hypomania with euphoric mood, that lithium, valproate, or carbamazepine may be used for mixed episodes or dysphoric mood, and that for mania with rapid cycling, either valproate or carbamazepine is the drug of first choice.[3] Patients with bipolar depression should receive antidepressants only if they are already taking lithium, valproate, or carbamazepine.[4]

Lithium. Lithium is classically used for bipolar disorders. It is effective in controlling acute mania, but the onset of this effect is delayed for 1 to 2 weeks and substantial improvement is usually not evident for 3 to 4 weeks. In practice, neuroleptics or benzodiazepines are usually added to the lithium to control the agitation and excessive activity of acute mania. In acute mania the usual dosage of lithium is 1200 to 1800 mg/day, whereas for maintenance therapy it is 900 to 1500 mg/day. When therapy is initiated, lithium is given twice or three times a day to minimize the adverse effects of nausea and tremor, but as soon as possible only a single daily dose should be given at bedtime. Aside from convenience, this is thought to decrease the risk of renal damage. Lithium is useful in cyclothymic disorder and as a potentiating agent for tricyclic or SSRI antidepressants in cases of refractory depression.[5]

The most common adverse effect of lithium is hand tremor, which occurs in one fourth to one half of patients.[5] This can be minimized by lowering the dose or by adding a beta-blocker.[4] Other side effects are leukocytosis, hypothyroidism, subclinical hypothyroidism, acne, and polyuria because of reduced urinary concentrating ability.[4,5] It has been estimated that between one fourth and one half of patients taking lithium for bipolar disease discontinue it, in large part because of adverse effects.[6] Patients taking lithium should be warned to drink plenty of fluids in hot weather.[5] Diuretics should be avoided. Concomitant use of nonsteroidal antiinflammatory agents may lead to lithium toxicity.[7]

Before lithium therapy commences, recommended laboratory investigations are complete blood count, urinalysis, electrocardiography if over age 50, TSH, BUN, and creatinine and electrolytes.[5]

During the initiation of therapy, lithium levels should be assessed every 5 to 7 days, as well as 5 to 7 days after any change in dosage. During maintenance therapy lithium levels should be checked every 1 to 2 months during the early period and every 6 to 12 months once the patient's condition is stable while receiving the drug. Lithium levels should be measured 10 to 12 hours after the last lithium dose. The therapeutic range for maintenance therapy is 0.6 to 1 mmol/L (0.6 to 1 mEq/L), whereas for acute mania the aim is 0.8 to 1.4 mmol/L (0.8 to 1.4 mEq/L). Toxic levels are 1.2 mmol/L (1.2 mEq/L) or greater. TSH and creatinine levels should be checked annually.[5]

Anticonvulsants. Carbamazepine (Tegretol) and valproic acid (Depakene) or divalproex (Depakote, Epival) have proved to be effective drugs for mania.[1,4,6] Adverse effects include nausea, weight gain, diarrhea, and tremor; the last can be treated with beta-blockers.[4] If patients are being treated with any of these drugs, they should have regular monitoring of serum levels, which should be maintained at the same level as for seizure control (see seizures).

REFERENCES

1. Werder SF: An update on the diagnosis and treatment of mania in bipolar disorder, *Am Fam Physician* 51:1126-1136. 1995
2. American Psychiatric Association: *Diagnostic and statistical manual of mental disorders,* ed 4, Washington, DC, 1994, American Psychiatric Association, pp 350-358.
3. Francis A, Docherty JP, Kahn DA: The expert consensus guideline series: treatment of bipolar disorder, *J Clin Psychiatry* 57 (suppl 12A):1-89, 1996.
4. Drugs for psychiatric disorders, *Med Lett* 39:33-40, 1997.
5. Price LH, Heninger GR: Lithium in the treatment of mood disorders, *N Engl J Med* 331:591-598, 1994.
6. Joffe RT: Valproate in bipolar disorder; the Canadian perspective, *Can J Psychiatry* 38(3 suppl 2):S46-S50, 1993.
7. Ragheb M: The clinical significance of lithium-nonsteroidal antiinflammatory drug interactions, *J Clin Psychopharmacol* 10: 350-354, 1990.

Depression

(See also adverse effects associated with low cholesterol levels; anxiety disorders; bipolar affective disorder; chest pain; cocaine; fibromyalgia; guns; homicide; insomnia; premenstrual syndrome; quitting smoking; serotonin syndrome; sexual abuse; sexual dysfunction)

Epidemiology

A community survey of depression in several different countries using DSM-III criteria found striking variations in prevalence rates. The highest incidence was in Beirut and Paris and the lowest in Taiwan and Korea. What was common to most countries was an association with substance abuse and anxiety disorders and a higher rate in females than in males and in divorced or separated individuals compared with married individuals. This survey found little variation in the prevalence of bipolar disorder.[1]

The incidence of smoking is much higher among individuals who have ever been depressed compared with those who have not, and the success rate in quitting among smokers who have ever been depressed is much lower than among those who have never been depressed.[2]

Suicide

Although the highest suicide rate is found among men over the age of 69,[3] the incidence of suicide among the young has been increasing in the Western world. This is particularly marked among aboriginal peoples.[4] The availability of guns appears to increase the risk of suicide. In a study involving 11 European nations, Canada, the United States, and Australia, overall rates of suicide, as well as rates of suicide carried out with a gun, correlated with the percentage of households containing guns.[5] In a U.S. study of 803 suicides the relative risk ratio for suicide in a home containing guns was 4.8, after controlling for other risk variables that included living alone, taking prescribed psychotropic medication, a history of being arrested, a history of drugs or alcohol abuse, and not graduating from high school.[6] Over 90% of individuals who commit suicide have a diagnosable psychiatric illness. Depression and alcoholism head the list, but other important disorders are bipolar affective disorder and schizophrenia.[3] Pregnancy seems to have a protective effect.[7]

Antidepressants

At present many physicians choose SSRIs as first-line antidepressants. This is not because they are more effective than tricyclics (they are not), but because they are reputed to have fewer adverse effects and therefore patient compliance should be better.[8,9]

Clinical response to antidepressants may take several weeks. However, the likelihood of response is much greater if some improvement is seen between 2 and 4 weeks. In a study of patients receiving a fixed dose of 20 mg of fluoxetine daily, only a third of the patients who showed no improvement at 2 weeks had responded by 8 weeks. Of those who showed no response at 4 weeks, only 19% had improvement at 8 weeks.[10]

What is the optimal duration of treatment of depression with antidepressants? For a first episode it should be at least 3 to 6 months, and for recurrent episodes, severe first depressions, or depressions that have not fully responded to therapy it should be for many years or for life. Current evidence suggests that full therapeutic doses should be used for maintenance therapy.[9]

Drug interactions with antidepressants, particularly those that involve inhibition of one or more of the 30 or so isoenzymes of the cytochrome P450 system, are a major concern. Many antipsychotics and antidepressants, including most of the SSRIs, do this, which could result in toxic elevations of the blood levels of concurrently taken medications. This is particularly notable with the combination of some of the SSRIs with tricyclics (toxic levels of tricyclics), but it is also reported when selected SSRIs are combined with certain antipsychotics or benzodiazepines, carbamazepine (Tegretol), theophylline, terfenadine (Seldane), and astemizole (Hismanal) among others.[11]

Treatment of depression is a complicated and rapidly changing field. At present family physicians would be well advised to look up drug interactions before prescribing another drug to a patient taking any of the newer antidepressants. If a second drug is to be prescribed that is inactivated through the P450 system, low doses should be given and when possible (as in case of tricyclics) serum levels should be monitored.

Tricyclics and related antidepressants. In most cases tricyclics are no longer the first therapeutic choice for depression (see antidepressants). Exceptions are made if the patient has previously been successfully treated with a drug from this class and did not suffer significant adverse reactions or if cost is an important consideration. In the elderly, low-dose desipramine (Norpramin, Pertofrane) or nortriptyline (Aventyl) is a good choice.[12] Some of the more frequently used tricyclics are listed in Table 59.

If tricyclics are used for young or middle-aged adult outpatients, the starting dose is usually 25 or 50 mg/day. It is increased by 25 mg every 3 to 5 days until a therapeutic level of 150 mg is reached. The exceptions are protriptyline (Triptil), which has a therapeutic dose range of 30 to 60 mg/day (it is three times as potent as amitriptyline), and nortriptyline (Aventyl), for which the usual therapeutic dose is 75 to 100 mg/day (it is twice as potent as amitriptyline). Tricyclic antidepressants can usually be given as a single daily dose, most commonly at bedtime. If side effects are distressing, divided doses can be tried. Some patients find that desipramine and protriptyline cause insomnia if given at bedtime.

Important adverse effects include urinary retention and, rarely, fatal arrhythmias. Because of the latter, use of the drugs should be avoided for patients with conduction abnormalities or recent myocardial infarctions.[13] Weight gain is a common adverse effect; the worst offender is amitriptyline (Elavil), whereas the drug least likely to induce this effect is desipramine.[12] These drugs, like the SSRIs, are associated

Table 59 Tricyclics and Related Antidepressants

Drugs	Usual doses
Tricyclics	
Amitriptyline (Elavil)	150 mg qhs
Amoxapine (Asendin)	150 mg qhs; has antipsychotic properties
Desipramine (Norpramin, Pertofrane)	150 mg qhs; half of this for elderly
Doxepin (Sinequan)	150 mg qhs
Imipramine (Tofranil)	150 mg qhs
Nortriptyline (Aventyl)	75-100 mg daily; half of this for elderly
Protriptyline (Triptil)	15-30 mg/day
Trimipramine (Surmontil)	150 mg qhs
Tetracyclic Derivatives	
Maprotiline (Ludiomil)	150 mg qhs
Modified Cyclic Derivatives	
Trazodone (Desyrel)	150-300 mg qhs

with a fairly high incidence of sexual dysfunction, usually in the form of anorgasmia or ejaculatory delay.[14]

Tricyclics should not be used or should be used with caution in children and adolescents because sudden cardiac deaths have been reported among children using these drugs.[12]

Amoxapine (Asendin) has antipsychotic properties and may be useful in cases of psychotic depression.[15] Two drugs closely related to the tricyclics are maprotiline (Ludiomil), which is a tetracyclic, and trazodone (Desyrel), which is a modified cyclic. Trazodone is sedative and has been used successfully in doses of 100 mg at bedtime as a hypnotic in depressed patients who had persistent, exacerbated, or new-onset insomnia when being treated with fluoxetine or bupropion.[16] Priapism is a rare complication of trazodone therapy.

Tricyclics have been used for a number of conditions other than depression, including insomnia, chronic pain, enuresis, urinary incontinence, panic disorder, phobic disorder, obsessive-compulsive disorder, premature ejaculation, and snoring. These issues are discussed elsewhere in the text.

Specific serotonin reuptake inhibitors. At present SSRIs are probably the drugs of first choice for treatment of depression. They have fewer reported adverse effects than tricyclics, and patients are more likely to continue taking the drugs or to reach full therapeutic levels than patients taking tricyclics. However, when outcomes were measured at 6 months, no difference was found between patients taking fluoxetine (Prozac) and those taking either desipramine (Norpramin, Pertofrane) or imipramine (Tofranil). Although the cost of fluoxetine was higher, total costs were the same because more frequent physician visits were required by patients taking tricyclics.[8]

In addition to their use in depression, SSRIs are effective for anxiety disorders, including panic disorder, phobic disorder, and obsessive-compulsive disorder, and in bulimia. Nausea is an important adverse effect that can be mitigated by giving the drug with meals.

A complication of SSRIs sometimes seen in the elderly is hyponatremia associated with the inappropriate secretion of antidiuretic hormone (SIADH).[17]

Sexual dysfunction is an adverse effect with all the SSRIs. It is often underreported because direct inquiry to the patient about this issue was not made. It may manifest itself as decreased libido, difficulty with arousal, or delayed or absent orgasm (anorgasmia). Anorgasmia occurs in about one fifth of men taking SSRIs, and this is independent of ejaculation.[14] Management of sexual dysfunction in patients taking SSRIs is controversial, and recommendations are often based on case reports. Suggested protocols include reducing the dosage of the SSRI, maintaining the dose and hoping that tolerance and return of orgasms will come with time, waiting until the SSRI can be discontinued, or switching to another class of antidepressants that is not reputed to cause this problem as frequently, such as nefazodone (Serzone) or bupropion (Wellbutrin).[13,18,19] One study of 30 outpatients taking fluoxetine (Prozac), paroxetine (Paxil), or sertraline (Zoloft) assessed the value of discontinuing the drug after the Thursday morning dose and restarting it on Sunday at noon. Improved sexual functioning during the weekend was noted by those taking paroxetine and sertraline but not by those taking fluoxetine (presumably because of the long half-life of the latter).[18] In another study 39 women with anorgasmia when taking fluoxetine (Prozac) were switched to bupropion (Wellbutrin), and 90% had complete or partial resolution of the problem.[19]

Other pharmacological interventions that have been tried include adding another drug such as yohimbine (Yocon), bethanechol (Urecholine), buspirone (Buspar), amantadine (Symmetrel), dexamphetamine (Dexedrine), pemoline (Cylert), and cyproheptadine (Periactin).[14,18] That so many drugs have been tried suggests that none works well.

If discontinuation of an SSRI and replacement with another antidepressant are desired, there is a washout period that varies with the half-life of the drug. It is long for fluoxetine (Prozac), and the patient must wait at least 2 weeks after discontinuing the drug until an antidepressant of another class can be started. For the other SSRIs the washout period is generally 3 or 4 days.

Other newer antidepressants. An increasing number of new classes of antidepressants have been developed, and several of these are listed in Table 61. Venlafaxine (Effexor) inhibits both serotonin and norepinephrine reuptake. It is chemically unrelated to the SSRIs. In higher doses it may cause diastolic hypertension.[13]

Nefazodone (Serzone) acts through the blockade of serotonin type 2 (5-HT_2) receptors, as well as the inhibition of serotonin reuptake. Drug interactions have been reported with astemizole (Hismanal), terfenadine (Seldane), cisapride

Table 60 Selective Serotonin Reuptake Inhibitors for Depression

Drugs	Usual doses
Fluoxetine (Prozac)	20-60 mg/day qam
Fluvoxamine (Luvox)	50-150 mg/day qhs
Paroxetine (Paxil)	20 mg/day qam
Sertraline (Zoloft)	50-200 mg/day with evening meal

Table 61 Other Newer Antidepressants

Drugs	Usual doses
Combined Serotonin and Norepinephrine Uptake Inhibitors	
Venlafaxine (Effexor)	75-375 mg/day in 3 divided doses
Phenylpiperazine Compounds	
Nefazodone (Serzone)	100-250 mg bid
Aminoketone	
Bupropion (Wellbutrin)	100 mg tid

(Prepulsid), and MAO inhibitors. Although nefazodone (Serzone) is chemically related to trazodone, it does not appear to cause priapism.[12,20,21] One of its advantages is that it is not associated with an increased incidence of sexual dysfunction.[12]

Bupropion is not chemically related to other antidepressants, and its mechanism of action is unknown. Its most serious adverse effect is seizures. Other adverse effects include agitation and insomnia. Bupropion does not appear to cause sexual dysfunction.[12,19]

MAO inhibitors. First-generation MAO inhibitors include phenelzine (Nardil) and tranylcypromine (Parnate). They are effective in the treatment of depression and panic disorder, but because of adverse effects they are rarely used at present. If these drugs are prescribed, the initial doses should be low and built up gradually at weekly intervals. Patients must be warned stringently to avoid all sympathomimetic drugs ("cold" remedies containing ephedrine or related drugs) and meperidine (Demerol). Foods to be avoided while taking these drugs include "natural" or "herbal" food supplements because they may contain ephedrine,[22] aged cheeses, pickled herring, chicken livers, yeast extracts, meat extracts such as Bovril or Oxo, broad bean pods, red wines, beer, and ripe bananas. A newer selective MAO-A inhibitor is moclobemide (Manerix). The drug can be started at its full therapeutic dose of 100 mg tid or 150 mg bid, and dietary restrictions are not required.[23]

Bipolar disease and antidepressants. When seeing a depressed patient, the physician should check carefully for a personal or family history of bipolar disorders. Antidepressants should not be prescribed for someone with a bipolar disorder unless the patient is first taking lithium or mania may be precipitated. A patient who is depressed but has a family history of bipolar disorder should be watched closely for mania if antidepressants are prescribed. A patient with bipolar disorder may become manic from the rapid withdrawal of antidepressants.

Relapses after treatment with antidepressants. Relapses after successful pharmacotherapy for depression are common. In one study of patients with diagnoses of depression alone, dysthymia alone, or dysthymia plus depression (double depression) who had responded to desipramine (Norpramin, Pertofrane), continuation of the drug over a 2-year period resulted in a relapse rate of 11% compared with those assigned at random to receive placebo, whose relapse rate was 52%. Most of the relapses occurred in the 6 months after stopping the active drug. The relapse rate was highest in patients with pure dysthymia or dysthymia plus depression.[24]

Table 62 MAO Inhibitors

Drugs	Usual doses
Nonselective MAO Inhibitors	
Phenelzine (Nardil)	30 mg qam, and 15-30 mg at noon
Tranylcypromine sulfate (Parnate)	20 mg qam and 10 mg in the afternoon
Selective MAO-A Inhibitors	
Moclobemide (Manerix)	150 mg bid or 100 mg tid

MAO, Monoamine oxidase.

Electroconvulsive therapy

Electroconvulsive therapy (ECT) is usually prescribed for severely depressed patients who do not respond to antidepressants. The usual course of therapy is three times a week for 6 to 12 treatments.[25] ECT is reported to be effective in 50% to 70% of such patients.[26] It is also effective in mania. However, if a patient who responds to ECT is not put on maintenance therapy with antidepressants or lithium, the relapse rate is high.[25] The occasional patient needs maintenance ECT at weekly or monthly intervals.[25]

REFERENCES

1. Weissman MM, Bland RC, Canino GJ, et al: Cross-national epidemiology of major depression and bipolar disorder, *JAMA* 276:293-299, 1996.
2. Glassman AH: Cigarette smoking: implications for psychiatric illness, *Am J Psychiatry* 150:546-553, 1993.
3. Hirschfeld RM, Russell JM: Assessment and treatment of suicidal patients, *N Engl J Med* 337:910-915, 1997.
4. Malchy B, Enns MW, Young TK, et al: Suicide among Manitoba's aboriginal people, 1988-94, *Can Med Assoc J* 156:1133-1138, 1997.
5. Killias M: International correlations between gun ownership and rates of homicide and suicide, *Can Med Assoc J* 148:1721-1725, 1993.
6. Kellermann AL, Rivara FP, Somes G, et al: Suicide in the home in relation with gun ownership, *N Engl J Med* 327:467-472, 1992.
7. Marzuk PM, Tardiff K, Leon AC, et al: Lower risk of suicide during pregnancy, *Am J Psychiatry* 154:122-123, 1997.
8. Simon GE, VonKorff M, Heiligenstein JH, et al: Initial antidepressant choice in primary care: effectiveness and cost of fluoxetine vs tricyclic antidepressants, *JAMA* 275:1897-1902, 1996.
9. Hirschfeld RM: Long-term drug treatment of unipolar depression, *Int Clin Psychopharmacol* 11:211-217, 1996.
10. Nierenberg AA, Mclean NE, Alpert JE, et al: Early nonresponse to fluoxetine as a predictor of poor 8-week outcome, *Am J Psychiatry* 152:1500-1503, 1995.
11. Nemeroff CB, DeVane Cl, Pollock BG: Newer antidepressants and the cytochrome P450 system, *Am J Psychiatry* 153:311-320, 1996.
12. Andrews JM, Nemeroff CB: Contemporary management of depression, *Am J Med* 97:24S-32S, 1994.
13. Drugs for psychiatric disorders, *Med Lett* 39:33-40, 1997.
14. Segraves RT: Antidepressant-induced orgasm disorder, *J Sex Marital Ther* 21:192-201, 1995.
15. Anton RF Jr, Burch EA Jr: Amoxapine versus amitriptyline combined with perphenazine in the treatment of psychotic depression, *Am J Psychiatry* 147:1203-1208, 1990.
16. Nierenberg AA, Adler LA, Peselow E, et al: Trazodone for antidepressant-associated insomnia, *Am J Psychiatry* 151:1069-1072, 1994.

17. Liu BA, Mittmann N, Knowles SR, et al: Hyponatremia and the syndrome of inappropriate secretion of antidiuretic hormone associated with the use of selective serotonin reuptake inhibitors: a review of spontaneous reports, *Can Med Assoc J* 155:519-527, 1996.
18. Rothschild AJ: Selective serotonin reuptake inhibitor-induced sexual dysfunction: efficacy of a drug holiday, *Am J Psychiatry* 152:1514-1516, 1995.
19. Walker PW, Cole JO, Gardner EA, et al: Improvement in fluoxetine-associated sex dysfunction in patients switched to bupropion, *J Clin Psychiatry* 54:459-465, 1993.
20. Robinson DS, Roberts DL, Smith JM, et al: The safety profile of nefazodone, *J Clin Psychiatry* 57(suppl)2:31-38, 1996.
21. Pecknold JC, Langer SF: Priapism: trazodone versus nefazodone, *J Clin Psychiatry* 57:547-548, 1996.
22. Centers for Disease Control and Prevention: Adverse events associated with ephedrine-containing products—Texas, December 1993–September 1995, *JAMA* 276:1711-1712, 1996.
23. Freeman H: Moclobemide, *Lancet* 342:1528-1532, 1993.
24. Kocsis JH, Friedman RA, Markowitz JC, et al: Maintenance therapy for chronic depression—a controlled clinical trial of desipramine, *Arch General Psychiatry* 53:769-774, 1996.
25. Banazak DA: Electroconvulsive therapy: a guide for family physicians, *Am Fam Physician* 53:273-278, 1996.
26. Depression Guideline Panel: *Depression in primary care.* Vol 2. *Treatment of major depression,* AHCPR Pub No 93-0551, Rockville, Md, Department of Health and Human Services, Public Health Service, Agency for health Care Policy and Research, 1993, pp 95-96.

Treatment-resistant depression

In general, 60% to 70% of depressed patients respond to the initial antidepressant used and a further 10% to 15% to a second antidepressant or ECT.[1]

A variety of strategies can be used for patients who do not respond to their initial antidepressants. These are the four main options outlined by Joffe[2]:

1. Optimization. The first step is always optimization, which is to ensure that an adequate dose of the initial antidepressant has been prescribed, that the patient has been compliant in taking it, and that it has been given for a sufficient duration, which is usually 6 weeks. In the case of tricyclic antidepressants blood levels may be helpful.[2]
2. Substitution. Substitution refers to the substitution of another antidepressant for the one that was ineffective. In most instances a drug from another class would be chosen (e.g., a tricyclic if the initial drug was an SSRI) because the literature suggests that the response rate after switching classes is about 50% to 60% as opposed to 20% to 30% when switching within the same class. However, preliminary evidence based on open trials suggests that this may not be the case with the SSRIs; the response rate from substituting a second SSRI has been reported to be 50% to 60%.[2-4]
3. Augmentation. Augmentation is the addition to an antidepressant of another drug that on its own is not known to have antidepressant effects. Examples are lithium, triiodothyronine or liothyronine (Cytomel), buspirone (Buspar), and psychostimulants such as dextroamphetamine (Dexedrine) or methylphenidate (Ritalin). Most of the studies to date have involved lithium and triiodothyronine.[2]
4. Combination. Combination refers to combining two antidepressants from two different classes, for example, an SSRI and a tricyclic.[2]

Which strategies should be used? Few controlled trials have been conducted in this area, so the data on which recommendations are based come mostly from open trials. Optimization is obviously the first step for all patients. The traditional second step has been substitution, which can be very effective; the main disadvantage is the time taken to discontinue the first antidepressant and build up the second one to a full therapeutic level. Augmentation has the advantage that time is not lost from stopping one drug and starting another and that if a response is to occur, it sometimes does so within days and usually within 2 to 3 weeks. Combinations of antidepressants can also be effective, and time is not lost; care must be taken that toxicity is not induced through one agent's interfering with the metabolism of the other (see discussion of antidepressants).[5]

The preceding discussion has been limited to drug therapy for treatment-resistant depression. ECT is an alternative that perhaps should be used at an earlier stage in the therapeutic regimen than is currently the practice.[6]

Until a family physician has gained some experience with treatment-resistant depression, getting a telephone consultation with a more experienced colleague is advisable before trying some of the newer modalities of therapy.

REFERENCES

1. Warneke L: Management of resistant depression, *Can Fam Physician* 42:1973-1980, 1996.
2. Joffe RT, Levitt AJ, Sokolov ST: Augmentation strategies—focus on anxiolytics, *J Clin Psychiatry* 57(suppl 7):25-33, 1996.
3. Joffe RT, Levitt AJ, Sokolov ST, et al: Response to an open trial of a second SSRI in major depression, *J Clin Psychiatry* 57:114-115, 1996.
4. Thase ME, Blomgern SL, Birkett MA, et al: Fluoxetine treatment of patients with major depressive disorder who failed initial treatment with sertraline, *J Clin Psychiatry* 58:16-21, 1997.
5. Joffe RT, Levitt AJ: Antidepressant failure: augmentation or substitution? (editorial), *J Psychiatry Neurosci* 20:7-9, 1995.
6. Joffe RT, Kellner CH: The role of ECT in refractory depression (editorial), *Convuls Ther* 11:77-79, 1995.

Dysthymic disorder

For dysthymic disorder to be diagnosed, the patient must experience a depressed mood almost continuously for 2 years (1 year for a child), as well as having two or more of the symptoms usually associated with depression such as changes in eating or sleeping patterns, poor concentration, fatigue, and low self-esteem or feelings of hopelessness.[1]

The diagnosis of dysthymic disorder cannot be made if during the initial 2 years (1 year for a child) the patient has had major depression. However, if a major depression occurs before or after this period, the patient is given both diagnoses (dysthymic disorder and major depressive disorder) or is referred to as having "double depression." Other conditions that exclude the diagnosis of dysthymic disorder are a diagnosis of mania, hypomania, a mixed episode, or cyclothymia.[1]

Antidepressants are often effective not only for controlling the depressive symptoms of dysthymic disorder,[2-4] but also for improving psychosocial functioning.[3] Although both tricyclics and SSRIs may be used, SSRIs are currently the preferred class of drugs.[2-4] According to one author, treatment should start with small doses and increase slowly. Response may take several weeks, and the maximum that may be achieved in some patients, especially those with comorbid personality disorders, is a 25% to 30% improvement.[2]

How long should patients with dysthymia be maintained on antidepressants? In a placebo-controlled study of dysthymic patients who responded to desipramine these patients were selected at random to continue the desipramine (Norpramin, Pertofrane) or to take a placebo for a 2-year period. The relapse rate was much higher in the placebo group, and most such events occurred during the first 6 months after stopping the drug.[5]

REFERENCES

1. American Psychiatric Association: *Diagnostic and statistical manual of mental disorders,* ed 4, Washington, DC, 1994, American Psychiatric Association, pp 345-349.
2. Sansone RA, Sansone LA: Dysthymic disorder: the chronic depression, *Am Fam Physician* 53:2588-2596, 1996.
3. Kocsis JH, Zisook S, Davidson J, et al: Double-blind comparison of sertraline, imipramine, and placebo in the treatment of dysthymia: psychosocial outcomes, *Am J Psychiatry* 154:390-395, 1997.
4. Thase ME, Fava M, Halbreich U, et al: A placebo-controlled, randomized clinical trial comparing sertraline and imipramine for the treatment of dysthymia, *Arch Gen Psychiatry* 53:777-784, 1996.
5. Kocsis JH, Friedman RA, Markowitz JC, et al: Maintenance therapy for chronic depression—a controlled clinical trial of desipramine, *Arch Gen Psychiatry* 53:769-774, 1996.

Postpartum depression

Postpartum depression occurs within 6 to 12 weeks of delivery in about 10% of pregnancies.[1,2] It should be distinguished from postnatal blues, which are experienced by 50% to 80% of women and are mild and self-limited, and postpartum or puerperal psychosis, which affects about 0.2% of pregnant women.[2] The probability of a recurrence of postpartum depression with each subsequent pregnancy is about 1 in 3, and the risk of a major depression unrelated to pregnancy is about 43%.[1]

Pharmacotherapy is the treatment of choice for postpartum depression even in nursing mothers, since the adverse effects on mother, baby, and other family members of not using it are great. First-choice drugs are SSRIs. Tricyclics are also effective, and ECT leads to rapid improvement in refractory cases.[1,2]

An open clinical trial in a small group of women with a past history of postpartum depression compared the effects of antidepressants given immediately after delivery with clinical monitoring only. The rate of recurrent postpartum depression was much higher in the group not receiving antidepressants.[3]

In a recent double-blind placebo-controlled study of 61 women with postpartum depression, recovery was much more rapid in women receiving 200 μg of estradiol-17ß daily from skin patches (equivalent of two 100 μg/day patches of Estraderm, Vivelle, or Climara) than in those receiving placebo. In this study the estrogen was given alone for the first 3 months and for the subsequent 3 months a progestogen was added in cyclical fashion monthly.[4] As pointed out in an editorial accompanying the report, this is an intriguing finding, but it would be premature to use estrogens as first-line therapy at this time.[2]

REFERENCES

1. Pearce P: Postpartum depression: more than "the blues," *Can J CME,* February 1997, pp 31-35.
2. Murray D: Oestrogen and postnatal depression (editorial), *Lancet* 347:918-919, 1996.
3. Wisner KL, Wheeler S: Prevention of recurrent postpartum major depression, *Hosp Commun Psychiatry* 45:1191-1196, 1994.
4. Gregoire AJ, Kumar R, Everitt B, et al: Transdermal oestrogen for treatment of severe postnatal depression, *Lancet* 347:930-933, 1996.

Seasonal affective disorder

Between 10% and 15% of patients with mood disorders are said to suffer from seasonal affective disorder (SAD). Patients with SAD usually have "atypical" symptoms of depression: overeating, carbohydrate craving, weight gain, and oversleeping. They show a marked lack of energy. Symptoms usually begin in October or November and are worst in January and February. Spontaneous recovery usually occurs in April or May. In most cases the disorder is unipolar, but 20% have a type II bipolar disorder.

Light therapy requires about 5000 lux-hours/day. Light boxes providing 10,000 lux of illumination are available. Light therapy works best if it is used in the morning, and the usual prescription is half an hour every morning at 7 AM. If no response occurs after 2 weeks, light exposure should be increased to 1 hour qam. Patients can read while in front of the lights. Ultraviolet light (greater than 400 nm) should be filtered out.[1] Whether light therapy is actually more effective than a placebo response has not been settled.[2]

Relatively few studies have considered the efficacy of medications for SAD; at present fluoxetine (Prozac) shows promise.[1,3]

REFERENCES

1. Tam EM, Lam RW, Levitt AJ: Treatment of seasonal affective disorder—a review, *Can J Psychiatry* 40:457-466, 1995.
2. Levitt AJ, Wesson VA, Joffe RT, et al: A controlled comparison of light box and head-mounted units in the treatment of seasonal depression, *J Clin Psychiatry* 57:105-110, 1996.
3. Lam RW, Gorman CP, Michalon M, et al: Multicenter, placebo-controlled study of fluoxetine in seasonal affective disorder, *Am J Psychiatry* 152:1765-1770, 1995.

Serotonin Syndrome

(See also neuroleptic malignant syndrome)

The serotonin syndrome is characterized by an excess of serotonin in the brainstem, which in most cases is precipitated by giving two or more serotonergic drugs concurrently. Symptoms are nonspecific, and the diagnosis is often missed; they involve cognition and behavior, the autonomic nervous system, and the neuromuscular system. Some of the symptoms include the following[1,2]:

1. Cognition-behavior—confusion, disorientation, agitation, irritability, anxiety
2. Autonomic—hyperthermia, diaphoresis, flushing, sinus tachycardia, hypertension, dilated pupils, lacrimation, nausea, diarrhea
3. Neuromuscular—restlessness, myoclonus, muscle rigidity, trismus, teeth chattering, tremor, opisthotonos

The onset of symptoms is often within 1 to 2 hours of taking the offending drug and almost always takes place within 24 hours. The drugs are usually those used to treat affective disorders, obsessive-compulsive disorders, and Parkinson's disease. Meperidine and dextromethorphan can also precipitate this syndrome. The disorder usually follows the addition of a second drug, for example, an SSRI given to a patient with Parkinson's disease being treated with selegiline (Eldepryl) or levodopa.

Some of the more frequently responsible drugs are SSRIs, MAO inhibitors, antiparkinsonian drugs (selegiline [Eldepryl], amantadine [Symmetrel], levodopa [Sinemet, Prolopa], bromocriptine [Parlodel]), dextromethorphan, meperidine (Demerol), cocaine, and amphetamines. Some other drugs that have been reported to cause the syndrome are tricyclics, especially clomipramine (Anafranil) and imipramine (Tofranil), lithium, fenfluramine (Pondimin, Ponderal), and bupropion (Wellbutrin).

The treatment of choice is to discontinue the offending drug and give supportive therapy. A variety of specific therapeutic agents have been mentioned in case reports, but no specific agent has been shown to be beneficial.[2]

REFERENCES

1. Mills KC: Serotonin syndrome, *Am Fam Physician* 52:1475-1482, 1995.
2. Martin TG: Serotonin syndrome, *Ann Emerg Med* 28:520-526, 1996.

PERSONALITY DISORDERS

(See also attention-deficit/hyperactivity disorder)

Classification

The major personality disorders or Axis II disorders are borderline personality disorder, antisocial personality disorder, narcissistic personality disorder, histrionic personality disorder, dependent personality disorder, avoidant personality disorder, schizotypal personality disorder, schizoid personality disorder, paranoid personality disorder, and obsessive-compulsive personality disorder.[1]

Antisocial personality disorder

A diagnosis of antisocial personality disorder can be made only in individuals over the age of 18. They must show a consistent disregard for the rights of others and violation of those rights from the age of 15, as well as a history of conduct disorder starting before the age of 15.[1]

The overall reported prevalence rate in the Western world is between 2% and 4%, and males outnumber females by a ratio of between 5 and 7:1.[2] A striking characteristic of persons with antisocial personality disorders is that they are often fearless. This means they rarely learn from negative experiences, but it may also lead them to be heroes in combat situations.[2] In most cases criminal behavior "burns out" by middle age but difficulties in interpersonal relationships persist.[2]

Studies in North America and Europe have not shown any racial differences in the prevalence rate of antisocial personality disorder. However, it is rare in certain cultures, particularly East Asian communities such as Taiwan and Japan. This is thought to be related to the cohesiveness of traditional families in these environments. Support comes from the observation that in Europe and North America important risk factors for the development of antisocial personality disorder are antisocial behavior in the father, parental alcoholism, childhood physical abuse, and separation from or loss of a parent. The common denominator is lack of parental supervision and discipline.[2]

To acquire an antisocial personality disorder, a person seemingly must have the genetic potential and then be exposed to an environment conducive to its development.[2]

The definition of antisocial personality disorder in DSM-IV[1] is based largely on behavior and does not fully embrace the concept of psychopathy that Frick and co-workers[3] point out is characterized by superficial charm and the absence of enduring relationships, empathy, guilt, and anxiety. The distinction is important because persons who meet the criteria of antisocial personality disorder often have low intelligence and adverse family backgrounds, whereas those defined by psychopathic traits are notable for their narcissism and striking lack of anxiety.[3]

A significant risk factor for the development of antisocial personality disorder is antecedent ADHD. In one longitudinal follow-up study 18% of adults with antecedent ADHD developed antisocial personality disorder and 16% drug abuse disorder (many patients had both disorders) compared with rates of 2% and 4% in the control group.[4]

Borderline personality disorder

Patients with borderline personality disorder are often the bane of physicians because none of the reasonable suggestions made by physicians work or are implemented by the patient. Borderline patients obtain a sense of control if they can effectively sabotage the interventions recommended by their physicians.[5]

According to Dawson,[5] an essential aspect of the management of borderline patients is for the physician to refuse to play the role of an ever more powerful paternal figure looking after an increasingly regressing child. The physician should make it clear that the patient is a competent adult who is capable of taking responsibility for his or her own life and health; the physician is a helper but is of secondary importance and cannot take responsibility for the patient's self-destructive behavior. This process of establishing and maintaining a different type of social contract with the patient is called relationship management. Dawson describes a variety of interviewing techniques that may be helpful in establishing and maintaining this contract. A key element is for the physician to refrain from jumping in with empathetic words or gestures when the patient begins to complain about the miseries of life. Silence or emotionally neutral responses often lead the patient to come up with his or her own solutions. Paradoxical therapy is also useful at times. For example, a patient might state that she thinks she is a hopeless case and the therapist replies that she is probably right. This is a powerful tool that can easily backfire and should be employed only by physicians who have been trained in its use.[5]

Other useful suggestions in the management of borderline patients in primary care are the following[6]:

1. Set and observe limits. A verbal contract is often useful in spelling out such items as fixed but limited appointments, necessity of coming on time and not canceling, limited number of telephone calls, and contingency plans for overwhelming suicidal ideation.
2. Follow a behavioral approach to psychotherapy. This entails helping the patients understand how to get on with their lives.
3. Recognize and treat concomitant Axis I disorders.
4. Arrange for judicious psychiatric consultations (not referrals).
5. If all the above are unsuccessful, inform the patient that you will not be able to continue being his or her physician.

REFERENCES

1. American Psychiatric Association: *Diagnostic and statistical manual of mental disorders,* ed 4, Washington, DC, 1994, The Association, pp 629-673.
2. Paris J: Antisocial personality disorder: a biopsychosocial model, *Can J Psychiatry* 41:75-80, 1996.
3. Frick PJ, O'Brien BS, Wootton JM, et al: Psychopathy and conduct problems in children, *J Abnorm Psychol* 103:700-707, 1994.
4. Mannuzza S, Klein RG, Bessler A, et al: Adult outcome of hyperactive boys: educational achievement, occupational rank, and psychiatric status, *Arch Gen Psychiatry* 50:565-576, 1993.
5. Dawson DF: Relationship management and the borderline patient, *Can Fam Physician* 39:833-839, 1993.
6. Paré M, Linehan MM, Oldham JM, et al: Dx: personality disorder . . . now what? *Patient Care Can,* September 1996, 7:63-85.

PSYCHOSES

(See also nausea and vomiting; serotonin syndrome; vitamin E)

Schizophrenia and Smoking

About three fourths of outpatients with schizophrenia smoke. One theory is that nicotine causes burst-firing of dopamine cells in a particular brain locus (nucleus accumbens) and this apparently helps to compensate for the lack of dopamine release that seems to occur in the brains of many schizophrenic patients.[1]

Transcultural Aspects of Psychoses

In a cohort study of persons with diagnosed psychoses, blacks of African or Caribbean background living in the United Kingdom were found to have a better prognosis than white British patients.[2] This tends to support other studies showing that psychotic disorders such as schizophrenia have a better prognosis in nonindustrialized countries.[3]

Neuroleptics

The classification and usual dosages of selected neuroleptics are recorded in Table 63.

As of this writing risperidone (Risperdal), olanzapine (Zyprexa), and clozapine (Clozaril) are the only antipsychotic drugs available that counter the negative symptoms of schizophrenia, such as apathy and lack of initiative, as well as countering the positive symptoms.

Clozapine (Clozaril) is a new antipsychotic that is indicated for schizophrenic patients who do not respond to the conventional neuroleptics. It has been found that 30% to 50% of such patients respond to this drug. The most serious adverse effect of clozapine is agranulocytosis, which occurs in 1% to 2% of patients. Patients taking the drug must have their white blood cell counts monitored at weekly intervals during treatment. Another significant adverse effect of clozapine treatment is seizures, which have been reported in up to 5% of patients after 1 year of treatment. There are virtually no extrapyramidal reactions with this agent, and the risk of tardive dyskinesia is negligible. Besides using clozapine, methods of controlling refractory schizophrenia include the addition of benzodiazepines, lithium, or ECT.[4]

Olanzapine is structurally related to clozapine but does not cause agranulocytosis and to date is not associated with a significantly increased seizure rate. The incidence of extrapyramidal reactions is low. In doses above 5 mg/day many

Table 63 Neuroleptics

Drugs	Usual doses
Butyrophenone Derivatives	
Haloperidol (Haldol)	5-20 mg/day
Phenothiazines, Aliphatic	
Chlorpromazine (Thorazine, Largactil)	25-400 mg/day
Methotrimeprazine (Nozinan)	6-75 mg/day
Phenothiazines, Piperazine	
Trifluoperazine (Stelazine)	6-20 mg/day
Prochlorperazine (Compazine, Stemetil)	5-10 mg tid or qid; usually used for nausea and vomiting
Fluphenazine enanthate (Prolixin Enanthate, Moditen)	25 mg (12.5-100 mg) IM q2 weeks
Fluphenazine decanoate (Prolixin Decanoate, Modecate)	25 mg (12.5-50 mg) IM q3 weeks
Phenothiazines, Piperidine	
Thioridazine (Mellaril)	25-400 mg/day
Tricyclic Dibenzoxazepine Derivatives	
Loxapine (Loxapac)	60-100 mg/day
Dibenzodiazepine Derivatives	
Clozapine (Clozaril)	300-600 mg/day
Thiobenzodiazepine Derivatives	
Olanzapine (Zyprexa)	10 mg/day
Benzisoxazole Derivatives	
Risperidone (Risperdal)	4-8 mg/day

patients gain weight. Like risperidone (Risperdal), olanzapine counters both the negative and positive symptoms of psychoses.[4]

Antipsychotic drugs have often been divided into two groups: low and high potency. The low-potency group, which includes such drugs as chlorpromazine (Thorazine, Largactil), tends to cause sedation and hypotension but to have relatively few extrapyramidal effects. High-potency drugs such as haloperidol (Haldol) are less sedating and cause less hypotension but are associated with more extrapyramidal effects.[5]

Patients with schizophrenic illnesses who are taking neuroleptics and who have been in remission for a year or more have a relapse rate of 75% within 12 to 18 months of discontinuing therapy. Current recommendations are to treat patients for 1 to 2 years after a first episode of schizophrenia and for 5 years or even indefinitely if they have had two or more episodes. The relapse rate during medication regimens is 15% to 20% per year.[5]

In outpatient settings the dosage of neuroleptics should be relatively low initially and should be increased gradually as necessary. There is a lag period of weeks or even months from the initiation of therapy until maximum control of psychotic thought processes is achieved.[5] To evaluate the efficacy of the drug in controlling psychotic thought processes, the physician should reevaluate the patient every 2 weeks. However, agitation may be controlled much more rapidly through the sedative effects of neuroleptics, and to assess the efficacy of this action, the patient should be reevaluated daily at first and the dose increased rapidly until an adequate response has been achieved.

In the past large doses of neuroleptics were used for some patients. The current view is that doses greater than 10 to 20 mg of haloperidol or its equivalent add little if any additional therapeutic benefit.[5,6]

Much or all of the neuroleptic dose can be given at bedtime if nocturnal sedation is required. However, if daytime agitation is a problem, the total daily dose may be divided so that a portion of it is given during the day.

The following are some of the more important adverse effects of neuroleptics:

1. Seizures. In general the neuroleptics lower the seizure threshold. The incidence of seizures is particularly high with clozapine (Clozaril).
2. Interaction with tricyclics. The neuroleptics inhibit the metabolism of tricyclics and so raise their blood levels.
3. Hypotension. All of the phenothiazines may cause a marked hypotensive effect through alpha-adrenergic blockade. Phenothiazines should be used with extreme caution in the elderly.
4. Anticholinergic effects. The anticholinergic effects of neuroleptics are most marked in the aliphatic phenothiazines (chlorpromazine [Thorazine, Largactil], methotrimeprazine [Nozinan]).
5. Sedation. All of the neuroleptics are sedative, but of those commonly used, the most sedative seem to be methotrimeprazine (Nozinan), chlorpromazine (Thorazine, Largactil), and thioridazine (Mellaril).
6. Prolactin elevation. Prolactin levels are elevated by neuroleptics. Galactorrhea may result.
7. Tardive dyskinesia. The risk of tardive dyskinesia is generally related to the dosage and duration of treatment with neuroleptics. Early tardive dyskinesia may be detected by having the patient sit with an open mouth while drawing a spiral. Watch the patient's tongue for abnormal movements. The most effective treatment is withdrawal of the drug, although recent studies have shown an amelioration with vitamin E in doses of 1200 to 1600 mg/day.[7,8] There is almost no risk of tardive dyskinesia with clozapine.[5]
8. Neuroleptic malignant syndrome. The cardinal features of the neuroleptic malignant syndrome are hyperpyrexia, muscle rigidity, altered mental status, and autonomic instability (variations in pulse and blood pressure). Patients may have elevated creatinine kinase levels, myoglobinuria from rhabdomyolysis, and acute renal failure. The mortality rate of untreated persons is 20%. The disorder usually occurs within the first few weeks of starting a neuroleptic or of increasing the dose. Treatment is discontinuation

of the neuroleptic, fluids, and administration of dantrolene (Dantrium), bromocriptine (Parlodel) or pergolide (Permax).[5] (See also the discussion of serotonin syndrome.)

9. Extrapyramidal effects. The extrapyramidal effects of neuroleptics include dystonias, opisthotonos, oculogyric crises, Parkinson-like symptoms, and akathisia. These adverse effects are common with the butyrophenone derivatives (haloperidol [Haldol]), are rare with the aliphatic phenothiazine derivatives (chlorpromazine [Thorazine, Largactil], methotrimeprazine [Nozinan]), and are relatively uncommon with the usual oral doses of the piperidine phenothiazine derivatives (thioridazine [Mellaril]). The incidence of extrapyramidal side effects with the piperazine phenothiazine derivatives depends on the dosage. These effects are uncommon with the usual outpatient doses of trifluoperazine (Stelazine) but very common with the long-acting intramuscular forms (fluphenazine enanthate [Prolixin Enanthate, Moditen] and fluphenazine decanoate [Prolixin Decanoate, Modecate]). Extrapyramidal reactions are relatively rare with clozapine and olanzapine.
10. Acute dystonic reactions. Acute dystonic reactions can be controlled by a single injection of diphenhydramine (Benadryl) 50 mg. Other extrapyramidal effects are controlled by benztropine (Cogentin) or procyclidine (Kemadrin). At usual outpatient doses, one rarely needs antiparkinsonian drugs with chlorpromazine, methotrimeprazine, trifluoperazine, or thioridazine. Most patients taking haloperidol require them on a regular basis, and patients taking the long-acting intramuscular formulations of fluphenazine enanthate or fluphenazine decanoate require them only during the first week or two after the injections. The usual dosage of benztropine is 1 to 4 mg/day as a single dose or in 2 divided doses, whereas that of procyclidine (Kemadrin) is 7.5 to 20 mg/day in 3 divided doses.
11. Akathisia. Akathisia is an extrapyramidal effect that causes the patient to feel extremely restless. The main modality of treatment is to lower the dose of the neuroleptic, but some patients respond to propranolol.[9]

REFERENCES

1. Glassman AH: Cigarette smoking: implications for psychiatric illness, *Am J Psychiatry* 150:546-553, 1993.
2. McKenzie K, van Os J, Fahy T, et al: Psychosis with good prognosis in Afro-Caribbean people now living in the United Kingdom, *BMJ* 311:1325-1328, 1995.
3. Keh-Ming 1, Kleinman AM: Psychopathology and clinical course of schizophrenia: a cross cultural perspective, *Shizophr Bull* 14:555-567, 1988.
4. Olanzapine for schizophrenia, *Med Lett* 38:5-6, 1997.
5. Kane JM: Schizophrenia, *N Engl J Med* 334:34-41, 1996.
6. Carpenter WT Jr, Buchanan RW: Schizophrenia, *N Engl J Med* 330:681-690, 1994.
7. Dabiri LM, Pasta D, Darby JK, et al: Effectiveness of vitamin E for treatment of long-term tardive dyskinesia, *Am J Psychiatry* 151:925-926, 1994.
8. Akhtar S, Jajor TR, Kumar S: Vitamin E in the treatment of tardive dyskinesia, *J Postgrad Med* 39:124-126, 1993.
9. Dilsaver SC: Antipsychotic agents: a review, *Am Fam Physician* 47:199-204, 1993.

PSYCHOTHERAPY

A study of brief psychotherapy from the Jewish General Hospital in Montreal concluded that it was effective for patients with a variety of psychiatric diagnoses and that the experience of the therapists did not seem to influence the outcomes.[1] The success rate was as good when psychotherapy was conducted by medical students, family medicine residents, and psychiatry residents under supervision as it was for staff psychiatrists.

REFERENCES

1. Propst A, Paris J, Rosberger Z: Do therapist experience, diagnosis and functional level predict outcome in short term psychotherapy? *Can J Psychiatry* 39:168-176, 1994.

SUBSTANCE-RELATED DISORDERS

(See also alcohol; anabolic steroids; serotonin syndrome)

Substance use has been increasing among adolescents in North America and the United Kingdom. A survey of high-school adolescents in the Canadian province of Nova Scotia found that approximately half of the students drank alcohol, a third smoked cigarettes, a third smoked cannabis, a fifth used all three agents, and a third used none of them. Use of all three drugs correlated with low academic achievement, older age, and a higher risk of "harm."[1] Traditional preventive interventions for substance abuse in schools aim for total abstinence and emphasize the harm that comes from use of these agents. None of these projects has been successful in altering long-term behavior.[2] Therefore it has been suggested that interventions emphasize "harm-reduction" rather than abstinence. Although this has theoretical merits, there are as yet no reported trials of its efficacy.[1,2]

Cocaine

A New York City study found that two thirds of deaths from cocaine were due to fatal injuries caused by homicide, suicide, traffic accidents, and falls and that one third were due to drug overdose.[3]

Marijuana

Most studies of the long-term cognitive effects of heavy marijuana use have methodological flaws, and whether long-term adverse effects on the central nervous system occur is simply not known. In contrast, numerous studies clearly indicate long-term cognitive deficits from prolonged heavy drinking.[4]

REFERENCES

1. Poulin C, Elliott D: Alcohol, tobacco and cannabis use among Nova Scotia adolescents: implications for prevention and harm reduction, *Can Med Assoc J* 156:1387-1393, 1997.
2. Erickson PG: Reducing the harm of adolescent substance use (editorial), *Can Med Assoc J* 156:1397-1399, 1997.
3. Parzuk PM, Tardiff K, Leon AC, et al: Fatal injuries after cocaine use as a leading cause of death among young adults in New York City, *N Engl J Med* 332:1753-1757, 1995.
4. Block RI: Does heavy marijuana use impair human cognition and brain function? (editorial), *JAMA* 275:560-561, 1996.

RESPIROLOGY

Topics covered in this section

Asthma
Bronchitis, Acute
Chronic Bronchitis and Emphysema
Cough
Lung Cancer
Pneumonia
Pneumothorax
Sarcoid

ASTHMA

(See also allergic rhinitis–environmental control; aspirin sensitivity; asthma in children)

Epidemiology

The prevalence of asthma in the United States is about 5%.[1] Between 1980 and 1987 both the prevalence rate and the mortality rate increased by a relative rate of approximately 30%.[2]

Asthma usually first manifests itself in children or young adults. Between 30% and 70% of children with asthma have marked improvement or resolution of symptoms by the time they become adults. Such resolution is seen more often in patients with milder forms of the disease.[3]

REFERENCES

1. American Thoracic Society: Standards for the diagnosis and care of patients with chronic obstructive pulmonary disease (COPD) and asthma, *Am Rev Respir Dis* 136:225-244, 1987.
2. National Asthma Education Program: *Guidelines for the diagnosis and management of asthma: expert panel report,* Bethesda, Md, 1991, National Heart, Lung, and Blood Institute, National Institutes of Health, NIH Pub No 91-3042.
3. O'Connor GT, Weiss ST, Speizer FE: The epidemiology of asthma. In Gershwin ME, ed: *Bronchial asthma,* ed 2, Orlando, Fla, 1986, Grune & Stratton.

Spirometry or Peak Flow Measurements

Clinical practice guidelines recommend that physicians use objective measurements of pulmonary function such as spirometry or peak expiratory flow rates (PEFR) in assessing the severity of asthma in ambulatory patients.[1] The arguments for this are the observation that wheezing on auscultation may be absent in the presence of significant airway obstruction[2] and reports that patients cannot accurately judge the severity of their own condition.[3] Are these guidelines being followed? A survey of family practices in the United States and Canada found that in over 50% of cases they were not.[4] This could be because of ignorance or plain pigheadedness, but there are alternative explanations. It is questionable whether the guidelines are based on evidence or are targeted toward the family practice setting,[5] and there are papers claiming that patient self-assessment diaries (of nocturnal symptoms, persistent morning dyspnea after bronchodilator inhalation, shorter duration of benefit after bronchodilator inhalation, and inability to go to work or school) are as accurate in detecting exacerbations as is the determination of peak flow rates.[6] Since it is unknown whether measurements of PEFR by patients themselves affect outcome,[7] physicians will have to decide for themselves whether the current guidelines best serve the interests of their patients.

REFERENCES

1. National Asthma Education Program Panel: *Guidelines for the diagnosis and management of asthma,* Washington, DC, 1991, US Department of Health and Human Services, Public Health Service, National Institutes of Health, Pub No 91-3042.
2. Shim CS, Williams H: Relationship of wheezing to the severity of obstruction in asthma, *Arch Intern Med* 143:890-892, 1983.
3. Cross D, Nelson HS: The role of the peak flow meter in the diagnosis and management of asthma, *J Allergy Clin Immunol* 87:120-128, 1991.
4. Fried RA, Miller RS, Green LA, et al: The use of objective measures of asthma severity in primary care: a report from ASPN, *J Fam Pract* 152:1107-1136, 1995.
5. Berg AO, Moy JG: Guidelines for the diagnosis and management of asthma, *J Am Board Fam Pract* 5:629-634, 1992.
6. Malo J-L, L'Archevêque J, Trudeau C, et al: Should we monitor peak expiratory flow rates or record symptoms with a simple diary in the management of asthma? *J Allergy Clin Immunol* 91:702-709, 1993.
7. Clark NM, Evans D, Mellins RB: Patient use of peak flow monitoring, *Am Rev Respir Dis* 145:722-725, 1992.

Delivery Systems for Inhaled Medications

(See also local side effects of inhaled steroids)

Delivery systems for inhaled medications used for outpatients are generally divided into two major categories: metered dose inhalers (MDIs) with propellants and dry powder inhalers (inspiratory flow–generated aerosols). If the patient cannot generate an adequate airflow, the latter devices are ineffective.[1]

Although traditional practice is to use nebulizers to deliver $beta_2$-agonists to hospitalized patients and young children, the supervised use of MDIs with spacer devices has proved as effective in the emergency setting for both adults[2] and children[3] as nebulizer therapy.

Metered dose inhalers

When MDIs are used, the open mouth technique is said to be more effective than the closed mouth technique. The open mouth technique is performed as follows[4]:

1. Remove the cap of the MDI.
2. Shake the MDI several times.
3. Hold the MDI vertically about 2.5 to 5 cm (1 to 2 inches) from the open mouth.
4. Tilt the head slightly backward.
5. Exhale normally (not a forced or maximum exhalation).
6. Breathe in at a moderate rate, and activate the MDI in the middle of inspiration.
7. Hold the breath for 10 seconds or more.

Whether an MDI is full or empty can be determined by placing it in a bowl of water. If it sinks, it is full, and if it floats sideways, it is empty.[4]

Not all patients are able to use MDIs correctly. In a study of elderly subjects with a mean age of 70, only about half used the devices properly 1 week after an extensive instructional session. Major determinants of failure have been shown to be cognitive impairments and weak hand strength.[5] These problems may be overcome with the use of spacers (see below).

Spacers

Spacers or aerochambers are designed to be used with MDIs. Large particles are precipitated out in the chamber, slightly higher effective doses reach the lungs, and much less drug is deposited in the oropharynx and therefore is swallowed and absorbed systemically (see the discussion of local side effects of inhaled steroids). Spacers require less coordination than MDIs alone, so they are particularly useful for children, the aged, the disabled, and the uncoordinated. Proper use of spacers requires that the MDI be activated only once for each inhalation and that the inhalation be started as soon as possible after the activation.[6]

Turbuhalers

Turbuhalers supply medications in the form of dry powder that is not adsorbed to lactose (as is the case with medications supplied by disk inhalers). Therefore the particle size is smaller. Medications available with Turbuhalers include terbutaline (Bricanyl) and budesonide (Pulmicort). Turbuhalers are small and easily transportable and provide good delivery to the lower airways. Steroids given by Turbuhalers are less likely to cause dysphonia than those delivered by MDIs.[7]

The dose of medication from a Turbuhaler is made accessible by turning the bottom of the device. The instructions that come with the apparatus are clear, and the pharmacist is a good resource if problems occur. The basic way of using a dry powder inhaler is as follows[4]:

1. Prepare the dose.
2. Expire fully (forced or maximum expiration).
3. Close the mouth tightly around the mouthpiece.
4. Inhale fully and rapidly.

The inhalation technique with a Turbuhaler differs from that of the MDI, in which expiration is not forced and inspiration is at a moderate rate. The patient using a Turbuhaler will not feel the medication going into the airways as is usually the case with MDIs.

Concentration of drugs reaching the lungs

Reports of concentrations of medications reaching the lungs from various delivery systems vary from one reference to another. All figures indicate that use of an MDI plus an aerochamber or use of a Turbuhaler leads to a greater concentration of medication deposition in the lungs than does an MDI alone. One report showed that a Turbuhaler delivers about twice as much steroid to the lungs as do standard MDIs.[8] Another study found that with a Turbuhaler a normal inhalation resulted in almost twice as much pulmonary delivery as did a slow inhalation.[9]

REFERENCES

1. Fong PM, Sinclair D: Inhalation devices for asthma, *Can Fam Physician* 39:2377-2382, 1993.
2. Turner MO, Patel A, Ginsburg S, et al: Bronchodilator delivery in acute airflow obstruction: a meta-analysis, *Arch Intern Med* 1736-1744, 1997.
3. Kelly HW, Murphy S: Beta-adrenergic agonists for acute, severe asthma, *Ann Pharmacother* 26:81-91, 1992.
4. Szefler SJ, Chambers CV: Diagnosis and management of asthma, *Am Fam Physician* Monogr No 2 1995, pp 1-25.
5. Gray SL, Williams DM, Pulliam CC, et al: Characteristics predicting incorrect metered-dose inhaler technique in older subjects, *Arch Intern Med* 156:948-988, 1996.
6. O'Callaghan C, Barry P: Spacer devices in the treatment of asthma: amount of drug delivered to the patient can vary greatly (editorial), *BMJ* 314:1061-1062, 1997.
7. Selroos SO, Backman R, Forsen K-O, et al: Local side effects during four years treatment with inhaled corticosteroids—a comparison between metered dose inhalers and Turbuhalers, *Allergy* 49:888-890, 1994.
8. Thorsson L, Edsbäcker S, Conradson TB: Lung deposition of budesonide from Turbuhaler is twice that from a pressurized metered-dose inhaler P-MDI, *Eur Respir J* 7:1839-1844, 1994.
9. Borgstrom L, Bondesson E, Moren F, et al: Lung deposition of budesonide inhaled via Turbuhaler: a comparison with terbutaline sulphate in normal subjects, *Eur Respir J* 7:69-73, 1994.

Pharmacotherapy of Asthma

The most important principle to remember about the pharmacotherapy of asthma is that the disease is caused by inflammation of the airways and that the most effective therapeutic drugs are antiinflammatory agents. The most potent antiinflammatories are corticosteroids, and for most patients with stable moderate or severe asthma twice-daily use of inhaled formulations of these agents is the cornerstone of treatment (Table 64).[1-4] Other, less potent antiinflammatory agents that are sometimes used for mild or moderate asthma are inhaled formulations of cromolyn, also called disodium or sodium cromoglycate (Intal) or nedocromil (Tilade),[1-4] and oral formulations of leukotriene receptor antagonists such as zafirlukast (Accolate)[5] and zileuton (Zyflo).[6] Oral corticosteroids are used primarily (and liberally) for acute flare-ups of asthma,[2-4] and unless the patient is extremely ill, the oral route is just as effective as the parenteral one (see the section on emergency treatment of asthma).[4,7] Once-a-day morning doses of prednisone 40 to 60 mg/day for adults and 0.6 mg/kg for children for 1 to 2 weeks without tapering are usually adequate.[3,4] Inhaled steroids should be given concurrently with oral steroids and continued after the oral steroids have been stopped.[8]

Bronchodilators, primarily the short-acting $beta_2$-adrenergic agonists, should be used alone only for mild asthma and for exercise-induced asthma (Table 64). If a person with mild asthma needs more than one or two inhalations of a $beta_2$-agonist daily, he or she probably needs to begin receiving inhaled steroids.[4] Patients with mild asthma do as well taking $beta_2$-agonists on an as-needed basis as they do taking regularly scheduled doses.[9] Large doses of $beta_2$-agonists along with steroids are used for the emergency treatment of asthma (see below).

A more complete discussion of the emergency treatment of asthma, the various drug classes used in asthma, the role of immunotherapy in asthma, and exercise-induced asthma may be found in the ensuing paragraphs. Some aspects of the epidemiology and management of asthma in children are discussed in the pediatrics section.

Table 64 Inhaled Medications for Asthma

Names	Delivery systems
$Beta_2$-Adrenergic Agonists, Nonselective	
Metaproterenol or <u>orciprenaline</u> (Alupent)	MDI
$Beta_2$-Adrenergic Agonists, Selective, Short-Acting	
Albuterol or <u>salbutamol</u> (Proventil, Ventolin)	MDI
Fenoterol (Berotec)	MDI
Pirbuterol (Maxair)	MDI
Terbutaline (Bricanyl, Brethaire)	Turbuhaler
$Beta_2$-Adrenergic Agonists, Selective, Long-Acting	
Salmeterol (Serevent)	MDI
Anticholinergics	
Ipratropium bromide (Atrovent)	MDI
Steroids	
Beclomethasone dipropionate (Beclovent)	MDI
Budesonide (Pulmicort)	Turbuhaler
Fluticasone propionate (FloVent)	MDI
Flunisolide (AeroBid, <u>Bronalide</u>)	MDI
Triamcinolone acetonide (Azmacort)	MDI
Antiallergic Agents	
Cromolyn or <u>sodium cromoglycate</u> (Intal)	MDI
Nonsteroidal Antiinflammatory Agents	
Nedocromil sodium (Tilade)	MDI

REFERENCES

1. Barnes PJ. Inhaled glucocorticoids for asthma, *N Engl J Med* 332:868-875, 1995.
2. Drugs for asthma, *Med Lett* 37:1-4, 1995.
3. Szefler SJ, Chambers CV: Diagnosis and management of asthma, *Am Fam Physician*, Monogr No 2, 1995, pp 1-25.
4. Bai TR: Glucocorticosteroid treatment of asthma, *Can Fam Physician* 41:1921-1927, 1995.
5. Zafirlukast for asthma, *Med Lett* 38:111-112, 1996.
6. Zileuton for asthma, *Med Lett* 39:18-19, 1997.
7. Grunfeld AF, Ho K: Emergency management of acute adult asthma, *Can Fam Physician* 41:1909-1916, 1995.
8. Beveridge RC, Grunfeld AF, Hodder RV, et al (CAEP/CTS Asthma Advisory Committee): Guidelines for the emergency management of asthma in adults, *Can Med Assoc J* 155:25-37, 1996.
9. Drazen JM, Israel E, Boushey HA, et al: Comparison of regularly scheduled with as-needed use of albuterol in mild asthma, *N Engl J Med* 335:841-847, 1996.

Emergency Treatment of Asthma

(See also steroids and osteoporosis)

$Beta_2$-agonists are the drugs of choice for the initial emergency treatment of asthma (Table 64). According to guidelines published by the Canadian Association of Emergency Physicians, the Canadian Thoracic Society, and the Association des Médecins d'Urgence du Québec, metered dose inhalers are more effective than wet nebulization for the emergency treatment of asthma and should be used whenever possible. In severe asthma a spacer is recommended, but for moderate asthma it is optional. The suggested dosage is 4 to 8 puffs every 15 to 20 minutes. In severe cases 1 puff may be given every minute up to a maximum of 20 puffs. Anticholinergic therapy (ipratropium bromide [Atrovent]) is recommended for severe asthma and may be useful in moderate asthma. Patients should receive systemic steroids, unless contraindicated, and these should be started as soon as possible. The oral route is as efficacious as an IV infusion. Oral steroids such as prednisone in doses of 30 to 60 mg/day should be continued for 7 to 14 days, and tapering is not required for this duration of treatment. Inhaled steroids should be prescribed on discharge and given concomitantly with the oral steroids.[1]

Although the preceding guidelines recommend that anticholinergic drugs be used in the emergency treatment of severe asthma, evidence supporting this is tenuous. In a series of 384 asthmatic adults treated in the emergency room of a New York hospital either with nebulized albuterol or, as it is called in Canada, salbutamol (Ventolin, Proventil) or with nebulized albuterol plus ipratropium bromide (Atrovent), no differences in outcome were detectable.[2] A similar study from Cleveland also failed to show any benefit from ipratropium.[3]

REFERENCES

1. Beveridge RC, Grunfeld AF, Hodder RV, et al (CAEP/CTS Asthma Advisory Committee): Guidelines for the emergency management of asthma in adults, *Can Med Assoc J* 155:25-37, 1996.
2. Karpel JP, Schacter EN, Fanta C, et al: A comparison of ipratropium and albuterol vs albuterol alone for the treatment of acute asthma, *Chest* 110:611-616, 1996.
3. Mcfadden ER, Elsanadi N, Strauss L, et al: The influence of parasympatholytics on the resolution of acute attacks of asthma, *Am J Med* 102:7-13, 1997.

Inhaled steroids

(See also glaucoma, open angle; oral steroids)

A number of the available inhaled steroids are listed in Table 64.

Systemic side effects. Systemic side effects from inhaled steroids in adults are usually observed only if the daily dose is greater than 800 μg.[1] Budesonide (Pulmicort) has less systemic bioavailability than beclomethasone (Beclovent) because the rate of biotransformation on first pass in the liver is greater with budesonide and because budesonide does not have active metabolites. Whether these findings are of clinical significance is uncertain. Choosing budesonide for patients requiring higher doses seems reasonable, since no important systemic effects have been noted with daily doses of 1600 to 2000 μg.[2]

A report from Montreal suggests that daily doses of inhaled steroids greater than 1500 μg of flunisolide (Bronalide, AeroBid) or 1600 μg of other inhaled steroids taken continuously for more than 3 months are associated with a slightly increased risk of ocular hypertension or open angle glaucoma. No such association was found among patients taking lower doses of inhaled steroids either intermittently or continuously or among patients taking nasal steroids.[3]

Do inhaled steroids inhibit growth in children? In one study of children aged 6 to 16 the cohort given beclomethasone 84 μg qid (336 μg/day) showed growth velocity suppression, especially the boys,[4] but the ultimate effect on height was not assessed. In another study no decrease in growth was observed in children taking 200 μg of budesonide daily for periods of 3 to 5 years,[5] while a metaanalysis of the effects of both oral and inhaled corticosteroids in children did not detect growth impairment.[6]

No adverse effects of inhaled steroids have been found in pregnancy, labor, or delivery.[1]

Local side effects. Local side effects of inhaled steroids include thrush and dysphonia or hoarseness, which is probably due to steroid myopathy of laryngeal muscles. These adverse effects, particularly the dysphonia, occur less frequently when spacers, disk inhalers, or Turbuhalers are used.[1] In one study the incidence of dysphonia with Turbuhalers was 6% compared with 21% with MDIs.[7] With the spacer or aerochamber many large particles are precipitated out in the chamber, so fewer fall on the buccal or pharyngeal mucosa. With the disk inhalers and Turbuhalers the drug is delivered by rapid active inhalation, which causes partial closure of the false cords, thus giving some protection to the larynx. The Turbuhaler is particularly useful, at least in theory, because the medication is not adsorbed to lactose so there are fewer large particles to precipitate out in the mouth and pharynx. In addition to using spacer devices, rinsing out the mouth and gargling with water after steroid inhalation are said to decrease the incidence of thrush.[1]

REFERENCES

1. Barnes PJ, Pedersen S: Efficacy and safety of inhaled corticosteroids in asthma: report of a workshop held in Eze, France, October 1992, *Am Rev Respir Dis* 148:S1-S26, 1993.
2. Bai TR: Glucocorticosteroid treatment of asthma, *Can Fam Physician* 41:1921-1927, 1995.
3. Garbe E, LeLorier J, Boivin J-F, et al: Inhaled and nasal glucocorticoids and the risks of ocular hypertension or open-angle glaucoma, *JAMA* 277:722-727, 1997.
4. Tinkelman DG, Reed CE, Nelson HS, et al: Aerosol beclomethasone dipropionate compared with theophylline as primary treatment of chronic, mild to moderately severe asthma in children, *Pediatrics* 92:64-77, 1993.
5. Volovitz B, Amir J, Malik H, et al: Growth and pituitary-adrenal function in children with severe asthma treated with inhaled budesonide, *N Engl J Med* 329:1703-1708, 1993.
6. Allen DB, Mullen M, Mullen B: A meta-analysis of the effect of oral and inhaled corticosteroids on growth, *J Allergy Clin Immunol* 93:967-976, 1994.
7. Selroos SO, Backman R, Forsen K-O, et al: Local side effects during four years treatment with inhaled corticosteroids—a comparison between metered dose inhalers and Turbuhalers, *Allergy* 49:888-890, 1994.

Oral steroids

(See also inhaled steroids; steroids and osteoporosis)

An important part of the management of severe asthmatic crises is the use of oral steroids for 1 to 2 weeks. A Toronto study of patients with asthma attacks treated in the emergency room compared patients given a discharge regimen of prednisone 40 mg/day that was tapered to zero over 8 days with a placebo-matched control group. The prednisone group did much better in terms of symptom scores, use of bronchodilators, and relapses requiring further medical attention.[1]

When oral steroids are used, a 10- to 14-day course of 0.6 mg/kg/day as a single morning dose (about 40 mg/day for most patients) can be safely given without tapering. Patients have no higher incidence of rebound asthma than with tapering regimens and do not have clinically significant adrenal suppression.[2,3]

Several studies have shown that oral steroids in doses of 40 to 60 mg/day are as effective as IV corticosteroids for acute asthmatic attacks.[4,5]

REFERENCES

1. Chapman KR, Verbeek PR, White JG, et al: Effect of a short course of prednisone in the prevention of early relapse after the

emergency room treatment of acute asthma, *N Engl J Med* 324: 788-794, 1991.
2. Bai TR: Glucocorticosteroid treatment of asthma, *Can Fam Physician* 41:1921-1927, 1995.
3. O'Driscoll BR, Kalra S, Wilson M, et al: Double-blind trial of steroid tapering in acute asthma, *Lancet* 341:324-327, 1993.
4. Grunfeld AF, Ho K: Emergency management of acute adult asthma, *Can Fam Physician* 41:1909-1916, 1995.
5. Ratto D, Alfaro C, Sipsey J, et al: Are intravenous corticosteroids required in status asthmaticus? *JAMA* 260:527-529, 1988.

Noncorticosteroid antiinflammatory agents

Cromolyn, which is also called sodium or disodium cromoglycate (Intal), may be useful for mild asthma in children and as a prophylactic agent for exercise and cold-induced asthma. It is supplied as an MDI, and the usual dose is 2 puffs qid. Up to 6 weeks may be necessary to determine whether the drug is effective.[1] Nedocromil sodium (Tilade) is also supplied as an MDI. The usual dosage for adults and children over the age of 6 is two activations qid. Both cromolyn and nedocromil are less effective than inhaled corticosteroids in moderate or severe asthma.[1]

Two leukotriene inhibitors have recently been marketed, zafirlukast (Accolate) and zileuton (Zyflo). Leukotrienes are some of the mediators of the inflammatory response in asthma, so in theory blocking them would alleviate asthmatic symptoms.[1] According to the *Medical Letter,* no trials comparing either drug with inhaled steroids have been conducted.[2,3] In the trials that have been done, the drugs are better than placebo and are moderately effective in the management of chronic asthma. Zafirlukast and zileuton inhibit the cytochrome P450 isoenzyme 2C9 (CYP2C9), and therefore interact with a number of drugs.[2,3] The bioavailability of zafirlukast is markedly diminished by food,[2] whereas that of zileuton is not.[3] The usual dose of zafirlukast (Accolate) for adults and children age 12 or older is 20 mg bid 1 hour before or 2 hours after a meal. The usual dose of zileuton (Zyflo) for adults is 600 mg qid. Patients taking zileuton should be monitored for hepatic toxic effects.[3]

REFERENCES

1. Drugs for asthma, *Med Lett* 37:1-4, 1995.
2. Zafirlukast for asthma, *Med Lett* 38:111-112, 1996.
3. Zileuton for asthma, *Med Lett* 39:18-19, 1997.

Beta$_2$-adrenergic agonists, short-acting

(See also emergency treatment of asthma; exercise-induced asthma; overview of the pharmacotherapy of asthma)

Beta$_2$-adrenergic agonists such as albuterol, or as it is called in Canada, salbutamol (Proventil, Ventolin), are potent bronchodilators. A number of the available agents that are administered by inhalation are listed in Table 64. They are used in large doses for the emergency management of asthma in conjunction with steroids (see section on emergency treatment of asthma), for the management of exercise- or cold-induced asthma (see section on exercise-induced asthma), and as adjunctive treatment for patients with moderate or severe asthma on inhaled steroids. For a few patients with mild asthma, they may be used as sole therapy provided no more than one or two doses a day is required (see the introductory paragraphs concerning pharmacotherapy of asthma).

Oral forms of beta$_2$-agonists may be used for children who cannot take the inhaled agents. Metaproterenol (orciprenaline in Canada) (Alupent) is available not only in an MDI but as a syrup and tablets. The usual oral dose for children aged 4 to 12 is 10 mg tid prn, and for children over 12 it is 20 mg tid prn.

Beta$_2$-adrenergic agonists, long-acting

Salmeterol (Serevent) is a long-acting beta$_2$-selective adrenergic agonist with a usual dose of 50 µg (2 puffs) bid. A number of studies, each spanning a period of a few months, have shown it to be effective[1-5] and to have no more side effects than short-acting beta$_2$-agonists. The conservative view is that it should be given only to patients who are taking maintenance steroids and continue to have symptoms. In a British trial asthmatic patients who were taking regular inhaled steroids and who were following a detailed protocol for adjusting their steroid doses according to symptoms and peak expiratory flow measurements were chosen at random to take salmeterol 50 µg bid or placebo for 6 months. Salmeterol was associated with better symptom control and lung function.[5]

Salmeterol would seem to be especially useful for preventing nocturnal asthma attacks and exercise-induced asthma.[6] If salmeterol is used, short-acting beta$_2$-agonists may still be needed for acute exacerbations. The drug is not recommended for children under the age of 12. It is important that salmeterol not be used to treat an acute asthmatic attack; fatalities have resulted from doing so.[7]

REFERENCES

1. Drugs for asthma, *Med Lett* 37:1-4, 1995.
2. Cheung D, Timmers MC, Zwinderman AH, et al: Long-term effects of a long-acting beta 2-adrenoceptor agonist, salmeterol, on airway hyperresponsiveness in patients with mild asthma, *N Engl J Med* 328:665-666, 1993.
3. D'Alonzo GE, Nathan RA, Henochowicz S, et al: Salmeterol xinafoate as maintenance therapy compared with albuterol in patients with asthma, *JAMA* 271:1447-1448, 1994.
4. Juniper EF, Johnston PR, Borkhoff CM, et al: Quality of life in asthma clinical trials: comparison of salmeterol and salbutamol, *Am J Respir Crit Care Med* 151:66-70, 1995.
5. Wilding P, Clark M, Thompson J, et al: Effect of long term treatment with salmeterol on asthma control: a double blind, randomised crossover study, *BMJ* 314:1441-1446, 1997.
6. Nelson HS: β-Adrenergic bronchodilators, *N Engl J Med* 333: 499-506, 1995.
7. Bone RC: Another word of caution regarding a new long-acting bronchodilator (editorial), *JAMA* 273:967-968, 1995.

Theophylline salts

Theophylline preparations are occasionally helpful in asthma or chronic obstructive pulmonary disease. They are indicated for patients unable (such as toddlers) or unwilling to use inhaled agents and as additive therapy for patients whose disease is not well controlled with adequate doses of inhaled steroids. Aside from producing bronchodilation, theophylline products may have some antiinflammatory and bronchoprotective effects and they are reputed to decrease diaphragmatic muscle fatigue. Toxicity is an ever present hazard. Therapeutic blood levels are between 55 and 110 μmol/L (10 and 20 μg/mL). For monitoring of serum concentrations, levels should be assessed 4 to 8 hours after the last dose once a steady state is achieved. A steady state is reached about 3 days after the initiation of therapy or a change in dose, provided the medications are taken regularly.[1]

Two of the sustained-release theophylline preparations are Theo-Dur, which is usually started at 200 to 300 mg q12h, and Uniphyl, which is usually started at 400 to 600 mg as a single dose in the evening with or within 1 to 2 hours of a meal. Oxtriphylline (Choledyl) is short acting and is usually prescribed as 200 mg qid for adults. The usual dosage for children under 5 is 24 to 36 mg/kg/day divided into 3 equal doses given at 8-hour intervals. The dosage for children over the age of 5 is 22 mg/kg/day divided into 4 equal doses.

REFERENCES

1. Weinberger M, Hendeles L: Theophylline in asthma, *N Engl J Med* 334:1380-1388, 1996.

Immunotherapy

Immunotherapy for asthma is controversial although it has been used for over 70 years.[1] One study showed minimal benefits for seasonal allergic asthma to ragweed as measured by skin test sensitivity, bronchoconstrictor response to ragweed, and peak expiratory flow and reduction of medications in the first year, but this was not sustained during the second year.[2] Few asthmatic patients are allergic to only one allergen; many are allergic to house dust mites, cat dander, molds, and cockroaches, and there is little evidence that immunotherapy with these agents has any value.[1] A double-blind, placebo-controlled trial of multiple-allergen immunotherapy in children with moderate to severe year-round asthma demonstrated no beneficial effect after at least 18 months of therapy.[3]

The British Thoracic Society does not recommend immunotherapy for asthma under any circumstances,[4] whereas the National Heart, Lung, and Blood Institute considers it acceptable when drug therapy is ineffective or allergens are unavoidable.[5]

REFERENCES

1. Barnes PJ: Is immunotherapy for asthma worthwhile? (editorial), *N Engl J Med* 334:531-532, 1996.
2. Creticos PS, Reed CE, Norman PS, et al: Ragweed immunotherapy in adult asthma, *N Engl J Med* 334:501-506, 1996.
3. Adkinson NF Jr, Eggleston PA, Eney D, et al: A controlled trial of immunotherapy for asthma in allergic children, *N Engl J Med* 336:324-331, 1997.
4. British Thoracic Society: Guidelines on the management of asthma, *Thorax* 48(suppl):S1-S24, 1993.
5. National Heart, Lung, and Blood Institute: National Asthma Education Program Expert Panel report: guidelines for the diagnosis and management of asthma, *J Allergy Clin Immunol* 88:425-534, 1991.

Exercise-Induced Asthma

The prevalence of exercise-induced asthma in patients with known asthma has been variously reported as between 40% and 90%. Factors likely to aggravate exercise-induced asthma are intense exercise, low temperature, and low humidity. For symptoms to occur, exercise must be maintained for more than 2 minutes.[1]

In patients with exercise-induced asthma, symptoms usually develop shortly after they stop exercising. Spontaneous recovery is usually complete within half an hour to an hour.[1] A few individuals experience a late response (6 to 10 hours after exercise).[2]

An interesting feature of exercise-induced asthma is that a preliminary bout of mild to moderate exercise decreases the degree of bronchoconstriction during subsequent strenuous exercise (tachyphylaxis). This protective effect lasts for about 40 minutes and can be used therapeutically by athletes if they make a point of doing moderate warm-up exercises before participating in strenuous exercise. The warm-up should last 15 to 30 minutes and be followed by a 15-minute rest before vigorous exercise.

Aside from warm-up exercises, management of exercise-induced asthma usually involves taking an inhaled $beta_2$-adrenergic agonist such as albuterol or salbutamol (Proventil, Ventolin) 10 to 15 minutes before the exercise. This is usually effective for a 2-hour period.[2] Alternatives are salmeterol (Serevent),[3] sodium cromoglycate (Intal), or nedocromil sodium (Tilade). In some cases both albuterol and sodium cromoglycate can be used together.

REFERENCES

1. McFadden ER Jr, Gilbert IA: Exercise-induced asthma, *N Engl J Med* 330:1362-1367, 1994.
2. D'Urzo AD: Exercise-induced asthma: what family physicians should do, *Can Fam Physician* 41:1900-1906, 1995.
3. Nelson HS: ß-Adrenergic bronchodilators, *N Engl J Med* 333: 499-506, 1995.

BRONCHITIS, ACUTE

(See also antibiotic resistance; asthma; cough)

Acute bronchitis may be defined as cough and sputum developing in previously healthy individuals, usually after an upper respiratory tract infection. Other diseases, especially asthma, should be ruled out. Treatment with antibiotics is generally not indicated, but if symptoms persist unduly long, many physicians prescribe a macrolide because if bacterial pathogens are involved, they are usually *Mycoplasma pneumoniae, Chlamydia pneumoniae,* or *Streptococcus pneumo-*

niae.[1] A recent study from the United States showed that albuterol (salbutamol) helped control cough in cases of acute bronchitis, but that erythromycin gave no added benefit.[2]

REFERENCES

1. Proceedings from the Canadian Bronchitis Symposium, Toronto, Ontario, Canada, February 18-19, 1994: recommendations on the management of chronic bronchitis, *Can Med Assoc J* 151 (suppl):S1-S23, 1994.
2. Hueston WJ: Albuterol delivered by metered-dose inhaler to treat acute bronchitis, *J Fam Pract* 39:437-440, 1994.

CHRONIC BRONCHITIS AND EMPHYSEMA

(See also asthma; delivery systems for inhaled medications; inhaled steroids; metered dose inhalers; steroids and osteoporosis; theophylline salts)

An excellent comprehensive review of this confusing and controversial subject is the proceedings from the Canadian Bronchitis Symposium held in Toronto in February 1994.[1] Inhaled medications and their delivery systems are discussed above in the section on asthma.

The definition of chronic bronchitis is a clinical one. Patients have excessive cough, productive of sputum on most days, for at least 3 months a year during at least 2 consecutive years.[2]

Epidemiology

Important risk factors for chronic bronchitis are tobacco smoke, atmospheric pollution, and recurrent respiratory tract infections, especially in infancy.[3] The risk of chronic bronchitis in smokers depends on the amount smoked. The risk for nonsmokers is 15%, for those smoking a half pack to a pack a day it is 40% to 50%, and for those smoking two packs a day it is 70% to 80%. The risk for pipe and cigar smokers is 33%.[4]

Differential Diagnosis

The differential diagnosis of chronic cough is extensive. Conditions that may be difficult to differentiate from COPD are asthma and bronchiectasis. The diagnosis of the latter may require computed tomography of the lungs.[1]

Management of Stable Chronic Obstructive Pulmonary Disease

Patients with COPD who stop smoking often show a marked improvement in symptoms. Coughing stops in 77% of those who quit and improves in another 17%. The effect is seen in about half the patients within 4 weeks.[5]

Respiratory rehabilitation for patients with COPD is defined as an exercise training program of at least 4 weeks' duration. A metaanalysis of 14 studies of this intervention concluded that it reduced the amount of dyspnea and improved the patients' ability to cope with the disease.[6]

Inhaled beta-agonists and inhaled anticholinergics give symptomatic relief to many patients with COPD. The failure of pulmonary function testing to show a bronchodilator response does not mean the patient will not respond clinically.[7] Patients with mild or moderate COPD may require these agents only during exercise or cold exposure, whereas those with more severe cases may need regular use of the agents. Anticholinergics (ipratropium bromide [Atrovent]) have been reported to produce greater bronchodilation in patients with COPD and cause fewer side effects than do beta-agonists,[9] but other studies have found no difference.[10] A practical approach is to let patients try both drugs and decide for themselves.[8] If a clinical response occurs, these drugs should be continued indefinitely.[7] An MDI containing both ipratropium bromide and salbutamol (Combivent) is available.

Oral theophylline may have a role for some patients who remain symptomatic while receiving inhaled bronchodilators. Theophylline increases respiratory muscle strength and endurance and perhaps mucociliary clearance.[11] Toxicity is always a risk with this drug. Theophylline preparations are discussed above in the section on asthma.

Except in periods of exacerbation, the role of corticosteroids in COPD is controversial.[1] Only about 10% to 20% of patients respond to these drugs.[12] To determine who might benefit, a steroid trial must be performed when the patient's condition is stable and he or she is taking maximum doses of bronchodilator drugs. This is accomplished by measuring the forced expiratory volume (FEV_1) before and after a 2-week course of oral prednisone at a dose of 30 to 40 mg/day. Between 10% and 20% of patients with COPD demonstrate a 20% or greater improvement in FEV_1. Half of those whose FEV_1 improves can maintain this state with inhaled steroids, but the remainder require maintenance doses of oral steroids, preferably on alternate days.[12] Formulations of inhaled steroids are discussed above in the section on asthma.

Whether prophylactic antibiotics are useful for patients with stable COPD is unresolved. Most studies have shown little positive effect, but evidence suggests that patients with the largest number of exacerbations may gain some benefit.[1]

Home oxygen therapy has proved useful for selected patients with advanced COPD. Criteria for this therapy are that the patient be clinically stable and have a resting arterial partial pressure of oxygen (Pao_2) of 55 mm Hg or less, or of 60 mm Hg or less if there is polycythemia or cor pulmonale indicating tissue hypoxia.[1] When properly selected patients have used home oxygen therapy for 18 hours a day on a regular basis, life expectancy has increased by 6 to 7 years.[13] Home oxygen therapy should be continuous for at least 15 hours a day and adjusted to maintain the Pao_2 between 65 and 80 mm Hg and an arterial oxygen saturation of 90%. Oxygen concentrators give a maximum flow rate of 4 L/min.

Management of Exacerbations

Controversy exists as to the need for chest x-ray examination in flare-ups of COPD. That they are probably indicated in all cases is suggested by the authors of one retrospective study that reported the finding of significant abnormalities in 16% of

685 emergency room visits. These were 88 infiltrates, 20 episodes of pulmonary edema, 2 new lung masses, and 1 pneumothorax. About one fourth of these abnormalities would not have been detected if the x-ray studies had been ordered on the basis of previously determined "high-yield criteria."[14]

There is good evidence that IV and oral steroids are beneficial during a flare-up of COPD.[15,16] The usual oral dose is 30 to 40 mg of prednisone daily for 7 to 10 days.[16]

Whether antibiotics are useful in exacerbations of COPD is controversial. Viral infections are associated with about one third of exacerbations, but the data on the role of bacteria are less clear.[1] Murphy and associates[17] reviewed six randomized prospective placebo-controlled trials and found that three showed a beneficial effect from antibiotics and three did not. Anthonisen and colleagues[18] from Winnipeg demonstrated a clear benefit of antibiotics in patients with severe exacerbations but no definite benefit in cases of milder exacerbation. A 1995 metaanalysis of randomized trials found a small but statistically significant improvement when antibiotics were given for exacerbations.[19]

The bacteria most frequently associated with exacerbations are *Streptococcus pneumoniae, Haemophilus influenzae,* and *Moraxella catarrhalis.* Although many strains of the organisms associated with exacerbations of COPD are resistant to aminopenicillins, trimethoprim-sulfamethoxazole, or tetracyclines in vitro, this does not seem to have made much difference in clinical trials. A practical algorithm for the use of antibiotics in patients with COPD exacerbations categorizes patients according to risk factors as follows[1]:

1. Patients under age 65 with no or only moderate impairment of pulmonary function and fewer than four exacerbations annually. If antibiotics are used, the choices should be amoxicillin, trimethoprim-sulfamethoxazole, or tetracyclines.
2. Patients who are over the age of 65, or who have an FEV_1 less than 50%, or who have four or more exacerbations annually, or who have comorbid medical illnesses (congestive heart failure, diabetes, chronic renal failure, chronic liver disease). If antibiotics are used, the choices should be second- or third-generation cephalosporins, trimethoprim-sulfamethoxazole, or amoxicillin-clavulanic acid (Augmentin, Clavulin).

In special circumstances quinolones or newer macrolides might also be considered for this group. However, the macrolides have little effect against *H. influenzae* and the quinolones are not very effective against *S. pneumoniae.*

REFERENCES

1. Proceedings from the Canadian Bronchitis Symposium Toronto, Ontario, Canada, February 18-19, 1994: recommendations on the management of chronic bronchitis, *Can Med Assoc J* 151(suppl):S1-S23, 1994.
2. Medical Research Council: Definition and classification of chronic bronchitis for clinical and epidemiological purposes, *Lancet* 1:775-779, 1965.
3. Sherrill DL, Lebowitz MD, Burrows B: Epidemiology of chronic obstructive pulmonary disease, *Clin Chest Med* 11: 375-387, 1990.
4. Burrows B, Lebowitz MD: Quantitative relationships between cigarette smoking and chronic productive cough, *Int J Epidemiol* 6:107-113, 1977.
5. Wynder EL, Kaufaman PL, Lesser RL: A short-term follow-up study on ex-cigarette smokers: with special emphasis on persistent cough and weight gain, *Am Rev Respir Dis* 96:645-655, 1967.
6. Lacasse Y, Wong E, Guyatt GH, et al: Meta-analysis of respiratory rehabilitation in chronic obstructive pulmonary disease, *Lancet* 348:1115-1119, 1996.
7. Guyatt G, Townsend M, Nogradi S, et al: Acute response to bronchodilator: an imperfect guide for bronchodilator therapy in chronic airflow limitation, *Arch Intern Med* 148:1949-1952, 1988.
8. Mellor J: Goals of treatment of COPD, *Can J CME,* August 1995, 7:33-40.
9. Gross NJ, Shorodin MS: Anticholinergic antimuscarinic bronchodilators, *Am Rev Respir Dis* 129:856-870, 1984.
10. Blosser SA, Maxwell SL, Reeveshoche MK, et al: Is an anticholinergic agent superior to a beta (2)-agonist in improving dyspnea and exercise limitation in COPD, *Chest* 108:730-735, 1995.
11. Miller MA, Fragoso CAV: Review of the clinical efficacy of theophylline in the treatment of chronic obstructive pulmonary disease, *Am Rev Respir Dis* 147:S40-S47, 1993.
12. Callahan CM, Dittus RE, Katz BP: Oral corticosteroid therapy for patients with stable chronic obstructive pulmonary disease: a meta-analysis, *Ann Intern Med* 114:216-223, 1991.
13. Cooper CB, Waterhouse J, Howard P: Twelve-year clinical study of patients with hypoxic cor pulmonale given long-term domiciliary oxygen therapy, *Thorax* 42:105-110, 1987.
14. Emerman CL, Cydulka RK: Evaluation of high-yield criteria for chest radiography in acute exacerbation of chronic obstructive pulmonary disease, *Ann Emerg Med* 22:680-684, 1993.
15. Murata GH, Gorby MS, Chick TW, et al: Intravenous and oral corticosteroids for the prevention of relapse after treatment of decompensated COPD: effect on patients with a history of multiple relapses, *Chest* 198:845-849, 1990.
16. Hudson LD, Monti CM: Rationale and use of corticosteroids in chronic obstructive pulmonary disease, *Med Clin North Am* 174:661-690, 1990.
17. Murphy TF, Sethi S: Bacterial infection in chronic obstructive pulmonary disease, *Am Rev Respir Dis* 146:1067-1083, 1992.
18. Anthonisen NR, Manfreda J, Warren CP, et al: Antibiotic therapy in exacerbations of chronic obstructive pulmonary disease, *Ann Intern Med* 106:196-204, 1987.
19. Saint S, Bent S, Vittinghoff E, et al: Antibiotics in chronic obstructive pulmonary disease exacerbations: a meta-analysis, *JAMA* 273:957-960, 1995.

COUGH

(See also asthma; bronchitis, acute; esophageal reflux; pain; pertussis; serotonin syndrome)

In a study by Mello and co-workers,[1] over 99% of patients who had persistent troublesome cough of longer than 3 weeks' duration, who were nonsmokers, who were not taking angiotensin-converting enzyme inhibitors, and who had normal or stable x-ray findings had one or a combination of three diagnoses: asthma, postnasal drip, and gastroesophageal reflux. They also found that the character of the cough (paroxysmal, barking, dry or productive) was not helpful in making the diagnosis.[1] According to some workers, cough may be the sole symptom of gastroesophageal reflux in up to 75% of cases.[2] The pathogenesis of cough secondary to reflux is thought to be reflex bronchoconstriction as a result of acidification of the esophageal mucosa, not from aspiration of gastric contents.[3] An often unrecognized cause of prolonged coughing in adults is pertussis (see pertussis).

Treatment of chronic cough depends on the diagnosis. Recommended treatment for gastroesophageal reflux includes prokinetic agents such as cisapride (Prepulsid) or proton pump inhibitors such as omeprazole (Prilosec, Losec).[2] Postnasal drip often responds well to topical steroids,[4] but if antihistamines are used, a first-generation H_1-blocker such as chlorpheniramine (Chlor-Trimeton, Chlor-Tripolon) should be chosen because second-generation drugs have less anticholinergic activity and are less effective for this condition.[2]

Cough suppressants are sometimes used for patients whose lives are made miserable by spasms of coughing caused by an upper respiratory tract infection. The usual treatment has been dextromethorphan, 15 to 30 mg q4-6h or sometimes codeine (usually as a syrup containing 10 mg/5 ml), 20 to 30 mg q4-6h.[5] Many cold remedies contain dextromethorphan (DM) but usually in combination with sympathomimetics such as pseudoephedrine and often analgesics. By and large the physician should prescribe nothing or dextromethorphan or codeine alone. Each physician should find a commercial product that contains only dextromethorphan and stick to it. A rare but important adverse effect of dextromethorphan is induction of the serotonin syndrome (see discussion of serotonin syndrome). This is most likely to occur in patients already taking selective serotonin reuptake inhibitors, monoamine oxidase inhibitors, or antiparkinsonian drugs.

A recent trial of albuterol (salbutamol) for "acute bronchitis" from two family medicine centers in the United States showed that albuterol therapy with an MDI was more effective than erythromycin in controlling the cough. Adding erythromycin to the albuterol regimen gave no added benefit.[6]

Oxycodone (Percocet, Percodan, Roxicodone, Roxicet, Roxiprin) should not be prescribed for cough. Although it works, it is a narcotic that is as potent as morphine and in many areas is a popular drug of abuse.

REFERENCES

1. Mello CJ, Irwin RS, Curley FJ: Predictive values of the character, timing and complications of chronic cough in diagnosing its cause, *Arch Intern Med* 156:997-1003, 1996.
2. Irwin RS, French CF, Curley FJ, et al: Chronic cough due to gastroesophageal reflux: clinical, diagnostic, and pathogenetic aspects, *Chest* 104:1511-1517, 1993.
3. Pope CE II: Acid-reflux disorders, *N Engl J Med* 331:656-660, 1994.
4. Balter MS: The cough that won't go away, *Ontario Thorac Rev* 9:1-5, 1997.
5. Irwin RS, Curley FJ, Bennett FM: Appropriate use of antitussives and protussives: a practical review, *Drugs* 46:80-91, 1993.
6. Hueston WJ: Albuterol delivered by metered-dose inhaler to treat acute bronchitis, *J Fam Pract* 39:437-440, 1994.

LUNG CANCER

(See also length bias; screening)

Smoking accounts for 90% of cases of lung cancer, and the disease will develop in 20% of smokers.[1] Thin smokers are reported to be at greater risk of lung cancer than are better endowed puffers.[2] The overall prognosis of the disease is abysmal; about 90% of patients are dead within a year of the diagnosis.[1]

A chest roentenogram showing an isolated pulmonary nodule is one method of presentation of lung cancer. About two thirds of such nodules are benign (usually granulomas or hamartomas). Malignancy is more likely if the lesion is large, spiculated, or in the upper lobe and if the patient is older, smokes, or has a past history of cancer.[3]

Surgery is considered the treatment of choice for patients with non-small-cell lung cancer who can undergo an operation, but according to a 1990 report less than one third of patients who have had "curative" resections are alive at 5 years.[4] A more recent report concerning resectable non-small-cell carcinomas found the 5-year survival of patients with stage I tumors to be 71% while that of stage II tumors was 41%.[5] Although most studies have shown an increased 5-year survival in surgically treated patients, this may be an artifact of length bias. The argument is that resectable tumors are indolent tumors and therefore the patients would have done relatively well even without surgery.[6]

Morbidity and mortality from lung cancer surgery may be considerable. Overall surgical mortality rates in California between 1983 and 1986 were reported as 5%. The death rate for segmental resections was 4% and for pneumonectomy 11.6%.[7] Major complications occur in 10% of patients,[8] and half of the patients have persistent incisional pain 1 to 4 years after the operation.[9]

Preliminary studies of newer treatment modalities for non-small-cell lung cancer show a significantly increased median life expectancy. These protocols include combination chemotherapy with a variety of new agents for widespread disease and chemotherapy plus surgical resection for lung tumors with early extension to the pleura, pericardium, or diaphragm (stage IIIA).[10]

Small-cell lung cancer is rarely treated by surgical resection. At the time of diagnosis most patients have extensive disease. With chemotherapy median survival is 8 to 9 months, whereas without it survival is less than 6 weeks.[11]

REFERENCES

1. Sethi T: Lung cancer, *BMJ* 314:652-655, 1997.
2. Kark JK, Yaari S, Rasooly I, Goldbourt U (Israel Civil Servant Cancer Study): Are lean smokers at increased risk of lung cancer? *Arch Intern Med* 155:2409-2416, 1995.
3. Swensen SJ, Silverstein MC, Ilstrup DM, et al: The probability of malignancy in solitary pulmonary nodules: application to small radiologically indeterminate nodules, *Arch Intern Med* 157:849-855, 1997.
4. Humphrey EW, Smart CR, Winchester DP, et al: National survey of the pattern of care for carcinoma of the lung, *J Thorac Cardiovasc Surg* 100:837-843, 1990.
5. Shah R, Sabanathan S, Richardson J, et al: Results of surgical treatment of stage I and II lung cancer, *J Cardiovasc Surg (Torino)* 37:169-172, 1996.
6. Lederle FA, Niewoehner DE: Lung cancer surgery: a critical review of the evidence, *Arch Intern Med* 154:2397-2400, 1994.
7. Romano PS, Mark DH: Patient and hospital characteristics related to in-hospital mortality after lung cancer resection, *Chest* 101:1332-1337, 1992.
8. Deslauriers J, Ginsberg RJ, Dubois P, et al: Current operative morbidity associated with elective surgical resection for lung cancer, *Can J Surg* 32:335-339, 1989.
9. Dajczman E, Gordon A, Kreisman H, et al: Long-term post-thoracotomy pain, *Chest* 99:270-274, 1991.
10. Hainsworth JD: Chemotherapy in the treatment of non-small cell lung cancer, *Am Fam Physician* 55:2265-2272, 1997.
11. Aisner J: Extensive-disease small-cell lung cancer: the thrill of victory; the agony of defeat, *J Clin Oncol* 14:658-665, 1996.

PNEUMONIA

(See also pneumonia in children)

Diagnosis and Investigation

Symptoms of pneumonia are usually less frequent and severe in elderly patients than in younger ones.[1] Fever occurs in 80% of patients with pneumoni, and crackles are heard in 80%; most have a respiratory rate greater than 20 breaths/min, but only 30% have signs of consolidation.[2]

Traditionally "atypical pneumonia" caused by organisms such as *Chlamydia* was said to be characterized by a viral-type prodrome, a nonproductive cough, and lack of lobar consolidation on x-ray examination. These criteria turn out to be quite nonspecific. It is not possible to determine which of the five most common organisms causing community-acquired pneumonia in adults *(Streptococcus pneumoniae, Haemophilus influenzae, Legionella* species, *Chlamydia pneumoniae,* or gram-negative rods) is responsible for the disease on the basis of history, physical examination, laboratory investigations (such as white blood cell count), or chest x-ray examination.[3,4] The clinical and radiological presentations seem to be more a matter of host response than the nature of the infecting organisms.[5] Sputum culture and Gram's stain are not helpful in most cases of community-acquired pneumonia; one third of patients cannot produce sputum, a third have already been treated with antibiotics, and a fourth are infected with organisms not easily cultured.[2] False-positive results of sputum cultures are common because of colonization of organisms in the oropharynx, and the false-negative rate in pneumococcal infections approaches 50%.[5] However, sputum cultures and Gram's stain may detect unusual organisms such as *Histoplasma, Pneumocystis carinii,* and *Mycobacterium tuberculosis.*[5] Blood cultures are positive in no more than 25% of cases; the positivity rate is greatest if the organism is *Streptococcus pneumoniae.*[2,5] The main indication for sputum cultures, Gram's staining of sputum, or more invasive procedures such as transtracheal aspiration or bronchoalveolar lavage is severely ill patients. For the majority of patients with community-acquired pneumonia, treatment is empirical.[5]

The finding of bilateral pleural effusions on the roentgenogram of a patient with community-acquired pneumonia is associated with an increased mortality rate.[6]

Prognosis

Prognosis is an important factor in determining whether patients with pneumonia require admission. Criteria for determining this have not been standardized, as is evident from the variability of admission rates for this condition from one geographical location to another.[1] Fine and associates[7] have developed a series of prediction rules that separate patients with good prognoses who can generally be treated at home from those with poor prognoses who should be admitted to the hospital. Predictors of increased risk of death based on the history and physical examination are as follows:

1. Age over 50
2. Coexisting illnesses (neoplasia, congestive heart failure, cerebrovascular disease, renal disease, and liver disease)
3. Altered mental status
4. Pulse ≥125/min
5. Respiratory rate ≥30 breaths/min
6. Systolic blood pressure <90 mm Hg
7. Temperature <35° C or ≥40° C

Management

Recommended treatment regimens for pneumonias treated on an outpatient basis vary from one author to another and from one country to another.[1] The pathogenic organisms tend to vary with age and with the presence of comorbid illnesses. Common to all groups are *Streptococcus pneumoniae* and *Haemophilus influenzae.* Otherwise well patients under the age of 65 tend to have a number of infections caused by *Mycoplasma pneumoniae* and *Chlamydia pneumoniae.* Individuals with comorbid illnesses or over the age of 65 are also at risk of infections caused by oral anaerobes, gram-negative rods, *Staphylococcus aureus,* and *Legionella.*[8]

Both American and Canadian guidelines suggest that the treatment of choice for pneumonia in otherwise well patients under the age of 60 to 65 is a macrolide (erythromycin, clarithromycin [Biaxin] or azithromycin [Zithromax]), with tetracycline an acceptable alternative. For patients over the age of 60 to 65, or for anyone with a comorbid illness, acceptable treatment options are a second-generation cephalosporin such as cefaclor (Ceclor) or cefuroxime axetil (Ceftin), trimethoprim-sulfamethoxazole (Septra, Bactrim), or a penicillin plus a beta-lactamase inhibitor (amoxicillin plus clavulanate potassium [Augmentin, Clavulin]), with the addition of a macrolide to any of these regimens if *Legionella* is suspected.[8,9] Although these recommendations make sense, a number of experienced clinicians would consider macrolides as the drug of first choice for otherwise healthy individuals over the age of 60 to 65.

Although *Legionella pneumoniae* may occur in epidemics, 2% to 15% of community-acquired pneumonias are caused by this organism; patients with the disease are usually sick enough to require admission. Aside from respiratory symptoms and fever, gastrointestinal problems, especially diarrhea, are common. Macrolides are the treatment of first choice, but there are case reports that ciprofloxacin, rifampin, tetracyclines, and trimethoprim-sulfamethoxazole are effective.[10]

Do all patients with pneumonia serious enough to require hospital admission require intravenous antibiotics? In a study from Dublin hospitalized patients with pneumonia were assigned at random to receive either intravenous or oral antibiotics; the outcome was equally good in both cases. Patients were excluded from the study if they were immunocompromised or if they had life-threatening infections.[11]

REFERENCES

1. Bartlett JG, Mundy LM: Community-acquired pneumonia, *N Engl J Med* 333:1618-1624, 1995.
2. Marrie TJ: Community-acquired pneumonia, *Clin Infect Dis* 18:502-515, 1994.
3. Fang G-D, Fine M, Orloff J, et al: New and emerging etiologies for community-acquired pneumonia with implications for therapy: a prospective multicenter study of 359 cases, *Medicine* 69: 307-316, 1990.
4. Kauppinen MT, Laehde S, Syrjaelae H: Roentgenographic findings of pneumonia caused by *Chlamydia* pneumonia: a comparison with *Streptococcus* pneumonia, *Arch Intern Med* 156:1851-1856, 1996.
5. Antoniou M, Grossman RF: Etiological diagnosis of pneumonia: a goal worth pursuing? *Can J Infect Dis* 6:281-283, 1995.
6. Hasley PB, Albaum MN, Li Y-H, et al: Do pulmonary radiographic findings at presentation predict mortality in patients with community-acquired pneumonia? *Arch Intern Med* 156: 2206-2212, 1996.
7. Fine MF, Auble TE, Yealy DM, et al: A prediction rule to identify low-risk patients with community acquired pneumonia, *N Engl J Med* 336:243-250, 1997.
8. Treatment of community acquired pneumonia in adults—conference report, *Can J Infect Dis,* January/February 1993, vol 4, no 1.
9. Niederman MS, Bass JB Jr, Campbell GD, et al: American Thoracic Society Guidelines for the initial management of adults with community-acquired pneumonia: diagnosis, assessment of severity, and initial antimicrobial therapy, *Am Rev Respir Dis* 148:1418-1426, 1993.
10. Stout JE, Yu VL: Legionellosis, *N Engl J Med* 337:682-687, 1997.
11. Chan R, Hemeryck L, O'Regan M, et al: Oral versus intravenous antibiotics for community acquired lower respiratory tract infection in a general hospital: open, randomised controlled trial, *BMJ* 310:1360-1362, 1995.

PNEUMOTHORAX

(See also aviation medicine)

Spontaneous pneumothorax is traditionally treated by inserting a thoracostomy tube. A British study has demonstrated that simple aspiration of air with a 16- or 18-gauge needle resulted in less discomfort and a shorter hospital stay than thoracostomy tube placement. In this series aspiration technique was successful in 28 of 35 patients. In 7 patients the aspiration technique failed and tube placement was required.[1]

An emergency treatment for tension pneumothorax is to create a one-way valve with an 18-gauge needle and a portion of a latex glove. An 18-gauge needle is inserted into the pleural space through the second intercostal space. The tip of one finger of a latex glove is cut off and fitted over the hub of the needle, and portions of the cut edges are taped to the proximal shaft of the needle without making an airtight seal between these edges and the needle shaft. This creates a one way valve, allowing egress but not ingress of air through the needle.[2]

REFERENCES

1. Harvey J, Prescott RJ: Simple aspiration versus intercostal tube drainage for spontaneous pneumothorax in patients with normal lungs, *BMJ* 309:1338-1339, 1994.
2. Earp-Jones A: Lifesaving finger, *Patient Care Can,* June 1996, 7:18.

SARCOID

Sarcoid is a worldwide disease affecting both sexes, all races, and all ages. It is more common and more aggressive in blacks than in whites and most frequently occurs in persons under the age of 40.[1]

A common clinical presentation of sarcoid is peripheral arthritis, often associated with erythema nodosum. Almost all patients have involvement of the ankles, and other frequently affected joints are the knees, wrists, and elbows. The arthritis is rarely monarticular, and it does not cause joint destruction. Chest x-ray examination usually shows hilar adenopathy.[1,2] Between 20% and 50% of cases of sarcoid are manifested as arthralgias, erythema nodosum, and bilateral hilar adenopathy, a constellation of findings known as Löfgren's syndrome. Löfgren's syndrome has the best prognosis of any of the variants of sarcoid.[1] In one study of this form of clinical presentation the mean duration of the arthropathy was about 4 months, recurrence of arthritis after resolution of the initial episode occurred in 4%, and chronic pulmonary sarcoidosis developed in 8% of cases. Except for cases with pulmonary involvement in which corticosteroids are indicated, the treatment of choice is nonsteroidal antiinflammatory drugs.[2]

Most cases of sarcoid are probably asymptomatic; a number of these are identified by finding hilar adenopathy on chest roentgenograms taken for other reasons. Among patients with only hilar adenopathy the disease remits spontaneously in 60% to 80% of cases. For patients with hilar adenopathy plus pulmonary infiltrates, spontaneous remission occurs in 50% to 60% of cases, whereas if there are only pulmonary infiltrates without hilar adenopathy, spontaneous remission is seen in less than 30%. The prognosis is worse in patients over 40, blacks, and those whose symptoms last longer than 6 months.[1]

No specific laboratory investigations are used for sarcoidosis. The serum level of angiotensin-converting enzyme (ACE) may be elevated, but this finding has little diagnostic value because it is nonspecific; the Kveim-Siltzbach test is of historical interest only.[1]

In most patients who do not have deteriorating lung disease or serious extrapulmonary disease, treatment with corticosteroids may be withheld for 6 months because about 40% of patients have spontaneous improvement.[1]

REFERENCES

1. Newman LS, Rose CS, Maier LA: Sarcoidosis, *N Engl J Med* 336:1224-1234, 1997.
2. Gran JT, Bohmer E: Acute sarcoid arthritis: a favourable outcome? A retrospective survey of 49 patients with review of the literature, *Scand J Rheumatol* 25:70-73, 1996.

SMOKING

(See also detrimental effects of alcohol; smoking in pregnancy)

Topics covered in this section

Epidemiology
Beneficial Effects of Smoking
Detrimental Effects of Smoking
Quitting Smoking
Tobacco Industry

EPIDEMIOLOGY

(See also detrimental effects of alcohol; poverty)

The prevalence of smoking among Americans over the age of 17 fell from 42.4% in 1965 to 25.5% in 1990. In 1992 the prevalence was 26.5%. The increase was partly explained by a change in definition to include intermittent as well as daily smokers.[1]

The highest rates of smoking in 1992 were in the 25- to 44-year-old group (31%) and among those below the poverty line (35%). Slightly more men (29%) than women (25%) smoked, and smoking incidence declined with years of education.[1] Persons who had not started smoking during adolescence were unlikely ever to become smokers.[2]

Although smoking rates have fallen in the developed world, they have been increasing in the developing world and represent a major public health problem in these regions.[3] For example, in the district of Shanghai, China, 67% of males and 2% of females smoke.[4] The cost of smoking represents 60% of personal income and 17% of household income.[4] Physicians in China are heavy smokers as well; in a 1989 survey in Beijing, 68% smoked.[5]

Alcohol abusers tend to be heavy smokers.[6,7] In fact, a history of heavy smoking may alert the clinician to unacknowledged alcohol abuse.[7]

REFERENCES

1. Cigarette smoking among adults—United States, 1992, and changes in the definition of current cigarette smoking, *MMWR* 43:342-346, 1994.
2. Department of Health and Human Services: *Preventing tobacco use among young people: a report of the Surgeon General,* Washington, DC, 1994, US Government Printing Office, pp 5, 58.
3. World Bank: *World development report 1993,* New York, 1993, Oxford University Press.
4. Cigarette smoking in China: prevalence, characteristics, and attitudes in Minhang District, *JAMA* 274:1232-1234, 1995.
5. Skolnick AA: Answer sought for "tobacco giant" China's problem, *JAMA* 275:1220-1221, 1996.
6. Hurt RD, Offord KP, Croghan IT, et al: Mortality following inpatient addictions treatment: role of tobacco use in a community-based cohort, *JAMA* 275:1097-1103, 1996.
7. Valiant GE, Schnurr PP, Baron JA, et al: A prospective study of the effects of cigarette smoking and alcohol abuse on mortality, *J Gen Intern Med* 6:299-304, 1991.

BENEFICIAL EFFECTS OF SMOKING

Epidemiological evidence has been presented that smoking is "good" for ulcerative colitis. The disease is more common in nonsmokers than in smokers, the initial onset of the disease often correlates with discontinuing smoking, and smoking may control the symptoms of the disease.[1] These apparently beneficial effects are not seen in Crohn's disease. In a randomized, double-blind study of 72 patients with ulcerative colitis, nicotine patches improved the symptoms in the treated patients.[2] An editorial accompanying the report cautions against general use of such therapy at this time.[1] The use of nicotine patches to help maintain remission in ulcerative colitis has not proved beneficial.[3]

The incidence of Parkinson's disease has been reported to be less in smokers than in nonsmokers.[4] The reason may be that the brains of smokers have a very low level of monoamine oxidase B (MAO B), which causes the breakdown of dopamine.[5]

In a case-control study the incidence of endometrial cancer was found to be lower in postmenopausal smokers than in postmenopausal nonsmokers. This is thought to occur because smoking has the ability to inactivate estrogens to some degree.[6]

REFERENCES

1. Hanauer SB: Nicotine for colitis—the smoke has not yet cleared (editorial), *N Engl J Med* 330:856-857, 1994.
2. Pullan RD, Rhodes J, Ganesh S, et al: Transdermal nicotine for active ulcerative colitis, *N Engl J Med* 330:811-815, 1994.
3. Thomas GAO, Mani V, Williams GT, et al: Transdermal nicotine as maintenance therapy for ulcerative colitis, *N Engl J Med* 332:988-992, 1995.
4. Doll R, Peto R, Wheatley K, et al: Mortality in relation to smoking: 40 years' observations on male British doctors, *BMJ* 309: 901-911, 1994.
5. Fowler JS, Volkow ND, Wang GJ, et al: Inhibition of monoamine oxidase B in the brains of smokers, *Nature* 379:733-736, 1996.
6. Lesko SM, Rosenberg L, Kaufman DW, et al: Cigarette smoking and the risk of endometrial cancer, *N Engl J Med* 313:593-596, 1985.

DETRIMENTAL EFFECTS OF SMOKING

(See also smoking in pregnancy)

Smoking contributes to increased mortality rates from multiple causes. McGinnis and colleagues[1] estimate that smoking accounts for 19% of U.S. deaths, which puts it ahead of all other causes of preventable deaths. Diet/activity patterns came second, accounting for 14% of deaths.[1] In a 40-year study of British physicians the excess total mortality of continuing smokers between the ages of 45 and 64 was three times that of nonsmokers, while for continuing smokers aged 65 to 84 it was twice that of nonsmokers. The authors of this study concluded that half of all regular smokers are likely to die from their habit.[2] Extrapolating from a 15-year follow-up of the British Regional Heart Study, Phillips and colleagues[3] concluded that only 42% of 20-year-old smokers who continued to smoke all their lives would still be alive by age 73 compared with 78% of 20-year-old nonsmokers who never took up the habit.[3]

In the United States smoking is responsible for about 30% of all cancer deaths.[4] The overall cancer death rates in smokers is twice that of nonsmokers, and the cancer death rate for heavy smokers is four times that of nonsmokers. Cancers related to smoking include those of the lung, oral cavity, larynx, esophagus, stomach, pancreas, colon, uterine cervix, bladder, ureter and kidney, and breast. In addition, about 14% of leukemias are thought to be caused by smoking.

Cardiovascular diseases associated with smoking are coronary artery disease, myocardial infarction, sudden death, strokes, subarachnoid hemorrhages, peripheral vascular disease, and aortic aneurysms. Smoking is known to decrease the oxygen-carrying power of the blood because of carbon monoxide production, to activate platelets, and to foster the development of atherosclerosis. In one study of women smokers, even one to four cigarettes per day more than doubled the risk of coronary artery disease.[5] Nonsmokers exposed to secondhand smoke have an increased incidence of both fatal and nonfatal cardiac events.[6,7]

Respiratory diseases in adults caused by smoking include chronic obstructive pulmonary disease and pneumonia. Smokers have an increased death rate from influenza. Smoking even as few as five cigarettes a day in adolescence diminishes the normal growth of lung function, particularly in girls.[8]

Passive smoke affects children, who when exposed have a higher incidence of asthma, bronchitis, pneumonia, middle ear effusions, tonsillectomies, adenoidectomies, and deaths (usually from lower respiratory tract infections or fires).[9] Exposure of infants to cigarette smoke has also been associated with an increased risk of sudden infant death syndrome.[10]

Smoking during pregnancy is associated with intrauterine growth retardation, low-birth-weight infants, preterm births, placenta previa, abruptio placentae, and a higher incidence of miscarriages of viable infants.[11] Smokers have been reported to have a lower fertility rate than nonsmokers.[12]

Smoking has been reported to increase the risk of acquiring non-insulin-dependent diabetes.[13] It also adversely affects thyroid function.[14-16] It is associated with an increased incidence of Graves' disease and even more so with Graves' ophthalmopathy[14] and may also be a contributing factor to the development of subclinical hypothyroidism even if it does not aggravate the clinical manifestations.[15]

The relapse rate of Crohn's disease is greater in smokers than nonsmokers.[17] The risk of age-related macular degeneration is increased in both male[18] and female[19] smokers, and it is likely that smoking is also a risk factor for cataracts.[20] Sun-exposed smokers have a higher incidence of wrinkles and skin cancers than sun-exposed nonsmokers.[21] There is an association between smoking and low back pain, but whether this is a causal relationship is uncertain.[22] Cigarettes are the leading cause of fire fatalities.[23]

Pipe and cigar smokers have lower mortality rates for ischemic heart disease, lung cancer, and chronic obstructive pulmonary disease than do cigarette smokers, in large part because they smoke less tobacco but also because they tend to inhale less. Cigarette smokers who switch to cigars or pipes achieve a decreased mortality rate for these diseases, but to a lesser degree than cigar and pipe smokers who have never smoked cigarettes. This is probably because the switchers inhale more.[24]

REFERENCES

1. McGinnis JM, Foege WH: Actual causes of death in the United States, *JAMA* 270:2207-2211, 1993.
2. Doll R, Peto R, Wheatley K, et al: Mortality in relation to smoking: 40 years' observations on male British doctors, *BMJ* 309:901-911, 1994.
3. Phillips AN, Wannamethee SG, Walker M, et al: Life expectancy in men who have never smoked and those who have smoked continuously: 15 year follow up of large cohort of middle aged British men, *BMJ* 313:907-908, 1996.

4. Bartecchi CE, MacKenzie TD, Schrier RW: The human costs of tobacco use (first of two parts), *N Engl J Med* 330:907-912, 1994.
5. Willett WC, Green A, Stampfer JM, et al: Relative and absolute excess risks of coronary heart disease among women who smoke cigarettes, *N Engl J Med* 317:1303-1309, 1987.
6. Glantz SA, Parmley WW: Passive smoking and heart disease: mechanisms and risk, *JAMA* 273:1047-1053, 1995.
7. Kawachi I, Colditz GA, Speizer FE, et al: A prospective study of passive smoking and coronary heart disease, *Circulation* 95: 2374-2379, 1997.
8. Gold DR, Wang X, Wypij D, et al: Effects of cigarette smoking on lung function in adolescent boys and girls, *N Engl J Med* 335:931-937, 1996.
9. Difranza JR, Lew RA: Morbidity and mortality in children associated with the use of tobacco products by other people, *Pediatrics* 97:560-568, 1996.
10. Klonoff-Cohen HS, Edelstein SL, Lefkowitz ES, et al: The effect of passive smoking and tobacco exposure through breast milk on sudden infant death syndrome, *JAMA* 273:795-798, 1995.
11. Brosky G: Why do pregnant women smoke and can we help them quit? (editorial), *Can Med Assoc J* 152:163-166, 1995.
12. deMouzan J, Spira A, Schwartz D: A prospective study of the relation between smoking and fertility, *Int J Epidemiol* 17:378-384, 1988.
13. Rimm EB, Chan J, Stampfer MJ, et al: Prospective study of cigarette smoking, alcohol use, and the risk of diabetes in men, *BMJ* 210:545-546, 1995.
14. Prummel MF, Wiersinga WM: Smoking and risk of Graves' disease, *JAMA* 269:479-482, 1993.
15. Müller B, Zulewski H, Huber P, et al: Impaired action of thyroid hormone associated with smoking in women with hypothyroidism, *N Engl J Med* 333:964-969, 1995.
16. Utiger RD: Cigarette smoking and the thyroid (editorial), *N Engl J Med* 333:1001-1002, 1995.
17. Duffy LC, Zielezny MA, Marshall JR, et al: Cigarette smoking and risk of clinical relapse in patients with Crohn's disease, *Am J Prevent Med* 6:161-166, 1990.
18. Christen WG, Glynn RJ, Manson JE, et al: A prospective study of cigarette smoking and risk of age-related macular degeneration in men, *JAMA* 276:1147-1151, 1996.
19. Seddon JM, Willett WC, Speizer FE, et al: A prospective study of cigarette smoking and age-related macular degeneration in women, *JAMA* 276:1141-1146, 1996.
20. West S: Does smoke get in your eyes? (editorial), *JAMA* 268: 1025-1026, 1992.
21. Gilchrest BA: A review of skin ageing and its medical therapy, *Br J Dermatol* 135:867-875, 1996.
22. Leboeufyde C, Yashin A: Smoking and low back pain—is the association real, *J Manip Physiolog Therapeut* 18:457-463, 1995.
23. McGuire A: Cigarettes and fire deaths, *NY State J Med* 83: 1296-1298, 1983.
24. Wald NJ, Watt HC: Prospective study of effect of switching from cigarettes to pipes or cigars on mortality from three smoking related diseases, *BMJ* 314:1860-1863, 1997.

QUITTING SMOKING

(See also behavioral changes for prevention; detrimental effects of smoking; nicotine replacement therapy)

What techniques should a family physician use to help patients give up smoking? Guidelines based on an extensive literature review have been developed by the U.S. Agency for Health Care Policy and Research (AHCPR). Some of the essential points of these guidelines are that smoking status should be determined for every patient at every visit and that for smokers the desire to quit or not quit should be assessed. For smokers who do not plan to quit, an attempt should be made to motivate them to do so, and for those who want to quit, a detailed plan should be worked out.[1]

A systematic review of 188 randomized controlled trials of smoking cessation found that personal advice from a physician during a single consultation resulted in a 2% success rate measured 1 year later. Additional support such as follow-up letters or visits had a positive but variable benefit. Patients at high risk (pregnant patients and those with coronary artery disease) had a cessation rate of about 8%. Behavior modification techniques in individual or group sessions with a psychologist had a 2% success rate. No data were given for hypnosis, and acupuncture was not effective. Nicotine replacement therapy led to a 13% success rate. There was no evidence supporting the efficacy of other pharmacological interventions.[2]

A common consequence of quitting smoking is weight gain. In one study the average excess weight gain at 10 years among persons who had quit smoking compared with control subjects who had never smoked was 4.4 kg (10 lb) for men and 5 kg (11 lb) for women.[3]

Nicotine gum and nicotine patches have proved valuable in helping patients quit smoking; this is discussed in the subsections below. Nicotine is thought to stimulate the release of dopamine in the brain, and it is this neurotransmitter that leads to "feeling good" after a cigarette. Recent work suggests that the brains of smokers have low levels of MAO B, which normally breaks down dopamine, and this too would contribute to the good feeling experienced by having a smoke.[4] It is logical to think that quitting might be facilitated by antidepressants, particularly MAO B inhibitors such as moclobemide (Manerix), and this has apparently been documented by some French workers.[5] A relationship between smoking and depression is supported by the observation that smokers with a history of major depression have a high recurrence rate if they quit successfully. In a 3-month follow-up of 126 individuals who had quit smoking successfully, the incidence of major depression was 2% among those with no history of depression, 17% among those with a history of a single episode of depression, and 30% for those with a history of recurrent depressions.[6]

Two major factors that predict success in quitting are low nicotine dependence and successful abstinence during the first 2 weeks of quitting.[7,8] One study has even shown that success on the first day of quitting correlates with improved long-term success.[9]

Persons making life-style changes such as quitting smoking pass through several stages, and it is important for patients to deal with the particular stage they are in.[10] This is discussed in the section on behavioral changes for prevention.

If all endeavors to give up smoking fail, encouraging the patient to switch to cigars or pipes might be worthwhile (see discussion of detrimental effects of smoking).[11]

REFERENCES

1. Fiore MC, Wetter DW, Bailey WC, et al (Smoking Cessation Clinical Practice Guideline Panel and Staff): The Agency for Health Care Policy and Research Smoking Cessation clinical practice guideline, *JAMA* 275:1270-1280, 1996.
2. Law M, Tang JL: An analysis of the effectiveness of interventions intended to help people stop smoking, *Arch Intern Medicine* 155:1933-1941, 1995.
3. Flegal KM, Troiano RP, Pamuk ER, et al: The influence of smoking cessation on the prevalence of overweight in the United States, *N Engl J Med* 333:1165-1170, 1995.
4. Fowler JS, Volkow ND, Wang GJ, et al: Inhibition of monoamine oxidase B in the brains of smokers, *Nature* 379:733-736, 1996.
5. Stephenson J: Clues found to tobacco addiction, *JAMA* 275: 1217-1218, 1996.
6. Covey LS, Glassman AH, Stetner F: Major depression following smoking cessation, *Am J Psychiatry* 154:263-265, 1997.
7. Kenford SL, Fiore MC, Jorenby DE, et al: Predicting smoking cessation: who will quit with and without the nicotine patch? *JAMA* 271:589-594, 1994.
8. Gourlay SG, Forbes A, Marriner T, et al: Prospective study of factors predicting outcome of transdermal nicotine treatment in smoking cessation, *BMJ* 309:842-846, 1994.
9. Westman EC, Behm FM, Simel DL, et al: Smoking behavior on the first 1997 day of a quit attempt predicts long-term abstinence, *Arch Intern Med* 157:335-340, 1997.
10. Prochaska JO: Why do we behave the way we do? *Can J Cardiol* 11(suppl A):20A-25A, 1995.
11. Wald NJ, Watt HC: Prospective study of effect of switching from cigarettes to pipes or cigars on mortality from three smoking related diseases, *BMJ* 314:1860-1863, 1997.

Nicotine Replacement Therapy

(See also ulcerative colitis)

Nicotine replacement therapy is available in the form of 2- and 4-mg nicotine-containing chewing gum (Nicorette), nicotine-containing transdermal patches with various concentrations of nicotine (Habitrol, Nicoderm, Nicotrol, and ProStep), and more recently a nicotine-containing nasal spray (Nicotrol NS) (Table 65).

Nicotine chewing gum

An analysis of the results of 28 randomized trials of chewing gum containing 2 mg of nicotine, 6 trials of chewing gum containing 4 mg of nicotine, and 6 trials of nicotine transdermal patches showed that both the gum and patches decreased smoking rates measured after 1 year. The 4-mg gum was effective in about one third of "high-dependence" smokers and the 2-mg chewing gum in 6% of smokers (11% of self-referred subjects and 3% of invited subjects).[1] This study supports the findings of a previous Danish report that among highly dependent smokers, gum containing 4 mg of nicotine resulted in abstinence rates of 44% at 1 year and 33% at 2 years, whereas they were only 12% and 6% for those taking gum containing 2 mg of nicotine.[2] In a short-term study of "high-dependence" smokers told to chew 12 pieces of gum a day, the abstinence rate at 6 weeks was 59% for the 4-mg gum, 30% for the 2-mg gum, and 39% for the placebo group.[3]

Table 65 Nicotine Replacement Therapy

Drug names	Drug concentrations
Nicotine Polacrilex Chewing Gum	
Nicorette	2 mg
Nicorette DS, Nicorette Plus	4 mg
Nicotine Transdermal Systems	
Habitrol	21, 14, 7 (mg absorbed/24 hr)
Nicoderm	21, 14, 7 (mg absorbed/24 hr)
Nicotrol	15, 10, 5 (mg absorbed/16 hr)
ProStep	22, 11 (mg absorbed/24 hr)
Nicotine Nasal Spray	
Nicotrol NS	0.5 mg per activation

For patients who smoke fewer than 20 cigarettes a day, the initial dose is approximately one 2-mg dose for every two cigarettes. For those who smoke 20 or more cigarettes a day, one 4-mg dose should be prescribed for every three or four cigarettes. The nicotine intake from such doses is still considerably below the total daily intake of most smokers. Nicotine polacrilex should not be chewed like ordinary gum. The gum should be chewed a few times and then held in the mouth for a minute or so before repeating the cycle. This prevents nicotine rushes. Each piece should be used for about 30 minutes.[4] Most patients should have the gum available for 3 to 6 months.

Nicotine patches

A metaanalysis of 17 studies using nicotine patches showed them to be effective. At a 6-month follow-up patch users were three times more likely to be abstaining from cigarettes than were the placebo control subjects. No difference was observed between 16-hour and 24-hour patches, intensive behavioral therapy had only a modest effect on discontinuation rates, and extending treatment beyond 8 weeks resulted in no additional benefit.[5]

A group in California used a 16-hour patch for 12 weeks plus a 6-week tapering period. No special counseling was done. At the end of a year nearly three times as many nicotine patch users were abstinent as were those using control patches.[6]

Nicotine patches are safe in patients with known stable coronary artery disease.[7,8]

The nicotine plasma levels in patients using the patch are usually less than are found in a pack-a-day smoker. In general, patients smoking more than 10 cigarettes a day should be started on the highest dose patch, while those who smoke less may be started on midrange patches. For very heavy smokers who do not respond to conventional therapy, using two patches simultaneously appears safe. Weaning to lower doses is tried every 1 to 2 months.[4]

Patches should be applied to hairless areas of the skin and the site changed daily to prevent irritation. Habitrol, Nicoderm, and ProStep are changed every 24 hours, whereas Nicotrol is applied first thing in the morning and removed at bedtime (16 hours of use).

Nicotine nasal spray

The usual dose of the nicotine nasal spray (Nicotrol NS) is two activations in each nostril (a total of 4 mg) with a maximum of 5 doses an hour or 40 doses an day.

REFERENCES

1. Tang JL, Law M, Wald N: How effective is nicotine replacement therapy in helping people to stop smoking? *BMJ* 308:21-26, 1994.
2. Tonnesen P, Fryd V, Hansen M, et al: Effect of nicotine chewing gum in combination with group counseling on the cessation of smoking, *N Engl J Med* 318:15-18, 1988.
3. Sachs DP: Effectiveness of the 4-mg dose of nicotine polacrilex for the initial treatment of high-dependent smokers, *Arch Intern Med* 155:1973-1980, 1995.
4. Henningfield JE: Nicotine medications for smoking cessation, *N Engl J Med* 333:1196-1203, 1995.
5. Fiore MC, Smith SS, Jorenby DE, Baker TB: The effectiveness of the nicotine patch for smoking cessation: a meta-analysis, *JAMA* 271:1940-1947, 1994.
6. Sachs DP, Sawe U, Lleischow SJ: Effectiveness of a 16-hour transdermal nicotine patch in a medical practice setting, without intensive group counseling, *Arch Intern Med* 153:1881-1890, 1994.
7. Working Group for the Study of Transdermal Nicotine in Patients with Coronary Artery Disease: Nicotine replacement therapy for patients with coronary artery disease, *Arch Intern Med* 154:989-995, 1994.
8. Joseph AM, Norman SM, Ferry LH, et al: The safety of transdermal nicotine as an aid to smoking cessation in patients with cardiac disease, *N Engl J Med* 335:1792-1798, 1996.

TOBACCO INDUSTRY

Between 1990 and 1991, U.S. cigarette manufacturers increased their advertising budgets by 16% to $4.6 billion per year.[1] There is persuasive circumstantial evidence that much of the industry's advertising has been aimed at children. In 1988 RJR Nabisco introduced a marketing campaign featuring Old Joe Camel.[2] Fischer and associates[3] found that 80% of 6-year-olds and 30% of 3-year-olds were able to associate a picture of Old Joe Camel with a pack of cigarettes.[3] Between the introduction of the campaign in 1988 and 1990 the proportion of smokers under the age of 18 who smoked Camels increased from 0.5% to 32%.[4]

It has long been suspected that the tobacco industry has known that nicotine is addictive and that smoking causes numerous serious diseases. The industry has spent huge sums on lobbying efforts. The evidence for this has been cumulative, but the most damning was the publication of the "Brown and Williamson Documents" (Brown and Williamson Tobacco Corporation) and the statements of a one-time tobacco lobbyist, Victor L Crawford, in whom metastatic squamous cell carcinoma of the tongue developed, almost certainly as a result of smoking. Most of the July 19, 1995, issue of *JAMA* is devoted to this subject,[5] which has been further elaborated in the 1996 book *The Cigarette Papers*.[6]

One of the arguments put forward in support of the tobacco industry is that economic benefits derive from producing and marketing the product. On a global basis this accounts for jobs estimated at between 16 and 140 million.[7] However, according to a World Bank study the net global economic effect of tobacco is a loss of $200 billion.[8] A computer simulation of the economic effects of eliminating the tobacco industry in the United States concluded that although many jobs would be lost in the Southeast, these would be offset by new jobs developed in the rest of the country because of the increased discretionary spending of all the former smokers.[9]

REFERENCES

1. Cigarette smoking among adults—United States, 1992, and changes in the definition of current cigarette smoking, *MMWR* 43:342-346, 1994.
2. MacKenzie TD, Bartecchi CE, Schrier RW: The human costs of tobacco use (second of two parts), *N Engl J Med* 330:975-980, 1994.
3. Fischer PM, Schwartz MP, Richards JW Jr, et al: Brand logo recognition by children aged 3 to 6 years: Mickey Mouse and Old Joe the Camel, *JAMA* 266:3145-3148, 1991.
4. DiFranza JR, Richards JW, Paulman PM et al: RJR Nabisco's cartoon camel promotes Camel cigarettes to children, *JAMA* 266:3149-3153, 1991.
5. The Brown and Williamson documents, *JAMA* 274:199-202, 219-258, 1995.
6. Glantz SA, Slade J, Bero LA, et al: *The cigarette papers,* Berkeley, 1996, University of California Press.
7. Phillips A, deSavigny D, Law MM: As Canadians butt out, the developing world lights up (editorial), *Can Med Assoc J* 153: 1111-1114, 1995.
8. Barnum H: The economic burden of the global trade in tobacco, *Tobacco Control* 3:358-361, 1994.
9. Warner KE, Fulton GA, Nicolas P, et al: Employment implications of declining tobacco product sales for the regional economies of the United States, *JAMA* 275:1241-1246, 1996.

UROLOGY

Topics covered in this section

BLADDER CANCER

(See also hematuria; urinalysis)

One of the rationales sometimes given for performing office urinalyses is the early detection of bladder cancer. However, there is no evidence that early diagnosis improves survival.[1,2] Therefore the Canadian Task Force on the Periodic Health Examination[3] and the U.S. Preventive Services Task Force[4] give urinalysis for the detection of bladder cancer in the general population a "D" recommendation. For similar reasons they give a "D" recommendation for urine cytology screening for bladder cancer in the general population.[3,4]

REFERENCES

1. Mommosen S, Aagaard J, Sell A: Presenting symptoms, treatment delay and survival in bladder cancer, *Scand J Urol Nephrol* 17:163-167, 1983.
2. Gulliford MC, Petruckevich A, Burney PGI: Survival with bladder cancer, evaluation of delay in treatment, type of surgeon, and modality of treatment, *BMJ* 303:437-440, 1991.
3. Canadian Task Force on the Periodic Health Examination: *Canadian guide to clinical preventive health care,* Ottawa, 1994, Canada Communication Group—Publishing, pp 826-836.
4. US Preventive Services Task Force: *Guide to clinical preventive services,* ed 2, Baltimore, 1996, Williams & Wilkins, pp 181-186.

CATHETERS, LONG-TERM INDWELLING

(See also urinalysis; bacteriuria and pyuria in the elderly; urinary tract infections)

Permanent indwelling Silastic catheters are usually changed every 3 to 12 weeks. Bacteriuria develops in virtually all patients with long-term urinary catheters, but despite this no evidence has been found that changing the catheters leads to sepsis.[1] The Canadian Task Force on the Periodic Health Examination gives an "E" rating to screening and treatment of asymptomatic bacteriuria in patients with indwelling catheters.[2]

REFERENCES

1. Bregenzer T, Frei R, Widmer AF, et al: Low risk of bacteremia during catheter replacement in patients with long-term urinary catheters, *Arch Intern Med* 157:521-525, 1997.
2. Canadian Task Force on the Periodic Health Examination: *Canadian guide to clinical preventive health care,* Ottawa, 1994, Canada Communication Group—Publishing, pp 966-967.

HEMATURIA

(See also acute exertional rhabdomyolysis; bladder cancer; diarrhea and hematochezia in runners; IgA nephropathy; urinalysis)

In a study from the Mayo Clinic, microscopic hematuria (defined as presence of any red blood cells in a high-power field) occurred in 13% of asymptomatic men and postmenopausal women. Younger women were excluded from the study because of the high rate of contamination of the urine with menstrual flow. After a 3½-year follow-up, only 0.5% of the patients were found to have renal cell cancer or bladder cancer.[1]

In a recent study from a British "hematuria clinic" no diagnosis was reached in 20% of the cases.[2] In the same clinic infections accounted for the most cases (25%), followed by benign prostatic hyperplasia (22%).

Not all red urine is caused by blood. Aside from myoglobinuria and hemoglobinuria, a variety of ingested substances can give a reddish urine. These include beets, berries, food coloring, cascara-containing laxatives, ibuprofen (Motrin, Advil), pyridium, phenytoin (Dilantin), quinine, sulfamethoxazole (Septra, Bactrim), chloroquine (Aralen), and rifampin.[3]

Exercise-Induced Hematuria

Exercise-induced hematuria is a common condition that is usually microscopic but may be macroscopic.[3,4] It affects both sexes and is associated with both contact sports such as boxing and football and noncontact sports such as swimming, track, and rowing. There are a variety of pathophysiological explanations—ischemic damage to the nephrons from renal vessel constriction, more marked constriction of the efferent than the afferent glomerular arterioles, and repeated trauma to the bladder mucosa caused by the posterior wall slapping against the base.[4]

The differential diagnosis includes exercise-induced rhabdomyolysis and march hemoglobinuria. In neither of these cases are red blood cells found in the urine. In exercise-induced hematuria, a urine dipstick test is positive for blood and the urinalysis reveals red blood cells. The diagnosis can be safely made in asymptomatic individuals under the age of 40 with microscopic hematuria if there are red blood cells, no red blood cell casts, and clearance of hematuria within 72 hours of the precipitating physical activity.[3,5] The presence of gross hematuria raises the question of urothelial neoplasm, and the presence of red blood cell casts suggests a glomerular disease. Patients with exercise-induced hematuria will not damage their kidneys if they continue participating in the activities that elicit the phenomenon.[3]

REFERENCES

1. Mohr DN, Offord KP, Owen RA, et al: Asymptomatic microhematuria and urologic disease: a population-based study, *JAMA* 256:224-229, 1986.
2. Paul AB, Collie DA, Wild SR, et al: An integrated haematuria clinic, *Br J Clin Pract* 47:128-130, 1993.
3. Gambrell RC, Blount BW: Exercise-induced hematuria, *Am Fam Physician* 53:905-911, 1996.
4. Abarbanel J, Benet AE, Lask D, Kimche D: Sports hematuria, *J Urol* 143:887-890, 1990.
5. Cianflocco AJ: Renal complications of exercise, *Clin Sports Med* 11:437-451, 1992.

INCONTINENCE

Classification

Urinary incontinence may be classified as transient or longstanding.[1] The two most common causes of persistent urinary incontinence are stress incontinence and detrusor overactivity (detrusor instability, detrusor hyperreactivity, urge incontinence).[1] Although overflow incontinence accounts for only 5% to 10% of cases of urinary incontinence, it should be ruled out in all cases.[1,2]

Transient urinary incontinence

The following are important causes of transient incontinence[1]:

1. Delirium
2. Urinary tract infections (not asymptomatic bacteriuria)
3. Atrophic urethritis and vaginitis
4. Medications (sedatives, hypnotics, anticholinergics such as antipsychotics and tricyclic antidepressants, narcotics, alpha-adrenergic antagonists, dihydropyridine calcium channel blockers, diuretics)
5. Excess urine output
6. Restricted mobility
7. Fecal impaction

Stress incontinence

Stress incontinence is one of the major causes of incontinence in women, and its diagnosis can often be made with reasonable certainty on the basis of the history.[1] If the patient is mentally competent and denies that incontinence occurs instantaneously with a stress maneuver, the diagnosis of stress incontinence can be ruled out with 90% certainty.[1] An important aggravating factor in some cases of stress incontinence is the treatment of hypertension with alpha-adrenergic blockers such as terazosin (Hytrin), doxazosin (Cardura), labetalol (Trandate), methyldopa (Aldomet), and clonidine (Catapres). These drugs inhibit the alpha-adrenergic receptors of the internal sphincter, which stimulate its closure. If possible they should be discontinued.[2]

The first-line pharmacological treatment for stress incontinence is probably estrogens.[2] These should be given in the usual doses for hormonal replacement therapy, and when indicated progestins should be added. Beneficial effects may be delayed for several weeks. Estrogen acts by thickening the mucosa of the urethra and trigone and also seems to increase the sensitivity and numbers of alpha-adrenergic receptors, which supply and cause contraction of the internal urethral sphincter.[2] In one study 56% of women with stress incontinence noted improvement or resolution of symptoms after 3 months of Kegel exercises (perineal muscle contraction exercises) and Premarin therapy.[3] Such a beneficial effect has not been found in all studies. A randomized double-blind placebo-controlled study found no improvement in a group of postmenopausal women with stress incontinence or detrusor instability treated with equine estrogens (Premarin) 0.625 mg and medroxyprogesterone (Provera) 10 mg given cyclically over 3 months.[4] A behavioral technique for controlling stress incontinence is to have patients cross their legs before coughing. A report of elderly women with stress incontinence found that three fourths became continent when they followed this procedure.[5]

Detrusor overactivity

Detrusor overactivity or urge incontinence is characterized by sudden onset of an intense desire to void or even a sudden gush of urine unrelated to a stress maneuver without any urge to void.[1] It is a common problem in the elderly and is caused by failure of cortical centers to inhibit detrusor activity or by spontaneous premature contractions of the detrusor muscle. Exacerbating factors are excessive caffeine intake, beta-blockers (beta-adrenergic stimulation inhibits the detrusor muscle), and sedatives.[2]

Bladder training is helpful for many patients with detrusor overactivity. The intervals between periods of incontinence are recorded, and the patient is instructed to void before that interval. For example, if incontinence occurs after 3 hours, the patient should void after 2 hours and consciously suppress any voiding urges during those first 2 hours. After this routine is established and the incontinence is controlled, the intervals between voidings are gradually lengthened.[1]

Pharmacotherapy for detrusor overactivity may be tried if behavioral approaches and removal of exacerbating factors fail. Commonly used drugs are those with anticholinergic or smooth muscle relaxation effects because they relax the detrusor muscle.[1,2] Examples are oxybutynin (Ditropan) 5 mg bid or tid, flavoxate (Urispas) 200 mg tid to qid, dicyclomine (Bentyl, Bentylol) 10 to 30 mg qid, and low doses of imipramine (Tofranil) and desipramine (Norpramin, Pertofrane). Care should be taken not to induce urinary retention.[2]

Eradicating bacteriuria in incontinent nursing home residents did not improve the degree of incontinence.[6]

Overflow Incontinence

Overflow incontinence may be due to obstructive lesions, to neurological disorders such as multiple sclerosis or diabetic neuropathy with denervation of the detrusor muscle, or to the secondary effects of medications such as the tricyclic antidepressants (the anticholinergic actions inhibit detrusor muscle contraction).[1] Abdominal assessment for a distended bladder is thus an essential part of the examination of a patient complaining of incontinence. The presence of a distended bladder points to overflow incontinence, although the absence of this finding does not rule it out.

Pharmacotherapy for inadequate detrusor muscle function is not very effective, but the cholinergic drug bethanechol (Urecholine) 10 to 25 mg tid or qid may be tried. Adverse effects include diarrhea and abdominal cramps, bradycardia, hypotension, and bronchospasm.[1]

REFERENCES

1. Resnick NM: An 89-year-old woman with urinary incontinence, *JAMA* 276:1832-1840, 1996.
2. Mold JW: Pharmacotherapy of urinary incontinence, *Am Fam Physician* 54:673-680, 1996.
3. Elia G, Bergman A: Pelvic muscle exercises: when do they work? *Obstet Gynecol* 81:283-286, 1993.
4. Fantl JA, Bump RC, Robinson D, et al (Continence Program for Women Research Group): Efficacy of estrogen supplementation in the treatment of urinary incontinence, *Obstet Gynecol* 88:745-749, 1996.
5. Norton PA, Baker JE: Postural changes can reduce leakage in women with stress urinary incontinence, *Obstet Gynecol* 84: 770-774, 1994.
6. Ouslander JG, Schapira M, Schnelle JF, et al: Does eradicating bacteriuria affect the severity of chronic urinary incontinence in nursing home residents? *Ann Intern Med* 122:749-754, 1995.

INFERTILITY, MALE

(See also infertility, female)

An estimated 15% of couples have fertility problems. The problem rests exclusively with the male in 30% of cases and partly with the male in another 20%. Unfortunately, the causes of the male abnormalities usually remain unknown even after a thorough workup.[1]

Factors known to adversely affect spermatogenesis include medications (cimetidine, sulfasalazine, nitrofurantoin), illicit drugs (marijuana, cocaine, anabolic steroids), cigarette smoking, excessive heat exposure from hot tubs or saunas, and varicocele.

According to Howards,[1] infection is a rare cause of male infertility even though considerable literature supports such a relationship. Antisperm antibodies may be associated with male infertility, but the role of corticosteroid treatment under these circumstances is controversial.[2]

Intracytoplasmic sperm injection of the ovum is used in many centers when infertility is related to sperm dysfunction in the male. To date no increase in the incidence of congenital anomalies has been found in children born as a result of this procedure.[3]

REFERENCES

1. Howards SS: Treatment of male infertility, *N Engl J Med* 332: 312-317, 1995.
2. Haas GG Jr: Antisperm antibodies in infertile men, *JAMA* 275: 885, 1996.
3. Palermo GD, Colombero LT, Schattman GL, et al: Evolution of pregnancies and initial follow-up of newborns delivered after intracytoplasmic sperm injection, *JAMA* 276:1893-1897, 1996.

INTERSTITIAL CYSTITIS

Interstitial cystitis is a disease of unknown etiology and uncertain management. It usually affects middle-aged women and is characterized by urinary frequency (more than eight times during the day and twice at night), urgency, and perineal, suprapubic, or pelvic pain that is relieved in part by voiding. The diagnosis can be made only if other diseases such as bacterial urinary tract infection or bladder cancer are ruled out and if, on cystoscopy, multiple mucosal glomerulations or pinpoint hemorrhages are seen. There are no specific findings on bladder biopsy.[1]

REFERENCES

1. Keller MS, McCarthy DO, Neider RS: Measurement of symptoms of interstitial cystitis: a pilot study, *Urol Clin North Am* 21: 67-71, 1994.

PENIS

Pearly Penile Papules

Pearly penile papules are normal anatomical structures found around the corona of the penis in up to 20% of young men. They are smooth whitish elevations and are said to be more common in blacks and in the uncircumcised. Treatment is reassurance.

PROSTATE

Benign Prostatic Hyperplasia

Symptoms

The major symptoms of benign prostatic hyperplasia are found in the American Urological Association questionnaire, which was developed to give a quantitative estimate of symptomatic distress.[1] The seven symptoms of significance are:

1. Sensation of incomplete bladder emptying
2. Increased daytime urinary frequency (less than 2-hour intervals)
3. Increased frequency of nighttime urination
4. Urinary urgency
5. Involuntary interruptions of stream when urinating
6. Weak stream
7. Straining to begin urination

Surgical treatment

The standard surgical treatment of benign prostatic hyperplasia is transurethral resection. For patients with moderate to severe symptoms, immediate results are excellent.[2,3] However, 20% to 25% of patients do not have long-term satisfactory outcomes, and the reoperation rate in men followed for 10 or more years is 15% to 20%. Reported complications of surgery include retrograde ejaculation in about three fourths of the patients, impotence in 5% to 10%, some degree of urinary incontinence in 2% to 4%, postoperative urinary tract infections in 5% to 10%, and blood transfusions in 5% to 10%.[2] Independent of problems with ejaculation or impotence are alterations in orgasm. In one study of men who were sexually active both before and after transurethral resection of the prostate, about half reported absent or altered orgasm.[4] Because of the potential complications of surgery, and because there is now good evidence that benign prostatic hypertrophy is not always a progressive disease, watchful waiting is a reasonable therapeutic option for many patients with mild or moderate symptoms (see section on watchful waiting below).[3]

Aside from transurethral and retropubic prostatectomy, a surgical option for treating benign prostatic hyperplasia is a transurethral incision of the prostate. This is a relatively simple intervention that is effective in many instances. It is used particularly for men with small prostate glands, for those who want to avoid retrograde ejaculation, and for those who are debilitated and therefore not good candidates for more extensive procedures. Another option for some patients is a permanently indwelling prostatic stent. Procedures under development include microwave and laser therapies.[2,5] A commercial device for delivering microwaves is the Prostatron. It is used in 1-hour outpatient therapy. It is not as effective as transurethral resection. Urinary retention requiring prolonged catheterization is the major adverse reaction.[5,6]

Medical treatment

Three $alpha_1$-adrenergic blocking agents, terazosin (Hytrin),[7-9] doxazosin (Cardura),[10,11] and prazosin (Minipress),[12] have been shown to relieve the symptoms of benign prostatic hyperplasia by relaxing the smooth muscles within the prostate. Most of the studies to date have involved terazosin, which improved urine flow rates and symptoms in 50% to 70% of patients. The usual dose of terazosin is 5 to 10 mg qhs, while that of doxazosin is 4 to 8 mg qhs.

Finasteride (Proscar) inhibits 5-alpha-reductase, an intracellular enzyme that metabolizes testosterone into the more potent dihydrotestosterone. Use of this drug (usual dose is 5 mg daily) causes atrophy of the prostate.[13] About 50% of men improve, but it takes 6 to 12 months of therapy before this is evident. Furthermore, how much of the benefit is due to the drug, how much to placebo effect, and how much to a spontaneous remission is unclear.[14] A 1996 Canadian multicenter trial found that two thirds of finasteride-treated men had clinical improvement but that 7.7% of them experienced ejaculatory problems compared with 1.7% of control subjects and 15.8% suffered impotence compared to 6.3% of the control group.[15]

A 1996 Veterans Administration study compared placebo to finasteride (Proscar), terazosin (Hytrin) and a combination of terazosin and finasteride. Finasteride was no more effective than placebo, terazosin resulted in significant symptom relief, and the addition of finasteride to terazosin gave no additional benefit.[9] A plausible explanation for the fact that finasteride was ineffective in this study but was effective in two previous randomized controlled studies,[16,17] as well as in at least one subsequent study,[15] is that in the investigations that reported benefits the subjects had much larger prostates than was the case in the Veterans Administration trial. Relatively small prostates may respond to the muscle relaxation of an $alpha_1$-adrenergic antagonist such as terazosin, whereas larger prostates may respond only if epithelial elements are caused to atrophy through the use of a 5-alpha-reductase drug such as finasteride.[13,15,18]

Watchful waiting

The simplest form of treatment is no treatment. A review of five studies on the natural history of moderately symptomatic benign prostatic hyperplasia concluded that over time, 40% of the men improve, 45% have no change in symptoms, and 15% deteriorate.[2] A recent collaborative study from nine U.S. centers compared transurethral resection with watchful waiting for 800 men with benign prostatic hypertrophy. At the end of 3 years 24% of those who were in the watchful waiting group underwent surgery.[3]

REFERENCES

1. Barry MJ, Fowler FJ Jr, O'Leary MP, et al (Measurement Committee of the American Urological Association): The American Urological Association symptom index for benign prostatic hyperplasia, *J Urol* 148:1549-1557, 1992.
2. Oesterling JE. Benign prostatic hyperplasia: medical and minimally invasive treatment options, *N Engl J Med* 332:99-109, 1995.
3. Wasson JH, Reda DJ, Bruskewitz RC, et al: A comparison of transurethral surgery with watchful waiting for moderate symptoms of benign prostatic hyperplasia, *N Engl J Med* 332:75-79, 1995.
4. Dunsmuir WD, Emberton M, Neal DE (Steering Group of the National Prostatectomy Audit): There is significant sexual dissatisfaction following TURP, *Br J Urol* 77:161A, 1996.
5. Hicks RJ, Cook JB: Managing patients with benign prostatic hyperplasia, *Am Fam Physician* 52:135-142, 1995.
6. de la Rosette JJ, D'Ancona FC, Debruyne FM: Current status of thermotherapy of the prostate, *J Urol* 157:430-438, 1997.
7. Terazosin for benign prostatic hyperplasia, *Med Lett* 36:15-16, 1994.
8. Lepor H, Auerbach S, Pras-Baez A, et al: A randomized placebo-controlled multicenter study of the efficacy and safety of terazosin in the treatment of benign prostatic hyperplasia, *J Urol* 148:1467-1474, 1992.
9. Lepor H, Williford WO, Barry MJ, et al: The efficacy of terazosin, finasteride, or both in benign prostatic hyperplasia, *N Engl J Med* 335:533-539, 1996.
10. Chapple CR, Carter P, Ghristmas TJ, et al: A three month double-blind placebo controlled study of doxazosin as treatment for benign prostatic bladder outlet obstruction (abstract), *J Urol* 147(suppl):366A, 1992.

11. Gillenwater JY, Mobley DL: A sixteen week, double-blind, placebo-controlled, dose-titration study using doxazosin tablets for the treatment of benign prostatic hyperplasia (BPH) in normotensive males, *J Urol* 144:908-912, 1990.
12. Hedlund H, Andersson KE, Ek A: Effects of prazosin in patients with benign prostatic obstruction, *J Urol* 130:275-278, 1983.
13. Farmer A, Noble J: Drug treatment for benign prostatic hyperplasia: decreasing muscle tone within the prostate gland may be more effective than reducing the size of the prostate (editorial), *BMJ* 4:1215-1216, 1997.
14. Rittmaster RS: Finasteride, *N Engl J Med* 330:120-125, 1994.
15. Nickel JC, Fradet Y, Boake RC, et al: Efficacy and safety of finasteride therapy for benign prostatic hyperplasia: results of a 2-year randomized controlled trial (the PROSPECT Study), *Can Med Assoc J* 155:1251-1259, 1996.
16. Gormley GJ, Stoner E, Bruskewitz RC, et al: The effect of finasteride in men with benign prostatic hyperplasia, *N Engl J Med* 327:1185-1191, 1992.
17. Finasteride Study Group: Finasteride (MK-906) in the treatment of benign prostatic hyperplasia, *Prostate* 22:291-299, 1993.
18. Walsh PC: Treatment of benign prostatic hyperplasia (editorial), *N Engl J Med* 335:586-587, 1996.

PROSTATE CANCER

(See also detrimental effects of investigations; prevention; screening; vasectomy and prostate cancer)

Methods of detecting and managing prostate cancer are controversial. Many American urologists are strong proponents of case finding by PSA determinations and digital rectal examinations, and believe that radical prostatectomy will save lives in patients with localized prostate cancer. Elsewhere in the world, enthusiasm for such interventions is muted or nonexistent.

Staging and Histological Grading

The two main methods of staging prostate cancer are Whitmore staging and the TNM system.These are outlined in Tables 66 and 67. Two ways of grading prostate cancer by histological features are shown in Table 68.

Epidemiology

(See also screening and apparent prevalence rates; management of prostate cancer; vasectomy)

Excluding skin cancer, prostate cancer is the most common cancer in the United States.[1] According to 1993 U.S. statistics, prostate cancer was the second leading cause of cancer death in men; a quarter of men with prostate cancer die of their disease.[2] Among cancers in the United States, breast cancer kills 1.3 times as many people as prostate cancer and lung cancer 4.2 times as many.[3] Other causes of death also exceed those of prostate cancer; for every prostate cancer death in the United States there are 3 accidental deaths, 5 deaths from strokes, and 20 deaths from heart disease.[4,5]

In the period 1989-1991 the incidence of prostate cancer in United States increased by more than 40%.[6] Much of this

Table 66 Whitmore Staging of Prostate Cancer

Classification	Description
A1	Single nonpalpable microscopic focus (<5% of gland)
A2	Single nonpalpable focus (>5% of gland)
B1	Palpable localized nodule limited to one lobe
B2	Palpable localized nodules involving both lobes
C	Localized disease extending beyond the capsule
D	Distant metastases

Table 67 TNM Classification of Prostate Cancer (Tumor Only)

Classification	Description
T1	Clinically inapparent; not palpable or visible on imaging
T1a	Incidental histological finding ≤5% of tissue resected
T1b	Incidental histological finding >5% of tissue resected
T1c	Identified by blind biopsy done because of elevated prostate specific antigen
T2	Confined to the prostate
T2a	Involves half a lobe or less
T2b	Involves more than half a lobe but not both lobes
T2c	Involves both lobes
T3	Extends through prostate capsule
T4	Fixed or invades structures other than seminal vesicles

Table 68 Histological Grading of Prostate Cancer

Degree of differentiation	Gleason score
Well differentiated (grade 1)	2-4
Moderately differentiated (grade 2)	5-7
Poorly differentiated (grade 3)	8-10

is almost certainly because of an epidemic of PSA testing.[7-9] Of more concern than the skyrocketing incidence is a 23% increase in mortality rate from this disease in the United States over the last two decades.[6] Although the reasons for this are not known with certainty, at least part of the increase is probably a result of an increased longevity of the population and perhaps of an increased likelihood of recording prostate cancer as a cause of death on death certificates.[7]

The widespread use of PSA screening has led to a dramatic increase in the rate of radical prostatectomies in North America. For example, the number of radical prostatectomies performed under Medicare in the United States in 1987 was 7028, whereas by 1992, 39,157 such operations were performed; this is a 5.6-fold increase over 5 years.[10] Not only has the overall rate of prostatectomies of Medicare recipients in the United States increased nearly 6-fold, but this degree of increase has involved all age groups, including the very elderly.[11] The rate of radical prostatectomy is not evenly distributed across the United States; in the Pacific Northwest it is over twice that of New England and the Mid-Atlantic regions.[11]

Prostate cancer incidence has a large geographical and racial variation. The disease is very rare in Asia and highly prevalent in Northern Europe and North America.[12] Within the United States the incidence in blacks is about twice that of whites.[1,13] The incidence in Japanese-Americans rises in the second and subsequent generations.[13]

A family history of prostate cancer increases the odds ratio of acquiring the disease about twofold.[14] The more family members who have had prostate cancer, the greater the relative risk of acquiring it. A rare form of "hereditary prostate cancer" accounts for 9% of all prostate cancers but 43% of prostate cancers in men less than 55 years of age. This form appears to have a dominant mode of inheritance with high penetrance.[15] The presence of this syndrome in a family may be a good argument for PSA screening of all family members.[15,16]

An increased incidence of prostate cancer in patients who have had a vasectomy has been reported. The validity of these findings is controversial (see section on vasectomy).

REFERENCES

1. Litwin MS, Hays RD, Fink A, et al: Quality-of-life outcomes in men treated for localized prostate cancer, *JAMA* 273:129-135, 1995.
2. Boring CC, Squires TS, Tong T: Cancer statistics, 1993, *CA Cancer J Clin* 43:7-26, 1993.
3. American Cancer Society: *Cancer facts and figures, 1993,* Atlanta, 1993, The Society.
4. National Center for Health Statistics: *Advance report of final mortality statistics, 1990,* Monthly Vital Statistics Report, Hyattsville, Md, 1993, US Public Health Service, suppl, vol 41, No 7.
5. Woolf SH: Public health perspective: the health policy implications of screening for prostate cancer, *J Urol* 152:1685-1688, 1994.
6. Ries LA, Miller BA, Hankey BF, et al, eds: *SEER cancer statistics review 1973-1991: tables and graphs,* Bethesda, Md, 1994, National Cancer Institute, NIH Pub No 94-2789.
7. Meyer F: Rising incidence rate of prostate cancer (letter), *Can Med Assoc J* 149:1375-1376. 1993.
8. Potosky AL, Miller BA, Albertsen PC, et al: The role of increasing detection in the rising incidence of prostate cancer, *JAMA* 273:548-552, 1995.
9. Corder EH, Chute CG, Guess HA, et al: Prostate cancer in Rochester, Minnesota (USA), from 1935 to 1989: increases in incidence related to more complete ascertainment, *Cancer Causes Control* 5:207-214, 1994.
10. Olsson CA, Goluboff ET: Detection and treatment of prostate cancer: perspective of the urologist, *J Urol* 152:1695-1699, 1994.
11. Lu-Yao GL, McLerran D, Wasson J, et al (Prostate Patient Outcomes Research Team): An assessment of radical prostatectomy: time trends, geographic variation, and outcomes, *JAMA* 269:2633-2636, 1993.
12. Meikle AW, Smith JA Jr: Epidemiology of prostate cancer, *Urol Clin North Am* 17:709-718, 1990.
13. Gittes RF: Carcinoma of the prostate, *N Engl J Med* 324:236-245, 1995.
14. Aprikian AG, Bazinet M, Plante M, et al: Family history and the risk of prostatic carcinoma in a high risk group of urological patients, *J Urol* 154:404-406, 1995.
15. McLellan DL, Norman RW: Hereditary aspects of prostate cancer, *Can Med Assoc J* 153:895-900, 1995.
16. Nickel JC: The dilemma of hereditary prostate cancer (editorial), *Can Med Assoc J* 153:935-938, 1995.

Digital Rectal Examination

(See also clinical practice guidelines for screening; informed consent; prevention; prostate specific antigen)

Scardino and associates[1] reviewed several series of screening programs for prostate cancer using digital rectal examination (DRE). Detection rates varied from 0.8% to 1.4%. The positive predictive value of DRE for detecting prostate cancer was between 22% and 36%, which means that 64% to 78% of men with suspect findings on DRE did not have cancer. Of the cancers found, between 12% and 47% had clinically evident spread and were not candidates for curative therapy. Clinically localized tumors were present in between 53% and 88% of detected cases; however, since 63% of such tumors (in Scardino's series) were found to have capsular invasion on pathological examination, the rate of truly localized tumors detected by DRE is probably between 20% and 32%. Put another way, 68% to 80% of prostate cancers detected by DRE are incurable.

The U.S. Preventive Services Task Force gives DRE for prostate screening a "D" recommendation,[2] while the Canadian Task force on the Periodic Health Examination gives it a "C."[3] A 1994 decision analysis by Krahn et al[4] supports the views of the two task forces. According to this study, screening unselected men between the ages of 50 and 70 with DRE alone would not reduce mortality at any age.[4]

REFERENCES

1. Scardino PR, Weaver R, Hudson MA: Early detection of prostate cancer, *Hum Pathol* 23:211-222, 1992.
2. US Preventive Services Task Force: *Guide to clinical preventive services,* ed 2, Baltimore, 1996, Williams & Wilkins, pp 119-134.
3. Canadian Task Force on the Periodic Health Examination: *Canadian guide to clinical preventive health care,* Ottawa, 1994, Canada Communication Group—Publishing, pp 817-823.
4. Krahn MD, Mahoney JE, Eckman MH, et al: Screening for prostate cancer. a decision analytic view, *JAMA* 272:773-880, 1994.

Prostate Specific Antigen

(See also digital rectal examination; informed consent; prevention screening; surrogate outcomes; prevention; radical prostatectomy)

History

PSA was discovered in 1979, and PSA testing became widely available in North America in the mid-1980s.

Causes of elevated prostate specific antigen and setting of normal values

PSA is secreted by the normal prostate, the hypertrophied or hyperplastic prostate, and carcinoma of the prostate. Prostate cancer cells raise the PSA level 10 times more than do the cells of benign prostatic hyperplasia.[1,2] Aside from prostate cancer the diseases most commonly causing elevation of PSA are benign prostatic hyperplasia and prostatitis.[3] Of particular clinical importance is the finding that PSA levels in patients without prostate cancer increase markedly with age. According to one study, if the cutoff value for a normal PSA is considered to be ≤4 ng/ml, the false-positive rate varies from none among patients under 50 years of age to 26% for those 70 or older.[4] This phenomenon is the basis for recommending changes to the range of normal values according to age. A group from the Mayo Clinic designed a system in which the upper limits of normal would be 2.5 ng/ml for ages 40 to 49 and 6.5 ng/ml for ages 70 to 79.[5]

Aside from age-specific PSA reference ranges discussed above, several methods aimed at increasing the specificity of PSA determinations are under active investigation. These include PSA velocity, which is a measurement of the rate of change of PSA over time; PSA density, which correlates prostatic gland volume as determined by ultrasound with PSA levels; and the percentage of free serum PSA (patients with prostate cancer have relatively less free PSA than do patients with normal glands or benign prostatic hypertrophy).[6] These are all experimental procedures and at present have no general clinical application.

DRE before a PSA test may cause a small (0.26 μg/L) but statistically significant increase in PSA levels. This is of no clinical significance.[7] Ejaculation can cause a temporary elevation of PSA levels; if the test is to be ordered, the patient should refrain from ejaculation for 48 hours before its performance.[8]

Early detection of prostate cancer by prostate specific antigen

Does PSA screening result in the detection of more localized and therefore operable prostate cancers? The answer is clearly yes, since the rate of pathologically advanced cancers detected by initial or serial PSA screening is about half that found in a referral population in which the disease is detected by other means.[9] The overall rate of pathologically advanced cancers detected by PSA in one series was about a third. If the PSA level was 4.1 to 9.9 ng/ml, one fourth of the cancers were advanced, whereas if it was over 10 ng/ml, over half of the cancers had extended beyond the capsule.[10]

If a PSA screening program is undertaken, how many men will have "positive" results requiring further investigations? The answer is many. Smith and associates[10] reviewed numerous studies and concluded that in initial screenings of men with PSA, between 10% and 15% have values above 4 ng/ml and about the same number of men have suspect findings on DRE. Since many of these men have both abnormal DRE findings and an abnormal PSA level, between 15% and 25% of men participating in an initial prostate cancer screening program are advised to have further investigations such as transrectal ultrasonographies and prostate biopsies.[10] As expected, the percentage of men with abnormal PSA concentrations on repeat screenings decreases somewhat; in the series of Smith and co-workers[10] it dropped from 10% (at the initial screening) to between 6% and 7%.

Only a few men with "positive" PSA tests actually have cancer. A 10-year prospective study of PSA for the detection of clinically significant prostate cancer (using archival blood samples from the Physicians' Health Study) reported an overall sensitivity of 46% (73% within the first 4 years) and a false-positive rate of 9%[11]; the positive predictive value was calculated to be just under 13% over the 10-year period.[12] In another study using archival blood samples, Parkes and colleagues[4] found the positive predictive value of a positive PSA (using the upper limit of normal as 4 ng/ml) to be about 9% to 10%. Figures for the positive predictive value of a positive PSA test from other reports ranged from 8% to 33%.[13]

Benefits and harm of prostate specific antigen screening

Prostate screening programs clearly cause considerable psychological and physical morbidity among men who do not have the disease but have positive test results. What is still unknown is whether such a screening program will save lives. That PSA screening results in a "stage shift" to less advanced tumors does not necessarily mean that treatment will improve mortality. Small tumors are surrogate endpoints for decreased mortality, and apparent short-term beneficial results of treatment may be spurious because of lead time and length bias (see section on prevention). This is important because no randomized controlled studies have been reported to show a decrease in mortality from PSA screening or from radical prostatectomy (see discussion of radical prostatectomy).

The current debate about PSA screening and radical prostatectomy has been likened to the one that went on in the 1960s and 1970s with respect to screening for lung cancer with chest x-ray examination and sputum cytology.[14] These screening procedures led to the detection of more small operable lung cancers and to an increased 5-year survival rate. However, this survival benefit proved to be entirely the result of length and lead time biases; long-term follow-up showed no decrease in mortality. It is now evident that chest x-rays and sputum cytology have no role as screening methods for lung cancer.[14]

Ordering a PSA test has far-reaching implications because it begins an almost irreversible diagnostic and treatment cascade that can result in significant harm (see discussion of prevention and screening).[15,16] Many patients have false-positive results and suffer the psychological consequences. Others are told that they have inoperable cancer and become subject to this psychological distress several months or years before they would have if the diagnosis had been based on clinical symptoms. Physical harm is inevitable for anyone with a positive PSA because the screening cascade involves rectal ultrasound, prostatic biopsies, and if localized cancer is found, prostatectomy with attendant morbidity and mortality. The adverse effects of surgery are discussed below under "Management of Clinically Localized Prostate Cancer."

Informed consent for prostate specific antigen screening

Clearly PSA screening is an experimental procedure, and its value will be determined only by randomized controlled trials as suggested by Parkes and associates.[4] In this context it is essential that patients understand the pros and cons of PSA testing and give informed consent before screening.[16-22] If this is done, many patients will probably decide not to have the test.[17,18]

Clinical practice guidelines

Both the U.S. Preventive Services Task Force[23] and the Canadian Task Force on the Periodic Health Examination[24] give a "D" recommendation to PSA screening. The American College of Physicians does not recommend routine screening but advises its members to discuss the pros and cons with their patients and decide on an individual basis.[25]

The American Cancer Society recommends annual PSA testing and DRE for all men aged 50 or over.[26] Both the American Urological Association[27] and the Canadian Urological Association initially recommended screening all men between 50 and 70 for PSA, but in 1994 the Canadian association reversed its stand.[28]

The American Urological Association guidelines for PSA screening recommend that this not be done for men over the age of 70.[23] The life expectancy of men over that age is such that even if radical prostatectomy does decrease prostate cancer deaths, they would be far more likely to die of other diseases. Nevertheless, widespread screening of elderly men for PSA is conducted in the United States. A recent survey of U.S. primary care physicians found that PSA screening was ordered routinely for 65% of men aged 70 to 74, 58% of men aged 75 to 79, and 53% of men aged 80 or over.[29] It is no wonder that about one third of all radical prostatectomies are performed in men over the age of 70.[30]

REFERENCES

1. Stamey TA, Yang N, Hay AR, et al: Prostate-specific antigen as a serum marker for adenocarcinoma of the prostate, *N Engl J Med* 317:909-916, 1987.
2. Partin AW, Carter HB, Chan DW, et al: Prostate-specific antigen in the staging of localized prostate cancer: influence of tumor differentiation, tumor volume and benign hyperplasia, *J Urol* 143:747-752, 1990.
3. Nadler RB, Humphrey PA, Smith DS, et al: Effect of inflammation and benign prostatic hyperplasia on elevated serum prostate specific antigen levels, *J Urol* 154:407-413, 1995.
4. Parkes C, Wald NJ, Murphy P, et al: Prospective observational study to assess value of prostate specific antigen as screening test for prostate cancer, *BMJ* 311:1340-1343, 1995.
5. Oesterling JE, Jacobsen SJ, Chute CH, et al: Serum prostate-specific antigen in a community-based population of healthy men: establishment of age-specific reference ranges, *JAMA* 270:860-864, 1993.
6. Catalona WJ, Smith DS, Wolfert RL, et al: Evaluation of percentage of free serum prostate-specific antigen to improve specificity of prostate cancer screening, *JAMA* 274:1214-1220, 1995.
7. Internal Medicine Clinic Research Consortium: Effect of digital rectal examination on serum prostate-specific antigen in a primary care setting, *Arch Intern Med* 155:389-392, 1995.
8. Tchetgen M-B, Song JT, Strawderman M, et al: Ejaculation increase the serum prostate-specific antigen concentration, *Urology* 47:511-516, 1996.
9. Smith DS, Catalona WJ: The nature of prostate cancer detected through prostate specific antigen based screening, *J Urol* 152: 1732-1736, 1994.
10. Smith DS, Catalona WJ, Herschman JD: Longitudinal screening for prostate cancer with prostate-specific antigen, *JAMA* 276:1309-1315, 1996.
11. Gann PH, Hennekens CH, Stampfer MJ: A prospective evaluation of plasma prostate-specific antigen for detection of prostatic cancer, *JAMA* 273:289-294, 1995.
12. Marshall KG: The utility of prostate-specific-antigen for detecting prostate cancer (letter), *JAMA* 274:607, 1995.
13. Feightner JW: The early detection and treatment of prostate cancer: the perspective of the Canadian task force on the periodic health examination, *J Urol* 152:1682-1684, 1994,
14. Collins MM, Barry MJ: Controversies in prostate cancer screening: analogies to the early lung cancer screening debate, *JAMA* 276:1976-1979, 1996.
15. Albertsen P: A 72-year-old man with localized prostate cancer, *JAMA* 274:69-74, 1995.
16. Marshall KG: Screening for prostate cancer: how can patients give informed consent? *Can Fam Physician* 39:2385-2390, 1993.
17. Wolf A, Nasser JF, Wolf AM, et al: The impact of informed consent on patient interest in prostate-specific antigen screening, *Arch Intern Med* 156:1333-1336, 1996.
18. Mazur DJ, Hickam DH: Patient preferences for management of localized prostate cancer, *West J Med* 165:26-30, 1996.
19. Lee JM: Screening and informed consent, *N Engl J Med* 328: 438-440, 1993.
20. Marshall KG: Prevention: how much harm? how much benefit? II. Ten potential pitfalls in determining the clinical significance of benefits, *Can Med Assoc J* 154:1837-1843, 1996.
21. Marshall KG: Prevention: how much harm? how much benefit? III. Physical, psychological and social harm, *Can Med Assoc J* 155:169-176, 1996.
22. Marshall KG: Prevention: how much harm? how much benefit? IV. The ethics of informed consent for preventive screening programs, *Can Med Assoc J* 155:377-383, 1996.
23. US Preventive Services Task Force: *Guide to clinical preventive services,* ed 2, Baltimore, 1996 ,Williams & Wilkins, pp 119-134.
24. Canadian Task Force on the Periodic Health Examination: *Canadian guide to clinical preventive health care,* Ottawa, 1994, Canada Communication Group—Publishing, pp 812-823.
25. Gunby P: Prostate cancer's complexities of causation, detection, and treatment challenge researchers (medical news and perspectives), *JAMA* 277:1580, 1582, 1997.

26. Mettlin C, Jones G, Averett H, et al: Defining and updating the American Cancer Society guidelines for the cancer-related checkup: prostate and endometrial cancers, *CA Cancer J Clin* 43:42-46, 1993.
27. American Urological Association: Early detection of prostate cancer and use of transrectal ultrasound. In *American Urological Association 1992 policy statement book,* Baltimore, Md, 1992, The Association, vol 4, p 20.
28. Collins JP: Detection of prostate cancer (letter), *Can Med Assoc J* 152:328-329, 1995.
29. Barry MJ, Roberts RG, Oesterling JE, et al: Differences in how primary care physicians and urologists approach early detection of prostate cancer (abstract), *J Gen Intern Med* 1(suppl): 62, 1996.
30. Murphy GP, Mettlin C, Menck H, et al: National patterns of prostate cancer treatment by radical prostatectomy: results of a survey by the American College of Surgeons Commission on Cancer, *J Urol* 152:1817-1819, 1994.

Transrectal Ultrasound

Transrectal ultrasound was developed in 1986 and is the initial investigative tool used when a PSA concentration is elevated or a prostate lesion is felt on DRE. It is reported to cause pain in only 5% of patients.[1] It is not a good screening tool for prostate cancer and has received a "D" recommendation for this purpose from both the Canadian Task Force on the Periodic Health Examination[2] and the U.S. Preventive Services Task Force.[3]

REFERENCES

1. Hermansson CG, Hugosson J, Pedersen KV: Transrectal ultrasound examination of the prostate: complications and acceptance by patients, *Br J Urol* 71:457-459, 1993.
2. Canadian Task Force on the Periodic Health Examination: *Canadian guide to clinical preventive health care,* Ottawa, 1994, Canada Communication Group—Publishing, pp 812-823.
3. US Preventive Services Task Force: *Guide to clinical preventive services,* ed 2, Baltimore, 1996, Williams & Wilkins, pp 119-134.

Biopsy of Prostate

The incidence of pain from needle biopsies of the prostate is variously reported as being between 8%[1] and 31%.[2] Hematuria and hemospermia combined occur in over half of patients who have had needle biopsies.[2,3] Infection rates vary from about 1% to 6% and are lower in those given prophylactic antibiotics.[1,3] In a very few cases septicemia and even death have been reported.[4] Another rare complication is acute urinary retention.[2]

REFERENCES

1. Hermansson CG, Hugosson J, Pedersen KV: Transrectal ultrasound examination of the prostate: complications and acceptance by patients, *Br J Urol* 71:457-459, 1993.
2. Webb JA, Shanmuganathan K, McLean A: Complications of ultrasound-guided transperineal prostate biopsy: a prospective study, *Br J Urol* 72:775-777, 1993.
3. Gustafsson O, Norming U, Nyman CR, et al: Complications following combined transrectal aspiration and core biopsy of the prostate, *Scand J Urol Nephrol* 24:249-251, 1990.
4. Brewster SF, Rooney N, Kabala J, et al: Fatal anaerobic infection following transrectal biopsy of a rare prostatic tumour, *Br J Urol* 72:977-978, 1993.

Management of Clinically Localized Prostate Cancer

(See also epidemiology of prostate cancer; staging and histological grading of prostate cancer)

Therapeutic options

The standard treatment options for patients with clinically localized prostate cancer are radical prostatectomy, external beam radiation therapy (brachytherapy through computer optimized transperineal implantation of radioactive material is a developing alternative[1]), and watchful waiting. The best option is uncertain because to this time the Veterans Administration Cooperative Urological Research Group (VACURG) study has been the only published prospective randomized trial comparing prostatectomy with watchful waiting.[2] It failed to show any benefit from surgery but has been criticized for a variety of methodological deficits.

Since no definitive evidence has shown that one treatment modality is better than another, patients with localized prostate cancer and their physicians must base their decisions on the available data. The 1995 guidelines of the American Urological Association included the following points[3]:

1. Life expectancy and overall health status are more important than age in determining suitability for surgery.
2. Patients should be informed of the accepted treatment modalities, including radical prostatectomy, radiation, and watchful waiting.
3. The estimated benefits and harm of each modality should be discussed with the patient.

What are the current data? This is difficult to answer. Articles of varying quality and complexity are scattered widely throughout the medical literature. Some of this information is summarized in the following paragraphs.

Prognostic indicators

To decide what kind of treatment is optimal, patients and physicians must know both the benefits and adverse effects of each treatment modality. To assess benefits, they must understand the significance of prognostic indicators, three of the most important of which are staging, histological grading, and comorbidity.

Staging. Small foci of well-differentiated prostate cancer found incidentally in specimens from a transurethral resection do not constitute a significant clinical risk; patients with this finding will almost certainly die of some other disease and no treatment for this "pathologist's cancer" is required. On the other hand, curative treatment is not successful for patients with metastatic disease, pelvic lymph node disease (even one microscopic focus of cancer in a lymph node has the same prognostic significance as more widespread metastases), or locally invasive disease (T3 or C) even in the absence of lymph node or distant metastases.[4]

Grading. Histological grading significantly affects the prognosis regardless of treatment modality.[5-9] Chodak[5,6] found that in patients with prostate cancer followed for 10 years by watchful waiting, mortality from prostate cancer for patients with grade 1 (well-differentiated) or 2 (moderately well-differentiated) disease was 13%, whereas for those with grade 3 (poorly differentiated) disease it was 66%. By 10 years after diagnosis metastases had occurred in 19% of patients with grade 1 disease, 42% of those with grade 2 disease, and 74% of those with grade 3 disease. Survival at 10 years for patients with grade 1 or grade 2 tumors followed by watchful waiting approximated that of the general population; those with grade 3 tumors had a much higher mortality rate.[5,6] Similar results have been reported by Johansson,[7] Albertsen,[8] and Lu-Yao[9] and their associates in patients followed by watchful waiting. High-grade tumors also have a much worse prognosis in patients treated with radical prostatectomy or radiation therapy.[9]

Comorbidity. Another important prognostic indicator is comorbidity.[8,10] In the watchful waiting series of Albertsen and co-workers it was nearly as powerful a predictor of increased death rates as high Gleason scores. These authors point out that most studies of management strategies have not assessed comorbidity; it may be that the most healthy patients are treated by radical surgery, whereas the sickest have radiation therapy or are followed by watchful waiting. If this occurs, surgery would appear more beneficial than it really is because few of the patients treated by surgery would die of competing diseases within the next 10 years.[8] On the other hand, data on prostate cancer–specific mortality rates derived from older patients with high comorbidity rates cannot necessarily be applied to younger patients with low comorbidity rates. Aus and associates[10] developed a model that estimated that after 15 years of watchful waiting, the prostate cancer–specific mortality for older patients with high comorbidity would be 12.3%, whereas that for younger patients without high comorbidity would be 35.5%. According to this model, those most likely to benefit from radical prostatectomy would be younger healthier patients.

Benefits of radical prostatectomy

Certain biases in the published reports of radical prostatectomy may make this procedure appear better than radiation therapy or watchful waiting. One such bias is the tendency to perform surgery on younger healthier patients while those who are older or have significant comorbidity are more likely to be offered radiation therapy or watchful waiting. A second bias is that most reports of radical prostatectomy outcomes are based on "treatment received," not "intention to treat." If a surgeon finds positive lymph nodes or other evidence of tumor extension at the time of surgery, radical prostatectomy is not performed and statistics are based only on patients with more favorable prognoses. Obviously, this kind of selection bias is not possible with radiation therapy or watchful waiting. The importance of this issue is documented in a population-based study by Lu-Yao and associates[9]; the 10-year prostate cancer mortality for radical prostatectomy was 60% higher when calculated on the basis of "intention to treat" than on the basis of "treatment received."

As indicated previously, there is only one long-term published prospective study of radical prostatectomy and it did not show an advantage over no treatment.[2] Fowler and associates[11] found that after radical prostatectomy, recurrent prostate cancer was detected in 16% of patients by 2 years, 22% by 3 years, and 28% by 4 years.

Histological grading is an important factor in determining prognosis after radical prostatectomy.[9] Patients with low-grade tumors (Gleason grades 2 to 4) had no increased mortality compared with age-matched cohorts (equally good results for this grade of tumor were obtained with radiation therapy or watchful waiting), while it was much worse with high-grade tumors (Gleason grades 8 to 10). However, the prognosis for high-grade tumors was considerably better after radical prostatectomy than with radiation therapy or watchful waiting.

Adverse effects of radical prostatectomy and radiation therapy

What are the adverse effects of radical prostatectomy and radiation therapy? Initial estimates of the complication rates of radical prostatectomy were lower than in more recent reports.[11,12] In 1993 Fowler and associates[11] from Boston found that about 60% of patients had no erections after surgery and only 11% had erections sufficient for intercourse in the month before their survey. More than 40% of patients were wearing pads, diapers, or clamps to deal with urinary leakage, and over 40% reported dripping of urine when they coughed or had a full bladder. In addition, 20% were treated for a urethral stricture. Similar results were found in a survey of the outcomes of 2122 patients operated on in 484 institutions in the United States in 1990.[12] The operative mortality rate was 0.7%, and 56.6% of men who were potent before the surgery were left impotent. In regard to continence, 3.6% became completely incontinent, 4.1% required more than two pads daily, 11.2% required two or fewer pads daily, 23.1% had occasional incontinence but did not use pads, and 58% were totally continent.[12]

In early 1995 a report by Litwen and associates[13] from UCLA carefully evaluated the health-related quality of life in a group of men with localized prostate cancer treated by radical prostatectomy, radiation, or simple observation, as well as in a control group without cancer. They concluded that patients treated with surgery or radiation therapy had more urinary and sexual dysfunction than did control subjects or patients followed with observation only. The incidence of side effects was high (e.g., 40% of patients treated surgically had daily urine leakage), but many men were not bothered by "minor dysfunctions." An interesting additional finding was that patients treated by observation alone had a higher degree of emotional problems than did the control subjects or patients treated with surgery or radiation. The authors postulate that this is because these patients may have been anxious about the evolution of their disease and felt that nothing was being done for them.[13]

Lim and associates[14] compared patients who had radical prostatectomy with those who had external beam radiation therapy. Incontinence and impotence were much more common in the surgery group, whereas bowel dysfunction (diarrhea, urgency, and sometimes hematochezia) was more common in the radiation therapy group. As in Litwin's study the majority of patients in both groups stated that they would undertake the same treatment if they had to do it over again.[14] An accompanying editorial pointed out that patients will accept considerable morbidity in exchange for an extension of survival.[15] Unfortunately, undergoing radical prostatectomy or radiation therapy is no guarantee of survival extension, but cognitive consistency seems to prevent most patients and perhaps many physicians from acknowledging this.

Balancing the pros and cons

In 1993 Flemming and associates[16] pointed out regarding the three standard therapeutic modalities (radical prostatectomy, radiation therapy, and watchful waiting) that there is no conclusive evidence that one is superior to another, that complications of invasive treatment occur much sooner than any potential benefits, and that complications of invasive treatment will affect those who obtain no benefits as well as those who achieve benefits.

After carefully reviewing the literature on the treatment of prostate cancer, Chodak[5,6] concluded that for men over 70, particularly those with low-grade tumors, benefits of treatment by radical prostatectomy or radiation were slight in comparison to the risks. For men with longer life expectancies, benefits of radical treatment might well be increased. Support for this view comes from population models developed by Aus and associates.[10] The data from the study of Lu-Yao and colleagues[9] suggest that the 17% or so of men with high-grade tumors might benefit from surgery and that for men with low-grade tumors 10-year life expectancy is essentially normal regardless of treatment modality.

In 1996 the National Cancer Institute issued a press release stating that the mortality rate from prostate cancer fell 6.3% from the period 1971-1990 to 1991-1995.[17] Proponents of radical prostatectomy quote this as probable evidence that surgery is effective.[18] This is tenuous evidence. The numbers are small and may not reflect an ongoing trend. Even if radical prostatectomy turns out to decrease mortality, a lag time of 10 years would be expected before this is demonstrable, and whether this has occurred is questionable. More important, cancer mortality rates may change for unknown reasons. A good example is the dramatic decrease in the incidence and mortality of gastric cancer in North America over the last few decades.[19]

Informed consent for management of prostate cancer

Should patients with clinically localized prostate cancer have radical prostatectomy? There is no correct answer. They must have adequate information about the benefits and harm of each treatment option so that they can make a truly informed decision (see section on prevention and informed consent).[3]

REFERENCES

1. Zelefsky MJ, Whitmore WF Jr: Long-term results of retropubic permanent ^{125}iodine implantation of the prostate for clinically localized prostatic cancer, *J Urol* 158:23-30, 1997.
2. Iversen P, Madsen PW, Corle D: Radical prostatectomy versus expectant treatment for early carcinoma of the prostate: twenty-three year follow-up of a prospective randomized study, *Scand J Urol Nephrol* 172(suppl):65-72, 1995.
3. Middleton RG, Thompson IM, Austenfeld MS, et al (Prostate Cancer Clinical Guidelines Panel, American Urological Association): Summary report on the management of clinically localized prostate cancer, *J Urol* 154:2144-2148, 1995.
4. Scardino PT: Early detection of prostate cancer, *Urol Clin North Am* 16:635-655, 1989.
5. Chodak GW, Thisted RA, Gerber GS, et al: Results of conservative management of clinically localized prostate cancer, *N Engl J Med* 330:242-248, 1994.
6. Chodak GW: The role of watchful waiting in the management of localized prostate cancer, *J Urol* 152:1766-1768, 1994.
7. Johansson J-E: Expectant management of early stage prostatic cancer: Swedish experience, *J Urol* 152:1753-1756, 1994.
8. Albertsen PC, Fryback DG, Storer BE, et al: Long-term survival among men with conservatively treated localized prostate cancer, *JAMA* 274:626-631, 1995.
9. Lu-Yao GL, Yao S-L: Population-based study of long-term survival in patients with clinically localised prostate cancer, *Lancet* 349:906-910, 1997.
10. Aus G, Pileblad E, Hugosson J: Impact of competing mortality on the cancer-related mortality in localized prostate cancer, *Urology* 46:672-675, 1995.
11. Fowler FJ Jr, Barry MJ, Lu-Yao G, et al: Patient-reported complications and follow-up treatment after radical prostatectomy: the national Medicare experience, 1988-1990 (updated June 1993), *Urology* 42:622-629, 1993.
12. Murphy GP, Mettlin C, Menck H, et al: National patterns of prostate cancer treatment by radical prostatectomy: results of a survey by the American College of Surgeons Commission on Cancer, *J Urol* 152:1817-1819, 1994.
13. Litwin MS, Hays RD, Fink A, et al: Quality-of-life outcomes in men treated for localized prostate cancer, *JAMA* 273:129-135, 1995.
14. Lim AF, Brandon AH, Friedler J, et al: Quality of life: radical prostatectomy versus radiation therapy for prostate cancer, *J Urol* 154:1420-1425, 1995.
15. Mohler JL: Treatment issues in clinically localized prostatic carcinoma (editorial), *J Urol* 154:1433-1434, 1995.
16. Fleming C, Wasson JH, Albertsen PC, et al (Prostate Patient Outcomes Research Team): A decision analysis of alternative treatment strategies for clinically localized prostate cancer, *JAMA* 269:2650-2658, 1993.
17. Shalala DE: *Cancer death rate declined for the first time ever in the 1990s* (press release), Bethesda, Md, November 14, 1996, National Cancer Institute.

18. Walsh PC, Brooks JD: The Swedish prostate cancer paradox (editorial), *JAMA* 277:497-498, 1997.
19. National Cancer Institute of Canada: *Canadian cancer statistics 1997,* Toronto, 1997, The Institute.

Advanced Prostate Cancer

In a 1994 study by Chodak and associates[1] the median time from the detection of metastases to death from prostate cancer was 36 months. The 5-year survival rate for patients who have metastases at the time of diagnosis is 25%.[2]

Standard treatment protocols for advanced prostate cancer include castration, antiandrogens such as flutamide (Eulexin, Euflex) or nilutamide (Nilandron, Anandron), and inhibitors of gonadotropin secretion such as the gonadotropin-releasing hormone analogues leuprolide (Lupron) and goserelin (Zoladex). One study found that external radiation plus goserelin for locally advanced prostate cancer increased survival duration compared with that in control subjects who received only radiation therapy.[3]

REFERENCES

1. Chodak GW, Thisted RA, Gerber GS, et al: Results of conservative management of clinically localized prostate cancer, *N Engl J Med* 330:242-248, 1994.
2. American Cancer Society: *Cancer facts and figures, 1993,* Atlanta, 1993, The Society.
3. Bolla M, Gonzalez D, Dubois J, et al: Improved survival in patients with locally advanced prostate cancer treated with radiotherapy and goserelin, *N Engl J Med* 337:295-300, 1997.

RENAL CELL CARCINOMA

The highest incidence of renal cell carcinoma is in Scandinavia and North America. It is twice as common in men as in women and twice as common in smokers as in nonsmokers. Treatment is surgical with an overall cure rate of 58%. An occasional patient in whom a solitary metastasis develops after nephrectomy is cured by surgical removal of the metastasis. Chemotherapy has little value.[1]

REFERENCES

1. Motzer RJ, Bander NH, Nanus DM: Renal-cell carcinoma, *N Engl J Med* 335:865-875, 1996.

RENAL COLIC

High-Calcium Diet

High calcium intake is not associated with an increased risk of kidney stones. In fact, the reverse may be true. As calcium intake is reduced, oxalate absorption increases, leading to hyperoxaluria and the formation of calcium oxalate stones.[1]

Nonsteroidal Antiinflammatory Drugs in the Treatment of Renal Colic

In Europe parenteral nonsteroidal antiinflammatory drugs are commonly used to relieve the pain of acute renal colic.[2,3] The drugs most frequently reported are diclofenac (Voltaren) and indomethacin (Indocid). A recent metaanalysis of randomized controlled studies using these drugs via the parenteral route showed them to have excellent analgesic effect compared with placebo and to be equal to or better than analgesics for pain relief.[2] The only NSAID available for parenteral use in North America is ketorolac (Toradol). In one study 90 mg of ketorolac intramuscularly was as effective as 100 mg of meperidine intramuscularly.[3]

One British study found that a 100-mg rectal suppository of diclofenac was more effective than 100 mg of meperidine plus 12.5 mg of prochlorperazine (Compazine, Stemetil) intramuscularly.[4] Comparisons between 50 mg of indomethacin IV and 100 mg of indomethacin as a rectal solution (enema) found that both were effective but that quantitatively the IV route was better.[5,6]

High Water Intake

High water intake has been shown in a prospective study to decrease the incidence of recurrent nephrolithiasis in patients with idiopathic calcium stone disease.[7]

REFERENCES

1. Curhan GC, Willett WC, Rimm EB, et al: A prospective study of dietary calcium and other nutrients and the risk of symptomatic kidney stones, *N Engl J Med* 328:833-838, 1993.
2. Labrecque M, Dostaler L-P, Rousselle R, et al: Efficacy of nonsteroidal anti-inflammatory drugs in the treatment of acute renal colic, *Arch Intern Med* 154:1381-1387, 1994.
3. Oosterlinck W, Philp NH, Charig C, et al: A double-blind single dose comparison of intramuscular ketorolac tromethamine and pethidine in the treatment of renal colic, *J Clin Pharmacol* 30: 336-341, 1990.
4. Thompson JF, Pike JM, Chumas PD, et al: Rectal diclofenac compared with pethidine injection in acute renal colic, *BMJ* 299:1140-1141, 1989.
5. Nelson CE, Nylander C, Olsson AM, et al: Rectal versus intravenous administration of indomethacin in the treatment of renal colic, *Acta Chir Scand* 154:253-255, 1988.
6. Nissen I, Birke H, Olsen JB, et al: Treatment of ureteric colic: intravenous versus rectal administration of indomethacin, *Br J Urol* 65:576-579, 1990.
7. Borghi L, Meschi T, Amato F, et al: Urinary volume, water and recurrences in idiopathic calcium nephrolithiasis—a 5-year randomized prospective study, *J Urol* 155:839-843, 1996.

SEXUAL DYSFUNCTION

(See also hormone replacement therapy for postmenopausal genital atrophy; sexual dysfunction with selective serotonin reuptake inhibitors; tricyclic derivatives; radical prostatectomy; surgical treatment of benign prostatic hypertrophy; vaginismus)

Abnormalities of sexual function include problems with libido, erections, ejaculation, and orgasm. It is not always recognized that absence or altered sensations of orgasm may occur independent of erections or ejaculation. For example, normal ejaculation but anorgasmia or altered sensation of orgasm has been reported in some patients with multiple sclerosis and Parkinson's disease and in up to half of patients subjected to transurethral prostatic resection. Although patients who have had anterolateral cordotomy for the relief of chronic pain often become anorgasmic, one third of men with complete spinal cord transection report that they have normal orgasms.[1]

REFERENCES

1. Dunsmuir WD, Emberton M: Surgery, drugs, and the male orgasm: informed consent can't be assumed unless effects on orgasm have been discussed (editorial), *BMJ* 314:319-320, 1997.

Impotence

Erectile dysfunction is the inability to achieve and maintain an erection sufficient for satisfactory sexual coitus to occur.

Epidemiology

In one community study the incidence of complete impotence increased from 5% at age 40 to 15% at age 70.[1] In this study,[1] as well as others,[2] impotence is classified into degrees such as minimal, moderate, or complete. If all degrees of impotence are included, 40% of 40-year-olds and 67% of 70-year-olds have the disorder.[1,2] Unfortunately, degrees of impotence are not well defined, and indeed it is hard to imagine that they even exist if we accept the definition given above. From the context of some reports, degrees of impotence seem to be a measurement of patients' satisfaction with their sexual performance[1]; it appears that many of the physiological changes of aging are included in the categories of mild and moderate degrees of impotence (see below), and if this is so, a large percentage of normal men are being labeled as "ill."

Physiology of erections

Parasympathetic nerves cause arteriolar dilatation; as the corpora cavernosa and corpus spongiosum fill, outflow veins are compressed, augmenting the erection. Detumescence is brought about by sympathetic impulses, causing ejaculation and vasoconstriction along with diminished parasympathetic tone.[3]

Age-related changes in male sexual functioning

Normal changes with aging are reported to include these[1]:

1. Gradual decrease in sexual desire
2. More time and stimulation required to achieve erections. Achieving erections becomes more dependent on direct physical stimulation than on psychic stimulation.
3. Decline in the degree of penile rigidity when erection is achieved
4. More time required to achieve orgasm
5. Decreased semen volume
6. Increased latency between erections

One of the problems of defining the normal aging changes in sexual functioning is that data are often scanty or ancient. For example, in one 1995 review of the subject,[4] the only reference given to changes in penile rigidity during erections in the elderly was the famous 1948 Kinsey Report.[5]

Etiology of impotence

An estimated 80% of erectile dysfunction is physiological, and only 20% is psychological. Diseases associated with impotence include diabetes, hypertension, occlusive vascular disease, neurological disorders, and in a few cases hormonal disorders. Other important factors are alcohol abuse, smoking, illicit drugs, and a variety of pharmacological agents of which the most important are beta-blockers and diuretics, psychotropic agents, and H_2-blockers.[3,6]

Important psychological causes of erectile dysfunction are depression, a temporary failure as a result of drinking too much on a single occasion ("martini syndrome"), taking up with a casual partner, and a long period of abstinence ("widower syndrome"). Sudden onset of impotence or preservation of nocturnal erections and erections with masturbation suggests psychogenic causes.[3]

Impotence as a clue to medical illness

Impotence is often a measure of general health. Between 50% and 75% of diabetic men are impotent.[7] Untreated hypertensive men have a 20% risk of impotence compared with 7% in the control group,[8] and two thirds of elderly men with myocardial infarctions were impotent before the event.[9]

Investigations

There is little evidence that exhaustive investigations are useful. Grantmyre and co-workers[10] suggest that a complete blood cell count, urinalysis, fasting glucose measurement, liver function tests, and measurement of creatinine, testosterone, free testosterone, and prolactin levels are all that are required in most cases.

Oral medications

In a retrospective study from the Walter Reed Army Medical Center in Washington, D.C., 78% of impotent men with no known risk factors for erectile dysfunction had a positive response to trazodone (Desyrel). Positive responses were greatest in men who had symptoms for less than 12 months but were recorded in only 16% of those who had had symptoms for more than 5 years. Poor responses were found among smokers, men over the age of 60, and those with peripheral vascular disease.[11] A prospective study of psychogenic impotence from Milan found a positive response in 71% of the men treated with trazodone 50 mg/day plus yohimbine 15 mg/day.[12] Priapism is a rare but serious complication of trazodone and other drugs with alpha-adrenergic blocking attributes such as prazosin and several antipsychotics. Drugs of this nature should not be given to patients with a past history of priapism or prolonged erections.[13] The usual dose of trazodone is 50 to 300 mg qhs.

Yohimbine (Yocon, Yohimex) is a presynaptic alpha$_2$-adrenergic receptor antagonist. It has been reported to improve sexual function in patients with both psychogenic and organic dysfunction, including men whose problem can be attributed to serotonin reuptake inhibitors such as fluoxetine.[14] However, the 1996 guidelines of the American Urological Association for the management of impotence advise against the use of yohimbine on the grounds that in controlled studies it has been no more effective than placebo.[15] If the drug is used, it is usually built up to a maintenance dose of 5.4 to 6 mg tid.

Corpora cavernosa injections

A variety of pharmacological agents can be injected into the corpora cavernosa to cause erections.[6,16,17] The drugs act by inhibiting sympathetic tone and thus dilating the arterioles and relaxing the smooth muscle of the corpora cavernosa. Some of the regimens are alprostadil (prostaglandin E_1, Caverject, Prostin VR) alone; alprostadil plus papaverine and phentolamine; papaverine alone; and papaverine plus phentolamine mesylate (Rogitine) or alprostadil.[6,16]

Complications of intracavernosal injections are rare and, with the exception of priapism, usually mild. They include hematomas, temporary penile pain, prolonged erection (4 to 6 hours), priapism, fibrous nodules, and penile curvature.[17] According to the guidelines of the American Urological Association, alprostadil is the drug of choice for initial vasoactive drug injection therapy.[15]

Alprostadil, or prostaglandin E_1 (Caverject), is supplied as single-dose vials of 10 μg or 20 μg of alprostadil powder plus 1-ml syringes (and ½-inch no. 30 needles) prefilled with diluent. The usual dose is variable but in many patients is between 5 and 20 μg. Dosage is determined empirically during initial visits to the physician. At these initial visits the goal is to achieve an erection sufficient for intercourse but lasting less than 1 hour. The initial dose is usually 2.5 μg, and this is increased by increments of 5 μg if no response occurs and 2.5 μg if there is a partial response. When a response takes place, the patient should stay in the physician's office until detumescence has occurred.

Injections are made into one (not both) of the corpora cavernosa. The manufacturer suggests a 24-hour interval between injections and a maximum of three injections a week. Erection usually takes place within 5 to 10 minutes. Injection sites should be rotated around the corpora cavernosa.

Prolonged erections or priapism require treatment, which is usually instituted for erections lasting longer than 3 hours. A Vacutainer should be used to aspirate 40 to 60 ml of blood from one of the corpora cavernosa, and if detumescence does not occur, ice is applied for 20 minutes. If the erection still persists, 0.1 to 0.2 ml (50 to 100 μg) of phenylephrine (Neo-Synephrine) that has been diluted to 0.05% is injected into the corpora cavernosa every 2 to 5 minutes until detumescence occurs.

Transurethral medications

Alprostadil can be given by a transurethral route. In a study of 1511 men with organic impotence, 66% were able to achieve erections in the clinic through the intraurethral application of alprostadil in doses of 125 or 250 μg. The drug was applied by a proprietary device (MUSE, Vivus, Menlo Park, California) with a hollow stem 3.5 cm long that was fully inserted into the urethra. Men who achieved erections in the clinic were given home trials in which drug was compared with placebo. Among those taking the drug, about three quarters of applications resulted in intercourse or orgasm compared with only 15% among those receiving placebo.[18]

Tumescence devices

A penis ring or "cock ring" can be used for men who obtain an erection but fail to maintain it. The elastic ring has an adjustable tension and is placed over the base of the shaft of the penis once an erection is obtained. The tension is adjusted to be sufficient to prevent venous outflow and so maintain the erection, but not to be of such a degree that ejaculation is blocked because this might be painful.

Patients who are unable to obtain an erection may sometimes be assisted in doing so by applying a negative suction pump (vacuum tumescence device) over the penis that draws blood into the organ so that an erection is achieved. An elastic ring, similar to a penis ring, is then slipped over the base of the penis to maintain the erection. Pain on ejaculation has been a problem with some of these devices. One of the more recent products of this nature is the ErecAid system Esteem manufactured by Osbon Medical Systems.

REFERENCES

1. Feldman HA, Goldstein I, Hatzichristou DG, et al: Impotence and its medical and psychosocial correlates: results of the Massachusetts Male Aging Study, *J Urol* 151:54-61, 1994.
2. NIH Consensus Development Panel on Impotence: NIH Consensus Conference: impotence, *JAMA* 270:83-90, 1993.
3. Dewire DM: Evaluation and treatment of erectile dysfunction, *Am Fam Physician* 53:2101-2106, 1996.
4. Schiavi R, Rehman J: Sexuality and aging, *Urol Clin North Am* 22:711-726, 1995.
5. Kinsey AC, Pomeroy WB, Martin CE: *Sexual behaviour in human male,* Philadelphia, 1948, WB Saunders.
6. Grantmyre J, Keresteci AG: Impotence: treating erectile dysfunction, *Patient Care Can* 6:34-48, 1995.
7. Kaiser FE, Korenman SG: Impotence in diabetic men, *Am J Med* 85(suppl 5A):147-152, 1988.
8. Bauer GE, Hunmyor SN, Baker J: Clinical side effects during antihypertensive therapy: a placebo-controlled double-blind study (special report), *Postgrad Med Commun,* 1981, pp 49-54.
9. Wabrek AJ, Burchell RC: Male sexual dysfunction associated with coronary artery disease, *Arch Sex Behav* 9:69-75, 1980.
10. Grantmyre J, Drachenberg D: Erectile dysfunction: a guide to treatment, *Can J CME,* February 1997, 9:169-183.
11. Lance R, Albo M, Costabile RA, et al: Oral trazodone as empirical therapy for erectile dysfunction: a retrospective review, *Urology* 46:117-120, 1995.
12. Montorsi F, Strambi LF, Guazzoni G, et al: Effect of yohimbine-trazodone on psychogenic impotence: a randomized double-blind, placebo-controlled study, *Urology* 44:732-736, 1994.

13. Thompson JW Jr, Ware MR, Blashfield RK: Psychotropic medication and priapism: a comprehensive review, *J Clin Psychiatry* 51:430-443, 1990.
14. Yohimbine for male sexual dysfunction, *Med Lett* 36:115-116, 1994.
15. Guidelines for treating erectile dysfunction issued, *JAMA* 277: 7-8, 1997.
16. Intracavernous injection of alprostadil for erectile dysfunction, *Med Lett* 37:83-84, 1995.
17. Linet OI, Ogring FG: Efficacy and safety of intracavernosal alprostadil in men with erectile dysfunction, *N Engl J Med* 334: 873-877, 1996.
18. Padma-Nathan H, Hellstrom WJ, Kaiser FE, et al: Treatment of men with erectile dysfunction with transurethral alprostadil, *N Engl J Med* 336:1-7, 1997.

Premature Ejaculation

(See also selective serotonin reuptake inhibitors)

The tricyclic agent clomipramine (Anafranil) and the selective serotinin reuptake inhibitors fluoxetine (Prozac), sertraline (Zoloft), and paroxetine (Paxil) have all been effective in treating premature ejaculation.[1-4] Doses of clomipramine were 25 to 50 mg/day,[2] sertraline 50 to 200 mg/day,[3] and paroxetine 20 to 40 mg/day.[4]

An important cause of sexual dysfunction, particularly anorgasmia, is the use of antidepressants, particularly the selective serotonin reuptake inhibitors (see discussion of selective serotonin reuptake inhibitors).[5]

REFERENCES

1. Althof S: Pharmacological treatment for rapid ejaculation: preliminary strategies, concerns, and questions, *Sex Marital Ther* 10:247-251, 1995.
2. Althof SE, Levine SB, Corty EW, et al: A double-blind crossover trial of clomipramine for rapid ejaculation in 15 couples, *J Clin Psychiatry* 56:402-407, 1995.
3. Mendels J, Camera A, Sikes C: Sertraline treatment for premature ejaculation, *J Clin Psychopharmacol* 15:341-346, 1995.
4. Waldinger MD, Hengeveld MW, Zwinderman AH: Paroxetine treatment of premature ejaculation: a double-blind, randomized, placebo-controlled study, *Am J Psychiatry* 151:1377-1379, 1994.
5. Segraves RT: Antidepressant-induced orgasm disorder, *J Sex Marital Ther* 21:192-201, 1995.

TESTES

Testicular Cancer

(See also clinical practice guidelines for screening; prevention; screening)

Ninety-five percent of testicular tumors are germ cell tumors. They are more common in whites than blacks and in cryptorchid testes. The two major types of germ cell tumors are seminomas, with a peak incidence in the twenties, and nonseminomatous germ cell tumors (embryonal carcinoma, yolk cell carcinoma, teratoma, and choriocarcinoma) with a peak incidence in the thirties. A painless testicular mass is highly suggestive of testicular tumor, but in most cases men have pain and swelling or increased testicular induration. Both seminomas and nonseminomatous germ cell tumors may cause elevations of human chorionic gonadotropin levels, whereas only nonseminomatous germ cell tumors increase alpha-fetoprotein. The overall cure rate for all germ cell tumors is greater than 90%. Most cases of seminomas are treated with orchiectomy plus retroperitoneal and pelvic lymph node irradiation, whereas nonseminomatous germ cell tumors are usually treated with orchiectomy with or without pelvic lymph node resection. Recurrences or widespread disease can usually be cured by chemotherapy, although the prognosis is considerably worse if there are hepatic, cerebral, or osseous metastases.[1]

Recommendations as to when physicians should examine the testes for cancer detection vary tremendously. Some of these are listed in Table 69.[2]

Table 69 Recommendations for Testes Examinations by Physicians

Authority	Recommendation
Canadian Task Force on the Periodic Health Examination	Only if history of cryptorchidism, infertility, atrophic testes, or ambiguous genitalia
U.S. Preventive Services Task Force	Ages 13-39 only if history of cryptorchidism, orchiopexy, or testicular atrophy
National Cancer Institute	Routine as part of periodic health examination
American Cancer Society	Every 3 years from 20-39 and thereafter annually
American Urological Association	Regularly starting at age 15
American Academy of Family Physicians	Ages 13-18 if history of cryptorchidism, orchiopexy, or testicular atrophy; as part of periodic health examination for ages 19-39

REFERENCES

1. Bosl GJ, Motzer RJ: Testicular germ-cell cancer, *N Engl J Med* 337:242-259, 1997.
2. US Public Health Service: Cancer detection in adults by physical examination, *Am Fam Physician* 51:871-885, 1995.

URINARY TRACT INFECTIONS

(See also interstitial cystitis; urinary tract infections in children)

Bacteriuria and Pyuria in the Elderly

(See also catheter, long-term indwelling; urinalysis)

Asymptomatic bacteriuria and asymptomatic pyuria are common findings in elderly women. In a prospective observational study from Boston, 61 women from a long-care institution and community housing sites submitted monthly clean-catch urine specimens for a 6-month period; 28% of patients had at least one sample showing bacteriuria alone, and bacteriuria with pyuria was found in at least one sample from 26% of patients. Bacteriuria with symptoms occurred in only 10% of patients. Spontaneous clearance of both bacteriuria and pyuria was common. For patients with symptoms the sensitivity of urine dipstick (leukocyte esterase) and microscopic examination for bacteria and white blood cells was 80% or better and the negative predictive value of these tests approached 100%.[1]

The Canadian Task Force on the Periodic Health Examination has concluded that there is no evidence that the treatment of asymptomatic bacteriuria in the elderly is beneficial. It gives "E" ratings for screening elderly institutionalized men and women and individuals of either sex with indwelling catheters for bacteriuria, a "E" rating for such screening of ambulatory elderly men, and a "C" rating for such screening of ambulatory elderly women.[2] The U.S. Preventive Services Task Force also gives "E" ratings to screening for bacteriuria in institutionalized elderly patients and a "C" rating for such screening in ambulatory elderly women.[3]

REFERENCES

1. Monane M, Gurwitz JH, Lipsitz LA, et al: Epidemiologic and diagnostic aspects of bacteriuria: a longitudinal study in older women, *J Am Geriatr Soc* 43:618-622, 1995.
2. Canadian Task Force on the Periodic Health Examination: *Canadian guide to clinical preventive health care,* Ottawa, 1994, Canada Communication Group—Publishing, pp 966-967.
3. US Preventive Services Task Force: *Guide to clinical preventive services,* ed 2, Baltimore, 1996, Williams & Wilkins, pp 347-359.

Risk Factors for Urinary Tract Infections

(See also prophylaxis of urinary tract infections)

Commonly stated risk factors for urinary tract infections include the following:

1. Sexual intercourse
2. Diaphragm use
3. Spermicide use (including spermicide-coated condoms,[1] probably by changing the vaginal flora to favor the growth of *Escherichia coli*[2])
4. History of recurrent urinary tract infections
5. Delayed postcoital micturition
6. Genetics (non–blood group secretors said to have higher incidence)

A prospective study of sexually active young women found that only the first four factors independently contributed to risk. Postcoital voiding was not protective in this group, and no relationship was found to blood group secretion status. The frequency of urinary tract infections increased with the frequency of coitus and the frequency of diaphragm use.[3]

REFERENCES

1. Fihn SD, Boyko EJ, Normand EH, et al: Association between use of spermicide-coated condoms and *Escherichia coli* urinary tract infection in young women, *Am J Epidemiol* 144:512-520, 1996.
2. Hooton TM, Stamm WE: Urinary tract infections in young women (letter), *N Engl J Med* 336:381, 1997.
3. Hooton TM, Scholes D, Hughes JP, et al: A prospective study of risk factors for symptomatic urinary tract infection in young women, *N Engl J Med* 335:468-474, 1996.

Dipsticks and Cultures

(See also urinalysis)

Leukocyte esterase dipsticks have sensitivities of 75% to 96%. Dipstick tests may be positive even when the white blood cells have lysed and so cannot be seen by microscopy. Nitrites are present in urine in many urinary tract infections. This reaction depends on the bacteria converting nitrates to nitrites. This requires time, so false-negative results are frequent unless the patient has not voided for several hours before supplying the urine specimen.

In symptomatic women urine colony counts of 10^2 to 10^5 are accurate indicators of infection. Values less than 10^5 may be found in about one third of cases.[1]

REFERENCES

1. Latham RH, Wong ES, Larson A, et al: Laboratory diagnosis of urinary tract infection in ambulatory women, *JAMA* 254:333-336, 1985.

Treatment of Uncomplicated Urinary Tract Infections

As of 1993 one third of organisms causing uncomplicated urinary tract infections in the United States demonstrated in vitro resistance to amoxicillin and sulfonamides, 15% to 20% were resistant to nitrofurantoin, and 5% to 15% to trimethoprim-sulfamethoxazole. Resistance to fluoroquinolones remained below 5% in most places.[1]

Three-day treatment is optimal in young women with uncomplicated urinary tract infections. As good results are obtained with a 3-day course as with a 7-day course, and better cure rates and fewer recurrences are seen than with single-dose therapy. This is especially so if amoxicillin or quinolones are used for single-dose therapy because these drugs are rapidly excreted and are often ineffective if there is occult renal infection. Best results for single-dose therapy are reported with trimethoprim-sulfamethoxazole. Trimethoprim-sulfamethoxazole or ofloxacin has been shown to be the best choice for 3-day treatment regimens. The authors of this study suggested limiting the use of quinolones when possible to prevent the emergence of resistant strains.[2] A new antibiotic, fosfomycin (Monurol), given as a single 3-g dose has been effective in many cases of uncomplicated urinary tract infections in women.[3]

Seven-day treatment should be considered if symptoms have persisted for more than 7 days or if the patient is using a diaphragm, is pregnant, has diabetes, or is over 65.

Table 70 Pharmacotherapy for Uncomplicated Urinary Tract Infections

Drugs	Usual doses
Trimethoprim-sulfamethoxazole (Bactrim, Septra)	160-800 mg (1 DS tablet) bid × 3 days
Amoxicillin	250 mg tid × 3 days
Ciprofloxacin (Cipro)	100 mg bid × 3 days
Norfloxacin (Noroxin)	400 mg bid × 3 days
Ofloxacin (Floxin	200 mg bid × 3 days
Nitrofurantoin (Macrobid)	100 mg bid × 7 days
Fosfomycin (Monurol)	3 g as a single dose

In recent years the recommended doses for uncomplicated urinary tract infections have been lower than those suggested in the past.[3] Some of the suggested treatment regimens for uncomplicated urinary tract infections are listed in Table 70.

Phenazopyridine (Pyridium) is an azo dye that was first marketed in the United States in 1914 as a urinary antiseptic. It is not effective in this role but continues to be prescribed as a urinary analgesic. There are no good studies supporting this indication, and since antibiotics give rapid relief of symptoms and phenazopyridine can cause methemoglobinemia, its use has little justification.[4]

REFERENCES

1. Stamm WE, Hooton TM: Management of urinary tract infections in adults, *N Engl J Med* 329:1328-1334, 1993.
2. Hooton TN, Winter C, Tiu S, Stamm WE: Randomized comparative trial and cost-analysis of 3-day antimicrobial regimens for treatment of acute cystitis in women, *JAMA* 273:41-45, 1995.
3. Fosfomycin for urinary tract infections, *Med Lett* 39:66-68, 1997.
4. Zelenitsky SA, Zhanel GG: Phenazopyridine in urinary tract infections, *Ann Pharmacother* 30:866-868, 1996.

Prophylaxis of Urinary Tract Infections

(See also hormone replacement therapy; risk factors for urinary tract infections)

There are a variety of acceptable antibiotic prophylactic regimens for recurrent urinary tract infections in women:

1. Continuous prophylaxis with trimethoprim-sulfamethoxazole, trimethoprim, or nitrofurantoin. Prophylaxis may be daily or three times a week.[1] Quinolones may also be used for this purpose.[2]
2. One antibiotic tablet from the above list taken after each coitus.[1] In one study 125 mg of ciprofloxacin taken immediately after intercourse was as effective as a daily prophylactic regimen of 125 mg of ciprofloxacin.[3]
3. Prescription of repeated 3-day treatment regimens. In this way the patient can self-treat at the onset of symptoms.[1]

An Israeli study found that intravaginal estriol was effective in preventing recurrent urinary tract infections in postmenopausal women. Estrogens facilitate the colonization of lactobacilli in the vagina, which lowers the vaginal pH and inhibits the growth of coliform bacteria.[4] Estriol is not absorbed systemically. It is not available in Canada or the United States.

A study of elderly women found that those who drank 300 ml of cranberry juice daily had a decreased incidence of bacteriuria with pyuria compared with control subjects given placebo.[5] However, whether drinking cranberry or blueberry juice will prevent urinary tract infections in young women is unknown.[6]

REFERENCES

1. Stamm WE, Hooton TM: Management of urinary tract infections in adults, *N Engl J Med* 329:1328-1334, 1993.
2. Charendoff J: Shuffle Rx in recurrent UTI? *Patient Care Can* 7:9, 1996.
3. Post-intercourse versus daily ciprofloxacin prophylaxis for recurrent urinary tract infections in premenopausal women, *J Urol* 157:935-939, 1997.
4. Raz R, Stamm WE: A controlled trial of intravaginal estriol in postmenopausal women with recurrent urinary tract infections, *N Engl J Med* 329:753-756, 1993.
5. Avorn J, Monane M, Gurwitz JH, et al: Reduction of bacteriuria and pyuria after ingestion of cranberry juice, *JAMA* 27:751-754, 1994.
6. Ronald A: Sex and urinary tract infections (editorial), *N Engl J Med* 335:511-512, 1996.

Pyelonephritis in Young Women

Between 20% and 30% of organisms causing pyelonephritis in the United States show in vitro resistance to amoxicillin and to first-generation cephalosporins. If a patient with pyelonephritis is not in a toxic state and can tolerate oral medications, she may be treated as an outpatient for 10 to 14 days with one of the following: trimethoprim-sulfamethoxazole 160 to 800 mg (DS) q12h, ciprofloxacin 500 mg q12h, ofloxacin 200 to 300 mg q12h, or norfloxacin 400 mg q12h.[1]

Imaging of the urinary tract is not needed for a first episode of pyelonephritis in young women.

REFERENCES

1. Stamm WE, Hooton TM: Management of urinary tract infections in adults, *N Engl J Med* 329:1328-1334, 1993.

VASECTOMY

(See also tubal sterilization)

Vasectomy and Prostate Cancer

Some reports have noted an increased risk of prostate cancer among patients who have had a vasectomy[1,2]; other studies have not found such a relationship.[3,4] The reports of an association between vasectomy and carcinoma of the prostate have been criticized as methodologically flawed.[5-8] One possible explanation for the finding of an increased incidence of the disease in vasectomized men may be that this group of patients is more likely to seek preventive health care than others and therefore more prostate cancers are diagnosed.[9]

REFERENCES

1. Giovannucci E, Ascherio A, Rimm EV, et al: A prospective cohort study of vasectomy and prostate cancer in US men, *JAMA* 269:873-877, 1993.
2. Giovannucci E, Tosteson TD, Speizer FE, et al: A retrospective cohort study of vasectomy and prostate cancer in US men, *JAMA* 269:878-882, 1993.
3. Nienhuis H, Goldacre M, Seagroatt V, et al: Incidence of disease after vasectomy: a record linkage retrospective cohort study, *BMJ* 304:743-746, 1992.
4. Sidney S, Quesenberry CP Jr, Sadler MC, et al: Vasectomy and the risk of prostate cancer in a cohort of multiphasic health-checkup examinees: second report, *Cancer Causes Control* 2: 113-116, 1991.
5. Howards SS, Peterson HB: Vasectomy and prostate cancer: chance, bias, or a causal relationship (editorial), *JAMA* 269:913-914, 1993.
6. Guess HA: Is vasectomy a risk factor for prostate cancer? *Eur J Cancer* 29A:1055-1060, 1993.
7. DerSimonian R, Clemens J, Spirtas R, Perlman J: Vasectomy and prostate cancer risk: methodological review of the evidence, *J Clin Epidemiol* 46:163-172, 1993.
8. Skegg D: Vasectomy and prostate cancer: is there a link? *NZ Med J* 106:242-243, 1993.
9. Goldstein M: No-scalpel vasectomy: a kinder, gentler approach, *Patient Care Can,* June 1995, 6:29-43.

VASOVASOTOMY

A review of close to 1500 microsurgical procedures to reverse vasectomies found that if the procedure was performed within 3 years of vasectomy, the patency rate was 97% and the pregnancy rate 76%. If the procedure was performed 15 years after the vasectomy, the patency rate was 71% and the pregnancy rate 30%.[1]

REFERENCES

1. Belker AM, Thomas AJ Jr, Fuchs EF, et al: Results of 1,469 microsurgical vasectomy reversals by the Vasovasostomy Study Group, *J Urol* 145:505-511, 1991.

INDEX

Numerals in italics refer to tables.

N

O

Q

R